Clinically Applied Microcirculation Research

Edited by

John H. Barker
Gary L. Anderson
Michael D. Menger

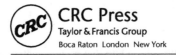

CRC Press
Taylor & Francis Group
Boca Raton London New York

CRC Press is an imprint of the
Taylor & Francis Group, an **informa** business

CRC Press
Taylor & Francis Group
6000 Broken Sound Parkway NW, Suite 300
Boca Raton, FL 33487-2742

Reissued 2019 by CRC Press

© 1995 by Taylor & Francis Group, LLC
CRC Press is an imprint of Taylor & Francis Group, an Informa business

No claim to original U.S. Government works

A Library of Congress record exists under LC control number:

Publisher's Note
The publisher has gone to great lengths to ensure the quality of this reprint but points out that some imperfections in the original copies may be apparent.

Disclaimer
The publisher has made every effort to trace copyright holders and welcomes correspondence from those they have been unable to contact.

ISBN 13: 978-0-367-20345-0 (hbk)
ISBN 13: 978-0-367-20411-2 (pbk)
ISBN 13: 978-0-429-26131-2 (ebk)

Visit the Taylor & Francis Web site at http://www.taylorandfrancis.com and the CRC Press Web site at http://www.crcpress.com

THE EDITORS

John H. Barker, M.D., Ph.D., is an Associate Professor of Surgery and is Research Director of the Division of Plastic and Reconstructive Surgery at the University of Louisville in Kentucky. He also holds the position of Associate Professor in the Departments of Anatomical Science/Neurobiology and Physiology at the University of Louisville and Scientific Director of the Jewish Hospital Research Grant Program.

Dr. Barker obtained his M.D. in 1984 from the National University of Córdoba in Argentina, and he earned his Doctor of Medicine degree in 1987 at the University of Heidelberg in Germany, where he was a fellow of the International Society of Microcirculation from 1986 through 1988.

Dr. Barker is a member of the European and American Societies for Microcirculation, the European Society for Surgical Research, the American Society for Reconstructive Microsurgery, the Wound Healing Society, and the Plastic Surgery Research Council. He is a scientific reviewer for the journals *Microvascular Research, Microcirculation, International Journal of Microcirculation, Microsurgery*, and the *International Journal of Vascular Research*.

Dr. Barker has received several national and international awards for his research, has made over 100 presentations at national and international meetings, has published over 40 original papers, and has authored over 10 book chapters.

Dr. Barker's current major research interests include skin and muscle flap pathophysiology, angiogenesis in wound healing, medical informatics, and the use of telecommunication techniques in medical education.

Gary L. Anderson, Ph.D., is an Associate Professor of Physiology and Biophysics and an Associate in Surgery at the University of Louisville School of Medicine. He obtained his B.S. degree in Animal Science from Washington State University and his Ph.D. degree in Physiology from the University of Arizona College of Medicine.

Dr. Anderson was a recipient of an institutional NIH Postdoctoral Fellowship at the Dalton Research Center at the University of Missouri and a recipient of an NIH New Investigator Award for Research at the University of Louisville. He has received four Golden Apple Teaching Awards at the University of Louisville School of Medicine, and he was awarded the 1991 Distinguished Teaching Professor Award by the University of Louisville.

Dr. Anderson is a member of the American Physiological Society and a member of the Microcirculation Society. He is also a member of Alpha Zeta National Agricultural Honor Society and Phi Kappa Phi National Honor Society.

Dr. Anderson's research interest is in the application of microcirculation research to clinical problems including thrombosis, emboli, and ischemia/perfusion injury associated with transplantation and reconstructive surgery.

Michael D. Menger, M.D., Ph.D., Prof. Dr. Med., is Chairman and Professor of the Institute for Clinical-Experimental Surgery, Faculty of Medicine at the University of Saarland (Homburg/Saar, Germany).

Dr. Menger received his M.D. and his Doctor of Medicine degree from the Albert-Ludwigs-University of Freiburg, Germany, in 1981 and 1983, respectively. In 1990, he received his board qualification for surgery at the University of Saarland. In 1992, he received his Ph.D. degree (Priv.-Doz.) from the Ludwig-Maximilians-University of Munich.

Dr. Menger is a member of the German Society of Surgery, the German Society of Thoracic and Cardiovascular Surgery, the Surgical Association for Clinical Studies, the

Surgical Association for Biomaterials, the European Society for Surgical Research, the European Society for Microcirculation, and the International Society for Oxygen Transport to Tissue.

Dr. Menger was the president of the Gesellschaft für Mikrozirkulation e.V. in 1993. He is a member of the Executive Committee of the Section of Experimental Surgery of the German Society of Surgery, the German delegate of the European Society for Surgical Research, and the delegate of the Scientific Committee of the Forum of the German Society of Surgery.

Among other awards, he has received the Bernhard-von-Langenbeck Award of the German Society of Surgery and the Steilmann-Award of the German Society for Transplantation. His work is supported by the German Research Council, the Wilhelm-Sander-Foundation, and the Friedrich-Baur-Foundation.

Dr. Menger has presented over 50 invited lectures at international meetings and seminars and over 25 invited lectures at national meetings and seminars. He has published approximately 170 research papers and has edited three books. His current major research interests include quantitative analysis of the microcirculation in endotoxemia/sepsis, shock/resuscitation and ischemia/reperfusion, analysis of angiogenesis and vascularization of benignant and malignant tissue, the microcirculation of solid organ transplants, and the *in vivo* analysis of molecular determinants in cell-cell interaction.

FOREWORD

In this book, we combine state-of-the-art modern microcirculation technology with present and potential applications in clinical medicine. To accomplish this goal, we invited experts in the field of microcirculation from both the clinical and research sectors to contribute their knowledge (23 clinicians and 35 basic researchers from 12 countries). We think that this conceptual design will provide a comprehensive guide for clinicians interested in applying microcirculation technology in their respective fields and a reference source for scientists studying the pathophysiology of disease at the microcirculatory level.

This volume consists of 34 chapters divided into 5 sections. Each chapter addresses the microcirculation from a clinical standpoint and at the same time critically assesses the latest ideas and techniques in basic microcirculation research. The first two sections of the volume analyze how the microcirculation is involved in pathological states. The third section contains the history of microcirculation as a science and presents the latest technological developments in the field. The third chapter in this section embodies the essence of the entire book, giving an example of how the science of microcirculation can be applied to the clinical practice of diagnosing, understanding, and treating disease. The fourth and largest section in the book uses 16 chapters to summarize the microcirculation in different organs/tissues and focuses on the physiological and pathological form and function of each. In addition, each of these chapters provides a description of the latest models and techniques being used to study the microcirculation in the respective tissues.

Finally, the last seven chapters (fifth section) describe important functional components of the microcirculation. This volume does not cover all of the topics that might have been included in this rapidly expanding field; however, we hope it will serve as a comprehensive guide for clinicians and researchers and will help to expand the application of microcirculation research into clinical medicine. We hope that this book offers an example of how cooperation between clinicians and scientists can lead to a better understanding of the mechanisms that cause disease.

DEDICATION

To my father, D. John Gosch-Barker. His example has made me a caring physician and an inquisitive scientist.

ACKNOWLEDGMENTS

There are a number of individuals who have contributed both directly and indirectly to this book. I would like to thank my parents who have always believed in and supported my projects and goals. I thank my early science teachers, Jodi Bennett and J. Stires, and clinical teachers, D. John Gosch-Barker and J. Norberto Allende, whose support and example have made me an inquisitive scientist and a caring physician. I owe a great deal to my teachers in microcirculation research, Karl E. Arfors, Alfred Bollinger, Peter Gaehtgens, Marcos Intaglietta, David H. Lewis, Konrad Messmer, Terence J. Ryan, Laurence H. Smaje, and Robert D. Acland. Most importantly, I would like to thank all of my students from whom I will never stop learning. It is their ever-fresh enthusiasm and constant thirst for learning that draws me to work each morning to endure the treacheries of academic medicine. Finally, I would like to thank John E. Tooke, Peter Gaehtgens, Gerry A. Meininger, Michael D. Menger, and Konrad Messmer for their advice on how to structure this work. Special thanks to Barbara Gilmore for her assistance in all aspects of coordinating the manuscripts in this book. Of course, a special thanks goes to the 62 authors whose work makes up this book. Undoubtedly, it is their high level of expertise and insight included herein that will make this work an important scientific contribution today and for years to come.

PREFACE

Many physicians, including myself, have tended to view the most peripheral part of the cardiovascular system, the microcirculation, as a foreign land in which mysterious events occur. Many view the researchers who are at home in this field as remote individuals who speak a strange tongue. This serious misconception stood in my way for years when I as a surgeon sought to address a straightforward question regarding the cause of failure in certain operations. The question concerned unexplained, patchy perfusion failure in tissue that had been surgically transplanted. The answer lay in understanding what was happening in the microcirculation. Even though I worked in the same building as a renowned team of microcirculation scientists, the distance between my world and theirs seemed infinite. When I finally got up the courage to take the short walk and the brief elevator ride to where they lived, I was greatly surprised. Here were individuals whose language was the same as mine. I readily understood their operating principles. Their seemingly formidable equipment opened a window to a world of vast interest and singular beauty. My question was regarded as welcome and interesting. By fusing my skills with theirs, we devised a way to address my question and arrived at a useful answer. I know that I am a safer and much more knowledgeable surgeon as a result.

This well-conceived book, written by a fusion of clinicians and basic scientists, is intended to lessen the distance between the fields of clinical practice and microcirculation science. I hope that many clinicians whose interests and questions border on the microcirculation will read this book. In doing so, I hope their experience will be as revealing and useful as mine was when I took my short walk and brief elevator ride.

Robert D. Acland, M.D.

CONTRIBUTORS

Jens L. Andresen
Research Laboratory for Biochemical
  Pathology
Aarhus University Hospital
Denmark

Toke Bek
Department of Ophthalmology
Aarhus University Hospital
Denmark

H. Glenn Bohlen
Department of Physiology
Indiana University Medical School
Indianapolis, Indiana

Alfred Bollinger
Angiology Division
Universitatsspital Zurich
Zurich, Switzerland

John R. Casley-Smith
Henry Thomas Laboratory
University of Adelaide
Adelaide, Australia

William M. Chilian
Department of Medical Physiology
Texas A&M University
College Station, Texas

Julio C. U. Coelho
Department of Surgery
Federal University of Parana
Curitiba, Brazil

John D. Conger
Veterans Affairs Medical Center
Denver, Colorado

Michael J. Davis
Department of Medical Physiology
Texas A&M University
College Station, Texas

Gary D. Dunn
Department of Surgery
Louisiana State University Medical
  Center
Shreveport, Louisiana

Bernhard Endrich
St. Elisabeth Hospital
Department of Surgery
Dillingen, Germany

Bengt Fagrell
Department of Medicine
Karolinska Hospital
Stockholm, Sweden

John Firrell
Christine M. Kleinert Institute for
  Hand and Microsurgery
Louisville, Kentucky

Johannes M. Frank
Department of Trauma Surgery
University of Saarland
Homburg/Saar, Germany

Peter Gaehtgens
Department of Physiology
Freie Universitat Berlin
Berlin, Germany

R. Neal Garrison
Department of Surgery
University of Louisville
Louisville, Kentucky

Harris Gellman
Orthopaedic Surgery
University of Arkansas
Little Rock, Arkansas

D. Neil Granger
Department of Physiology and
  Biophysics
Louisiana State University Medical
  Center
Shreveport, Louisiana

Alan C. Groom
Department of Medical Biophysics
University of Western Ontario
London, Ontario, Canada

James I. Harty
Department of Surgery
University of Louisville
Louisville, Kentucky

George A. Hedge
Research and Graduate Studies
West Virginia University School of
  Medicine
Morgantown, West Virginia

Michael A. Hill
Department of Physiology
Eastern Virginia Medical School
Norfolk, Virginia

Linda J. Huffman
Department of Physiology
West Virginia University School of
  Medicine
Morgantown, West Virginia

Marcos Intaglietta
Department of Bioengineering
University of California at San Diego
La Jolla, California

Alan J. Jaap
Department of Vascular Medicine
  (Diabetes Research)
University of Exeter
Exeter, England

Peter Koch Jensen
Department of Ophthalmology
Aarhus University Hospital
Denmark

Ronald J. Korthuis
Department of Physiology and
  Biophysics
Louisiana State University Medical
  Center
Shreveport, Louisiana

Lih Kuo
Department of Medical Physiology
Texas A&M University
College Station, Texas

Thomas Ledet
Research Laboratory for Biochemical
  Pathology
Aarhus University Hospital
Denmark

Hans-Anton Lehr
Department of Pathology
University of Washington
Seattle, Washington

Ian C. MacDonald
Department of Medical Biophysics
University of Western Ontario
London, Ontario, Canada

Ingo Marzi
Department of Trauma Surgery
University of Saarland
Homburg/Saar, Germany

Michael A. Matthay
Department of Medicine
Cardiovascular Research Institute
University of California at San
  Francisco
San Francisco, California

Gerald A. Meininger
Department of Medical Physiology
College of Medicine
Texas A&M University
College Station, Texas

Konrad Messmer
Institute for Surgical Research
Klinikum Grosshadern
Munich, Germany

Judy M. Muller
Department of Medical Physiology
Texas A&M University
College Station, Texas

Masaya Oda
Department of Internal Medicine
School of Medicine
Keio University
Tokyo, Japan

Mirjam G. A. oude Egbrink
Department of Physiology
Cardiovascular Research Institute
  Maastricht
University of Limburg
Maastricht, The Netherlands

Lars M. Rasmussen
Research Laboratory for Biochemical
 Pathology
Aarhus University Hospital
Denmark

Robert S. Reneman
Department of Physiology
Cardiovascular Research Institute
 Maastricht
University of Limburg
Maastricht, The Netherlands

Andrew M. Roberts
Department of Physiology
University of Louisville
Louisville, Kentucky

William I. Rosenblum
Neuropathology
Medical College of Virginia
Virginia Commonwealth University
Richmond Virginia

Terence J. Ryan
Department of Dermatology
The Churchill Hospital
Headington, Oxford, England

Una S. Ryan
T Cell Sciences
Needham, Massachusetts

Eric E. Schmidt
Department of Medical Biophysics
University of Western Ontario
London, Ontario, Canada

Dale A. Schuschke
Center for Microcirculatory Research
University of Louisville
Louisville, Kentucky

Dick W. Slaaf
Department of Biophysics
Cardiovascular Research Institute
 Maastricht
University of Limburg
Maastricht, The Netherlands

Laurence H. Smaje
Wellcome Trust
London, England

Geert Jan Tangelder
Department of Physiology
Cardiovascular Research Institute
 Maastricht
University of Limburg
Maastricht, The Netherlands

John E. Tooke
Department of Vascular Medicine
 (Diabetes Research)
Postgraduate Medical School
University of Exeter
Exeter, England

Peter Vaupel
Institute of Physiology and
 Pathophysiology
University of Mainz
Mainz, Germany

Eric Vicaut
Biophysics Department
Hopital F. Widal
Paris, France

Brigitte Vollmar
Institute for Clinical-Experimental
 Surgery
University of Saarland
Homburg/Saar, Germany

Mark A. Wilson
Department of Surgery
University of Louisville
Louisville, Kentucky

Howard Winet
Department of Orthopaedics
University of Southern California and
 Orthopaedic Hospital
Los Angeles, California

Yuan Yuan
Departments of Surgery and Medical
 Physiology
Texas A&M University
Temple, Texas

Benjamin W. Zweifach
Ames Bioengineering
University of California at San Diego
La Jolla, California

CONTENTS

Section IV: Specific Application of Microcirculation Research

Section I

Introduction

Chapter 1

The Microcirculation and Clinical Disease

John E. Tooke and Laurence H. Smaje

CONTENTS

I. INTRODUCTION

Most clinicians are interested primarily in the pathogenesis and pathophysiology of those disease processes that affect the organ system with which their specialty is concerned. Accordingly, the structure of this book is such that the specialist can focus attention on the anatomy, physiology, disease mechanisms, and investigative models in the microcirculation relevant to his or her discipline. However, as will be apparent from the Contents pages of this book, malfunction of the microcirculation is a feature of many disease states; and without a framework for thinking, it is difficult to build detailed organ-specific knowledge. The purpose of this chapter is to help create such a framework.

Common themes are emphasized: general functions expressed by most microcirculatory beds, the general structure of the microcirculation, and the broad principles that underlie microvascular failure. Some of these are illustrated by examples taken from only one microvascular bed or only one disease state, and caution must thus be exercised in extrapolation to the microcirculation in general. Nevertheless, we hope that consideration of the potential relevance of such observations in the context of a framework of knowledge of the physiology and pathophysiology of microcirculation will be of value to those dealing with day-to-day problems in clinical microvascular disease.

Cardiovascular disease is still the single most important cause of mortality and morbidity in the West and, increasingly, in urban areas of the third world, accounting for 40% of all deaths. And it is the impact on microcirculation and the consequent sequels that are responsible for these horrific statistics. The details of microvascular physiology,

0-8493-4870-6/95/$0.00+$.50
© 1995 by CRC Press, Inc.

pathophysiology, and disease follow in succeeding chapters; but here we attempt to provide a framework for thinking together with an encouragement to encompass the new techniques of molecular and cell biology while remembering that they are *techniques*. The important *questions* come from clinical medicine and whole-animal research.

An illustration of the interdependence of the new sciences as clinical observation is provided by the recognition that certain patients who suffered frequent and widespread infections had an abnormality of neutrophil mobility. It was subsequently discovered that neutrophils in a young boy suffering from a similar syndrome lacked a particular protein carried by normal neutrophils. A monoclonal antibody prepared against the normal protein was found to prevent normal leukocyte emigration in response to inflammation. We now know that the patient's neutrophils lacked a membrane glycoprotein which is essential for adhesion-related processes, and in the experimental situation, it was blocked by the monoclonal activity. Normal neutrophil adhesion and emigration was thus prevented (see Reference 1). Much remains to be learned about adhesion molecules, but answers will come from a combination of cell and molecular biology combined with careful observation in the clinic and experimental microcirculation laboratory — none of these alone is sufficient.

II. FUNCTION OF THE MICROCIRCULATION

By the middle of the 19th century, it was already apparent to perceptive observers that "The arteries and veins are mere machinery for conveying and reconveying the blood ... [to the microcirculation, where the capillaries serve] ... the office of bringing the fluid blood into contact with the material-tissues of the system, and here all the blood changes, and all nutrition and absorption of the material tissues are affected" (Hall, 1861.[2] See also Manuel, 1994[3] for details of Hall's work). This view of the importance of the microcirculation remains as true today as it was more than a century ago, and clinical scientists are becoming more and more concerned with developing an understanding of the fundamentals of microvascular biology and the pathophysiology of disease.

As is now well known, the microcirculation is principally concerned with the processes of transport, diffusion, and exchange of materials between blood and tissue for the purposes of metabolism, tissue defense, and repair. The specialization of animal organ systems also means that particular functions take precedence in certain vascular beds, e.g., careful control of the environment of the brain, heat exchange in the skin, rapid secretion of fluid in the salivary glands, excretion of water and waste products in the kidneys, and so on.

These processes depend in turn on a restricted number of factors that can be controlled by the organism — namely, the fluid pressure, the area for exchange, the size and electric charge of the pathways through which materials pass, the distance between distribution points, and the flow of exchangeable material. The physical nature of the important exchange materials cannot be controlled and can only be accommodated by the design of the microcirculation in response to evolutionary pressures.

Even now, however, it is possible to speculate on why the pressure in the systemic circulation is high in mammals. It is higher in the feet of man (and especially giraffes) than in mice because of simple hydrostatics and because the circulation has to accommodate.[4] But systemic arterial pressure is relatively high in all mammals, and capillary pressure is roughly similar at heart level. During activity, however, flow may increase several fold. In part, this is because the heart has the potential of increasing its output, and individual microcirculations have the ability to control their resistance to flow. Central mechanisms come into play to maintain systemic arterial pressure and thus maintain basic flow in the different parts of the circulation while allowing increased flow in the active area. This naturally becomes a serious problem during major physical exercise, because

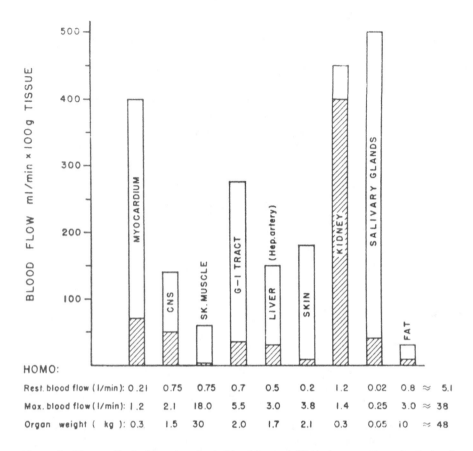

Figure 1 Diagram illustrating approximate blood flows of different organs at maximal vasodilation (*total areas*) and "at rest" (*hatched areas*) expressed in ml/min × 100 g tissue at perfusion pressure 100 mmHg (Ref.: 20, 46, 129, 159, 163, 264, 274, 298, 322). *Below:* Approximate figures for regional blood flows in a 70-kg man "at rest" and at maximal dilatation are deduced on the basis of organ weights. (The organs included comprise some 70% of total body weight.) (From Mellander, S. and Johansson, B., Control of resistance, exchange, and capitance functions in the peripheral circulation, *Pharmacolog. Rev.*, 20, 3, 117–196, 1968.)

some 50% of the body mass is composed of skeletal muscle. Despite variations of metabolism of several fold in different areas of the microcirculation during activity, control of pressure and flow through capillaries and adequate fluid and solute exchange can be maintained in the normal circulation (Figure 1).

An appreciation of integration of organ requirements with macrocirculatory control of central arterial and venous pressures, as well as the interdependence of microcirculatory pressure and flow at a local level, provides some insight into how finely balanced organ function is, and how dependent it is on intact microvascular function. Figure 2 illustrates the current view of the forces involved in fluid and solute exchange.

III. STRUCTURE OF THE MICROCIRCULATION

The microcirculation is usually defined as those vessels distal to the conduit arteries and before the veins; in addition, the prenodal lymphatics are conventionally also included. The blood microvessels comprise arterioles, the capillaries and venules, as well as

Blood flow

$$\text{FLOW} = \frac{\text{Pressure drop}}{\text{Resistance}} = \frac{P_a - P_v}{R}$$

R
⇓

P_a → FLOW → P_v

⇑
R

Transcapillary fluid flux

Fluid flux (Jv) depends on the water permeability of the wall (Lp), the surface area (A), the colloid osmotic (π) and hydrostatic (P) pressures inside (c) and outside (t) the vessel and the characteristics of the porous pathways (σ). When $\sigma = 0$, the osmotic pressure = 0 as solute goes through as easily as water. When $\sigma = 1$, the pathway is semi-permeable allowing only water to pass through.

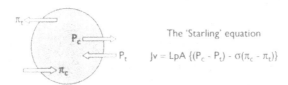

The 'Starling' equation

$$Jv = LpA \{(P_c - P_t) - \sigma(\pi_c - \pi_t)\}$$

Solute transport

Solute flux (Js) depends on diffusion and convection. Diffusive flux depends on the permeability of the vessel wall to the solute (P), the area available for exchange (A) and the concentration difference between the inside (C_c) and outside (C_t) of the capillary. The convective flux is determined by the amount of fluid that is flowing over (Jv), the reflexion coefficient (σ) and the average concentration in the capillary pore ($\bar{c}$).

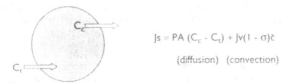

$$Js = PA (C_c - C_t) + Jv(1 - \sigma)\bar{c}$$

(diffusion)   (convection)

Figure 2a, b, c

specialized structures in some organ beds such as arteriovenous shunts. The lymphatics comprise terminal lymphatics, precollectors, and collectors. In certain animal models where detailed anatomical studies are possible, considerable attention has been paid to the size and branch order of the arterioles; as there is evidence that terminal arterioles may respond to a different range of stimuli than do more proximal resistance vessels,[5] such a distinction may be important. The arteriole is characterized by the presence of vascular smooth muscle cells in its wall, which may be several layers thick in the case of proximal vessels. In contrast, as arterioles approach the capillary bed, vascular smooth muscle cells become more sparse. The precapillary sphincter, which in most microvascular beds is a functional concept rather than a demonstrable anatomical entity, comprises the last, single vascular smooth muscle

Continuous, fenestrated and discontinuous capillaries

Definitions		Examples
Continuous basement membrane. Continuous layer of endothelium except for junctions	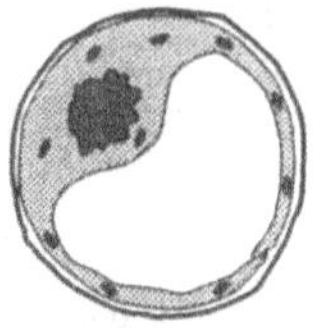 **Continuous**	Brain Muscle - skeletal, cardiac and smooth Mesentery Skin Lung
Continuous basement membrane. Attenuated endothelium with openings - fenestrae which may have internal structure.	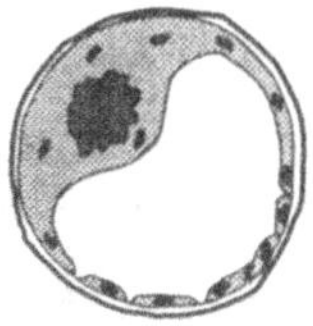 **Fenestrated**	Exocrine glands Endocrine glands Intestinal mucosa Renal glomerulae Choroid plexus Vasa rectae Synovium
Discontinuous basement membrane. Discontinuous endothelium	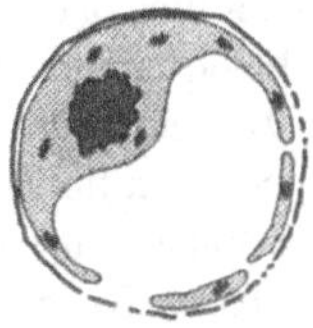 **Discontinuous**	Bone marrow Liver Spleen

Figure 3

cell encircling the endothelial tube that constitutes the capillary. Arterioles in general are characterized by relatively dense innervation that have nerve terminals possessing a wide range of neurotransmitters dependent upon the circulation studied.[6]

The capillary itself lacks a muscle layer and comprises endothelium with an outer sleeve of basement membrane. In some microcirculations, pericytes, which partially surround the endothelial tube and may be capable of contraction, are present. The precise configuration of the endothelial layer varies from organ to organ and defines the capillary type. There are three main types: continuous, fenestrated, and discontinuous. Figure 3 illustrates these and gives examples of each. It is important to emphasize that the simple transmission electron microscopic appearance does not necessarily indicate function. As can be seen from Table 1, brain, skeletal muscle, and heart all have continuous capillaries as judged by transmission electron microscopy, but their permeability to water and small molecules varies considerably. Similarly, fenestrated capillaries in the salivary gland and kidney have water and small solute permeabilities many times higher than those in continuous capillaries but have similar protein permeabilities. It would appear that these differences lie in the detailed structure of the junctions between continuous capillaries and the fact that all capillary endothelia are covered by a layer of "glycocalyx" composed of a mixture of glycoproteins, carbohydrates, and entrapped proteins. This "fiber matrix" almost certainly plays a crucial role in determining capillary permeability.[7,8]

The venules into which capillaries flow are somewhat wider and are loosely invested with vascular smooth muscle cells yet typically have a thicker adventitial coat.

A. THE LYMPHATICS

Lymphatic capillaries are usually arranged in networks within connective tissue or within the stroma of parenchymatous organs. From these networks' blind-ending sacs, the

Table 1 Capillary Permeability Coefficients and Hydraulic Conductivity
Determined for a Variety of Tissues According to Capillary Type

| | Continuous Capillaries | | | Fenestrated Capillaries | |
| | Skeletal | | | | |
	Muscle	Heart	Brain	Kidney	Stomach
Capillary Permeability Coefficient cm $s^{-1} \times 10^{-5}$					
Na+	5.1	4.6	0.04	—	>210
Sucrose	1.4	3.6	0.01	>150	140
Insulin	0.2	0.4	0.0005	70	70
Hydraulic Conductivity cm $s^{-1} \times$ (cm $H_2O)^{-1} \times 10^{-8}$	10	—	0.03	4000–6000	—

Adapted from *Recent Advances in Physiology*, Baker, P. F., Ed., Churchill Livingstone, Edinburgh, 1984, 125–162.

terminal lymphatics extend into the interstitial space. The wall of the terminal lymphatic and lymphatic capillaries consist of a continuous type of endothelium surrounded by basal lamina that may be discontinuous. In contrast to blood capillaries, open junctions between endothelial cells in terminal lymphatics are commonly observed.[9] Anchoring filaments from the abluminal surface of the endothelial cell fuse with collagen fibrils within the interstitium and arguably result in patency of the lymphatic network (rather than compression) if interstitial fluid volume is increased. For further detail, refer to Chapter 31 in this volume.

B. THE ENDOTHELIUM

The above treatise is the traditional approach to microvascular structure but fails to emphasize the importance of the roles played by the common component — the lining endothelium. In the last 2 decades, it has become clear that far from acting as a passive semipermeable membrane, the endothelium is a dynamic structure that has a major influence on the fluidity of the blood and vascular smooth muscle tone as well as the response to injury. Ultrastructural analysis of capillary endothelium reveals that certain endothelial cells contain actin filaments, suggesting they are capable of shape change and perhaps modification of interendothelial cell gaps. A review of the rapidly developing field of endothelial biology is beyond the scope of this chapter, and readers are referred to Chapter 30 in this volume and the following recent works: Rubanyi (1991),[10] Thiemermann (1991),[11] and Haynes and Webb (1993).[12]

IV. MALFUNCTION OF THE MICROCIRCULATION

Anything that interferes with the main functions of the microcirculation — transport and exchange — is likely to lead to disease. Microcirculatory disease occurs when the local adaptive mechanisms fail to cope with major changes in circulatory hemodynamics or the disease process itself leads to abnormal blood components, induces a change in the control of microvascular resistance, or leads to abnormalities in the endothelial barrier function.

This relatively simple and obvious statement encompasses a vast array of disease states, and it may be worth trying to create ways of categorizing them. One approach, which is extremely useful in many disease states, is to consider the pathogenesis. Is the disease primary or secondary? Is it acute or chronic? Is it structural or functional? Table 2 provides definitions and examples.

An alternative approach is to think pathophysiologically. In this case, one thinks in terms of the impact of the disease on the relevant components and the functions of the microcirculation.

Table 2 Simple Pathogenetic Classification of Microvascular Disease

1. Primary Microvascular Disease
   Where the microcirculation itself is damaged. A primary failure in one part may lead to a secondary change elsewhere.
   Examples of primary damage might include the following:
   a. Infection and septic shock
   b. Immune and autoimmune disease
   c. Metabolic disease: a) Diabetes
                          b) Scurvy
   d. Genetic disease such as angioneurotic edema
   e. Toxins from bacteria such as diphtheria, toxins from venomous animals such as snakes
2. Secondary Microvascular Disease
   Where the microcirculation is compromised secondary to changes elsewhere in the microcirculation or the blood.
   a. Hypertension
   b. Ischemia and reperfusion injury
   c. Hemorrhagic shock
   d. Hypoproteinemia secondary to liver disease, renal disease, kwashiorkor, etc.
   e. Autonomic neuropathy
   f. Blood cell pathology such as sickle cell disease, spherocytosis, adhesion molecule abnormalities, platelet pathology
3. Acute Microvascular Disease
   Where the disease is acute in onset and limited in duration. It may develop into a chronic situation.
   a. Acute inflammation including infections and immune and autoimmune responses
   b. Type I diabetes
4. Chronic Microvascular Disease
   a. Chronic inflammation (e.g., rheumatoid arthritis)
   b. Type I and Type II diabetes
   c. Hypertension
5. Structural
   Where the disease leads to structural damage to essential components of the microcirculation.
   a. Acute and chronic inflammation including immune and autoimmune disease
   b. Mechanical damage
   c. Scurvy
   d. Abnormal angiogenesis (e.g., diabetes, tumors)
   e. Hypertension
6. Functional
   Where the disease process leads to abnormal function of the components of the microcirculation and the blood.
   a. Abnormalities of flow, permeability, pressure, and surface area of the microvasculature
   b. Autonomic neuropathy
   c. Biochemical and genetic abnormalities leading to pathologically high or low release of endothelial mediators of vascular smooth muscle tone, platelet aggregation and/or white cell adhesion and migration

The account that follows utilizes the latter approach; but when considering microvascular disease, it may be as well to consider both approaches.

A. REDUCTION IN ARTERIAL PRESSURE

Microvascular beds possess differing capacities to cope with reduction in arterial feeding pressure. In human disease, this capacity has been best studied in the lower limb, chronic ischemia due to proximal atherosclerotic stenotic disease being the common cause. Microvascular function remains intact with moderate reduction in arterial pressure, greater reduction being associated with impaired maximal microvascular hyperemic capacity following, for example, a brief period of arterial occlusion.[13] With more profound reduction in arterial pressure, the resulting compensatory chronic vasodilatation of precapillary resistance vessels has a number of adverse consequences for integrated microvascular performance: dependent upon the precise geometry of the microvascular bed, certain areas will be rendered hypoxic before others; chronic vasodilatation in these areas will arguably affect a microvascular steal of blood flow, thus disturbing the normal spatial and temporal homogeneity of flow. Vasoparalysis in the presence of severe hypoxia also disturbs those mechanisms upon which the maintenance of local tissue fluid economy depends: vasomotion, the waxing and waning of precapillary resistance observed in health, allows for periods of filtration and reabsorption. Abolition of this process favors net filtration. Normally on dependency, the rise in intravascular pressure triggers precapillary vasoconstriction, thereby limiting the rise in capillary pressure, the venoarteriolar response. This posturally-induced vasoconstriction, which is thought to be an important edema prevention mechanism in health, is impaired in the presence of severe arterial insufficiency and explains the apparent paradox of the cold ischemic yet edematous foot in this condition.[14]

B. INCREASE IN ARTERIAL PRESSURE

A sustained increase in arterial blood pressure is encountered in the clinical condition hypertension. Although the origins of the common form of the condition, essential hypertension, remain obscure and are in all probability multifactorial, attention has centered upon cardiac, renal, and neurohumoral mechanisms. At a microvascular level, adaptive changes occur that involve structural modification of precapillary resistance. Such structural autoregulation of capillary pressure arguably sustains the increased peripheral vascular resistance,[15] which is a feature of established hypertension, although prospective studies are required of people at risk of developing hypertension (for example, through family history) to know whether structural limitation of vasodilatation antedates the emergence of high blood pressure.

Regardless of whether such changes in peripheral vascular resistance are primary or secondary, maximum vasodilatory capacity of the microcirculation is impaired in established arterial hypertension.[16] Despite adaptive structural change, the microvascular bed is not completely protected from the increased pressure head. Skin capillary pressure has shown to be elevated in essential hypertension;[17] similar systemic change probably accounts for the increased escape rate of albumin from the microcirculation in this condition.[18] (See Chapter 4 in this volume.)

C. LUXURY PERFUSION

Certain conditions are associated with increased organ blood flow in the absence of arterial hypertension resulting from a resetting of pre- and post-capillary resistance in the microvascular beds. Insulin-dependent diabetes is an example of such a condition, increased microvascular blood flow having been demonstrated in the early stages of the disease in the eye, kidney, and periphery.[19] Multiple theories have been put forward to explain this luxury perfusion, ranging from vasodilatory effects of intermediary metabolites, increased production of vasodilatory endothelial cell mediators in response to increased wall shear stress,[20] as well as the toxic effects of glucose upon cell responsiveness to vasoconstrictors.[21] The relevance of this malsetting of peripheral vascular resistance is that chronic capillary hypertension occurs, as has been confirmed in the rat glomerulus[22] and human skin.[23] High capillary pressure stimulates the production of the mesangium in the glomerulus,[24] and capillary basement membrane thickening.[25] The massive increase in basement membrane width, which is the ultrastructural hallmark of diabetic microangiopathy, ultimately leads to a structural limitation of perfusion and loss of autoregulatory capacity as well as perhaps altered permeability characteristics. (See Chapter 3 in this volume.)

D. REPERFUSION INJURY

In recent years, it has come to be recognized that restoration of blood flow following a period of circulatory arrest may result in further damage to organ function. Common circumstances where such processes may operate include thrombolytic therapy for coronary artery occlusion and removal of proximal arterial clamps following insertion of distal vascular prosthetic grafts.

Arrest of the circulation results in profound downstream vasodilatation and vasoparalysis alluded to in the section on chronic ischemia above. While such vasoparalysis lasts, capillary pressure regulation will be lost and edema will result when arterial pressure is restored. However, more sinister is the activation of the white blood cells reperfusing the ischemic area, resulting in the generation of toxic free radicals, possible white cell plugging of some venules, and endothelial cell damage.[26] (See Chapter 6 in this volume.)

E. ALTERED PERMEABILITY

The role of primary changes in permeability in clinical disease is very difficult to ascertain because of the absence of specific techniques to measure permeability that avoid the compounding influences of changes in microvascular pressure and flow. A few conditions are characterized by sporadic changes in generalized permeability and usually represent environmentally triggered activation of a generalized inflammatory response in individuals preprogrammed (either genetically or immunologically) to such stimuli.[27] Generalized increase in microvascular permeability appears to be an important component of shock states.[28] Chronic low-grade enhancement of permeability may reflect inherited differences in microvascular barrier function and may underlie the susceptibility of some individuals to microvascular complications of diabetes and/or the atherosclerotic process.[29] The endothelial exchange barrier is largely a function of the content of heparan sulfate proteoglycan, the derivation of which is enzymatically determined. It has been proposed that inherited differences in key enzymes involved in its production, such as glucosaminyl N-deacetylase, could determine differences in generalized endothelial barrier function.

F. IMPAIRED LYMPHATIC FUNCTION

Although in some clinical conditions (e.g., filiarisis) the consequences of impaired lymphatic function are easy to observe, the contribution of this part of the microvasculature to other disease processes is difficult to discern and may well be underestimated. This lack of clarity again reflects the paucity of techniques available to measure human microvascular function and the impact of other variables (principally Starling's forces and capillary permeability) upon lymphatic performance. The importance of knowledge of these confounding variables is illustrated by recent observations suggesting that tissue fluid in upper limb post-mastectomy "lymphedema" is actually relatively low in protein, suggesting that elevated capillary pressure may contribute to its occurrence.[30] (See Chapter 31 in this volume.)

G. ACTIVATION OF TISSUE DEFENSE SYSTEMS

The microcirculation plays important roles in tissue defense, particularly against infection. The inflammatory response to infection involves expression of adhesion receptors for leukocytes on the endothelial cell surface. Activated neutrophils release products including proteolytic enzymes and oxygen free radicals, that destroy both microorganisms and (inevitably) some tissue cells, prior to subsequent tissue repair.[31] Evidence suggests that in certain pathophysiological circumstances, this microvascular defense system may be activated to the overall disadvantage of tissue function. These concepts are best developed in relation to severe peripheral ischemia, although much remains theoretical and requires validation in man. Patients with severe arterial insufficiency of the limbs tend to have higher leukocyte counts than normal patients, and studies of white cell filterability[32] suggest that circulating white cells are more activated, particularly if blood is sampled from the ischemic limb. In distal arterioles, activation of white cells may shift the balance of vasoregulatory mediators away from vasodilatation (e.g., the generation of superoxide radicals by activated leukocytes results in the breakdown of EDRF) and toward (inappropriate) vasoconstriction (e.g., release of 5-HT and formation of TXA_2 by activated platelets, the activation of which is enhanced in the presence of activated leukocytes). In addition, it is argued that activation of the microvascular defense system will favor capillary obstruction by leukocyte and platelet aggregates, as well as endothelial cell damage (visible microscopically as blebs in the cell, widening of interendothelial cell gaps, and swelling that may contribute to capillary obstruction).

H. INAPPROPRIATE ANGIOGENESIS

The growth of new blood vessels is fundamental to embryological development and healing and tissue repair throughout life. However, in certain circumstances, uncontrolled or inappropriate angiogenesis can result in clinical disease. The classical example of this is the preretinal new vessel growth that follows retinal hypoxia. The most common setting for this occurrence is diabetes, patchy ischemia of the retina resulting in the release of a number of growth factors.[33] The new vessels that are stimulated by such factors are more permeable than normal and tend to grow forward into the vitreous rather than in the plane of the retina. As such, they are liable to bleed; vitreous hemorrhage obscures the light path to the retina, thus interrupting ocular function irrespective of any potential benefit of such new vessel growth in regard to retinal oxygen tension. (See Chapter 3 and 14 in this volume.)

V. IMPLICATIONS FOR CLINICAL MANAGEMENT

A. DIAGNOSIS OF MICROVASCULAR MALFUNCTION

As in any other area of clinical medicine, diagnosis is dependent upon symptoms, signs, and investigations. Symptoms are seldom specific for the microcirculation and may be organ related or systemic and general in nature. The signs of microvascular malfunction are more helpful and include at one end of the spectrum the classical combination of redness, swelling, and local heat that characterizes the inflammatory response, to pallor or mottling and cold in the presence of ischemia. Major disruption of microvascular integrity may be suggested by petechia along with edema; lymphedema is often referred to as brawny and relatively resistant to pitting.

More subtle or low-grade chronic derangement is usually only detectable by investigation, and the majority of these tests are clinical research tools rather than methods used in current clinical practice. Organ-specific methodologies in current use are referred to in the relevant chapters and examples only are summarized here. An estimation of pulmonary capillary pressure may be obtained from the pulmonary "wedge" pressure, obtained by advancing a catheter into the pulmonary artery until it wedges in a distal artery. An estimate of alveolar permeability may be obtained by measuring the transfer factor — the disappearance of carbon monoxide from inhaled air, a freely diffusible molecule with avidity for hemoglobin. Access to filtrate (urine) makes renal microvascular function more accessible to clinical investigation and techniques exist for estimating the clearance of various solutes, renal plasma flow, and glomerular filtration rates.[34] The selectivity of the glomerular barrier can be assessed both in terms of charge and molecular size using appropriate molecular probes. The retina is one of the few vascular beds that is routinely observed in clinical practice. The development of vitreous fluorophotometry provides the means to quantitative retinal vessel barrier function[35] and laser scanning ophthalmoscopy enables detailed analysis of microvascular perfusion in the macular region.[36]

B. PROGNOSIS

Detailed knowledge of the pathophysiological condition of an organ or tissue may permit the important clinical function of prognostication. Such capacity is generally poorly developed as far as the microvasculature is concerned, although knowledge of the preoperative derangement of peripheral microvascular hemodynamics may permit the prediction of those patients likely to develop postoperative edema following arterial reconstruction.[37] The most pressing prognostic requirement in the field of critical limb ischemia is the capacity to determine when tissue is no longer viable, a distinction that would help guide the vascular surgeon as to the wisdom of arterial reconstruction or the amputation level to choose. Transcutaneous oxygen tension measurements and laser Doppler flux determinations may have some future in this regard.[38] The latter technique applied to the skin may also be able to characterize diabetic patients at high risk of developing clinical microangiopathy, although the outcomes of long-term prospective studies are required to validate this assertion.[39]

C. TREATMENTS

Primary treatment of the microcirculation is in its infancy, and its development and application are likely to stem from a greater understanding of microvascular pathophysiology and its cellular and molecular basis. Nevertheless, attempts are being made to address the principle anomalies. Research workers are beginning to study the impact of hypotensive drugs on microvascular hemodynamics in hypertension, and initial steps to treat the sustained capillary hypertension observed in insulin-dependent diabetes are being made.[40] Exciting developments in the field of endotoxic shock suggest that blocking the endothelial product nitric oxide may increase blood pressure[41]; rutin derivatives may have a primary impact on enhanced microvascular permeability in a number of disease states; the capacity to restore vasomotion pharmacologically may lead to more homogeneous tissue perfusion despite no change in total organ blood flow.[42]

VI. SUMMARY AND CONCLUSIONS

It is hopefully clear from this introductory chapter that numerous disease processes in many different organs impact upon microvascular function. A knowledge of microvascular breakdown requires a sound understanding of microvascular function in health and the integrated control mechanisms involved. The development of specific techniques for studying such physiological processes in man in recent years is adding to our knowledge although we remain largely ignorant about many aspects of permeability and lymphatic function, particularly in inaccessible organs. There is nonetheless real prospect for developing tools that can be used in clinical practice to define microvascular function and will contribute to the processes of therapeutic monitoring and prognosis. The development of specific pharmacotherapy to correct microvascular malfunction is also becoming a plausible prospect. Given the ubiquity of microvascular involvement in common disease processes, the impact of such developments may be considerable for the future practice of clinical medicine.

REFERENCES

1. **Harlan, J. M.**, Leukocyte adhesion deficiency syndrome: insights into the molecular basis of leukocyte emigration, *Clin. Immunol. Immunopathol.*, 67, S16–S24, 1993.
2. **Hall, C.**, *Memoirs of Marshall Hall*, Richard Bentley, London, 1861, 76.

3. **Manuel, D. E.,** Marshall Hall on the structure and physiology of the capillaries, 1830; breaking the rules of the philosophical transactions, *Int. J. Microcirc.: Clin. Exp.*, 14(1–2), 83–90, 1994.

4. **Hargens, A. R.,** Gravitational cardiovascular adaptation in the giraffe, *The Physiologist*, 30, S15–S18, 1994.

5. **Mellander, S., Maspers, M., Bjornberg, J., and Andersson, L.-O.,** Autoregulation of capillary pressure and filtration in cat skeletal muscle in states of normal and reduced vascular tone, *Acta Physiol. Scand.*, 129, 337–351, 1987.

6. **Burnstock, G.,** Regulation of local blood flow by neurohumoral substances released from perivascular nerves and endothelial cells, *Acta Physiologica Scand.*, 571 (Suppl [JC:luf]), 53–59, 1988.

7. **Curry, F. R. E.,** Mechanics and thermodynamics of transcapillary exchange, in *Handbook of Physiology, The Cardiovascular System, Microcirculation*, Bethesda, MD, Am. Physiol. Soc., 1984, Sect. 2, Vol. VI, Part 1, Chap. 8, 309–374.

8. **Katz, M. A.,** Structural change in fiber matrix allows for enhanced permeability and reduced conductivity, *MVR*, 43, 1–6, 1992 .

9. **Hammersen, F. and Hammersen, E.,** On the fine structure of lymphatics, in *The Initial Lymphatics*, Bollinger, A., Portsch, H., and Wolfe, J. H. N., Eds., Georg Thieme Verlag, Stuttgart, 1985, 58–65.

10. **Rubanyi, G. M.,** Endothelium-derived relaxing and contracting factors, *J. Cell. Biochem.*, 46, 27–36, 1991.

11. **Thiemermann, C.,** Biosynthesis and interaction of endothelium derived vasoactive mediators, *Eicosanoids*, 4, 187–202, 1991.

12. **Haynes, W. G. and Webb, D. J.,** The endothelin family of peptides: Local hormones with diverse roles in health and disease?, *Clin. Sci.*, 84(5), 485–500, 1993.

13. **Schwartz, R. W., Freedman, A. M., Richardson, D. R., Hyde, G. L., Griffen, W. O., Vincent, D. G., and Price, M. A.,** Capillary blood flow: Videodensitometry in the atherosclerotic patient, *J. Vasc. Surg.*, 1, 800–808, 1984.

14. **Ubbink D. T., Jacobs M. J. H. M., Tangelder, G. J., Slaaf, D. W., and Reneman, R. S.,** Posturally induced microvascular constriction in patients with different stages of leg ischaemia: Effect of local skin heating, *Clin. Sci.*, 81(1), 43–49, 1991.

15. **Folkow, B.,** 'Structural autoregulation' — The local adaptation of vascular beds to chronic changes in pressure, in *Development of the Vascular System*, Pitman Books, London, 56–79, 1983.

16. **Williams, S. A. and Tooke, J. E.,** Noninvasive estimation of increased structurally based resistance to blood flow in the skin of subjects with essential hypertension, *Int. J. Microcirc. Clin. Exp.*, 11, 109–116, 1992.

17. **Williams, S. A., Boolell, M., MacGregor, G. A., Smaje, L. H., Wasserman, S. M., and Tooke, J. E.,** Capillary hypertension and abnormal pressure dynamics in patients with essential hypertension, *Clin. Sci.*, 79, 5–8, 1990.

18. **Parving, H.-H., Jensen, H. A. E., and Westrup, M.,** Increased transcapillary escape rate of albumin and IgG in essential hypertension, *Scand. J. Clin. Lab. Invest.*, 37, 223–227, 1977.

19. **Tooke, J. E.,** Microvascular haemodynamics in diabetes mellitus, *Clin. Sci.*, 70, 119–125, 1986.

20. **Tooke, J. E.,** Microvascular haemodynamics in diabetes, *Eye*, 7, 227–229, 1993.

21. **Williams, B., Tsai, P., and Schrier, R.W.,** Glucose-induced downregulation of angiotensin II and arginine vasopressin receptors in cultured rat aortic vascular smooth muscle cells, *J. Clin. Invest.*, 90, 1992–1999, 1992.

22. **Fujihara, C. K., Padilha, R. M., and Zatz, R.,** Glomerular abnormalities in long-term experimental diabetes — role of hemodynamic and nonhemodynamic factors and effects antihypertensive therapy, *Diabetes*, 41, 286–293, 1992.

23. **Sandeman, D. D., Shore, A. C., and Tooke, J. E.,** Relation of skin capillary pressure in patients with insulin-dependent diabetes mellitus to complications and metabolic control, *N. Engl. J. Med.*, 327, 760–764, 1992.

24. **Riser, B. L., Cortes, P., Zhao, X., Bernstein, J., Dumler, F., Narins, R. G., Hassett, C. C., Sastry, K. S. S., Atherton, J., and Holcomb, M. A.,** Intraglomerular pressure and mesangial stretching stimulate extracellular matrix formation in the rat, *J. Clin. Invest.*, 90, 1932–1943, 1992.

25. **Williamson, J. R. and Kilo, C.,** Current status of capillary basement-membrane disease in diabetes mellitus, *Diabetes*, 26, 65–73 , 1977.

26. **Green, M. A. and Shearman, C. P.,** Reperfusion injury in peripheral vascular disease, *Vasc. Med. Rev.*, 5(2), 97–106, 1994.

27. **Atkinson, J. P., Waldmann, T. A., Stein, S. F., Gelfand, J. A., MacDonald W. J., Heck, L. W., Cohen, E. L., Kaplan, A. P., and Frank, M. M.,** Systemic capillary leak syndrome and monoclonal IgG gammopathy: Studies in a sixth patient and a review of the literature, *Medicine*, 56 (3), 225–239, 1977.

28. **Fleck, A., Raines, G., Hawker, F., Trotter, J., Wallace, P. I., Ledingham, I. McA., and Calman, K. C.,** Increased vascular permeability: A major cause of hypoalbuminaemia in disease and injury, *Lancet*, 1(8432), 781–784, 1985.

29. **Deckert, T., Feldt-Rasmussen, B., Borch-Johnsen, K., Jensen, T., and Kofoed Enevoldsen, A.,** Albuminuria reflects widespread vascular damage: The Steno hypothesis, *Diabetologia*, 32, 219–226, 1989.

30. **Bates, D. O., Levick, J. R., and Mortimer, P. S.,** Macromolecular composition of interstitial fluid from swollen and normals arms following breast cancer treatment, implications for fluid exchange, *Clin. Sci.*, 85(6), 737–746, 1993.

31. **Lowe, G.,** Pathophysiology of critical leg ischaemia, in *Critical Leg Ischaemia*, Dormandy, J. A. and Stock, G., Eds., Springer Verlag, Berlin, 1990, Chap. 3.

32. **Nash, G. B., Thomas, P. R. S., and Dormandy, J. A.,** Abnormal flow properties of white cells in patients with severe ischaemia of the leg, *Br. Med. J.*, 296, 1699–1701, 1988.

33. **Arner, P., Sjoberg, S., Gjotterberg, M., and Skottner, A.,** Circulating insulin-like growth factor in type 1 (insulin-dependent) diabetic patients with retinopathy, *Diabetologia*, 32, 753–758, 1989.

34. **Namamura, Y. and Myers, B. D.,** Charge selectivity of proteinuria in diabetic glomerulopathy, *Diabetes*, 37, 1202–1211, 1988.

35. **Waltman, S. R., Oestrich, C., Krupin, T., Hanish, S., Ratzan, S., Santiago, J., and Kilo, C.,** Quantitative vitreous fluorophotometry a sensitive technique for measuring early breakdown of the blood-retinal barrier in young diabetic patients, *Diabetes*, 27, 85–87, 1978.

36. **Arend, O., Wolf, S., Jung, F., Bertram, B., Postgens, H., Toonen, H., and Reim, M.,** Retinal microcirculation in patients with diabetes mellitus: Dynamic and morphological analysis of perifoveal capillary network, *Br. J. Ophthalmol.*, 75, 514–518, 1991.

37. **Jacobs, M. J. H. M., Beckers, R. C. Y., Jorning, P. J. G., Slaaf, D. W., and Reneman, R. S.,** Microcirculatory hemodynamics before and after vascular surgery in severe limb ischemia — the relation to post-operative oedema formation, *Eur. J. Vasc. Surg.*, 4, 5, 525–529, 1990.

38. **Franzek, U. and Rayman, G. A.,** Assessment of microvascular function and tissue viability, *Textbook of Vascular Medicine*, Tooke, J. E. and Lowe, G. E., Eds., Edward Arnold, London, 1994.

39. **Shore, A. C., Price, K. J., Sandeman, D. D., Green, E. M., Tripp, J. H., and Tooke, J. E.,** Impaired microvascular hyperaemic response in children with diabetes mellitus, *Diabetic Med.*, 8, 619–623, 1991.

40. **Shore, A. C., Donohoe, M., Jaap, A. J., and Tooke, J. E.,** The effect of increasing doses of an angiotensin converting enzyme inhibitor on capillary pressure levels in patients with insulin-dependent diabetes mellitus and microalbuminuria, BDA 1–2 April 1993, University of Liverpool, *Diab. Med.*, 10, (Suppl. 1), A18, 55, 1993.

41. **Vallance, P.,** Clinical use of inhibitors of nitric oxide synthesis in septic shock, *Vasc. Med. Rev.*, 5(3), 185–189, 1994.

42. **Colantuoni, A., Bertuglia, S., and Intaglietta, M.,** The effects of alpha or beta-adrenergic receptor agonists and antagonists and calcium entry blockers on the spontaneous vasomotion, *Microvasc. Res.*, 28, 143–158, 1984.

Section II

Clinical Syndromes and the Microcirculation

Chapter 2

Atherosclerosis and the Microcirculation

Hans-Anton Lehr

CONTENTS

I. INTRODUCTION

Atherosclerosis is a disease process characterized by the formation of atheromas (fibrofatty intimal plaques) resulting in progressive hardening of the arterial wall and loss of vascular elasticity. Different segments of the vascular tree vary in their susceptibility to develop atherosclerotic lesions. Atheromas characteristically have been associated with middle- and large-sized muscular and elastic arteries. Aorta and iliac, coronary and cerebral arteries are considered the prime targets, and so peripheral artery disease, myocardial infarcts, and cerebral infarcts are the most prominent clinical manifestations of the disease.

This chapter will focus on the most distal part of the circulatory tree, the microcirculation. Here, its functional and morphological damage parallel or are subsequent to macrovascular atherosclerotic disease and often this is crucial for the clinical manifestations of the disease. It will become increasingly apparent as the reader scans the chapters of this book, that the microcirculation has a limited spectrum of responses to a wide variety of different challenges, ranging from localized or systemic ischemia/reperfusion, hypertension, inflammation, to metabolic and (auto-) immunologic disorders.

It is the aim of this chapter to avoid discussing specific trigger mechanisms other than the ones relevant to atherogenesis, and to reduce overlap with chapters dedicated specifically to the discussion of microcirculatory derangements during diabetes and hypertension, as well as individual organ systems.

II. PATHOPHYSIOLOGY

There does not exist one definite microcirculatory manifestation of atherosclerosis. Rather, there is an array of different microcirculatory involvements in distinct processes with relevance to atherosclerosis. For instance, the microcirculation shows functional

0-8493-4870-6/95/$0.00+$.50

alterations during atherosclerotic progression in larger feeding arteries that are not necessarily associated with morphological changes of the microcirculatory unit per se (downstream dysfunction). Beside diabetes and hypertension (resulting in various microvascular changes including hyaline arteriolosclerosis), the microcirculation may be affected by systemic pathophysiological challenges such as immunologic factors during acute and/or chronic rejection of transplanted organs (transplant-associated accelerated allograft atherosclerosis, AAA) as well as effects of drugs and surgical interventions (iatrogenic microvascular damage). Finally, one paragraph will cover the microcirculation as it becomes relevant in vaso vasorum of complicated atherosclerotic lesions from larger vessels.

A. GENERAL CONSIDERATIONS

Atherosclerosis is considered to be a disease process of multifactorial etiology and incompletely understood pathophysiology. Several concepts have been put forward, trying to combine as many aspects of the disease as possible into unifying hypotheses. The most popular and most widely accepted hypothesis is the "response to injury hypothesis" initially formulated by Ross and Glomset in 1973,[1] and later actualized and extended by Ross in 1986.[2] This hypothesis holds that the lesions of atherosclerosis are initiated as a response to some form of injury to the arterial endothelium. Without going into the details of this hypothesis — which is summarized in an overview written by Ross[2] in 1986 — the general message of relevance for the understanding of the microcirculatory changes associated with atherosclerosis is the concept of a balance between damaging mechanisms affecting the vessel wall on one hand and the protective defense mechanisms intrinsic to the vessel wall on the other. This concept covers both functional "regulatory" mechanisms (such as vasodilator/vasoconstrictor responses) and also morphological aspects (such as oxidative attacks to membrane lipids, leading to impaired endothelial cell homeostasis, breakdown of endothelial integrity, leakage of fluid and macromolecules, deposition of fat and extracellular matrix, etc.). In recent years, particular interest has been directed toward the mechanisms underlying the upregulation of adhesion receptors for leukocytes and platelets as well as their role in micro- and macrovascular injury associated with atherosclerosis.

B. DOWNSTREAM DYSFUNCTION

It has been shown both in clinical tests and by using various imaging techniques that the microcirculation is functionally affected in patients with atherosclerosis of large arteries. For instance, laser Doppler fluxmetry on toe pulp and leg skin has revealed marked retardation and complete loss of vasodilator response during postischemic reactive hyperemia in patients with lower limb atherosclerosis, contributing to intermittent claudication or critical ischemia.[3] In skeletal muscle of atherosclerotic rabbits, vasodilation to acetylcholine is impaired.[4,5] Similar effects have been observed in the coronary microcirculation, suggesting that while atherosclerotic lesions are confined to the major coronary arteries, the functional consequences extend into the microcirculation. Myocardial perfusion is regulated predominantly by resistance arterioles less than 200 μm in diameter.[6] More recently, Chilian et al. have demonstrated in atherosclerotic non-human primates a significantly augmented vasoconstrictor response to serotonin, not only in atherosclerotically affected coronary arteries, but also in morphologically unaffected downstream microvessels.[7] Several explanations have been put forward to explain these findings: inhibition of formation of vasodilator prostacyclin from endothelial cells in atherosclerotic patients has been proposed.[8] Comparative studies using various endothelium-dependent and endothelium-independent vasodilators in models of microvascular response have suggested that endothelium-dependent vascular relaxation is abnormal in the coronary microcirculation of atherosclerotic animals.[4,9] Further evidence supporting this concept was provided in an experiment in which the abnormal physiological and pharmacological response in arterioles of atherosclerotic pigs could be completely restored by administration of L-arginine, the precursor of nitric oxide or the so-called endothelial-derived relaxing factor (EDRF).[10] Similar findings have also been reproduced in patients with early atherosclerosis.[11]

While earlier studies have attributed the inhibited vasodilator response of microvessels in atherosclerotic subjects to the prevailing high levels of circulating lipid and circulating cholesterol,[12,13] Kugiyama et al. showed that oxidatively modified low-density lipoprotein (oxLDL), but not native low-density lipoprotein, inhibits endothelium-dependent arterial relaxation by inducing selective unresponsiveness to receptor-regulated endothelium-dependent vasodilators.[14] In addition, the fact that dietary fish oil has the capacity to improve endothelium-dependent responses in hypercholesterolemic and atherosclerotic porcine coronary arteries[13] indicates a role for arachidonic acid metabolites in mediating the impaired vasodilator response in coronary microvessels.

C. TRANSPLANT-ASSOCIATED ACCELERATED ALLOGRAFT ATHEROSCLEROSIS

Accelerated allograft atherosclerosis (AAA) was first described in an orthotopic heart dog model and later in human beings.[15] AAA affects the major epicardial vessels along their entire length, and — unlike naturally occurring "classic" atherosclerosis — includes small epicardial branches and even the intramyocardial microcirculation. Besides extending into the microcirculation, the histopathologic findings of AAA differ from "classical" atherosclerosis: typically, AAA is characterized by a concentric intimal proliferation and pronounced cellular infiltration, sparing the elastic lamina and leaving the media unaffected.[16-18] In earlier stages of intimal proliferation, clusters of subendothelial lymphocytes may be seen. Later, intimal proliferations consist of mononuclear cells, lipid-laden macrophages (foam cells), smooth muscle cells, and cholesterol clefts (reviewed in Reference 16). AAA develops over months or only a few years and seems to be largely independent of HLA ABC mismatch, of the immunosuppressive regimen, and of major risk factors for "classical" atherosclerosis, such as dyslipoproteinemia, sex, age, family disposition, or tobacco abuse (reviewed in Reference 17). These distinctions between classic atherosclerosis and AAA may imply important differences in the pathogenesis of these disorders. An important feature of AAA is selective involvement of the engrafted organ's arteries, but sparing of the host's own vessels. An immune mechanism for the pathogenesis of AAA could account for the localization of this process in transplanted arteries. Thus, the development of these lesions appears not merely a consequence of the transplanted state or administration of immunosuppressive therapy. However, the details of involvement of the immune system in this form of atherosclerosis remain obscure.[18] It has been proposed that the development of AAA may represent the response of the cells within the donor arteries to stimuli released by a chronic, localized form of delayed hypersensitivity to alloantigens on graft-derived vessel wall cells.[18] Evidence suggesting that AAA is immune mediated is supported by studies relating it to recurrent rejection episodes, cytotoxic B-cell antibodies, vascular immunoglobulin and complement deposition, and the presence of T-cell infiltrates in affected vessels (reviewed in Reference 19). Recently, cytomegalovirus infection has been implicated in the subsequent development of AAA.[20]

Similar histologic changes seen in the chronically rejecting heart have been observed in the chronically rejecting liver.[21] Loss of small arterioles, presumably due to immune-mediated cellular injury, induce the ischemic damage with loss of small bile ducts, resulting in the diagnosis of "ductopenic chronic rejection". As in the case of cardiac

AAA, the pathogenesis of chronic liver graft failure, or as some have termed it "graft atherosclerosis", remains obscure.

Epidemiologic observations and *in vitro* experiments have linked low-density lipoproteins, in particular after oxidative modification, with several steps in atherosclerotic lesion inception, including accumulation and adhesion of circulating leukocytes to endothelial cells, their transendothelial emigration, differentiation, and formation of foam cells and fatty streak lesions.[22-24] Using a dorsal skinfold chamber model for intravital microscopy in hamsters and mice, we have recently provided *in vivo* evidence for the chemotactic and leukocyte adhesion promoting action of oxidized low-density lipoprotein (oxLDL).[25,26] OxLDL stimulated leukocyte adhesion, not only to macrovascular endothelium of the aorta of the animals, but also to the endothelium of arterioles and postcapillary venules.[25,26] Although *in vivo*, oxLDL is rapidly cleared from the circulation via scavenger receptors in the liver, several authors have demonstrated the presence of oxLDL in plasma[27] and atherosclerotic lesions.[28]

Based on *in vitro* experiments[29,30] and inhibition studies on cholesterol-fed laboratory animals[31,32] demonstrating the role of oxygen-free radicals and lipoxygenase products in both the oxidative modification of LDL and the inception and progression of atherosclerotic lesions, we have injected oxLDL into animals in which the generation and action of leukotrienes and superoxide anions was blocked by pretreatment with either 5-lipoxygenase inhibitors and dietary fish oil[25,33] or with superoxide dismutase and antioxidant vitamins.[34,79] These pretreatment regimens resulted in a significant inhibition of oxidized LDL (oxLDL)-induced leukocyte/endothelium interaction, demonstrating a key mediator role for leukotrienes and oxygen free radicals in this event.

Leukotrienes, platelet activating factor, oxygen radicals, and numerous cytokines are generated in organ allografts in response to cold storage, reperfusion injury, and the confrontation of the donor organ with the recipient immune system, giving rise to a more or less dramatic acute or chronic allograft rejection and mimicking the morphologic appearance of cell-rich atherosclerotic lesions.[17,18] The tissue damage induced by reperfusion injury,[35,36] but also by acute[37] and chronic rejection[21] is characterized by accumulation and emigration of circulating leukocytes. While in reperfusion injury and acute rejection, infiltrating leukocytes — either directly or through the release of enzymes, inflammatory mediators, and oxygen free radicals — contribute to the breakdown of endothelial integrity and microvascular perfusion,[35-37] the release of leukocyte-derived mediators, growth factors, cytokines, and oxygen free radicals during chronic allograft rejection could contribute to peroxidative damage of endothelial cells and the proliferative response of various cell types within the vessel wall. The deleterious action of infiltrating leukocytes and oxygen free radicals has been documented extensively in various single organs, such as liver,[38] heart,[39] kidney,[40] islets of Langerhans,[41] and is thought to be responsible for the loss of function of these organs after transplantation.

Under normal conditions, tissues contain enough antioxidants and free radical scavengers to protect against oxygen free radical damage. A marked dysbalance between the generation of radicals and antioxidative defense mechanisms has been shown to precede the clinical manifestations of rejection episodes with high predictive values.[42,43] How oxidation of lipoproteins by oxygen free radicals or lipoxygenase products is involved in the peroxidative damage and the infiltration of inflammatory cells into these organs can only be speculated. Evidence for the involvement of lipid peroxidation in allograft rejection can be derived from a study demonstrating that a rise in conjugated dienes for free fatty acids in experimental cardiac transplantation in pigs is temporally associated with allograft rejection.[44] In addition to its effects on peroxidative damage and leukocyte infiltration, oxLDL, like interferon gamma and TNF,[18] could also contribute to the immune insult by inducing the upregulation of HLA-Dr antigens on donor endothelial cells.[23]

D. IATROGENIC MICROVASCULAR DAMAGE

Of minor importance in comparison to the above-described clinico-pathological involvement of the microcirculation in atherosclerosis is the damage to the microcirculation by the intake of analgetics, such as the capillarosclerosis observed after excessive phenacetin and paracetamol intake.[45]

Another rather rare complication of atherosclerosis with relevance for the microcirculation is the cholesterol emboli syndrome following diagnostic and/or therapeutic invasive procedures in atherosclerotic patients, resulting in a variety of clinical consequences, ranging from cutaneous manifestations, myalgias, retinal damage, acute renal and hepatic failure, splenic infarction and ischemic bowel syndromes to multiorgan failure and death (reviewed in Reference 46).

Finally, ionizing radiation therapy has been shown to induce endothelial cell swelling in capillaries and small arterioles, predisposing for the formation of platelet and fibrin thrombi, leading to microvessel occlusion and, ultimately, obliteration and fibrotic degeneration (reviewed in Reference 47).

E. VASO VASORUM

In normal arteries, vaso vasorum are present as an adventitial network, which extends into the outer media of only the very largest vessels such as the aorta and the pulmonary arteries.[48] With the development of atherosclerosis, however, adventitial vessels proliferate and penetrate the media to form a microvascular plexus in the diseased intima.[49,50] A correlation could be established between the extent of the vascular network of vaso vasorum and the degree of intimal thickening. Vaso vasorum originate from the adventitia, commonly from sites proximal to the atherosclerotic lesion, and in some instances from intramural branches or even from the lumen of the atherosclerotically affected vessel. To date, there is almost no information regarding the mechanism by which vasa vasorum are formed in the atherosclerotically affected vessel. Although some investigators have reported that oxygen consumption of atherosclerotic vessels exceeds that of their normal counterparts,[51] it is unknown whether increases in oxygen demand could account for this marked increase in vaso vasorum. On the other hand, current evidence suggests that isolated plaque fragments possess angiogenic activity per se. Alpern-Elran et al.[52] demonstrated that fragments of human plaque induced angiogenesis when implanted into rabbit corneas. Boiled plaque was not angiogenic. Later studies have identified elevated levels of growth factors in atherosclerotic plaques, such as fibroblast growth factor,[53] transforming growth factor beta,[54] and tumor necrosis factor.[55] In particular, fibroblast growth factor was found concentrated around vaso vasorum, suggesting a potential role in angiogenesis.[53]

III. CLINICAL CONSEQUENCES

A. DOWNSTREAM DYSFUNCTION

It is now generally accepted that atherosclerosis augments vasoconstrictor responses and impairs vasodilator responses to a variety of vasoactive compounds. In patients, atherosclerosis inhibits flow-induced vasodilation.[56] In this context, there are clinical studies that report augmented coronary constrictor responses to ergonovine in the absence of gross atherosclerotic lesions in epicardial coronary arteries.[57] The role of this abnormality in the pathogenesis of myocardial ischemia remains to be determined. For many years, clinicians have been intrigued with the fact that in some patients with electrocardiographic, scintigraphic, and biochemical signs of myocardial ischemia the coronary arteriogram fail to reveal a lesion that would account for the severity of the clinical symptoms. Accordingly, myocardial ischemia in these patients has been tentatively ascribed to a defect affecting small arteries not visualized by arteriography.[58] Also, coronary microvascular spasms, sufficient to result in demonstrable myocardial ischemia, have been implicated in patients with evidence of only minor coronary artery disease.[57,58] Of further importance for the clinical translation of the phenomenon of downstream dysfunction is the observation that patients with so-called "microvascular angina" exhibit impaired forearm vasodilator reserve,[59] suggesting a systemic manifestation of this phenomenon.

B. TRANSPLANT-ASSOCIATED ACCELERATED ALLOGRAFT ATHEROSCLEROSIS

Chronic vascular rejection constitutes a severe threat to the long-term benefit of organ transplantation. This is particularly true in cardiac transplantation, where AAA is the number one cause for mortality following the first few months after transplantation. While AAA has been detected angiographically in over 90% of cardiac allograft recipients at 5 years, it may cause death as early as 5 months after transplantation. The luminal occlusion of AAA results in the same myocardial changes as those of classic atherosclerosis, namely myocardial ischemia and infarction. The fact that the microcirculation is not spared as in "classic" atherosclerosis precludes coronary artery bypass operations and — in most cases — atherectomy or other interventional coronary artery procedures. Because small intramyocardial branches of the coronary tree are affected, they are often occluded before the luminal occlusion of major epicardial vessels, and this results in small, multiple stellate infarcts. This fact, together with the denervation that occurs at the time of transplantation, accounts for the lack of the normal anginal pain that often accompanies ischemia and infarcts. Sudden death, therefore, is not uncommon in these patients.

AAA is, however, not confined to cardiac transplantation. In liver transplantation, up to 50% of liver graft failures are attributed to chronic allograft rejection with features of arteriolar and bile duct loss.[21] Likewise, in renal transplantation, AAA accounts for a majority of late graft losses.[60] Finally, experimental data indicate a similar involvement of the allograft microvasculature by AAA in pulmonary transplantation.[61] While the advent of cyclosporine therapy has greatly improved early graft survival, this drug has at the same time not reduced, but rather increased the frequency and severity of AAA.[60]

C. VASO VASORUM

Vaso vasorum may play a crucial permissive role in plaque progression. In other words, the excessive oxygen demand of atherosclerotic lesions may imply that plaques require vaso vasorum to exceed growth beyond a certain critical mass. If vasa vasorum are required to sustain the viability of the plaque and underlying media, then the frequent occurrence of necrosis in advanced lesions may represent ischemia, resulting from the inability of the plaque vaso vasorum to meet the metabolic requirements of the enlarging lesion. Vaso vasorum could play a significant role in regulating the contractile properties of atherosclerotically affected vessels. In addition to eicosanoids like prostacyclin, it is now well established that endothelial production of nitric oxide (NO) from arginine by NO synthase is responsible for producing a variety of physiologic effects such as parasympathic coronary dilation and dilation in response to increased flow.[62] In addition to regulating smooth muscle contraction, NO inhibits smooth muscle proliferation, platelet aggregation and adhesion, as well as leukocyte adhesion and activation.[63,64] Thus, both the contractile properties of the vessels and factors involved in atherogenesis may be influenced by endothelium-derived NO. A recent report by Lamas et al.[65] has localized mRNA for the constitutive form of NO synthase in vaso vasorum. Given that the endothelial surface of the plaque vaso vasorum is likely many times that of the diseased vessel lumen, it is intriguing to speculate that the vaso vasorum-derived NO may contribute to the maintenance of lumen diameter. Conversely, dysfunction of the vaso vasorum or production of vasoconstrictors such as endothelin may result in vasospasm. Finally, rupture of the coronary vaso vasorum may play an important role in the onset or triggering of acute myocardial infarction.[50] Indeed, these authors have suggested that with the morning increase in blood pressure, fragile vaso vasorum may be more prone to rupture and may be responsible, in part, for the circadian variation in myocardial infarction.[50]

IV. THERAPEUTIC CONSEQUENCES

A. DOWNSTREAM DYSFUNCTION

Based on the knowledge of the pathophysiology of downstream dysfunction in atherosclerotic extremities, as well as the mediators involved in this problem, various pharmacological approaches have been tested to correct for these changes. For instance, one clinical study has used low-dose aspirin aimed at the distorted balance between vasodilator prostacyclin and vasoconstrictor thromboxane A2 in patients with atherosclerosis.[8] Although a favorable change in the balance of these vasoactive arachidonic acid metabolites was measured, no clinical data were presented, which might have suggested an improvement of the resulting vasodysregulation. Another promising approach that is suggested from experimental data is the use of dietary fish oil. Indeed, it has been shown that dietary fish oil has the capacity to improve endothelium-dependent relaxation responses in hypercholesterolemic and atherosclerotic porcine coronary arteries.[13] If these effects are due to inhibition of vasoconstrictor cyclooxygenase products of arachidonic acid or of leukocyte chemotactic and adhesion-promoting lipoxygenase products of arachidonic acid, this remains to be shown. However, the availability of dietary fish oil for use in patients and the low spectrum of side effects warrants the experimental use in selected patients suffering from downstream dysfunction, in particular for "microvascular angina". Furthermore, the demonstration that oxLDL limits endothelium-derived arterial relaxation[14] suggests that clinical trials with antioxidants (antioxidant vitamins, probucol, etc.) might prove beneficial in the management of patients with downstream dysfunction.

B. TRANSPLANT-ASSOCIATED ACCELERATED ALLOGRAFT ATHEROSCLEROSIS

Various pharmacological and dietary trials have been undertaken to attenuate AAA. Beside angiopeptin,[66,67] the mechanism of which is still incompletely understood, beneficial effects have been documented with the administration of stable prostacyclin analogs[67] and with dietary supplementation of n-3 fatty acids.[68,69] Although all these experimental approaches exert a variety of diverse actions, one common mechanism of all these drugs is a potent inhibitory effect on leukocyte chemotaxis and adhesion to endothelial cells.[67,70,71] The unequivocal demonstration that leukocytes contribute to tissue damage after ischemia/reperfusion has led to a host of experimental studies demonstrating that postischemic tissue damage can be attenuated by therapies directed against leukocyte adhesion[72] or toward the mediators of leukocyte/endothelium interaction such as oxygen free radicals,[73,74] leukotrienes,[36,75] or platelet activating factor.[76] Likewise, treatment of laboratory animals with the antioxidant probucol,[31] inhibition of leukotriene biosynthesis by dietary fish oil,[32] or administration of PAF receptor antagonists[77] have resulted in a significant protraction of atherogenesis. However, to our knowledge, not a single study either on laboratory animals or on human subjects has been published to date investigating the effect of antioxidants or free radical scavengers on the long-term allograft function. Although conclusive evidence for their protective effects on clinical atherogenesis remains to be established,[78] the availability of such treatment modalities for long-term oral use in patients (vitamins C and E, Ubiquinol, Probucol, etc.) and the negligible spectrum of adverse effects should warrant their experimental use either in laboratory animals or in prospective clinical trails.

REFERENCES

1. **Ross, R. and Glomset, J. A.,** Atherosclerosis and the arterial smooth muscle cell, *Science,* 180, 1332–1339, 1973.
2. **Ross, R.,** The pathogenesis of atherosclerosis — an update, *N. Engl. J. Med.,* 314, 488–500, 1986.
3. **Kvernebo, K., Slasgsvold, C. E., and Stranden, E.,** Laser Doppler flowmetry in evaluation of skin post-ischaemic reactive hyperaemia. A study in healthy volunteers and atherosclerotic patients, *J. Cardiovasc. Surg. Torino,* 30, 70–75, 1989.
4. **Yamamoto, H., Bossaller, C., Cartwright, J., and Henry, P. D.,** Videomicroscopic demonstration of defective cholinergic arteriolar vasodilation in atherosclerotic rabbit, *J. Clin. Invest.,* 81, 1752–1758, 1988.
5. **Henry, P. D. and Yokoyama, M.,** Supersensitivity of atherosclerotic rabbit aorta to ergonovine. Mediation by a serotoninergic mechanism, *J. Clin. Invest.,* 66, 306–313, 1980.
6. **Nellis, S. A., Liedtke, A. J., and Whitesell, L.,** Small coronary vessel pressure and diameter in an intact beating rabbit heart using fixed-position and free-motion techniques, *Circ. Res.,* 49, 342–353, 1981.
7. **Chilian, W. M., Dellsperger, K. C., Layne, S. M., Eastham, C. L., Armstrong, M. A., Marcus, M. L., and Heistad, D. D.,** Effects of atherosclerosis on the coronary microcirculation, *Am. J. Physiol.,* 258, H529–H539, 1990.
8. **Kyrle, P. A., Minar, E., Brenner, B., Eichler, H. G., Heistinger, M., Marosi, L., and Lechner, K.,** Thromboxane A2 and prostacyclin generation in the microvasculature of patients with atherosclerosis — effect of low-dose aspirin, *Thromb. Haemost.,* 61, 374–377, 1989.
9. **Sellke, F. W., Armstrong, M. L., and Harrison, D. G.,** Endothelium-dependent vascular relaxation is abnormal in the coronary microcirculation of atherosclerotic primates, *Circulation,* 81, 1586–1593, 1990.
10. **Kuo, L., Davis, M. J., Cannon, M. S., and Chilian, W. M.,** Pathophysiological consequences of atherosclerosis extend into the coronary microcirculation. Restoration of endothelium-dependent responsiveness by L-arginine, *Circ. Res.,* 70, 465–476, 1992.
11. **Zeiher, A. M., Drexler, H., Wollschläger, H., and Just, H.,** Endothelial dysfunction of the coronary microvasculature is associated with impaired coronary blood flow regulation in patients with early atherosclerosis, *Circulation,* 84, 1984–1992, 1991.
12. **Heistad, D. D., Armstrong, M. L., Marcus, M. L., Piegors, D. J., and Mark, A. L.,** Augmented responses to vasoconstrictor stimuli in hypercholesterolemic and atherosclerotic monkeys, *Circ. Res.,* 54, 711–718, 1984.
13. **Shimokawa, H. and Vanhoutte, P. M.,** Dietary cod liver oil improves endothelium-dependent responses in hyperecholesterolemic and atherosclerotic porcine coronary arteries, *Circulation,* 78, 1421–1430, 1988.
14. **Kugiyama, K., Kerns, S. A., Morrisett, J. D., Roberts, R., and Henry, P. D.,** Impairment of endothelium-dependent arterial relaxation by lysolecithin in modified low-density lipoproteins, *Nature,* 344, 160–162, 1990.
15. **Bieber, C. P., Hunt, S. A., and Schwinn, D. A.,** Complications in long-term survivors of cardiac transplantation, *Transplant. Proc.,* 13, 207–211, 1981.
16. **Billingham, M. E.,** Histopathology of graft coronary disease, *J. Heart Lung Transplant.,* 11, S38–S44, 1992.
17. **Foegh, M. L.,** Chronic rejection — graft arteriosclerosis, *Transplant. Proc.,* 22, 119–122, 1990.
18. **Libby, P., Salomon, R. N., Payne, D. D., Schoen, F. J., and Pober, J. S.,** Functions of vascular wall cells related to development of transplantation-associated coronary arteriosclerosis, *Transplant. Proc.,* 21, 3677–3684, 1989.
19. **Winters, G. L.,** The pathology of heart allograft rejection, *Arch. Pathol. Lab. Med.,* 115, 266–272, 1991.
20. **McDonald, K., Rector, T. S., Braulin, E. A., Kubo, S. H., and Olivari, M. T.,** Association of coronary artery disease in cardiac transplant recipients with cytomegalovirus infection, *Am. J. Pathol.,* 64, 359–362, 1989.
21. **Oguma, S., Belle, S., Starzl, T. E., and Demetris, A. J.,** A histometric analysis of chronically rejected human liver allografts: Insights into the mechanisms of bile duct loss: Direct immunologic and ischemic factors, *Hepatology,* 9, 204–209, 1989.

22. **Quinn, M. T., Parthasarathy, S., Fong, L. G., and Steinberg, D.,** Oxidatively modified low density lipoproteins: A potential role in recruitment and retention of monocyte/macrophages during atherogenesis, *Proc. Natl. Acad. Sci. U.S.A.*, 84, 2995–2998, 1987.

23. **Frostegard, J., Nilsson, J., Haegerstrand, A., Hamsten, A., Wigzell, H., and Gidlund, M.,** Oxidized low-density lipoprotein induces differentiation and adhesion of human monocytes and the monocytic cell line U937, *Proc. Natl. Acad. Sci. U.S.A.*, 87, 904–908, 1990.

24. **Steinberg, D., Parthasarathy, S., Carew, T. E., Khoo, J. C., and Witztum, J. L.,** Beyond cholesterol. Modifications of low-density lipoprotein that increase its atherogenicity, *N. Engl. J. Med.*, 320, 915–924, 1989.

25. **Lehr, H. A., Hübner, C., Finckh, B., Angermüller, S., Nolte, D., Beisiegel, U., Kohlschütter, A., and Messmer, K.,** Role of leukotrienes in leukocyte adhesion following systemic administration of oxidatively modified human low density lipoproteins in hamsters, *J. Clin. Invest.*, 88, 9–14, 1991.

26. **Lehr, H. A., Kröber, M., Hübner, C., Vajkoczy, P., Menger, M. D., Nolte, D., Kohlschütter, A., and Messmer, K.,** Stimulation of leukocyte/endothelium interaction by oxidized low-density lipoprotein in hairless mice: Involvement of CD11b/CD18 adhesion receptor complex, *Lab. Invest.*, 68, 388–395, 1993.

27. **Avogaro, P., Bittolo Bon, G., and Cazzolato, G.,** Presence of a modified low density lipoprotein in humans, *Arteriosclerosis*, 8, 79–87, 1988.

28. **Ylä-Herttuala, S., Palinski, W., Rosenfeld, M. E., Parthasarathy, S., Carew, T. E., Butler, S., Witztum, J. L., and Steinberg, D.,** Evidence for the presence of oxidatively modified low density lipoprotein in atherosclerotic lesions of rabbit and man, *J. Clin. Invest.*, 84, 1086–1095, 1989.

29. **Heinecke, J. W., Baker, L., Rosen, H., and Chait, A.,** Superoxide-mediated modification of low-density lipoprotein by arterial smooth muscle cells, *J. Clin. Invest.*, 77, 757–761, 1986.

30. **Parthasarathy, S., Steinbrecher, U. P., Barnett, J., Witztum, J. L., and Steinberg, D.,** Essential role of phospholipase A_2 activity in endothelial cell-induced modification of low density lipoprotein, *Proc. Natl. Acad. Sci. U.S.A.*, 82, 3000–3004, 1985.

31. **Carew, T. E., Schwenke, D. C., and Steinberg, D.,** Antiatherogenic effect of probucol unrelated to its hypocholesterolemic effect: Evidence that antioxidants *in vivo* can selectively inhibit low-density lipoprotein degradation in macrophage-rich fatty streaks and slow the progression of atherosclerosis in the Watanabe heritable hyperlipidemic rabbit, *Proc. Natl. Acad. Sci. U.S.A.*, 84, 7725–7729, 1987.

32. **Weiner, B. H., Ockene, I. S., Levine, P. H., Cuenoud, H. F., Fisher, M., Johnson, B. F., Daoud, A. S., Jarmolych, J., Hosmer, D., Johnson, M. H., Natale, A., Vaudreuil, C., and Hoogasian, J. J.,** Inhibition of atherosclerosis by cod-liver oil in a hyperlipidemic swine model, *N. Engl. J. Med.*, 315, 841–846, 1986.

33. **Lehr, H. A., Hübner, C., Finckh, B., Nolte, D., Beisiegel, U., Kohlschütter, A., and Messmer, K.,** Dietary fish oil reduces leukocyte/endothelium interaction following systemic administration of oxidatively modified low-density lipoprotein, *Circulation*, 84, 1725–1731, 1991.

34. **Lehr, H. A., Becker, M., Marklund, S. L., Hübner, C., Arfors, K. E., Kohlschütter, A., and Messmer, K.,** Superoxide-dependent stimulation of leukocyte adhesion by oxidatively modified LDL *in vivo*, *Arterioscler. Thromb.*, 12, 824–829, 1992.

35. **Menger, M., Sack, F. U., Barker, J. H., Feifel, G., and Messmer, K.,** Quantitative analysis of microcirculatory disorders after prolonged ischemia in skeletal muscle, *Res. Exp. Med.*, 188, 151–165, 1988.

36. **Lehr, H. A., Guhlmann, A., Nolte, D., Keppler, D., and Messmer, K.,** Leukotrienes as mediators in ischemia-reperfusion injury in a microcirculation model in the hamster, *J. Clin. Invest.*, 87, 2036–2041, 1991.

37. **Häyry, P., van Willebrand, E., Parthenais, E., Nemlander, A., Soots, A., Lautenschlager, I., Alfoldy, P., and Renkonen, A.,** The inflammatory mechanism of allograft rejection, *Immunol. Rev.*, 77, 85–142, 1984.

38. **Adams, D. H., Wang, L. F., Burnett, D., and Stockley, R. A.,** Neutrophil activation — an important cause of tissue damage during liver allograft rejection?, *Transplantation*, 50, 86–91, 1990.

39. **Rowe, G. T., Eaton, L. R., and Hess, M. L.,** Neutrophil-derived, oxygen free radical-mediated cardiovascular dysfunction, *J. Mol. Cell. Cardiol.*, 16, 1975–1979, 1984.

40. **Baud, L. and Ardaillou, R.,** Reactive oxygen species: Production and role in the kidney, *Am. J. Physiol.*, 251, F765–F776, 1986.

41. **Nomikos, I. N., Prowse, S. J., Carotenuto, P., and Lafferty, K. J.,** Combined treatment with nicotinamide and desferroxamine prevents islet allograft destruction in NOD mice, *Diabetes*, 35, 1302–1304, 1986.

42. **Rosenberg, L., Merion, R. M., Campbell, D. A., Dafore, D. C., Clarke, S., Rocher, L., and Turcotte, J. G.,** Peripheral blood catalase in patients undergoing renal transplantation, *J. Surg. Res.*, 44, 493–498, 1988.

43. **Kloc, M., Mailer, K., and Stepkowski, S.,** Superoxide dismutase decreases in cardiac transplants, *Transplantation*, 41, 794–796, 1986.

44. **Koike, K., Hesslein, P. S., Dasmahapatra, K. H., Wilson, G. J., Finlay, C. D., David, S. L., Kielmanowicz, S., and Coles, J. G.,** Telemetric detection of cardiac allograft rejection. Correlation of electrophysiological, histological, and biochemical changes during unmodified rejection, *Circulation*, 78, 1106–1112, 1988.

45. **Bethke, B. A. and Schubert, G. E.,** Capillarosclerosis of the lower urinary tract as a sign of analgesic abuse, *Dtsch. Med. Wschr.*, 110, 343–346, 1985.

46. **Freund, N. S.,** Cholesterol emboli syndrome following cardiac catheterization, *Postgrad. Med.*, 87, 55–60, 1990.

47. **Eldor, A., Fuks, Z., Matzner, Y., Witte, L. D., and Vlodavsky, I.,** Perturbation of endothelial functions by ionizing irradiation: Effects on prostaglandins, chemoattractants and mitogens, *Semin. Thromb. Hemost.*, 15, 215–225 1989.

48. **Wolinsky, H. and Glagov, S.,** Nature and species differences in the medial distribution of aortic vasa vasorum in mammals, *Circ. Res.*, 20, 409–421, 1967.

49. **Barger, A. C., Beeuwkes, R., and LeCompte, P. M.,** Vaso vasorum and neovascularization of human coronary arteries: A possible role in the pathophysiology of atherosclerosis, *N. Engl. J. Med.*, 310, 175–177, 1984.

50. **Barger, A. C. and Beeuwkes, R.,** Rupture of coronary vaso vasorum as a trigger of acute myocardial infarction, *Am. J. Cardiol.*, 66, 41G–43G, 1990.

51. **Whereat, A. F.,** Oxygen consumption of normal and atherosclerotic intima, *Circ. Res.*, 9, 571–575, 1961.

52. **Alpern-Elran, H., Morog, N., Robert, F., Hoover, F., Kalant, N., and Brem, S.,** Angiogenetic activity of the atherosclerotic carotid artery plaque, *J. Neurosurg.*, 70, 942–945, 1989.

53. **Brogi, E., Winkles, J. A., and Libby, P.,** Regional expression of acidic and basic fibroblast growth factor in human atheroma and non-atherosclerotic arteries, *Circulation*, 86, 185, 1992.

54. **Nikol, S., Isner, J. M., Pickering, J. G., Kearney, M., Leclerc, G., and Weir, L.,** Expression of transforming growth factor-beta 1 is increased in human vascular restenosis lesions, *J. Clin. Invest.*, 90, 1582–1592, 1992.

55. **Barath, P., Fishbein, M. C., Cao, J., Berenson, J., Helfant, R. H., and Forrester, J. S.,** Detection and localization of tumor necrosis factor in atheroma, *Am. J. Cardiol.*, 65, 297–302, 1990.

56. **Cox, D. A., Vita, J. A., Treasure, C. B., Fish, R. D., Alexander, R. W., Ganz, P., and Selwyn, A. P.,** Atherosclerosis impairs flow-mediated dilation of coronary arteries in humans, *Circulation*, 80, 458–465, 1989.

57. **Cannon, R. O., Watson, R. M., Rosing, D. R., and Epstein, S. E.,** Angina caused by reduced casodilator reserve of the small coronary arteries, *J. Am. Coll. Cardiol.*, 1, 1359–1367, 1983.

58. **Cannon, R. O. and Epstein, S. E.,** Microvascular angina as a cause of chest pain with angiographically normal coronary arteries, *Am. J. Cardiol.*, 61, 1338–1343, 1988.

59. **Sax, F. L., Cannon, R. O., Hanson, C., and Epstein, S. E.,** Impaired forearm vasodilator reserve in patients with microvascular angina, *N. Engl. J. Med.*, 317, 1366–1370, 1987.

60. **Rossmann, P., Jirka, J., Chadimova, M., Reneltova, I., and Saudek, F.,** Arteriolosclerosis of the human renal allograft: Morphology, origin, life history and relationship to cyclosporine therapy, *Virchows Arch. A. Pathol. Anat. Histopathol.*, 418, 129–141, 1991.

61. **Haverich, A., Dawkins, K. D., Baldwin, J. C., Reitz, B. A., Billingham, M. E., and Jamieson, S. W.,** Long-term cardiac and pulmonary histology in primates following combined heart and lung transplantation, *Transplantation*, 39, 356–360, 1985.

62. **Broten, T. P., Miyashiro, J. K., Moncada, S., and Feigl, E. O.,** Role of endothelium-derived relaxing factor in parasympathic coronary vasodilation, *Am. J. Physiol.*, 262, H1579–H1584, 1992.

63. **Bath, P. M., Hassall, D. G., Gladwin, A. M., Palmer, R. M., and Martin, J. F.,** Nitric oxide and prostacyclin: Divergence of inhibitory effects on monocyte chemotaxis and adhesion to endothelium *in vitro*, *Arterioscler. Thromb.*, 11, 254–260, 1991.

64. **Kubes, P., Suzuki, M., and Granger, D. N.,** Nitric oxide: An endogenous modulator of leukocyte adhesion, *Proc. Natl. Acad. Sci. U.S.A.*, 88, 4651–4655, 1991.
65. **Lamas, S., Tichel, T., Brenner, B. M., and Tarsden, P. A.,** Nitric oxide synthesis in endothelial cells: Evidence for a pathway inducible by the TNF-alpha, *Am. J. Physiol.*, 261, C634–C641, 1991.
66. **Foegh, M. L.,** Accelerated cardiac transplant atherosclerosis/chronic rejection in rabbits: Inhibition by angiopeptin, *Transplant. Proc.*, 25, 2095–2097, 1993.
67. **Fellström, B., Dimeny, E., Foegh, M. L., Larsson, E., Wanders, A., and Tufesson, G.,** Accelerated atherosclerosis in heart transplants in the rat stimulating chronic vascular rejection: Effect of prostacyclin and angiopeptin, *Transplant. Proc.*, 23, 525–528, 1991.
68. **Sweny, P.,** Use of dietary fish oils in renal allograft recipients with chronic vascular rejection, *Transplant. Proc.*, 25, 2089–2091, 1993.
69. **Homan van der Heide, J. J., Bilo, H. J. G., Donker, J. M., Wilmink, J. M., and Tegzess, A. M.,** Effect of dietary fish oil on renal function and rejection in cyclosposine-treated recipients of renal transplants, *N. Engl. J. Med.*, 329, 769–773, 1993.
70. **Boxer, L. A., Allen, J. M., Schmidt, M., Yoder, M., and Baehner, R. L.,** Inhibition of polymorphonuclear leukocyte adherence by prostacyclin, *J. Lab. Clin. Med.*, 95, 672–678, 1980.
71. **Kim, D. N., Schmee, J., and Thomas, W. A.,** Dietary fish oil added to a hyperlipidemic diet for swine results in reduction in the excessive number of monocytes attached to arterial endothelium, *Atherosclerosis*, 81, 209–221, 1990.
72. **Hernandez, L. A., Grisham, M. B., Twohig, B., Arfors, K. E., Harlan, J. M., and Granger, D. N.,** Role of neutrophils in ischemia-reperfusion-induced microvascular injury, *Am. J. Physiol.*, 253, H699–H703, 1987.
73. **Suzuki, M., Inauen, W., Kvietys, P. R., Grisham, M. B., Meininger, C., Schelling, M. E., Granger, H. J., and Granger, D. N.,** Superoxide mediates reperfusion-induced leukocyte-endothelial cell interactions, *Am. J. Physiol.*, 257, H1740–H1745, 1989.
74. **Menger, M. D, Pelikan, S., Steiner, D., and Messmer, K.,** Microvascular ischemia/reperfusion injury in striated muscle: Significance of reflow paradox, *Am. J. Physiol.*, 263, H1901–H1906, 1992.
75. **Zimmerman, B. J., Guillory, D. J., Grisham, M. B., Gaginella, T. S., and Granger, D. N.,** Role of leukotriene B4 in granulocyte infiltration into the postischemic feline intestine, *Gastroenterology*, 99, 1358–1363, 1991.
76. **Kubes, P., Ibbotson, G., Russell, J., Wallace, J. L., and Granger, D. N.,** Role of platelet-activating factor in ischemia/reperfusion-induced leukocyte adherence, *Am. J. Physiol.*, 259, G300–G305, 1990.
77. **Feliste, R., Perret, B., Braquet, P., and Chap, H.,** Protective effect of BN 52021, a specific antagonist of platelet-activating factor (PAF-acether) against diet-induced cholesteryl ester deposition in rabbit aorta, *Atherosclerosis*, 78, 151–158, 1989.
78. **Steinberg, D.,** Antioxidants and atherosclerosis: A current assessment, *Circulation*, 84, 1420–1425, 1991.
79. **Lehr, H. A., Frei, B., Olofsson, M., Carew, T. E., and Arfors, K. E.,** Protection from oxidized LDL-induced leukocyte adhesion to microvascular and macrovascular endothelium *in vivo* by vitamin C, but not by vitamin E, *Circulation*, 91, 1525–1532, 1995.

Chapter 3

Diabetes and the Microcirculation

Alan J. Jaap and John E. Tooke

CONTENTS

I. INTRODUCTION

Damage to the microcirculation plays a central role in the development of the long-term complications of diabetes, leading to a specific microangiopathy characterized by basement membrane thickening in capillaries, arterioles, and venules. Although classically affecting the retina and kidney, the histological features of microangiopathy are apparent in a wide variety of other microvascular beds including skin, adipose tissue, and skeletal and cardiac muscle. In addition, it is increasingly recognized that microvascular abnormalities are involved in the development of neuropathy and diabetic foot ulceration. Microvascular disease is responsible for a substantial amount of morbidity in the non-elderly in Western countries, with diabetic retinopathy and nephropathy being the most common causes of blindness and renal failure, respectively. Foot ulceration is also a major problem, accounting for a large proportion of diabetes-related hospital admissions and bed occupancy. This chapter will outline the pathogenesis of these microvascular complications, their clinical manifestations in different tissues, and the potential treatment options available to minimize the impact of microvascular disease.

0-8493-4870-6/95/$0.00+$.50
© 1995 by CRC Press, Inc.

32

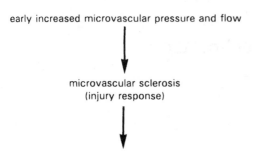

early increased microvascular pressure and flow

microvascular sclerosis
(injury response)

limited vasodilation and impaired autoregulation

Figure 1 The hemodynamic hypothesis for the development of diabetic microangiopathy.

II. PATHOGENESIS

It has been proposed that diabetic microangiopathy may be the end result of long-standing functional changes in the microcirculation,[1] such as increased pressure, blood flow, and permeability, which eventually lead to microvascular sclerosis perhaps via an injury response to repetitive endothelial damage (Figure 1). In turn, such structural changes could lead to further impairment of microvascular function by limiting flow reserve and the capacity for autoregulation. There is now a large amount of experimental evidence in favor of this hemodynamic hypothesis.[1-3] An important feature of such a chain of events is that the early functional changes are potentially reversible, in contrast to established microangiopathy, which is largely irreversible.

A. THE SKIN MICROCIRCULATION

Hemodynamic changes have been extensively characterized in the skin microcirculation, which is easily accessible to investigation using noninvasive techniques. Abnormalities of skin microcirculatory function may have direct clinical relevance in the pathogenesis of diabetic foot ulcers. Regardless of whether predominantly due to ischemia or neuropathy, this ulceration ultimately represents microcirculatory failure. In addition, abnormal microvascular function may have a profound effect on the healing of foot ulcers, e.g., limitation of vasodilation could depress the acute inflammatory response to infection and trauma.

1. Insulin-Dependent Diabetes

Increased microvascular blood flow is present in the skin at an early stage after diagnosis in patients with insulin-dependent diabetes mellitus (IDDM). Much of this increased flow occurs through arteriovenous shunt vessels, as suggested by both early experiments demonstrating histological arterialization of the venous system in the foot and partitioning of microspheres, and more recent studies showing high foot venous oxygen tension, abnormal forward flow in diastole on Doppler sonography, and high flow in the toe pulp — an area rich in arteriovenous anastomoses — using laser Doppler fluximetry (the experimental data on overperfusion is reviewed in Reference 2). There is also evidence for increased flow through the nutritive skin capillaries using direct videomicroscopy,[4] although it is unknown whether this is adequate to meet the increased metabolic demands of the tissues due to raised temperature and metabolic rate. Microcirculatory overperfusion is associated with poor glycemic control and the presence of neuropathy, and improvement in diabetic control using continuous subcutaneous insulin infusion, or intravenous insulin, has been shown to redistribute blood flow in favor of the nutritive microcirculation.[4,5]

Although microvascular overperfusion has been well characterized, capillary pressure measurements in patients with diabetes have only recently been reported. Studies in IDDM patients have demonstrated an increase in skin nailfold capillary pressure, which is present early in the course of the disease and is related to the degree of hyperglycemia.[6] Capillary pressure is elevated in patients with early evidence of nephropathy, in contrast to patients with a long disease duration but minimal evidence of microvascular complications who have capillary pressure values similar to those found in control subjects.[7]

Increased microvascular fluid permeability has been demonstrated in the tissues of the forearm in young IDDM patients with a short duration of diabetes even during acceptable glycemic control, suggesting a primary change in permeability.[8] In contrast, other early permeability changes, such as an elevated transcapillary escape rate of albumin, are improved with glycemic control.[9] Further increases in permeability to a variety of solutes are found in patients with longer disease duration.

In addition to such hemodynamic changes under resting conditions, there is evidence for impairment of postural responses, such as postural vasoconstriction, which is principally mediated by a local sympathetic axon reflex and which reduces blood flow in the distal limb on standing.[10] Ineffective postural vasoconstriction leads to increased microvascular pressure and flow on dependency, with increased fluid filtration from the microcirculation and ultimately edema formation. The postural vasoconstriction response is normally acquired during passage through puberty, yet children with diabetes fail to develop this protective reflex.[11] Loss of this and other protective mechanisms result in an increased hemodynamic burden during activity, which could further accelerate the rate of microvascular damage.

Despite microvascular overperfusion under resting conditions, there is limitation of maximum perfusion in response to a number of stimuli. Assessment of maximum vasodilatory capacity by laser Doppler fluximetry has shown a reduction in response to local heating in IDDM patients after several years of diabetes.[12] Similar reductions in maximum vasodilation have been demonstrated following minor skin trauma induced by a needle prick,[12] after arterial occlusion,[13] and in response to pharmacological agents.[14] Limited microvascular vasodilation has also been found in children who have had diabetes for several years,[15] despite the rarity of clinically detectable microangiopathy before puberty.

Finally, there is evidence for impaired microcirculatory autoregulation[13] in that there is poor maintenance of constant blood flow with varying perfusion pressure. This has been related to the amount of basement membrane thickening in terminal arteriolar walls,[16] supporting the idea that arteriolar sclerosis may contribute to limited vasodilation.

2. Non-Insulin-Dependent Diabetes

Although patients with non-insulin-dependent diabetes mellitus (NIDDM) develop the same spectrum of microvascular complications, the prevalence of some of these differs from that found in IDDM, e.g., maculopathy is a more common cause of sight-threatening retinopathy than proliferative retinopathy in patients with NIDDM. Such clinical observations are reflected by apparent differences in microvascular hemodynamic changes. Although microvascular overperfusion is present under resting conditions, the major functional abnormality found in NIDDM patients is a marked impairment of microvascular vasodilation. This has been found to be present at diagnosis in NIDDM,[17] in contrast to IDDM where a similar degree of vasodilatory impairment takes several years to become apparent. This may be due to difficulties in being certain about exact disease duration in NIDDM; however, preliminary work suggests that a similar limitation of vasodilation may be present in the prediabetic phase of NIDDM, that is, in subjects with impaired glucose tolerance.[18] Skin nailfold capillary pressure does not appear to be elevated in NIDDM[19] and no increase in forearm microvascular fluid permeability has been observed using a sensitive plethysmographic technique.[20] This spectrum of microcirculatory abnormalities suggests that there is an early rise in precapillary vascular resistance in NIDDM that protects the capillary bed from increased pressure and at the

increased capillary pressure

overperfusion at rest

limited maximal vasodilation

increased permeability

impaired autoregulation

Figure 2   Microvascular hemodynamic abnormalities present in diabetes.

same time limits vasodilatory capacity. Such a rise in peripheral vascular resistance may help to partly explain the high prevalence of hypertension in NIDDM.

The above functional abnormalities have been determined in studies of diabetic patients who are free from large vessel disease. As diabetes is also associated with a high prevalence of atherosclerosis, it is essential to consider the effects of large vessel disease on microvascular function. Studies in nondiabetic patients with peripheral vascular disease suggest that proximal arterial stenosis or occlusion can lead to a similar spectrum of microvascular functional abnormalities (reviewed in Reference 21), such as impaired postural vasoconstriction and limited vasodilation, thus compounding the effects of intrinsic microvascular disease.

B. FUNCTIONAL CHANGES IN OTHER TISSUES

There are considerable differences in the normal structure of individual microvascular beds in different tissues, allowing specialization of function, e.g., filtration in the glomerulus. Despite this, similar hemodynamic abnormalities to those already described are present in other tissues and organs affected by diabetic microangiopathy (Figure 2).

1. Kidney

In the kidney, an increase in glomerular filtration rate is present at diagnosis in IDDM, which relates to glycemic control. This glomerular hyperfiltration is due, in part, to increased renal plasma flow and an increase in filtration surface area.[22] There is also compelling indirect evidence in favor of a rise in intraglomerular hydrostatic pressure,[23] which is supported by the results of direct micropuncture studies in animal models. There is, at present, some controversy regarding the exact relationship of early glomerular hyperfiltration to the subsequent development of diabetic nephropathy. Glomerular permeability to macromolecules, as reflected by a rise in albumin excretion rate (AER), is also increased at this early stage.[8] Later in the course of the disease, a further variable rise in AER (microalbuminuria) heralds the onset of incipient diabetic nephropathy.[24] In advanced nephropathy, there is loss of autoregulation of glomerular filtration rate.[25] Renal hemodynamic changes may be different in NIDDM, as there does not appear to be glomerular hyperfiltration.[26] Abnormalities of tubular function may also contribute to diabetic nephropathy and could reflect generalized renal microcirculatory disease.

2. Retina

Studies of microvascular function have been more limited in the retina; however, once again, a rise in retinal blood flow has been detected at an early stage in IDDM,[27] along with increased capillary leakage observed in a proportion of fluorescein angiograms and on vitreous fluorophotometry, although the latter observation has not been confirmed in more recent studies.[28] There is also some evidence suggesting an elevation in retinal perfusion pressure.[29] At a later stage, there is maldistribution of retinal blood flow, with areas of nonperfusion adjacent to areas of overperfusion, and loss of autoregulation.[30] Pericytes are much more numerous in the retinal microcirculation than in other areas, and

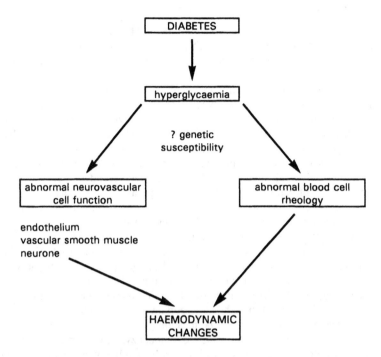

Figure 3 Proposed mechanisms for hemodynamic changes in diabetes.

pericyte loss, which is an early feature of diabetic retinopathy, may partly explain early retinal vasodilation.

3. Peripheral Nerve

In diabetic neuropathy, there is evidence for impaired nerve blood flow with a reduction in sural nerve oxygen tension, and for arteriovenous shunting supporting a pathogenetic role for microvascular hemodynamic abnormalities (reviewed in Reference 21). This is reinforced by finding at a more advanced stage of neuropathy that there is patchy fiber loss in sural nerve biopsies, suggesting local ischemia. In addition, studies demonstrating endothelial abnormalities and capillary closure in endoneurial vessels have been related to the severity of the neuropathy.[21]

C. THE MECHANISMS OF HEMODYNAMIC CHANGES

The exact molecular mechanisms underlying these hemodynamic abnormalities remain to be elucidated (Figure 3). Abnormal endothelial cell function seems likely to contribute, perhaps via an imbalance in the secretion of vasodilator and vasoconstrictor vascular mediators. Elevation of endothelium-derived relaxing factor (EDRF) early in the course of diabetes, due to increased shear stress acting on the endothelium, could lead to initial vasodilation and overperfusion; however, as endothelial damage accrues, limitation of EDRF production[31] could contribute to impaired maximal vasodilation. The situation is likely to be far more complex as there is evidence for alteration in the secretion and action of numerous other mediators in diabetes, such as catecholamines and components of the renin-angiotensin system. Abnormalities of prostaglandin secretion may be important in the development of glomerular hyperfiltration,[32] possibly via differential effects on afferent and efferent arteriolar tone. Altered endothelial cell and platelet function also contribute to the prothrombotic changes reported in patients with diabetes. These, along with changes in microvascular rheology, such as decreased red and white cell deformability, could contribute to disordered microcirculatory function; however, there is little evidence correlating such *in vitro* changes with early changes in microvascular blood flow, making it likely that such abnormalities are of more relevance in the presence of established microangiopathy.

The development of diabetic microangiopathy is closely linked with poor glycemic control. It therefore follows that hyperglycemia and its biochemical consequences, plus other metabolic changes associated with diabetes such as hyperinsulinemia, are likely to underlie the hemodynamic changes described. This is emphasized by the fact that microvascular complications are most marked in cells and tissues in which glucose uptake is largely independent of insulin action, so that cellular glucose concentration directly reflect blood levels. Hyperglycemia has a direct toxic effect on endothelial cells in culture and reduces the rate of cell division.[33] Such changes may relate to alterations in intracellular enzyme systems such as increased protein kinase C activity with subsequent widespread effects on cellular function.[34] Diabetes can be associated with peripheral hyperinsulinemia due to exogenous insulin therapy, and in NIDDM, increased endogenous insulin secretion due to insulin resistance. It has been demonstrated that insulin stimulates proliferation of capillary endothelial cells, pericytes, and smooth muscle cells in culture.[35] In addition, basement membrane-producing cells appear to be hypersensitive to the effects of insulin, leading to increased type IV collagen and decreased heparan sulfate synthesis,[36] the latter of these being important for the maintenance of the charge barrier that is a determinant of vascular permeability.[37]

A further result of hyperglycemia is increased nonenzymatic glycation of proteins,[38] such as the glycoproteins present in intercellular clefts and basement membrane, further altering charge or structural properties and therefore vascular permeability. Advanced glycation end products may also "quench" nitric oxide, providing a functional mechanism for limitation of vasodilation.

Lastly, increased activity of the enzymes of the polyol pathway as a consequence of hyperglycemia may alter cellular functions due to the osmotic effects of increased sorbitol concentrations, depletion of myoinositol, or altered sodium-potassium ATPase activity.[39] Increased polyol pathway activity is thought to be especially important in the pathogenesis of diabetic neuropathy, although it is also implicated in damage to other cell types, e.g., retinal pericytes.

In the presence of impaired autoregulation, further damage to the microcirculation may occur in the absence of hyperglycemia. Loss of flow regulation, accompanied by decreased perfusion following improved glycemic control, may compromise tissue nutrition, thus explaining the acute deterioration in microvascular disease observed under these circumstances ("glycemic re-entry" phenomenon). Likewise, during periods of hypoglycemia, loss of pressure autoregulation may allow transmission of increased systolic blood pressure directly to the capillary bed. This, along with the prothrombotic changes that accompany hypoglycemia, may further accelerate microvascular damage.[40]

Metabolic abnormalities alone are not sufficient to explain why some microvascular complications only affect a portion of patients (e.g., nephropathy), and there seems likely to be a genetic component also. The tendency to develop nephropathy may be linked to a genetic predisposition towards hypertension, as some studies have found a family history of hypertension, and also increased sodium-lithium countertransport activity in red blood cells both in patients with nephropathy and their parents.[41] Sodium-lithium countertransport is a marker for other cation exchange pumps in cell membranes and is elevated in essential hypertension. The role of putative candidate genes has still to be fully elucidated, but plausible candidates include those coding for enzymes or other proteins involved in any of the processes mentioned above. Of particular interest, in view of the therapeutic benefits of angiotensin converting enzyme (ACE) inhibitors in diabetic nephropathy is the recent discovery of a polymorphism for the ACE gene,[42] resulting in different tissue levels of angiotensin; and also possible genetic polymorphisms for the enzymes involved in the metabolism of heparan sulfate proteoglycan, e.g., N-deacetylase.[37]

III. CLINICAL FEATURES OF MICROVASCULAR DISEASE

A. RETINOPATHY

The earliest clinically detectable manifestations of diabetic retinopathy are microaneurysms, blot hemorrhages, and hard exudates on direct ophthalmoscopy (background retinopathy). Prior to the development of these, several abnormalities are apparent on fluorescein angiography, such as areas of capillary dilatation and leakage, as previously discussed. Background retinopathy is rare in the first few years of IDDM and before puberty, but increases in prevalence with increasing disease duration so that it is present in over 90% of patients after 25 years of diabetes.[43] In contrast, 21% of NIDDM patients already have background retinopathy at the time of diagnosis,[44] and although numbers subsequently increase, the overall prevalence of retinopathy in patients of long disease duration is lower in NIDDM than IDDM. Such background changes are rarely symptomatic, unless impinging on the macula, where they lead to macular edema and a decrease in visual acuity, which may become permanent visual loss if left untreated. As mentioned earlier, maculopathy is a particular problem in NIDDM, being present in over 15% of patients and, again, can already be present at diagnosis.[45] In the absence of microaneurysms and hard exudates, diabetic maculopathy is difficult to diagnose on direct ophthalmoscopy, as macular edema causes only subtle changes in the appearance of the area, such as a slight grey discoloration; however, significant maculopathy usually leads to a decrease in visual acuity that cannot be corrected by refraction.

A proportion of IDDM patients (especially those with hypertension or poor glycemic control) go on to develop more marked background retinopathy, with the development of numerous blot hemorrhages; venous abnormalities, such as beading, reduplication, and looping; variations in arteriolar caliber and arteriolar obstruction leading to "sheathing"; and cotton wool spots, indicating areas of retinal ischemia, which are visible as areas of nonperfusion on fluorescein angiography. At this time, proliferation of microvessels within the substance of the retina leads to intraretinal microvascular abnormalities (IRMAs). Such changes, indicating severe retinal ischemia, are termed preproliferative and herald the development of neovascularization, with proliferation of fragile new capillaries in association with fibrous tissue, growing forward from the surface of the retina (proliferative retinopathy). The presence of these neovascular membranes in association with retraction of the vitreous leads to sight-threatening vitreous hemorrhage from the fragile new vessels. Subsequently, further traction on the retina can cause retinal detachment. Neovascularization of the iris (rubeosis iridis) may lead to the development of a painful and intractable form of glaucoma. IDDM patients become susceptible to the development of proliferative retinopathy after several years of diabetes, with a rapid increase in the incidence of this problem between 10 and 15 years, and thereafter a relatively constant incidence. Around 50% of IDDM patients are affected after 25 years of diabetes,[43] and again, this is a less common problem in NIDDM, affecting around 20% of patients.[45]

B. NEUROPATHY

The prevalence of diabetic neuropathy is difficult to ascertain as there is no universally accepted definition of neuropathy. Prevalence rates vary from 10% in studies based on clinical findings, to greater than 90% in studies based on electrophysiology, and are probably similar in IDDM and NIDDM. Although there are a number of well-described clinical syndromes, e.g., peripheral neuropathy, autonomic neuropathy, painful neuropathy, and mononeuropathies, the most common is a symmetrical sensorimotor polyneuropathy, usually with autonomic involvement.[46] This is a typical peripheral neuropathy, which is first clinically apparent in the longest nerve fibers, with symptoms and signs first affecting the toes and then advancing proximally as the disease process develops, so that in severe cases the upper limb may eventually be involved. The patient may complain of numbness, although often sensory loss is poorly appreciated, or of painful symptoms such as burning and paresthesia.

All types of nerve fiber are affected by neuropathy and clinically there is loss of vibration sensation (large fiber), as detected by raised vibration sensory threshold using a biothesiometer. Thermal sensory thresholds are often raised at an early stage, reflecting small fiber involvement.[47] Damage to motor fibers causes an imbalance between the intrinsic and extrinsic extensor muscles of the foot and the development of clawed toes. This leads to altered weightbearing under the metatarsal heads, with increased plantar pressure, and subsequently the development of thick callus as a protective response. This callus acts as a foreign body traumatizing the underlying soft tissues, and in combination with the sensory loss and damage to the sudomotor nerves leading to dry, cracked skin, eventually may result in neuropathic foot ulceration. As already mentioned, microvascular disease appears to be important in the development and healing of diabetic foot ulcers, whether predominantly due to neuropathy or peripheral vascular disease.

C. NEPHROPATHY

The first detectable sign of impending diabetic nephropathy is an elevated AER (20–200 μg/min) or microalbuminuria,[24] although this appears to be less consistently associated with the development of nephropathy in NIDDM.[48] As renal disease progresses, the degree of proteinuria increases and glomerular filtration rate gradually decreases at a constant rate, which varies between individuals. Nephropathy is invariably associated with retinopathy, and the absence of the latter, or other atypical features, such as the presence of hematuria or rapid decline in GFR, should raise the possibility of nondiabetic renal disease as an alternative diagnosis. Again, nephropathy is related to disease duration in IDDM, being rare in the first 5 years after diagnosis and then increasing to reach a maximum prevalence of 30 to 40% after 15 years of IDDM and then declining.[49] The rate of decline of GFR in NIDDM may be slower than in IDDM,[48] and a smaller proportion reach end-stage renal failure; however, the majority of diabetic patients requiring renal replacement therapy are NIDDM as this is the more prevalent form of diabetes. Diabetic patients become symptomatic from uremia at lower serum creatinine levels than nondiabetic subjects, and are more prone to problems with fluid retention, necessitating the early introduction of renal replacement therapy.

D. OTHER CLINICAL MANIFESTATIONS

Diabetic microvascular disease has been implicated in the pathogenesis of some of the dermatological conditions associated with diabetes, such as necrobiosis lipoidica and diabetic dermopathy.[50] Both of these are most commonly found on the shins, with necrobiosis causing unsightly red/yellow plaques that may ulcerate and dermopathy causing asymptomatic small brown macules. Myocardial microangiopathy may be responsible for the development of diabetic cardiomyopathy, with the development of left ventricular dysfunction and cardiac failure in the absence of significant coronary artery disease.[51]

IV. TREATMENT

A. GENERAL MEASURES (Figure 4)
1. Improved Glycemic Control

There is now some evidence linking improved glycemic control with improved outcome of microvascular disease. As mentioned in the section on pathogenesis, many of the early

1. General	2. Specific
improved glycaemic control	laser photocoagulation (retinopathy)
antihypertensive medication	renal transplantation (nephropathy)
	renal dialysis (nephropathy)
?aldose reductase inhibitors	
?glycation inhibitors	
?capillary sealants	
?growth factor inhibitors (retinopathy)	
?prostaglandin inhibitors (nephropathy)	
?gamma-linoleic acid (neuropathy)	
?gangliosides (neuropathy)	

Figure 4 Treatment of microvascular disease.

hemodynamic abnormalities are closely associated with hyperglycemia. Near normoglycemia for 2 years has been shown to retard the progression of early retinopathy[52] and nephropathy[53] in IDDM, although this effect has not been found in all studies, probably reflecting the importance of disease duration and overall "glycemic burden". In a longer term study over a 7-year period, sustained lowering of glycated hemoglobin levels was, however, associated with reduced progression of established non-proliferative retinopathy.[54] In addition, a limited period of improved glycemic control may have a more prolonged benefit on rate of progression.[55] There is, however, conflicting evidence on whether normoglycemia following pancreatic transplantation may be associated with improvement of retinopathy.[56,57] The importance of hyperglycemia in the progression of established nephropathy remains unclear, due to the confounding effects of hypertension; however, pancreatic transplantation has been shown to prevent the development of diabetic nephropathy in combined renal and pancreas transplant recipients.[58] The effects of improved glycemic control on sensorimotor neuropathy are less consistent; and although some minor beneficial effects on nerve conduction and vibration sensation have been observed,[59] the lack of change in symptoms of sensory loss suggests that peripheral neuropathy is largely irreversible once established. This is supported by the lack of improvement in neuropathy following pancreatic transplantation.[60]

The role of optimal glycemic control in the primary prevention of microvascular complications awaits confirmation, with the results from two major long-term follow-up studies of newly diagnosed IDDM (Diabetes Control and Complications Trial) and NIDDM (U.K. Prospective Diabetes Study) patients, due to be reported in the next few years.

2. Antihypertensive Treatment

Control of hypertension has been shown to retard the progression of established nephropathy[61] in both IDDM and NIDDM. Although a variety of agents have proved to be effective, much attention has focused on the role of ACE inhibitors, due to their potential to lower raised intraglomerular pressure through a preferential effect on postglomerular vascular resistance, and these have been shown to reduce AER and the decline in glomerular filtration rate independent of their effects on systemic blood pressure in patients with nephropathy,[62] and in normotensive IDDM patients with microalbuminuria.[63] There is also preliminary evidence that subhypotensive doses of the ACE inhibitor, ramipril, can lower the elevated skin nailfold capillary pressure in patients with incipient nephropathy.[64] In NIDDM, there is an increased incidence of retinopathy in hypertensive patients,[65] suggesting that treatment of hypertension may also be beneficial in reducing the progression of retinopathy.

3. Potential Future Treatments

Several agents show promise for the future treatment of diabetic microvascular complications. The aldose reductase inhibitors, which inhibit polyol pathway activity, have shown marked benefits in experimental diabetes. In contrast, studies in human subjects have so far been disappointing and there have been problems with toxic side effects; however, most studies to date have looked at aldose reductase inhibitors in established microvascular disease and it may be that they are more effective in prevention. In neuropathy, regeneration and repair of myelinated fibers have been observed in sural nerve biopsy specimens from patients treated with sorbinil,[66] and decreased glomerular hyperfiltration has been seen with ponalrestat.[67] Another treatment that has shown great promise in experimental diabetes is inhibition of the advanced stages of protein glycation using aminoguanidine; however, no clinical trials have yet been reported using this agent.

Growth factors, such as insulin-like growth factor-1 (IGF-1), may be important in the development of proliferative retinopathy and the early renal hypertrophy that precedes the development of nephropathy. A study of IGF-1 inhibition, using the somatostatin analog octreotide, has shown reduction in glomerular hyperfiltration in IDDM.[68] Prostaglandin inhibitors, such as indomethacin, may also have beneficial effects on renal hemodynamics leading to reduced AER.[69] In neuropathy, dietary supplementation with the essential fatty acid gamma-linoleic acid may improve nerve conduction,[70] as may the intramuscular administration of gangliosides.[71] Hydroxymethyl rutosides (Paroven) may improve increased microvascular permeability.[72]

B. SPECIFIC TREATMENTS

Proliferative diabetic retinopathy and maculopathy can be treated using laser photocoagulation. The rationale behind this treatment in proliferative retinopathy is that destruction of large areas of ischemic retinal tissue reduces the stimulus for further new vessel formation; while in maculopathy, destruction of leaky microaneurysms leads to a subsequent reduction in hard exudates and macular edema, usually with some improvement in visual acuity. Laser photocoagulation can prevent severe visual loss in more than 50% of patients with proliferative retinopathy.[73] In more advanced diabetic eye disease, vitreoretinal microsurgery, to remove vitreous hemorrhage and repair retinal detachment, can result in the restoration of some degree of useful vision.

Dietary protein restriction is of known benefit in preventing the progression of nondiabetic renal failure, although whether it has similar effects in diabetic nephropathy remains controversial.[74] In any case, only moderate protein restriction is practical, however, as most patients find a low protein diet unacceptable. Once end-stage renal failure is reached, renal transplantation is the preferred choice of renal replacement therapy, with long-term transplantation results now approaching those in nondiabetic subjects. As transplantation is currently a limited option due to inadequate donor numbers, most patients with end-stage renal failure are treated with renal dialysis, at least for a period. Continuous ambulatory peritoneal dialysis is preferred to hemodialysis, as the latter is difficult in diabetic patients due to problems with vascular access, postural hypotension, and glycemic control. In addition, hemodialysis in elderly patients is associated with a higher mortality than other forms of renal replacement therapy.[75]

V. SUMMARY

Microvascular disease in diabetes is an important clinical problem leading to substantial morbidity. It is now accepted that early hemodynamic abnormalities precede the development of structural microangiopathy, although the exact mechanisms linking hyperglycemia and changes in microvascular function remain to be elucidated. Reversal of early functional abnormalities may be possible with achievement of near-normal blood glucose levels and control of hypertension. Such measures may also slow the rate of deterioration of established microangiopathy. The role of several other potential treatments again awaits the determination of the fundamental mechanisms underlying changes in microcirculatory function.

REFERENCES

1. **Parving, H.-H., Viberti, G. C., Keen, H., Christiansen, J. S., and Lassen, N. A.,** Haemodynamic factors in the genesis of diabetic microangiopathy, *Metabolism*, 32, 943–949, 1983.
2. **Tooke, J. E.,** Microvascular haemodynamics in diabetes mellitus, *Clin. Sci.*, 70, 119–125, 1986.
3. **Zatz, R. and Brenner, B. M.,** Pathogenesis of diabetic microangiopathy: The haemodynamic view, *Am. J. Med.*, 80, 443–453, 1986.
4. **Flynn, M. D., Edmonds, M. E., Tooke, J. E., and Watkins, P. J.,** Direct measurement of capillary blood flow in the diabetic neuropathic foot, *Diabetologia*, 31, 652–666, 1988.
5. **Tymms, J. A. and Tooke, J. E.,** The effect of continuous subcutaneous insulin infusion (CSII) on microvascular blood flow in diabetes mellitus, *Int. J. Microcirc.: Clin. Exp.*, 7, 347–356, 1988.
6. **Sandeman, D. D., Shore, A. C., and Tooke, J. E.,** Relation of skin capillary pressure in patients with insulin-dependent diabetes mellitus to complications and metabolic control, *N. Engl. J. Med.*, 327, 760–764, 1992.
7. **Shore, A. C., Jaap, A. J., and Tooke, J. E.,** Capillary pressure in insulin dependent diabetic patients of long disease duration with and without microangiopathy, *Diabet. Med.*, 9 (Suppl. 2), S11 (Abstr.), 1992.
8. **Jaap, A. J., Shore, A. C., Gartside, I. B., Gamble, J., and Tooke, J. E.,** Increased microvascular fluid permeability in young Type 1 (insulin-dependent) diabetic patients, *Diabetologia*, 36, 648–652, 1993.
9. **Parving, H.-H., Noer, I., Deckert, T., et al.,** The effect of metabolic regulation on microvascular permeability to small and large molecules in short-term juvenile diabetics, *Diabetologia*, 12, 161–166, 1976.
10. **Rayman, G., Hassan, A., and Tooke, J. E.,** Blood flow in the skin of the foot related to posture in diabetes mellitus, *Br. Med. J.*, 292, 87–90, 1986.
11. **Shore, A. C., Price, K. J., Sandeman, D. D., Tripp, J. H., and Tooke, J. E.,** Posturally induced vasoconstriction in diabetes mellitus, *Arch. Dis. Child.*, 70, 22–26, 1994.
12. **Rayman, G., Williams, S. A., Spencer, P. D., Smaje, L. H., Wise, P. H., and Tooke, J. E.,** Impaired microvascular hyperaemic response to minor skin trauma in type 1 diabetes, *Br. Med. J.*, 292, 1295–1298, 1986.
13. **Tooke, J. E., Lins, P.-E., Östergren, J., and Fagrell, B.,** Skin microvascular autoregulatory responses in Type 1 diabetes: The influence of duration and control, *Int. J. Microcirc.: Clin. Exp.*, 4, 249–256, 1985.
14. **Walmsley, D. and Wiles, P. G.,** Early loss of neurogenic inflammation in the human diabetic foot, *Clin. Sci.*, 80, 605–610, 1991.
15. **Shore, A. C., Price, K. J., Sandeman, D. D., Green, E. M., Tripp, J. H., and Tooke, J. E.,** Impaired microvascular hyperaemic response in children with diabetes mellitus, *Diabetic Med.*, 8, 619–623, 1991.
16. **Kastrup, J., Norgaard, T., Parving, H.-H., and Lassen, N. A.,** Decreased distensibility of resistance vessels of the skin in Type 1 (insulin-dependent) diabetic patients with microangiopathy, *Clin. Sci.*, 72, 123–130, 1987.
17. **Sandeman, D. D., Pym, C., Green, E. M., Seamark, C., Shore, A. C., and Tooke, J. E.,** Microvascular vasodilation in feet of newly diagnosed non-insulin dependent diabetic patients, *Br. Med. J.*, 302, 1122–1123, 1991.
18. **Jaap, A. J., Hammersley, M. S., Shore, A. C., and Tooke, J. E.,** Reduced microvascular hyperaemia in subjects at risk of developing Type 2 (non-insulin dependent) diabetes, *Diabetologia*, 37, 214–216, 1994.
19. **Shore, A. C., Jaap, A. J., and Tooke, J. E.,** Capillary pressure in patients with NIDDM, *Diabetes*, 43, 1198–1202, 1994.
20. **Jaap, A. J., Shore, A. C., Gamble, J., Gartside, I. B., and Tooke, J. E.,** Capillary filtration coefficient in Type 2 (non-insulin-dependent) diabetes, *J. Diab. Comp.*, 8, 111–116, 1994.

21. **Jaap, A. J. and Tooke, J. E.,** Is microvascular disease important in the diabetic foot? in *The Foot in Diabetes: Aetiology and Clinical Management,* Boulton, A. J. M., Connor, H., and Cavanagh, P. R., Eds., John Wiley & Sons, Chichester, UK, 1994, 49–56.

22. **Christiansen, J. S., Gammelgaard, J., Frandsen, M., and Parving, H.-H.,** Increased kidney size, glomerular filtration rate, and renal plasma flow in short-term insulin-dependent diabetics, *Diabetologia,* 20, 451–456, 1981.

23. **Zatz, R., Dunn, R., Meyer, T. W., Anderson, S., Rennke, H. G., and Brenner, B. M.,** Prevention of diabetic glomerulopathy by pharmacological amelioration of capillary hypertension, *J. Clin. Invest.,* 77, 1925–1930, 1986.

24. **Viberti, G. C., Hill, R. D., Jarrett, R. J., Argyropoulos, A., Mahmud, U., and Keen, H.,** Microalbuminuria as a predictor of clinical nephropathy in insulin-dependent diabetes mellitus, *Lancet,* i, 1430–1432, 1982.

25. **Parving, H.-H., Kastrup, H., Smidt, U. M., Andersen, A. R., Feldt-Rasmussen, B. F., and Sandahl Christiansen, J.,** Impaired autoregulation of glomerular filtration rate in Type 1 (insulin-dependent) diabetic patients with nephropathy, *Diabetologia,* 27, 247–252, 1984.

26. **Schmitz, A., Christensen, T., and Taagehoej Jensen, F.,** Glomerular filtration rate and kidney volume in normoalbuminuric non-insulin-dependent diabetics. Lack of glomerular hyperfiltration and renal hypertrophy in uncomplicated NIDDM, *Scand. J. Clin. Lab. Invest.,* 49, 103–108, 1989.

27. **Kohner, E. M., Hamilton, A. M., Saunders, S. J., Sutcliffe, B. A., and Bulpitt, C. J.,** The retinal blood flow in diabetes, *Diabetologia,* 11, 27–33, 1975.

28. **Chahal, P., Falon, T. J., Jennings, S. J., Chowienczyk, P. J., and Kohner, E. M.,** Vitreous fluorophotometry in patients with no or minimal diabetic retinopathy, *Diabetes Care,* 9, 134–139, 1986.

29. **Patel, V., Rassam, S., Newsom, S., Wiek, J., and Kohner, E.,** Retinal blood flow in diabetic nephropathy, *Br. Med. J.,* 305, 678–683, 1992.

30. **Grunwald, J. E., Riva, C. E., Sinclair, S. H., and Brucker, A. V.,** Altered retinal vascular response to 100% oxygen breathing in diabetes mellitus, *Ophthalmology,* 91, 1447–1452, 1984.

31. **Porta, M., La Selva, M., Molinatti, P., and Molinatti, G. M.,** Endothelial cell function in diabetic microangiopathy, *Diabetologia,* 30, 601–609, 1987.

32. **Viberti, G. C., Benigni, A., Bognetti, E., Remuzzi, G., and Wiseman, M. J.,** Glomerular hyperfiltration and urinary prostaglandins in Type 1 diabetes mellitus, *Diabetic Med.,* 6, 219–222, 1989.

33. **Lorenzi, M., Cagliero, E., and Toledo, S.,** Glucose toxicity for human endothelial cells in culture. Delayed replication, disturbed cell cycle, and accelerated death, *Diabetes,* 34, 621–627, 1985.

34. **Lee, T.-S., Saltsman, A., Ohashi, H., and King, G. L.,** Activation of protein kinase C by elevation of glucose concentration: Proposal for a mechanism in the development of diabetic vascular complications, *Proc. Natl. Acad. Sci. U.S.A.,* 86, 5141–5145, 1989.

35. **Stout, R. W.,** Insulin as a mitogenic factor: Role in the pathogenesis of cardiovascular disease, *Am. J. Med.,* 90(Suppl. 2A), 625–655, 1991.

36. **Ledbetter, S. R., Wagner, C. W., Martin, G. R., Rohrbach, D. H., and Hassel, J. R.,** Response of diabetic basement-membrane producing cells to glucose and insulin, *Diabetes,* 36, 1029–1034, 1987.

37. **Deckert, T., Feldt-Rasmussen, B., Borch-Johnsen, K., Jensen, T., and Kofoed-Enevoldsen, A.,** Albuminuria reflects widespread vascular damage: The Steno Hypothesis, *Diabetologia,* 32, 219–226, 1989.

38. **Brownlee, M., Vlassara, H., and Cerami, A.,** Non-enzymatic glycosylation and the pathogenesis of diabetic complications, *Ann. Intern. Med.,* 101, 527–537, 1984.

39. **Greene, D. A., Lattimer, S. A., and Sima, A. A. F.,** Sorbitol, phosphoinositides and sodium-potassium ATPase in the pathogenesis of diabetic complications, *N. Engl. J. Med.,* 316, 599–606, 1987.

40. **Frier, B. M. and Hilsted, J.,** Does hypoglycaemia aggravate the complications of diabetes?, *Lancet,* ii, 1175–1176, 1985.

41. **Mangili, R., Bending, J. J., Scott, G. S., Li, L. K., Gupta, A., and Viberti, G. C.,** Increased sodium-lithium countertransport activity in red cells of patients with insulin-dependent diabetes and nephropathy, *N. Engl. J. Med.,* 318, 146–149, 1988.

42. **Rigat, B., Hubert, C., Alhene-Gelas, F., Cambien, F., Corvol, P., and Soubrier, F.,** An insertion/deletion polymorphism in the angiotensin I converting enzyme gene accounting for half the variance of serum enzyme levels, *J. Clin. Invest.,* 86, 1343–1346, 1990.

43. **Klein, R., Klein, B. E. K., Moss, S. E., Davies, M. D., and DeMets, D. L.,** The Wisconsin Epidemiologic Study of Diabetic Retinopathy. II. Prevalence and risk of diabetic retinopathy when age of diagnosis is less than 30 years, *Arch. Ophthalmol.*, 102, 520–526, 1984.

44. **U.K. Prospective Diabetes Study 6.** Complications in newly diagnosed Type 2 diabetic patients and their associations with different clinical and biochemical risk factors, *Diabetes Res.*, 13, 1–11, 1990.

45. **Gall, M.-A., Rossing, P., Skøtt, P., et al.,** Prevalence of micro-and macroalbuminuria, arterial hypertension, retinopathy and large vessel disease in European Type 2 (non-insulin-dependent) diabetic patients, *Diabetologia*, 34, 655–661, 1991.

46. **Ward, J. D.,** Clinical aspects of diabetic somatic neuropathy, in *Textbook of Diabetes*, Pickup, J. and Williams, G., Eds., Blackwell Scientific, Oxford, 1991, 623–634.

47. **Guy, R. J. C., Clark, C. A., Malcolm, P. N., and Watkins, P. J.,** Evaluation of thermal and vibration sensation in diabetic neuropathy, *Diabetologia*, 28, 131–137, 1985.

48. **Fabré, J., Balant, L. P., Dayer, P. G., Fox, H. M., and Venert, A. T.,** The kidney in maturity onset diabetes mellitus: A clinical study of 510 patients, *Kidney Int.*, 21, 730–738, 1982.

49. **Andersen, A. R., Christiansen, J. S., Andersen, J. K., Kreiner, S., and Deckert, T.,** Diabetic nephropathy in Type 1 (insulin-dependent) diabetes: An epidemiological study, *Diabetologia*, 25, 496–501, 1983.

50. **Goodfield, M. J. D. and Millard, L. G.,** The skin in diabetes mellitus, *Diabetologia*, 31, 567–575, 1988.

51. **Shapiro, L. M.,** A prospective study of heart disease in diabetes mellitus, *Q. J. Med.*, 209, 55–68, 1984.

52. **Dahl-Jørgensen, K., Brinchmann-Hansen, O., Hanssen, K. F., et al.,** Effect of near normoglycaemia for 2 years on the progression of early diabetic nephropathy and neuropathy, *Br. Med. J.*, 293, 1195–1199, 1986.

53. **Feldt-Rasmussen, B., Mathiesen, E. R., and Deckert, T.,** Effect of 2 years of strict metabolic control on the progression of incipient nephropathy in insulin-dependent diabetes, *Lancet*, ii, 1300–1304, 1986.

54. **Brinchmann-Hansen, O., Dahl-Jørgensen, K., Sandvik, L., and Hanssen, K. F.,** Blood glucose concentrations and progression of diabetic retinopathy: The seven year results of the Oslo study, *Br. Med. J.*, 304, 19–22, 1992.

55. **Feldt-Rasmussen, B., Mathiesen, E. R., Jensen, T., et al.,** Effect of improved metabolic control on loss of kidney function in Type 1 (insulin-dependent) diabetic patients: an update of the Steno studies, *Diabetologia*, 34, 164–170, 1991.

56. **Ramsay, R. C., Goetz, F. C., Sutherland, D. E. R., et al.,** Progression of diabetic retinopathy after pancreas transplantation for insulin dependent diabetes mellitus, *N. Engl. J. Med.*, 318, 208–214, 1988.

57. **Ulbig, M., Lampik, A., Landgraf, R., and Land, W.,** The influence of combined pancreatic and renal transplantation on advanced diabetic retinopathy, *Transplant. Proc.*, 19, 3554–3556, 1987.

58. **Bohman, S. O., Tyden, G., Wilezek, H., et al.,** Prevention of kidney graft diabetic nephropathy by pancreas transplantation in man, *Diabetes*, 34, 306–308, 1985.

59. **Service, F. J., Rizza, R. A., Daube, J. R., O'Brien, P. C., and Dyck, P. J.,** Near normoglycaemia improves nerve conduction and vibration sensation in diabetic neuropathy, *Diabetologia*, 28, 722–727, 1985.

60. **Solders, G., Wilczek, R., Gunnasson, R., Tyden, G., Persson, A., and Groth, G. C.,** Effects of combined pancreatic and renal transplantation on diabetic neuropathy: a two-year follow-up study, *Lancet*, ii, 1232–1235, 1987.

61. **Parving, H.-H., Andersen, A. R., Smidt, U., Hommel, E., Mathiesen, E. R., and Svendsen, P. A.,** Effect of anti-hypertensive treatment on kidney function in diabetic nephropathy, *Br. Med. J.*, 294, 1443–1447, 1987.

62. **Björck, S., Mulec, H., Johnsen, S. A., Nordén, G., and Aurell, M.,** Renal protective effect of enalapril in diabetic nephropathy, *Br. Med. J.*, 304, 339–343, 1992.

63. **Mathiesen, E. R., Hommel, E., Giese, J., and Parving, H.-H.,** Efficacy of captopril in postponing nephropathy in normotensive insulin dependent diabetic patients with microalbuminuria, *Br. Med. J.*, 303, 81–87, 1991.

64. **Shore, A. C., Donohoe, M., Jaap, A. J., and Tooke, J. E.,** The effect of increasing doses of an angiotensin converting enzyme inhibitor on capillary pressure levels in patients with insulin-dependent diabetes mellitus and microalbuminuria, *Diabetic Med.*, 10(Suppl. 1), S5 (Abstr.), 1993.

44

65. **Knowler, W. C., Bennett, P. H., and Ballintine, E. J.,** Increased incidence of retinopathy in diabetics with elevated blood pressure. A six-year follow-up study in Pima Indians, *N. Engl. J. Med.*, 302, 645–650, 1980.

66. **Sima, A. A. F., Bril, V., and Nathaniel, V., et al.,** Regeneration and repair of myelinated fibers in sural nerve biopsy specimens from patients with diabetic neuropathy treated with sorbinil, *N. Engl. J. Med.*, 319, 542–548, 1988.

67. **Mau Pedersen, M., Christiansen, J. S., and Mogensen, C. E.,** Reduction of glomerular hyperfiltration in nomoalbuminuric IDDM patients by 6 months of aldose reductase inhibition, *Diabetes*, 40, 527–531, 1991.

68. **Serri, O., Beauregard, H., Brazeau, P., et al.,** Somatostatin analogue, octreotide, reduces increased glomerular filtration rate and kidney size in insulin-dependent diabetes, *JAMA*, 265, 888–892, 1991.

69. **Mathiesen, E. R., Hommel, E., Olsen, U. B., and Parving, H.-H.,** Elevated urinary prostaglandins and the effect of indomethacin on kidney function in incipient diabetic nephropathy, *Diabetic Med.*, 5, 145–149, 1988.

70. **Jamal, G. A. and Carmichael, H.,** The effect of gamma-linoleic acid on human diabetic peripheral neuropathy: A double-blind placebo-controlled study, *Diabetic Med.*, 7, 319–323, 1990.

71. **Crepaldi, G., Fedele, D., Tiengo, A., et al.,** Ganglioside treatment in diabetic peripheral neuropathy, *Acta Diabetol. Lat.*, 20, 265–276, 1983.

72. **Allen, A. and Tooke, J. E.,** Effects of hydroxyethyl-rutosides in diabetes mellitus, *Phlebology*, 5, 27–31, 1990.

73. **The Diabetic Retinopathy Study Research Group,** Photocoagulation treatment of proliferative diabetic retinopathy. Clinical application of the DRS findings, Report No. 8, *Ophthalmology*, 88, 583–600, 1981.

74. **Walker, J. D., Bending, J. J., Dodds, R. A., et al.,** Restriction of dietary protein and progression of renal failure in diabetic nephropathy, *Lancet*, ii, 1411–1415, 1989.

75. **Matson, M. and Kjellstrand, C. M.,** Long-term follow-up of 369 diabetic patients undergoing dialysis, *Arch. Intern. Med.*, 148, 600–604, 1988.

Chapter 4

Hypertension and the Microcirculation

Eric Vicaut and Gary L. Anderson

CONTENTS

I. INTRODUCTION

This chapter is intended to acquaint the reader with the main ideas about the involvement of the microcirculation in hypertension. Hypertension can result from increased cardiac output, increased blood volume, increased blood viscosity, or increased total peripheral resistance to blood flow. Only the latter two directly concern the microcirculation.

The exploration of microcirculation in hypertensive patients has been very limited by methodological difficulties. Indeed, *in vivo* capillaroscopy in hypertensive patients has mainly explored conjunctival and nailfold microcirculation. By contrast, considerable progress in the description of microvascular alterations during hypertension has been made possible by techniques of intravital microscopy in animals.[1,2] These works have permitted extensive discussion of the role of microcirculation in hypertensive states and will be described below. However, as stressed by Shore and Tooke,[3] it must be reminded that there is no precise animal model of human hypertension. In addition, most animal studies imploy surgical procedures that can influence the measured parameters. Consequently, care must be taken when extrapolating results obtained in different animal models to hypertensive patients.

II. PENETRATION OF SYSTEMIC BLOOD PRESSURE INTO THE MICROVASCULATURE

The evaluation of the relative part of the pressure gradient localized upstream from the microvascular network (i.e., in the resistance arteries) and that localized in the arteriolar network per se is still highly controversial. In normotensive conditions, several groups found values of blood pressure at the entrance of the microcirculation in a range between 50 and 70 mmHg,[4-7] and few groups found values as high as 80 to 90 mmHg.[8-10] In these

0-8493-4870-6/95/$0.00+$.50
© 1995 by CRC Press, Inc.

studies, most of the pressure drop occurs strictly within the microcirculation. Conversely, others reported blood pressure values in a range between 35 and 45 mmHg at the entrance to the microcirculation,[11-15] thus suggesting that a large part of the pressure drop occurred in the small arteries. Some of these discrepancies are explained by methodological limitations of the techniques used in intravital microscopy (i.e., use of anesthesia, surgical procedures, etc.).[3,8] It is also likely that the shape of the pressure profile is greatly affected by the topographical arrangement of the microvascular network, which differs between the different species or organs studied. However, taken together, most studies led us to consider that, in normotensive conditions, despite a certain heterogeneity in the shapes of pressure gradients among the different vascular trees, a large part of the pressure drop (at least >50%) takes place within the microcirculation. It may be stressed that this does not automatically imply that the microcirculation is responsible for the largest part of the increase in pressure during the passage from normotensive to hypertensive states. It is generally admitted that, in hypertension, the elevation of blood pressure is limited to the arteriolar side of the microvascular network.[4,7,16-19] This increased precapillary resistance prevents elevation of capillary or venular pressure which usually is found unchanged in hypertension. It may be stressed that this is an important role of the elevated precapillary resistance because it shields the tissues from the deleterious consequences that a high hydrostatic pressure could have on transcapillary fluid exchange.

The contribution of the microcirculation to the increased resistance in hypertension may be expressed by the ratio of the pressure measured at the entrance of the microvascular network to the systemic pressure. When comparisons were made between normotensive and hypertensive animals, this ratio was found to be lower in hypertensive rats than in their controls, in several studies indicating a greater role of resistance arteries in hypertensive than in normotensive states — i.e., 78 vs. 80% in spinotrapezius in spontaneous hypertension,[7] 36 and 38 vs. 51% in cremaster during renovascular and high salt diet hypertension.[12] However, other studies found higher ratios in hypertensive than in normotensive animals — i.e., 67 vs. 58% in intestine from genetic hypertensive rats,[4] 45 vs. 52% in spinotrapezius during high-salt diet hypertension.[20] Therefore, no unequivocal conclusion can be made on this aspect.

Regarding the effect of hypertension on the shape of the pressure profiles within the microcirculation, some differences also exist between experimental models of hypertension. Indeed, when normalized by systemic pressure, some pressure profiles of normotensive and hypertensive animals are found to be almost similar[7,19] or may exhibit marked difference as shown in Figure 1 for pressure profiles measured in skeletal muscle during renovascular or high-salt diet hypertension.[12] However, despite the differences among species or organs, a common finding in these studies is that all types of arterioles experience increased wall forces during hypertension and microvascular resistance is increased by mechanisms discussed in the following paragraphs.

III. POSSIBLE MECHANISMS FOR INCREASED PERIPHERAL RESISTANCE

A. CHANGES IN VASCULAR REACTIVITY

One way to view the many mediators that affect blood pressure is as countervailing systems. The constrictive/antinatriuretic systems include: renin-angiotensin system, sympathoadrenal system, endothelin, vasopressin, thromboxane/leukotrienes, and serotonin. The vasodilating/natriuretic systems include: atrial natriuretic peptide, prostaglandins E2 and I2, endothelium-derived relaxing factor (nitric oxide), kallikrein-kinin system, and dopamine. Either an increase in constrictor stimuli or a decrease in dilator stimuli can lead to increased peripheral resistance and hypertension.

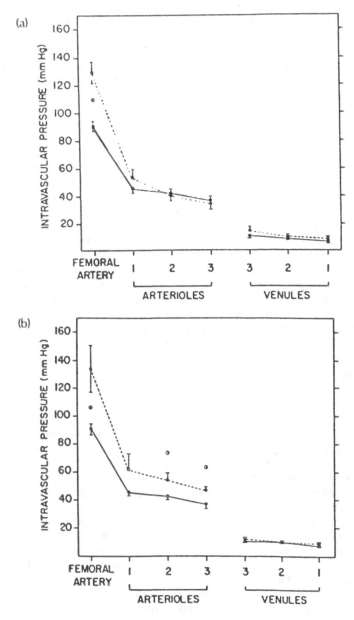

Figure 1 Pressure gradients along the vascular network measured on the cremaster muscle in renovascular or deoxycorticosterone-salt hypertensive rats (dashed lines) and in their normotensive controls (solid lines). It may be noted that the shapes of the pressure gradient and, in particular, the penetration of high blood pressure in the arteriolar network are different in the two types of hypertension. (From Meininger, G. A., Harris, P. D., and Joshua, I. G., *Hypertension*, 6, 27, 1984.)

1. Response to Vasoconstrictive Substances

Alterations that can result in an increased microvascular resistance may involve local changes in the vascular smooth muscle-receptor complex that lead to increased sensitivity of the arterioles to vasoconstrictive substances. In genetic hypertensive rats, such an increase in sensitivity was found for norepinephrine.[21,22] Increased reactivity to angiotensin II, norepinephrine, and potassium has also been found in renovascular hypertension.[23,24] The occurrence of these changes in reactivity is rapid since in renovascular hypertension, sensitivity to angiotensin II, norepinephrine, and potassium chloride have been found increased only 8 days after the onset of hypertension. Increased sensitivity of skeletal muscle arterioles to arginine vasopressin was also found in renovascular hypertension.[25]

Possible differences in receptor or post-receptor properties have been evoked, but very few experimental results are available to support this concept in the microvascular network. Increased reactivity to vasoconstrictors also may be explained by changes in the hydrostatic pressure at which arterioles are subjected to in hypertension. Indeed, Gore and Bohlen considered that in some arteriolar segments, hypertension can act directly on arteriolar smooth muscle by increasing transmural pressure and, thus, wall stress.[14] However, this explanation is not valid for all microvessels.

Calcium sensitivity also may be involved in the increased microvascular reactivity found in hypertension since calcium sensitivity of small mesenteric arterioles was also found higher in genetic hypertensive rats than in controls.[26] How other various electrolytes, including sodium, potassium, and calcium, can influence hypertension has been reviewed.[27] In addition to the obvious volume expansion aspects, the direct effects of these electrolytes on vascular smooth muscle can affect arteriole diameters by changing resting membrane potentials. It has been noted that enhanced sodium-proton exchange is a frequently seen ion transport abnormality in essential hypertension[28] that could be associated with enhanced sensitivity to vasoconstrictors and ultimately affect structural changes in arterioles. Many aspects of salt and its relationship to hypertension have also been recently reviewed.[29]

2. Local Microvascular Renin-Angiotensin System

It is now well recognized that the renin-angiotensin system is not only an endocrine system, but that some of its components are generated or activated in several tissues, including the wall of large arteries. The possibility that angiotensin II may be locally formed within the vasculature led some authors to test the hypothesis that the local renin-angiotensin system and especially local angiotensin converting enzyme activity can be different in hypertensive states. The local renin-angiotensin system has been recently studied at the microvascular level.[30] Local angiotensin converting enzyme activity was found to be effective in arterioles and could induce almost complete closure of terminal arterioles in the presence of angiotensin I, even in normotensive rats.[30] However, this microvascular angiotensin converting enzyme activity was found to be considerably higher in genetic hypertensive rats than in their normotensive controls[31] (Figure 2). In genetic hypertensive rats but not in normotensive controls, a significant local renin activity was found at the microvascular level, but it was shown that this renin was of renal origin. in both normotensive and genetic hypertensive rats, no local angiotensinogen was found.[31]

It is likely that, besides its direct effects, the increase in local production of angiotensin II may also amplify the responses to adrenergic stimuli.

3. Endothelium-Mediated Responses

Alterations of endothelium have been found in hypertensive patients and can provide an additional reason for increased microvascular reactivity in hypertension.[32,33] Vascular responses to vasoconstrictors such as norepinephrine have been consistently found to be amplified when production of relaxing factors by the endothelium was impaired. As shown in Figure 3, such a situation was found in cerebral arterioles in stroke-prone

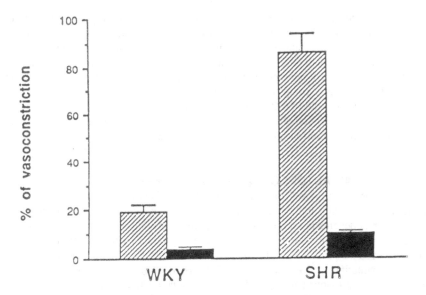

Figure 2 Response to topical administration of 0.1 nmol/ml angiotensin I (hatched columns) in rat cremaster terminal arterioles of genetic hypertensive rats (SHR) and normotensive controls (WKY). As the circulating renin-angiotensin system was excluded in this experimental model, the responses observed reflected local conversion of angiotensin I to angiotensin II. In both strains, local converting enzyme activity was largely diminished by the angiotensin converting enzyme inhibitor lisinopril (10 nmol/ml, black columns). (Derived from Vicaut, E. and Hou, X., *Hypertension*, 24, 70, 1994.)

genetic hypertensive rats for which the endothelium-dependent dilatation to acetylcholine was completely abolished, whereas the endothelium-independent dilation obtained with adenosine was similar in genetic hypertensive rats and in control.[34] Basal release of nitric oxide (one of the endothelial-derived relaxing factors) has also been found to decrease in cremaster muscle arterioles from renovascular hypertensive rats[35] and is responsible for

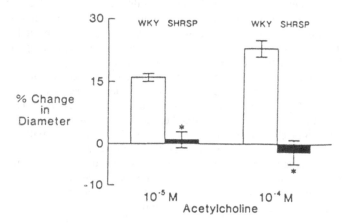

Figure 3 In response to acetylcholine, an endothelium-dependent reactivity was abolished in terminal cerebral arterioles of stroke prone genetic hypertensive rats. This finding demonstrates the decreased synthesis or liberation of endothelium-derived relaxing factors during hypertension. (From Mayhan, W. G., Faraci, F. M., and Heistad, D. D., *Am. J. Physiol.*, 253, H1435, 1987.)

attenuation of the vasodilatory response to acetylcholine. In addition, it cannot be excluded that, as found in kidney, the decrease of nitric oxide synthesis may interfere with the local vascular renin-angiotensin system. The hypothesis that in hypertension the balance between endothelial-derived relaxing and contracting factors may be disturbed,[32] or that locally produced angiotensin II may increase production of prostanoids,[36] was demonstrated by several groups in resistance arteries. In addition, enhanced synthesis of the constrictive prostanoid PGH2 has been recently demonstrated in arterioles of skeletal muscle.[37] Concerning endothelin (considered as the main endothelium-derived contracting factor), its implication in microvascular disorders associated with hypertension has not been demonstrated.

B. FUNCTIONAL AUTOREGULATORY MECHANISMS

Several authors[38,39] proposed that the origin of the increased peripheral resistance in hypertension might be simply an initial increase in cardiac output (the cause of this latter phenomenon is dependent on the cause of hypertension) that would initiate the raise of pressure. This initial increased pressure in arterioles induces a myogenic vasoconstriction[40] related to the properties of the intrinsic smooth muscle cells, but is also influenced by neural, paracrine, and endocrine factors. This mechanism does not exclude those described in the previous paragraph. Indeed, this functional autoregulation of flow can amplify the hormonal and/or neural vasoconstrictor stimuli and be an additional explanatory factor for the difference in sensitivity between microvessels from hypertensive and normotensive animals. Such an amplification was clearly demonstrated by Meininger and Trzeciakowski,[41] who suggested that, in hypertension, autoregulation could raise the resistance to levels higher than those caused directly by the phenylephrine or angiotensin II. Such an amplification in myogenic response in genetic hypertensive rats was also recently found by Huang et al.,[37] who demonstrated that this phenomenon was due to the enhanced production of endothelium-derived constrictor factors (Figure 4).

Besides this myogenic autoregulation of flow, the early increase in microvascular resistances could be due to the metabolic autoregulation of microvascular blood flows. This autoregulatory process is based on the possibility that tissues regulate their oxygen delivery to achieve an adequate oxygen tension at the cellular level. In this hypothesis, the initial increase in cardiac output would induce an increase in local blood flows, then oxygen delivery in excess of oxygen demand, and thus an increase in local O_2 tension. Several studies demonstrated that increased O_2 tension induces arteriolar vasoconstrictions by stimuli on vascular or tissue sensors.[42] This response was amplified in terminal arterioles of genetic hypertensive rats.[43] Several mechanisms have been reported for this vasoconstriction, including cyclooxygenase pathways, lipoxygenase,[44] or other endothelial regulatory mechanisms.[45] These different pathways have been reported to be disturbed in hypertension and thus these alterations can explain an increased responsiveness to high O_2 tension. This increased sensitivity to O_2 tension could amplify the autoregulation of blood flow in hypertensive animals and thus cause excessive vasoconstriction.

Autoregulation of O_2 delivery also can interact with vascular reactivity. Indeed, the high O_2 tension due to the initial increase in cardiac output may amplify the vasoconstrictor stimuli since oxygen may affect cell membrane transport of calcium.[46] In this connection, Ledingham evoked the possibility that a crucial genetic factor in genetic hypertensive rats may be a particular sensor for oxygen in the cell membrane that controls the permeability to, or the active transport of, calcium.[47]

C. MODIFICATIONS OF VASCULAR STRUCTURE
1. Wall Thickness

Folkow[48] described the "long-term counterpart of functional autoregulation" that is the rapid adjustment of resistance vessel structure. In this view, maintenance of the increased

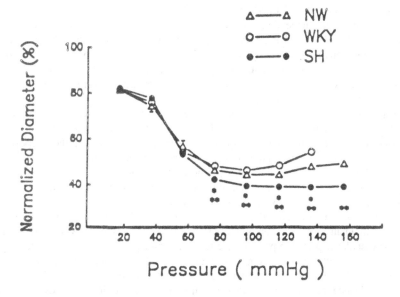

Figure 4 Comparison of pressure-induced changes in arteriole diameter (normalized to the corresponding passive diameter) of spontaneously hypertensive rats (SH) and normotensive controls, i.e., normal Wistar (NW) and Wistar-Kyoto (WKY). Arterioles from the hypertensive rats have an enhanced constriction in response to step increases in perfusion pressure compared with arterioles of normotensive rats. The authors suggest that this difference could be due to an enhanced production of endothelium-derived constrictor factors, primarily prostaglandin H_2. (From Huang, A., Dong, S., and Koller, A., *Hypertension*, 22, 913, 1993.)

peripheral resistance is due to arterial or arteriolar wall hypertrophy (cell enlargement) or hyperplasia (increase in cell number) reflected by an increase in wall thickness. This leads the resistance to flow to be raised even at normal levels of smooth muscle tone and smooth muscle shortening and accentuates luminal reductions compared to normotensive vessels.[49]

In arteries, hypertrophy or hyperplasia has been consistently found in almost all types of hypertension; conversely, in arterioles, the increase of wall thickness or wall cross-sectional area is highly dependent on the type of hypertension or organ. Such alterations were observed in muscles during hypertension due to aortic coarctation in rat,[50] but not in muscles from genetic hypertensive rats[7,51,52] nor in renovascular hypertension where wall thickness was changed but not wall area.[53,54] In renovascular hypertension, the changes in wall/lumen ratios observed from the 1st to the 9th week after induction of hypertension were demonstrated to be due to a failure of the arterioles to enlarge their diameter as the animal aged and were not due to changes in vascular mass.[53]

When present, structural changes in vessel wall structure in hypertension were generally considered to be the result of pressure-dependent mechanisms. However, the role of nonpressure-related factors have been more recently emphasized. In this connection, sympathoadrenergic influences have been demonstrated by the finding that sympathetic denervation strongly impaired the proliferation of vascular smooth muscle in the ear artery of growing rabbit[55] or in the cerebral vasculature of stroke-prone genetic hypertensive rats.[56] However, thickening of arteriolar wall in cremaster muscle was also reported in a model hypertension by aortic coarctation in rats that were also submitted to a peripheral sympathectomy.[50] Since, in such a model, intraarterial pressure distal to the aortic constriction (and consequently in cremaster muscle) remains normal, these findings suggest that humoral factors also may play an important role in the changes in microvascular wall associated with hypertensive states.

2. Resting Arteriolar Diameter

Controversial results have been found concerning the resting arteriolar diameter in hypertension. Capillary and arteriolar narrowing has been described in the conjunctiva of essential hypertensive patients by some authors,[57-59] but others reported no significant changes or an even larger diameters in young borderline hypertensive patients.[60] These opposite findings suggest that, in patients, arteriolar constriction is only associated with long time established hypertension.[3]

In animals, narrowing of arteriolar diameter of cremaster muscle was consistently found in renovascular hypertension for all types of arterioles[12,53,54,61] and in salt-induced hypertension for large arterioles.[62] In spontaneous hypertension, most authors reported no difference in diameter between hypertensive and normotensive animals in muscles[63-66] or brain,[67] but others observed a narrowing of some arteriolar segments in skeletal muscle,[13,68,69] intestine,[4] and cerebral cortex.[17] Schmid-Schonbein[19] opportunely stressed that some methodological difficulties must be kept in mind when interpreting these diverging results. This author calculated that a 13% average arteriolar narrowing would be sufficient to explain an elevated mean pressure of 48 mmHg at constant flow. If modifications of microvascular density are present (see following paragraphs), an even smaller degree of narrowing would be sufficient. Since there is a large heterogeneity of arteriolar diameter within every class of arterioles, because the vascular cross-sections are not circular and since the accuracy in intravital microscopy can be limited in several tissues, it is difficult technically to document very small modifications in vessel diameter.

In both normotensive and hypertensive rats, microvascular tone (related to the variation between resting and maximally dilated diameter) is consistently found to be higher in distal than in proximal arterioles. For most of the muscle arterioles studied, this tone was found to be higher in genetic hypertensive rats and in renovascular hypertension than in controls.[43,53,70] However, as suggested by Hashimoto et al.,[53] the contribution of the increased tone to the elevated resistance may vary during the evolution of hypertension and may decrease when structural changes appear in the microvascular network such as the reduction of microvessel density, described in the following paragraphs.

3. Arteriolar and Capillary Density

Reducing the number of parallel circuits increases the total resistance to blood flow in a vascular bed. Arterioles that either don't develop during growth, or arterioles that close and eventually atrophy, both result in arteriole rarefaction and contribute to hypertension.

In patients, the possibilities to explore microvessel density is limited to a few number of organs. In conjunctival microcirculation, capillary microscopy in vivo has found a decrease in arteriolar density in patients with essential established hypertension[58] and a decrease in capillary density in patients with either established or borderline hypertension.[58,72] A significant reduction in capillary density was also found in nailfold microcirculation under basal conditions in patients with essential hypertension,[72] and during hyperemia in sodium-resistant borderline hypertensive patients.[73] Histological findings also suggested a reduction in capillary density in skeletal muscle, myocardium, and stomach in hypertensive patients.[74,75]

In animals, several authors found a reduction in the number of arterioles perfusing muscular tissues in both spontaneous and renovascular hypertension. This concept of arteriolar rarefaction involves a functional aspect that is realized by the temporary closure of some terminal arterioles. For hypertensive animals, the basal inside diameter of these arterioles is so small that it does not allow the entrance of red blood cells, and thus does not allow a vizualization of the arterioles by intravital microscopy techniques. However, when a potent dilator is administered to the preparations, a dilation of the terminal arterioles is induced allowing perfusion by blood red cells, and their visualization. Functional rarefaction has been reported in muscles in both spontaneous[21,52,63,64] and

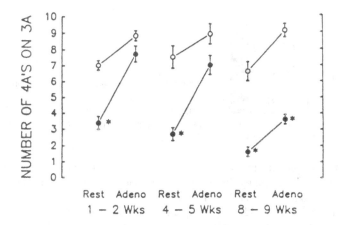

Figure 5 Changes in the number of cremasteric terminal arterioles (4A) visualized at different times after the onset of renovascular hypertension in rat. It may be noted that administration of adenosine abolished or reduced the difference between normotensive and hypertensive rats during the first weeks, but not after 8 weeks. This finding demonstrated the progression from functional to structural arteriolar rarefaction. (From Hashimoto, H., Prewitt, R. L., and Efaw, C. W., *Am. J. Physiol.*, 253, H933, 1987.)

renovascular hypertension.[53,54] The possibility that adrenaline originating from a sympathetic nervous system could be involved in temporary vessel closure, because of a higher reactivity in hypertension, has been demonstrated in cremaster muscle by Bohlen.[21] This author showed that the effect of denervation on the number of closed arterioles was almost three times higher in genetic hypertensive rats than in normotensive controls. It may be speculated that, because of the interaction between angiotensin II and sympathetic reactivity, the higher vascular angiotensin converting enzyme activity can have a role in this mechanism. However, it may be stressed that the closure of the terminal arterioles is certainly not related to a unique mechanism since Prewitt et al. found only a very little effect of denervation alone on functional rarefaction.[64] It is likely that the interactions between increased reactivity, myogenic and oxygen-dependent autoregulatory mechanisms, and/or humoral factors are required to induce a significant amount of complete arteriolar closures.

Another aspect of arteriolar rarefaction is structural (i.e., anatomical). At this stage of rarefaction, the number of arterioles perfused is decreased even after maximal dilation. Such a rarefaction has been demonstrated to be an early characteristic of spontaneous hypertension in the rat where the number of terminal arterioles was reduced by almost a factor of 2, as compared with normotensive controls.[65,66] In cremaster muscle during renovascular hypertension, it was clearly demonstrated that structural rarefaction takes the place of functional rarefaction after several weeks of hypertension (see Figure 5). In this latter case, the number of terminal arterioles branching from more proximal arterioles was 3 times lower in hypertensive animals than in the controls after 9 weeks of hypertension.[53]

The hypothesis that altered microvascular pressure could provide the stimulus for arteriolar rarefaction has been proposed.[76] However, a recent study by Boegehold et al.[77] reported a 20% rarefaction of distal arterioles in the rat cremaster muscle in coarcted hypertension. Since in this type of hypertension, pressure in the feeding artery of the muscle is not elevated (femoral pressure was even lower than controls in this study), these findings showed that pressure-independent mechanisms are also involved in the rarefaction process. Concerning the possible role of sodium in rarefaction, it still remains controversial since Hernandez et al.[78] reported that high salt intake can affect microvessel density independently of changes in pressure, but such changes in arteriolar density were

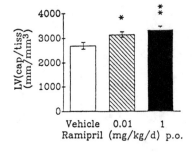

Figure 6 Effect of early onset long-term treatment with two oral doses of the angiotensin converting enzyme inhibitor ramipril on myocardial capillary length density (LV cap/tiss). (From Unger, T., Mattfeldt, T., et al., *Hypertension*, 20, 478, 1992.)

not found by Boegehold[62] in another model of salt-induced hypertension. Another hypothesis, recently discussed by Struijker et al.[79] is that primary hypertension is the result of a depressed angiogenesis at the arteriolar and capillary level.

Despite the number of studies reporting arteriolar rarefaction in hypertensive animals, very little was known until recently concerning the exact structural and ultrastructural changes that occur during arteriolar rarefaction. Very interesting observations on these aspects were recently reported by Hansen-Smith et al.[80] in cremaster muscle in chronic reduced renal mass hypertension. The authors found atrophy and degeneration of both endothelial cells and vascular smooth muscle cells. These ultrastructural changes were similar to those occurring after ischemic injury in muscle. This similarity between microvascular damages due to hypertension and ischemia might suggest that local hypoxic damages due to the arteriolar closure might have been the cause of degeneration. However, contrasting with what occurs after ischemia, no phagocytic response was observed in hypertension even 4 weeks after the inducement of hypertension. The cited authors suggested that the microvascular degeneration might occur too gradually to induce phagocytosis. Since phagocytosis is the first step for subsequent repair of microvascular structure, this might explain why such a process of repair cannot take place in hypertension and why the deleterious consequences of temporary closure (functional rarefaction) might induce a permanent structural rarefaction. But, it may be stressed that the exact cause of the vascular degeneration was not determined in this study and still remains hypothetical.

Despite this phenomenon being reported in many studies, the exact role arteriolar rarefaction has in increasing peripheral resistance is still controversial for several reasons. As mentioned previously, some authors consider that the major site of vascular resistance is upstream from the arterioles in the larger vessels and that, consequently, changes in arteriolar network morphology would not affect vascular resistance.[81] This point has been discussed previously. Others consider that because of anastomotic channels and alternative pathways, the arteriolar rarefaction would not affect total blood flow resistance.[19] However, in conditions of simulated rarefaction using 50-micron microspheres to block capillaries, a 50% increase in resistance occurred.[82] Mathematical modeling of rarefaction indicates that loss of 42% of the resistance arterioles can account for the resistance changes seen in hypertension.[83]

As regards the effects of drug therapy on microvessel density, some authors reported that antihypertensive drugs such as calcium blockers[84] or angiotensin converting enzyme inhibitors can prevent the arteriolar or capillary rarefaction in myocardium[85] (see Figure 6) and muscle,[86] but others reported an opposite effect of angiotensin converting enzyme inhibitors.[87]

D. BLOOD RHEOLOGY

Blood and plasma viscosity and hematocrit have been reported to be elevated in hypertensive patients.[87-90] Membrane properties of erythrocytes are also modified in hypertension, as shown by the increase in erythrocyte rigidity and aggregability.[87,90,91]

Relative frequency [%]

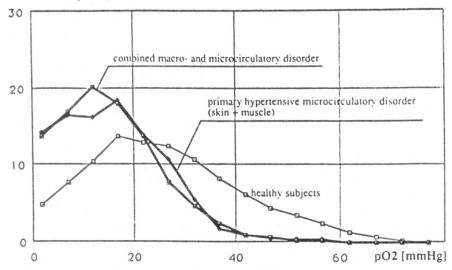

Figure 7 Intramuscular pO_2 in healthy subjects and in patients with primary hypertensive microcirculatory disorder of skin and muscle, and combined microcirculatory disorder and macroangiopathy. (From Jung, F. et al., *Clin. Invest.*, 71, 132, 1993.)

IV. HYPERTENSION AND TISSUE PERFUSION

In patients, conflicting results have been described concerning a possible decrease in capillary blood velocity associated with hypertension.[3]

In experimental studies, reduction of blood flow in different organs has been reported in renovascular or high-salt diet hypertension,[12] but such a reduction is far from being always associated with high blood pressure. In genetic hypertension, some groups found a large reduction in blood flow in cremaster muscle;[13,68] others found flow to be similar in genetic hypertensive rats and in controls,[7,17] with no differences in mean blood cell velocities.

However, it must be stressed that the total amount of blood flow entering tissues is not the only factor that determines the quality of tissue perfusion. The homogeneity of blood flow within the tissue is also a key factor to prevent the appearance of areas of local tissue hypoxia. Several authors reported that the degree of blood flow dispersion is larger in hypertensive animals.[7] As suggested by Schmid-Schonbein,[19] the elevated tone in some arterioles associated with hypertension may increase the heterogeneity of blood flow and red cell distribution at the diverging bifurcations. Such a mechanism would induce a higher degree of plasma skimming, as found in genetic hypertensive rats.[92] In addition, it may be remembered that the increased microvascular blood flow heterogeneity found in hypertension can certainly be considerably aggravated by rheological changes, such as changes in red cell or white cell membrane properties that are associated with hypertension or with possible associated diseases (diabetes, hyperlipidemia, etc.).

Changes in microvascular structures, regulatory mechanisms, and abnormal rheology can explain why the frequency of low values of intramuscular pO_2 were found more often in hypertensive patients than in normotensive controls[93] (see Figure 7).

V. CONCLUDING REMARKS

Despite the considerable amount of experimental results relating to hypertension-induced alterations in the microcirculation, the exact role of the microcirculation in the pathophysiology of hypertension is still unknown. It seems likely that the microvascular network plays a significant role in both the gradient of blood pressure in normal conditions and in the elevation of pressure in hypertension. However, the relative part of the modification of arteriolar network and resistance arteries upstream from the arterioles in the increase of peripheral resistance is probably dependent on the organ considered. In contrast to the findings regarding resistance arteries, the alterations in arteriole wall structure associated to hypertension are dependent on the type of hypertension. Some recent findings confirmed that, at the microvascular level, the trigger for the induction of such changes can be another factor other than the elevated pressure per se, but the reasons for which the arterioles did not exhibit the same changes in vascular wall in the different forms of hypertension is not known.

A key phenomenon that appears in microvascular networks during hypertension is temporary closure of some terminal arterioles. This phenomenon is likely due to amplification of some autoregulatory processes by alterations of microvascular reactivity by neurohumoral vasoconstrictors. Many alterations of regulatory mechanisms have been reported to be associated to hypertension and may be involved in this amplification, such as alterations in the balance between endothelium-derived relaxing and constricting factors, alterations in cyclooxygenase products, or alteration in the local renin-angiotensin system. However, it is not known whether altering only one of these pathways is sufficient to explain the microvascular changes found in hypertension, or if the simultaneous alteration of several pathways is required. The development of new transgenic models will allow more specific exploration of individual biochemical pathways and thus facilitate the identification of the most important regulatory mechanisms in the microcirculation.

Another crucial yet largely unexplored mechanistic aspect is the passage from functional to structural rarefaction. This passage is a crucial step in the evolution of hypertensive disease, since it represents the appearance of a real structural injury of the tissues. It is not known whether some specific immunologic alterations are present and/or necessary at this step of the disease to produce anatomical rarefaction and to impede a process of vascular repair.

Most microvascular studies have been carried out to examine the role of microcirculation in the elevation of pressure (as shown by this brief review); but, more than its causal role in the elevation of systemic pressure, we would like to emphasize the importance of the microcirculation as a crucial target of hypertension. Since the integrity of the microvascular system is essential for adequate O_2 supply and adaptation to metabolic changes in the tissues, hypertension-induced tissue injury is an important part of the disease to be considered. With this in mind, the association between hypertension-induced microcirculatory alterations and increased risk of organ failure and mortality becomes clear. In our view, the microvascular alterations seen in hypertension warrant characterizing hypertension as a tissue disease. Moreover, the presence of these microvascular alterations explain why, in spite of pressure decreases obtained with different drugs, these do not necessarily eliminate the damage done to the microvasculature. Finally, how different therapies alter the structure of the microcirculation and how these alterations can be reversed are perhaps the most important questions that microcirculation research can answer for the clinician.

REFERENCES

1. **Bohlen, H. G.,** The microcirculation in hypertension, *Hypertension,* 7, S117, 1989.
2. **Zweifach, B. W.,** The microcirculation in experimental hypertension, *Hypertension,* 5, 110, 1983.
3. **Shore, A. C. and Tooke, J. E.,** Microvascular function in human essential hypertension, *J. Hypertens.,* 12, 717, 1994.

4. **Bohlen, H. G.,** Intestinal microvascular adaptation during maturation of spontaneously hypertensive rats, *Hypertension,* 5, 739, 1983.

5. **Hill, M. A., Simpson, B. E., and Meininger, G. A.,** Altered cremaster muscle hemodynamics due to disruption of the deferential feed vessel, *Microvasc. Res.,* 39, 349, 1990.

6. **Meininger, G. A., Fehr, K. L., Yates, M. B., Borders, J. L., and Granger, H. J.,** Hemodynamic characteristics of the intestinal microcirculation in renal hypertension, *Hypertension,* 8, 66, 1986.

7. **Zweifach, B. W., Kovalcheck , S., DeLano, F., and Chen, P.,** Micropressure-flow relationships in a skeletal muscle of spontaneously hypertensive rats, *Hypertension,* 3, 601, 1981.

8. **DeLano, F. A., Schmid-Schonbein, G. W., Skalad, T. C., and Zweifach, B. W.,** Penetration of the systemic blood pressure into the microvasculature of rat skeletal muscle, *Microvasc. Res.,* 41, 92, 1991.

9. **Gore, R. W.,** Pressures in cat mesenteric arterioles and capillaries during changes in systemic arterial blood pressure, *Circ. Res.,* 34, 581, 1974.

10. **Zweifach, B. W. and Lipowski, H.,** Quantitative studies of microvascular structure and function III microvascular hemodynamics of cat mesentery and rabbit omentum, *Circ. Res.,* 41, 380, 1977.

11. **Bohlen, H. G., Gore, R. W., and Hutchins, P. M.,** Comparison of microvascular pressures in normal and hypertensive rats, *Microvasc. Res.,* 13, 125, 1977.

12. **Meininger, G. A., Harris, P. D., and Joshua, I. G.,** Distributions of microvascular pressure in skeletal muscle of one-kidney, one-clip, two-kidney, one-clip and deoxycorticosterone-salt hypertensive rats, *Hypertension,* 6, 27, 1984.

13. **Roy, J. W. and Mayrovitz, H. N.,** Microvascular pressure, flow and resistance in spontaneously hypertensive rats, *Hypertension,* 6, 877, 1984.

14. **Gore, R. W. and Bohlen, H. G.,** Microvascular pressure in rat intestinal muscle and mucosal villi, *Am. J. Physiol.,* 233, H685, 1977.

15. **Davis, M. J., Ferrer, P. M., and Gore, R. W.,** Vascular anatomy and hydrostatic pressure profile in the hamster cheek pouch, *Am. J. Physiol.,* 250, H291, 1986.

16. **Bohlen, H. G., Gore, R. W., and Hutchins, P. M.,** Comparison of microvascular pressure in normal and hypertensive rats, *Microvasc. Res.,* 13, 125, 1977.

17. **Harper, S. L. and Bohlen, H. G.,** Microvascular adaptation in the cerebral cortex of adult spontaneously hypertensive rats, *Hypertension,* 6, 408, 1984.

18. **Joyner, W. L., Davis, M. J., and Gilmore, J. P.,** Intravascular pressure distribution and dimensional analysis of microvessels in hamsters with renovascular hypertension, *Microvasc. Res.,* 22, 190, 1981.

19. **Schmid-Schonbein, G. W., Skalak , T. C., and Firestone, G.,** The microvasculature in skeletal muscle. V. The microvascular arcades in normotensive and hypertensive rats, *Microvasc. Res.,* 34, 385, 1987.

20. **Boegehold, M. A.,** Effect of salt-induced hypertension on microvascular pressures in skeletal muscle of Dahl rats, *Am. J. Physiol.,* 260, H1819, 1991.

21. **Bohlen, H. G.,** Arteriolar closure mediated by hyperresponsiveness to norepinephrine in hypertensive rats, *Am. J. Physiol.,* 5(1), H157, 1979.

22. **Wilmoth, F. R. and Price, J. M.,** Increased sensitivity of the cremaster microvasculature in spontaneously hypertensive rats with elevated body temperature, *Microvasc. Res.,* 41, 133, 1991.

23. **Click, R. L., Gilmore, J. P., and Joyner, W. L.,** Differential response of hamster cheek pouch microvessels to vasoactive stimuli during the early development of hypertension, *Circ. Res.,* 44, 512, 1979.

24. **Myers, T. O., Joyner, W. L., and Gilmore, F. P.,** Angiotensin reactivity in the cheek pouch of the renovascular hypertensive hamster, *Hypertension,* 12, 373, 1988.

25. **Joyner, W. L., Mohama, R. E., and Gilmore, J. P.,** Specificity of arginine vasopressin and angiotensin II for microvessels in the hamster cheek pouch after the induction of renovascular hypertension, *Microvasc. Res.,* 35, 8, 1988.

26. **Mulvany, M. J. and Nyborg, N.,** An increased calcium sensitivity of mesenteric resistance vessels in young and adult spontaneously hypertensive rats, *Br. J. Pharmacol.,* 71, 585, 1980.

27. **Haddy, F.,** Roles of sodium, potassium, calcium, and natriuretic factors in hypertension, *Hypertension,* 18(5), 179, 1991.

28. **Rosskopf, D., Dusing, R., and Siffert, W.,** Membrane sodium-proton exchange and primary hypertension, *Hypertension,* 21(5), 606, 1993.

29. **Folkow, B.,** Critical review of studies on salt and hypertension, *Clin. Exp. Hypertens.*, 14(1–2), 1, 1992.

30. **Vicaut, E. and Hou, X.,** Arteriolar constriction and local renin-angiotensin system in microcirculation, *Hypertension*, 21(4), 491, 1993.

31. **Vicaut, E. and Hou, X.,** The local renin-angiotensin system in the microcirculation of spontaneously hypertensive rats, *Hypertension*, 24, 70, 1994.

32. **Luscher, T. F.,** Endothelial vasoactive substances and cardiovascular disease, *Am. J. Cardiol.*, 60, 110, 1987.

33. **Panza, J. A., Quyyumi, A. A., Brush, J. E., and Epstein, S. E.,** Abnormal endothelium-dependent vascular relaxation in patients with essential hypertension, *N. Engl. J. Med.*, 323, 22, 1990.

34. **Mayhan, W. G., Faraci, F. M., and Heistad, D. D.,** Impairment of endothelium-dependent responses of cerebral arterioles in chronic hypertension, *Am. J. Physiol.*, 253, H1435, 1987.

35. **Nakamura, T. and Prewitt, R. L.,** Effect of NG-monomethyl L-arginine on endothelium-dependent relaxation in arterioles of one-kidney, one clip hypertensive rats, *Hypertension*, 17, 875, 1991.

36. **Lin, L. and Nasjletti, A.,** Contribution of vascular prostanoids to angiotensin II-induced vasoconstriction in hypertension, *FASEB*, 5, 3885, 1991.

37. **Huang, A., Dong, S., and Koller, A.,** Endothelial dysfunction augments myogenic arteriolar constriction in hypertension, *Hypertension*, 22, 913, 1993.

38. **Ledingham, J. M.,** Extrarenal factors in the pathogenesis of hypertension, in *Symposium on Hypotensive Drugs*, Harrington, M., Ed., Pergamon Press, London, 1956, 183.

39. **Ledingham, J. M. and Cohen, R. D.,** Circulatory changes during the reversal of experimental hypertension, *Clin. Sci.*, 22, 69, 1962.

40. **Folkow, B.,** Intravascular pressure as a factor regulating the tone of small vessels, *Acta Physiol. Scand.*, 17, 289, 1949.

41. **Meininger, G. A. and Trzeciakowski, J. P.,** Vasoconstriction is amplified by autoregulation during vasoconstrictor-induced hypertension, *Am. J. Physiol.*, 254, H709, 1988.

42. **Hutchins, P. M., Bond, R. F., and Green, H. D.,** Participation of oxygen in the local control of skeletal muscle microvasculature, *Circ. Res.*, 34, 85, 1974.

43. **Lombard, J. H., Hess, M. E., and Stekiel, W. J.,** Neural and local control of arterioles in SHR, *Hypertension*, 6, 530, 1984.

44. **Jackson, W. F.,** Lipoxygenase inhibitors block O_2 responses of hamster cheek pouch arterioles, *Am. J. Physiol.*, 255, H711, 1988.

45. **Vicaut, E. and Hou, X.,** Role of endothelium in the response of small terminal arterioles to hyperoxia, in *Biology of Nitric Oxide*, Moncada, S. et al., Eds., Pergamon, London, 79, 1993.

46. **Ebeige, A. B.,** Influence of hypoxia on contractility and calcium uptake in rabbit aorta, *Experientia*, 38, 935, 1982.

47. **Ledingham, J. M.,** Autoregulation in hypertension: A review, *Hypertension*, 7, S97, 1989.

48. **Folkow, B.,** Structural, myogenic, humoral and nervous factors controlling peripheral resistance, *Hypotensive Drugs*, 163, 1956.

49. **Folkow, B.,** Functional and structural "autoregulation" — some personal considerations concerning the century-old development of these microvascular concepts, *Microvasc. Res.*, 37, 243, 1989.

50. **Plunkett, W. C. and Overbeck, H. W.,** Arteriolar wall thickening in hypertensive rats unrelated to pressure or sympathoadrenergic influences, *Circ. Res.*, 63, 937, 1988.

51. **Bohlen, H. G. and Lobach, D.,** *In-vivo* study of microvascular wall characteristics and resting control in young and mature spontaneously hypertensive rats, *Blood Vessel*, 15, 322, 1978.

52. **Chen, I. I. H., Prewitt, R. L., and Dowell, R. F.,** Microvascular rarefaction in spontaneously hypertensive rat cremaster muscle, *Am. J. Physiol.*, 241, H306, 1981.

53. **Hashimoto, H., Prewitt, R. L., and Efaw, C. W.,** Alterations in the microvasculature of one-kidney, one-clip hypertensive rats, *Am. J. Physiol.*, 253, H933, 1987.

54. **Wang, D. H. and Prewitt, R. L.,** Captopril reduces aortic and microvascular growth in hypertensive and normotensive rats, *Hypertension*, 15, 68, 1990.

55. **Bevan, R. D.,** Effect of sympathetic denervation on smooth muscle cell proliferation in the growing rabbit ear artery, *Circ. Res.*, 37, 14, 1975.

56. **Hart, M., Heistad, D. D., and Brody, M. J.,** Effect of chronic hypertension and sympathetic denervation on wall/lumen ratio of cerebral arteries, *Hypertension*, 2, 419, 1980.

57. **Landau, J. and Davis, E.,** Capillary thinning and high capillary blood pressure in hypertension, *Lancet*, i, 1327, 1957.

58. **Harper, R. N., Moore, M. A., Marr, M. C., Watts, L. E., and Hutchins, P. M.**, Arteriolar rarefaction in the conjonctiva of human hypertensives, *Microvasc. Res.*, 16, 369, 1978.

59. **Korber, N., Jung, F., Kiesewetter, H., Wolf, S., Prunte, C., and Riem, M.**, Microcirculation in the conjunctival capillaries of healthy and hypertensive patients, *Klin. Wochenschr.*, 64, 953, 1986.

60. **Sullivan, J. M., Prewitt, R. I., and Josephs, J. A.**, Attenuation of the microcirculation in young patients with high-output borderline hypertension, *Hypertension*, 5, 844, 1983.

61. **Joshua, I. G., Wiegman, D. L., Harris, P. D., and Miller, F. N.**, Progressive microvascular alterations with the development of renovascular hypertension, *Hypertension*, 6, 61, 1984.

62. **Boegehold, M. A.**, Microvascular changes associated with high salt intake and hypertension in Dahl rats, *Int. J. Microcirc.: Clin. Exp.*, 12, 143, 1993.

63. **Hutchins, P. M. and Darnell, A. E.**, Observation of a decreased number of small arterioles in spontaneously hypertensive rats, *Circ. Res.*, 34/35 (Suppl. 1), 161, 1974.

64. **Prewitt, R. L., Chen, I. I. H., and Dowell, R.**, Development of microvascular rarefaction in the spontaneously hypertensive rat, *Am. J. Physiol.*, 243, H243, 1982.

65. **LeNoble, J., Tangelder, G. J., Slaaf, D. W., Essen, H. V., Reneman, R. S., and Struyker-Boudier, A. J.**, A functional morphometric study of the cremaster muscle microcirculation in young spontaneously hypertensive rats, *Hypertension*, 8, 741, 1990.

66. **Struyker-Boudier, H. A. J., Le Noble, J., Slaaf, D. W., Smits, J. F. M., and Tangelder, G. J.**, Microcirculatory changes in cremaster muscle during early spontaneous hypertension in the rat, *Hypertension*, 6, S185, 1988.

67. **Lin, S. Z., Sposito, N., Rybacki, P. L., McKenna, E., and Pettigrew, K.**, Cerebral capillary bed structure of normotensive and chronically hypertensive rats, *Microvasc. Res.*, 40, 341, 1990.

68. **Roy, J. W. and Mayrovitz, H. N.**, Microvascular blood flow in the normotensive and spontaneously hypertensive rat, *Hypertension*, 4, 264, 1982.

69. **Le Noble, J., Smith, T. L., Hutchins, P. M., and Struyker-Boudier, H. A. J.**, Microvascular alterations in adult conscious spontaneously hypertensive rats, *Hypertension*, 15, 415, 1990.

70. **Schmid-Schonbein, G. W., Zweifach, B. W., DeLano, F. A., and Chen, P. C. Y.**, Microvascular tone in a skeletal muscle of spontaneously hypertensive rats, *Hypertension*, 9, 164, 1987.

71. **Duprez, D., De Buyzere, M., De Bavker, T., Vercammen, J., Kaufman, J. M., Van Hoecke, M., Vermeulen, A., and Clement, D. L.**, Influence of nonhemodynamic factors on the microcirculation in moderate essential arterial hypertension, *Am. J. Hypertens.*, 4, 885, 1991.

72. **Gasser, P. and Bühler, F. R.**, Nailfold microcirculation in normotensive and essential hypertensive subjects, as assessed by video-microscopy, *J. Hypertens.*, 10, 83, 1992.

73. **Draaijer, P., De Leeuw, P. W., Van Hooff, J. P., and Leunissen, K. M.**, Nailfold capillary density in salt-sensitive and salt-resistant boderline hypertension, *J. Hypertens.*, 11, 1195, 1993.

74. **Henrich, H. A., Romen, W., Heimgartner, W., Hartung, E., and Baumer, F.**, Capillary rarefaction characteristic of the skeletal muscle of hypertensive patients, *Klin. Wochenschr.*, 66, 54, 1988.

75. **Fischer, P., Heimgartner, W., Hartung, E., and Henrich, H. A.**, Capillary rarefaction in different organ tissues of hypertensive patients (abstract), *Int. J. Microcirc.*, 4, 106, 1984.

76. **Hogan, R. D. and Hirschmann, L.**, Arteriolar proliferation in the rat cremaster muscle as a long-term autoregulatory response to reduced perfusion, *Microvasc. Res.*, 27, 290, 1984.

77. **Boegehold, M. A., Johnson, M. D., and Overbeck, H. W.**, Pressure-independent arteriolar rarefaction in hypertension, *Am. J. Physiol.*, 261, H83, 1991.

78. **Hernandez, I., Cowley, J. R. A. W., Lombard, H., and Greene, A. S.**, Salt intake and angiotensin II alter microvessel density in the cremaster muscle of normal rats, *Am. J. Physiol.*, 263, H664, 1992.

79. **Struijker, H. A. J., Le Noble, J. L. M. L., Messing, M. W. J., Huijberts, M. S. P., Le Noble, F. A. C., and Van Essen, H.**, The microcirculation and hypertension, *J. Hypertens.*, 10(S7), S147, 1992.

80. **Hansen-Smith, F., Greene, A. S., Cowley, A. W., Jr., and Lombard, J. H.**, Structural changes during microvascular rarefaction in chronic hypertension, *Hypertension*, 15, 922, 1990.

81. **Bohlen, H. G.**, Localization of vascular resistance changes during hypertension, *Hypertens. Dallas*, 8, 181, 1986.

82. **Hallback, M. G., Gothberg, S., Lundin, S.-E., Ricksten, and Folkow, B.**, Hemodynamic consequences of resistance vessel rarefaction and of changes in smooth muscle sensitivity, *Acta Physiol. Scand.*, 97, 233–240, 1976.

83. **Greene, A., Tonellato, P., Lui, J., Lombard, J., and Cowley, A., Jr.,** Microvascular rarefaction and tissue vascular resistance in hypertension, *Am. J. Physiol.,* 256, H126–H131, 1989.

84. **Turek, Z., Kubat, K., Kazda, S., Hoofd, L., and Rakusan, K.,** Improved myocardial capillarisation in spontaneously hypertensive rats treated with nifedipine, *Cardiovasc. Res.,* 21, 725, 1987.

85. **Unger, T., Mattfeldt, T., Lamberty, V., Bock, P., Mall, G., Linz, W., Scholkens, B., and Gohlke, P.,** Effect of early onset angiotensin converting enzyme inhibition on myocardial capillaries, *Hypertension,* 20, 478, 1992.

86. **Vicaut, E. and Hou, X.,** Early onset angiotensin converting enzyme inhibition prevents arteriole and capillary rarefaction in muscle of spontaneously hypertensive rats, *Am. J. Hypertens.,* 7 (Abstr.), 4, 88A, 1994.

87. **Leschke, M., Vogt, M., Motz, W., and Strauer, B.,** Blood rheology as a contributing factor in reduced coronary reserve in systemic hypertension, *Am. J. Cardiol.,* 65, 56G, 1990.

88. **Koenig, W., Sund, M., Ernst, E., Matrai, A., Keil, U., and Rosenthal, J.,** Is increased plasma viscosity a risk factor for high blood pressure?, *Angiology,* 40, 153, 1989.

89. **Hossmann, V., Aukl, H., Bonner, G., Wambach, G., Laaser, U., Allhoff, P., et al.,** Haemorrheology in adolescent hypertensives, *J. Hypertens.,* 3 (Suppl. 3), S331, 1985.

90. **Puniyani, R. R., Ajmani, R., and Kale, P. A.,** Risk factors in some cardiovascular diseases, *J. Biomed. Eng.,* 13, 441, 1991.

91. **Razavian, S. M., Del Pino, M., Simon, A., and Levenson, J.,** Increase in erythrocyte disaggregation shear stress in hypertension, *Hypertension,* 20, 247, 1992.

92. **Baker, C. H., Wuklitg, F. R., Syttib, E. T. N., and Takach, K.,** Red blood cell and plasma distribution in SHR cremaster muscle microvessels, *Am. J. Physiol.,* 242, H381, 1982.

93. **Jung, F., Kolepke, W., Sptizer, S., Kiesewetter, H., Ruprecht, K. W., Bach, R., Schieffer, H., and Wenzel, E.,** Primary and secondary microcirculatory disorders in essential hypertension, *Clin. Invest.,* 71, 132, 1993.

Chapter 5

Shock and Multiple-Organ Dysfunction and the Microcirculation

Mark A. Wilson and R. Neal Garrison

CONTENTS

I. INTRODUCTION

The clinical syndromes of systemic sepsis, shock, and multiple organ dysfunction or failure are typically initiated by other conditions, such as traumatic injury, prolonged hemorrhage, ischemia/reperfusion, and invasive infection. In most instances, these primary conditions can be adequately treated with conventional therapies, such as volume resuscitation and control of hemorrhage, debridement of nonviable tissue, drainage of infectious foci, and administration of antimicrobial agents. In spite of these standardized treatments, a significant number of patients with these disorders develop clinical evidence of vital organ dysfunction,[1-5] which is refractory to standard critical care supportive therapies.[2-4] This organ dysfunction most often occurs at sites that are remote from the initial infectious or traumatic focus.[6,7] As technologies to support critically ill patients have developed, the syndrome of multiple organ dysfunction (MOD) has become a leading cause of morbidity and mortality.[8-10]

Pathophysiologic alterations of cellular metabolism, cellular and humoral immune function, and microvascular perfusion are all postulated to be factors in both the development and maintenance of MOD.[2,4,10-13] Many researchers currently hypothesize that excessive or uncontrolled systemic activation of endogenous inflammatory cells and mediators is the central mechanism that results in the initiation and maintenance of MOD (Table 1).[10-13] Hemorrhagic shock, the sepsis syndrome, and the syndrome of multiple organ dysfunction each have complicated and multifactorial etiologies, but the microcirculation appears to be a common component. In fact, researchers increasingly recognize that the microcirculation is not only a vascular conduit that is affected by many mediators, but that it is also a functional system that elaborates cytokines and vasoactive substances and dynamically interacts with circulating leukocytes, platelets, and tissue mast cells. Activation, altered function, and injury of microvascular endothelial cells may occur from ischemia, from direct effects of mediators such as cytokines and eicosanoids, or as the result of neutrophil adherence and transendothelial migration. Subsequent endothelial activation or damage may result in altered fluid and macromolecular fluxes with an increase in interstitial edema. Furthermore, alterations of vascular tone and responsiveness to vasoactive compounds may affect regional nutrient blood flow and tissue oxygen delivery. The specific role(s) of the microcirculation in the development of human MOD (multiple organ dysfunction) is largely unconfirmed due to a lack of animal models that simulate the human syndrome and to technical limitations for study of the visceral microcirculation in human patients. However, the role of the microcirculation during

0-8493-4870-6/95/$0.00+$.50

Table 1 Potential Mediators of
Microvascular Alterations During Sepsis

Endotoxins
Interleukins
Tumor necrosis factor
Nitric oxide
Oxygen free radicals
Fibronectin
Phagocytic proteinases
Corticosteroids
Biogenic amines
  Histamine
  Catecholamines
  5-Hydroxytryptamine
Fatty acid metabolites
  Leukotrienes
  Platelet-activating factor
  Prostanoids
  Thromboxanes
Oligo/polypeptides
  Kinins
  Vasopressin
  Vasoactive intestinal polypeptide
  Endogenous opiates
  Complement
  Neuropeptide Y
  Endothelin
  Angiotensin

experimental hemorrhage and sepsis is more clearly characterized, and this chapter will therefore focus on the microvascular pathophysiology of experimental shock and sepsis.

II. MICROCIRCULATORY ALTERATIONS ASSOCIATED WITH HEMORRHAGIC SHOCK

The primary function of the microcirculation is the delivery of an adequate amount of oxygen and nutrients to tissues for the maintenance of cellular respiration by the mitochondrial respiratory chain. This supply of nutrients is dependent upon a complex set of interrelated factors that determine cardiac output, regional blood flow, distribution of blood flow within organs, and the oxygen and nutrient content of arterial blood. However, the final matching of nutrient blood flow to metabolically active, functional cellular units is accomplished at the microvascular level. This process of matching delivery to consumption is influenced by intrinsic factors such as the inherent properties of microvessels and the local production of vasoactive substances, as well as by multiple extrinsic factors such as circulating hormones and the autonomic nervous system.

Numerous mechanisms have been demonstrated to contribute to alterations of cellular and organ function following shock. These include direct cellular injury due to reactive oxygen species and the release of neutrophil enzymes, functional modulation by cytokines and/or lipid mediators, and altered availability of some substrates necessary for cellular metabolism. However, the initial and primary defects during hemorrhage are an overall decrease in oxygen delivery as well as a mismatch of nutrient delivery to metabolically active cells. These defects are mediated in part by the microcirculation. As oxygen delivery at the capillary level decreases, oxygen extraction initially increases such that oxygen consumption is preserved. With further impairment of oxygen delivery, oxygen consumption is compromised and becomes flow dependent,[14-16] resulting in cellular ischemia and impairment of adenosine triphosphate (ATP) production by the tricarboxylic acid cycle and oxidative phosphorylation. When ATP depletion reaches a critical level,[17] membrane integrity and organelle function are impaired, resulting in the influx of extracellular sodium, calcium, and fluid, and the activation of autocatalytic proteases. Similar impairment of oxygen delivery and cellular metabolism also occur during other low-flow states such as cardiogenic shock. In some tissues, such as skeletal muscle, tissue pO_2 decreases even before arterial hypotension occurs.[18]

The degree of cellular injury that results from this generalized ischemia is tissue dependent. Skin and muscle are more tolerant of impaired perfusion compared to the heart, brain, and visceral organs.[17,19] This variability is in part due to a higher metabolic rate in these susceptible organs, to the density of capillary perfusion within individual organs, and to the reserve energy stores in striated muscle (creatine phosphate). Certain organs, particularly the splanchnic bed, have been shown to have persistent hypoperfusion even after "adequate" resuscitation to normal central hemodynamics[20-23] and the return of skin and muscle perfusion to normal levels. Additionally, once tissue is injured, it may continue to be inadequately perfused following resuscitation even when adjacent noninjured tissue is well perfused.[24]

Organs vary in the relative degree to which they are controlled by intrinsic (autoregulation) vs. extrinsic factors. For instance, the conductance of the cerebral vasculature increases with progressive hypotension, indicating a progressive loss of vascular tone and suggesting that the primary control mechanism is intrinsic, serving to preserve cerebral blood flow.[25] Similarly, the myocardial microcirculation is regulated to a significant extent by locally secreted mediators. During progressive hemorrhage, myocardial vascular conductance increases to a greater extent than observed with local hypotension.[26] This suggests that a metabolically linked loss of vascular tone, secondary to compensatory tachycardia from baroreceptor stimulation, is the cause of this effect.[26]

Conversely, the mesenteric microcirculation is strongly influenced by extrinisic controls such as sympathetic neural tone, and autoregulation appears to be less pronounced than in the cerebral or renal circulations. Due to extensive innervation with sympathetic neural fibers, hemorrhagic hypotension causes baroreceptor-mediated intestinal vasoconstriction and a decrease in conductance to 50% at 40 mmHg.[25,27,28] Intravital microscopy of the small intestinal microcirculation during hemorrhagic hypotension demonstrates vasoconstriction of inflow (first-order) and premucosal (third-order) arterioles, but compensatory dilation of seromuscular arterioles (fourth-order).[20,29,30] Although intestinal arteriolar vasoconstriction can be prevented during hemorrhage and resuscitation with α-adrenergic receptor blockade, impaired microvascular blood flow is not reversed (unpublished data). Myers and others have provided convincing evidence that local production of vasodilator prostanoids is an important compensatory mechanism to microvascular vasoconstriction during hemorrhage.[30-32]

In addition to alterations of vascular tone during shock, two anatomical characteristics of the intestinal microcirculation may also contribute to its susceptibility to mucosal ischemia. First, the nutrient arterioles of the mucosa arise as right angle branches that enhance "plasma skimming."[33] This phenomenon results in a decreased hematocrit, and thus a decrease in oxygen-carrying capacity, in villous capillaries compared to the systemic circulation. Second, the arrangement of mucosal villous microvessels results in a countercurrent exchange of oxygen.[34] This countercurrent diffusion of oxygen from the central villous arteriole to villous capillaries and venules seems to decrease the pO_2 at the terminus of the central arteriole.[35,36] Because the transit time of villous blood is increased during low-flow states, countercurrent oxygen diffusion may be more pronounced and further exacerbate mucosal ischemia.[37]

Renal blood flow is regulated both by intrinsic and extrinsic controls. The renal microcirculation exhibits excellent autoregulation during hemorrhage, with an increase in vascular conductance to a perfusion pressure of about 60 to 70 mmHg. Below this pressure, renovascular conductance decreases to a greater extent than observed in other regional beds, suggesting that the vasculature is strongly influenced by extrinsic control mechanisms.[38,39] Hemorrhage reduces the total amount of blood flow to the kidneys,[40-42] but there is also redistribution of intrarenal blood flow, with the outer cortical areas sustaining the most marked reduction in flow.[43,44] In fact, in some models, outer medullary flow is preserved while cortical flow is markedly decreased.[45] Sympathetic neural stimulation and angiotensin II are probably both key mediators of hemorrhage-induced redistribution of intrarenal blood flow. Renal nerve stimulation without hypotension causes a decrease in outer cortical perfusion,[46] and increased sympathetic tone induced by carotid sinus ablation also redistributes blood away from the outer cortex.[47] Some studies have demonstrated complete reversal of outer cortical hypoperfusion with administration of α-adrenergic receptor antagonists,[48] although other studies report incomplete reversal unless angiotensin antagonists are also used.[49,50] Still other reports indicate that angiotensin II antagonists, but not α-adrenergic blockers, ameliorate decreased cortical blood flow.[45] Inhibition of renal prostaglandin synthesis during hemorrhage worsens arteriolar constriction and blood flow, indicating that prostaglandins are an important compensatory mechanism.[51]

In the liver, hemorrhagic shock induces impairment of microvascular and nutrient blood flow that persists despite resuscitation.[52-54] Both hemorrhagic hypotension and regional ischemia-reperfusion result in progressive loss of perfused sinusoids with vascular plugging.[55,56] Furthermore, the adhesion of leukocytes to the endothelium is increased following resuscitation from hemorrhage and is largely independent of sinusoidal diameter.[57] In contrast to skeletal muscle,[58] leukocytes are not simply trapped in occluded capillaries of the liver.[57] Kupffer cell swelling and focal ischemic changes are observed and thought to be mediated by both reactive oxygen intermediates and neutrophils.[59]

The microvascular response of striated muscle to hemorrhage is heterogenous and is characterized by large vessel (A1) constriction and small vessel (A4) dilation. During decompensation, there is further dilation of A4 arterioles, loss of vasomotion, and attenuation of venular constriction, implying a loss of vascular smooth muscle tone.[60,61] This loss of vascular tone in precapillary vessels is the probable explanation for the decrease in skeletal muscle microvascular resistance that is observed in the later phases of hemorrhage. There is also a differential reactivity of arterioles to norepinephrine during hemorrhage.[62] Large arterioles do not constrict further, probably due to maximal adrenergic stimulation mediated by increased sympathetic neural tone. Small arterioles constrict toward baseline and have return of vasomotion, suggesting that loss of skeletal muscle vascular tone during compensated shock is due to a selective impairment of adrenergic nerve transmission to small arterioles.[62] Tissue acidosis impairs the constrictor responses of large arterioles and venules during hemorrhage without altering the small arteriolar vasodilatory response.[63]

Many mediators may contribute to microvascular alterations during hemorrhage. Activation of the sympathetic nervous system, circulating catecholamines, local and systemic production of angiotensin, formation of reactive oxygen intermediates during resuscitation, inhibition of dilator prostanoid synthesis,[64] and activation of leukocytes[65] contribute to microvascular constriction, hypoperfusion, and endothelial injury. Leukotrienes,[66] thromboxanes,[67] and some cytokines[68,69] may also alter regional blood flow, but their specific roles in hemorrhage continue to be studied.

III. MICROCIRCULATORY ALTERATIONS OF SEPSIS

The central hemodynamic responses to severe infection or to systemic activation of inflammatory processes vary depending upon the severity of the insult and the adequacy of intravascular volume replacement, and may result in either a hyper- or hypodynamic condition. The hyperdynamic response to sepsis is characterized by increased cardiac output, peripheral vasodilation with warm, dry skin, increased oxygen consumption, and a decreased systemic vascular resistance. Hypodynamic septic shock is frequently manifested by hypotension, inadequate cardiac output, peripheral constriction, a decreased oxygen consumption, and variable changes in systemic vascular resistance.

Impaired cardiac function is prominent during the hypodynamic phase, but may also occur during the hyperdynamic phase. However, a central component of both of these phases of septic shock is maldistribution of blood flow among organs that appears to be mediated by the microcirculation. Much of the decrease in peripheral resistance that is observed during the hyperdynamic phase is due to vasodilation of skin and skeletal muscle.[70] The microvascular responses of striated muscle to hyper- and hypodynamic phases of experimental bacteremia are similar and are characterized by mild constriction of large arterioles and marked dilation of small arterioles.[71,72] The constriction of A1 arterioles is less pronounced than that observed during hemorrhage,[73] but is thought to be similarly mediated by sympathetic neural stimulation or circulating catecholamines. Small vessel dilation is due to vasodilator prostaglandins and to endothelial-derived relaxing factors such as nitric oxide,[74,75] and is thought to account for the overall decrease in skeletal muscle vascular resistance that is observed during sepsis. Large arteriolar constriction and small arteriolar dilation also occur during other sepsis models, including hyper- and hypodynamic endotoxemia[76] and systemic complement activation.[74] It appears that the dilation of small arterioles in muscle contributes to the redistribution of cardiac output, which decreases flow to visceral organs and increases flow to skeletal muscle during sepsis. The marked small arteriolar vasodilation and resulting increase in muscle vascular conductance are believed to be a primary cause of the decreased systemic vascular resistance that is observed during hyperdynamic human sepsis.

Blood flow alterations in the visceral circulation are less well characterized than those in striated muscle. In some infection models, total blood flow to the liver is increased during the earlier stages of sepsis[77] and is associated with an increase in microvascular blood flow.[78] Later in sepsis, decreased microvascular flow is observed.[79] Despite increases in cardiac output and microvascular blood flow as assessed by laser Doppler flowmetry and carbon-perfusion, hepatocellular function is impaired.[78] This cellular dysfunction has been postulated to not be the result of altered microvascular blood flow, but to be due to other events such as hepatic cytokine secretion. More sensitive measurement of hepatic microvessels using intravital microscopy demonstrates differential responses with some vessels that constrict and others that dilate.[80] Thus, total hepatic microvascular blood flow may be increased, but focal areas may be hypoperfused even during the early, hyperdynamic phase of shock. This postulate is supported by the well-described observation that sepsis-induced hepatic dysfunction is often characterized by focal ischemic changes with adjacent areas that appear normal.

Systemic or intraportal administration of endotoxin results in several hepatic microcirculatory disturbances as assessed by intravital microscopy. Leukocytes and platelets mechanically obstruct some microvessels, and Kupffer cell swelling results in increased tortuosity of vessels.[81-83] Further, endotoxin results in increased adhesion of leukocytes to the hepatic microvascular endothelium.[84] Leukocytes appear to adhere preferentially in periportal areas, particularly with lower doses of endotoxin; and at higher doses, there is also margination in midzonal and pericentral regions.[84] These observations are consistent with the concept that LPS-stimulated Kupffer cells secrete inflammatory mediators that regulate leukocyte adhesion to the endothelium.

Experimental hyperdynamic bacteremia[85] and systemic complement activation[86] both cause small intestinal microvascular hypoperfusion with constriction of inflow and premucosal arterioles. This microvascular hypoperfusion is associated with decreased mucosal blood flow as measured by laser Doppler flowmetry in spite of superior mesenteric artery blood flow being maintained.[87] The mechanisms that mediate splanchnic constriction are not completely defined. Treatment with leukotriene C4 and D4 receptor antagonists improves intestinal perfusion during endotoxemia,[88] and inhibition of endothelins reverses arteriolar constriction during bacteremia.[89] Administration of tumor necrosis factor elicits segmental intestinal ischemia with necrosis and hemorrhage,[90] but the relevance of this observation is uncertain because of the large doses required to cause these effects. Other cytokines, lipid mediators such as platelet activating factor, and eicosanoids are also probably involved, but their specific roles are not well defined. It is likely that adrenergic receptor stimulation due to sympathetic neural activation and to circulating catecholamines is also important in constriction of large intestinal arterioles that are densely innervated.

Sepsis is frequently associated with severe renal vasoconstriction despite normal or hyperdynamic central hemodynamics. Intravital microscopy demonstrates that hyperdynamic bacteremia induces preglomerular constriction of afferent and intralobular arterioles that is associated with microvascular hypoperfusion.[91,92] Interestingly, efferent arteriolar diameters are not affected in this sepsis model.[91,92] Several vasoconstrictors have been implicated in the genesis of renal vasoconstriction during experimental sepsis and include endothelins, thromboxanes, leukotrienes, and noncyclooxygenase-derived prostaglandins (e.g., PGF_2). Systemic endotoxemia results in impaired glomerular filtration that is restored by local arterial infusion of endothelin antiserum,[93] and specific endothelin receptor antagonists blunt renal vasoconstriction during bacteremia (unpublished data). Selective antagonism of thromboxane A_2 contributes to preservation of renal blood flow during nonhypotensive endotoxemia,[94] and TXA_2 may also be responsible for nonenzymatic generation of certain constrictor prostanoids that are PGF2-like compounds.[95] Leukotriene inhibition with nonspecific[94] or LTD_4-selective[96] antagonists improves renal blood flow during endotoxemia, but does so only during the later phases of sepsis. This implies that renal constriction may be temporally regulated by different mediators.

A prominent feature of sepsis is the impairment of vascular responsiveness to vasopressors including catecholamines, bradykinin, and angiotensin II. Clinically, this is observed as progressive vasodilation and hypotension despite increasing doses of pressors. This phenomenon is well described in experimental models of endotoxemia[97-99] and chronic polymicrobial sepsis.[100] Nitric oxide is produced from L-arginine by a family of enzymes termed "nitric oxide synthases," one of which is constitutively expressed in endothelial cells. Other isoforms are expressed following induction in many cell types including vascular smooth muscle and parenchymal cells of visceral organs. Recent studies with isolated rings of muscular arteries demonstrate that nitric oxide elaboration is a central effector of impaired vascular responsiveness,[97,98] although arachidonic acid metabolites may also be involved.[99] Whether nitric oxide or eicosanoids mediate similar responses in microvessels has not been determined. With regard to the microcirculation, nitric oxide also appears to contribute to regulation of regional blood flow and leukocyte-endothelial cell interactions.[101] Maldistribution of microvascular blood flow due to altered secretion of vasoactive compounds is central to the sepsis syndrome. However, other mechanisms such as microvascular plugging, interstitial edema with endothelial cell swelling, and possibly arteriovenous shunting in some organs also contribute to blood flow maldistribution. Other microvascular sequelae of sepsis include increased permeability and enhanced leukocyte-endothelial cell adhesion.[102-104] This adhesion process requires activation of both neutrophils and endothelial cells with enhanced cell surface expression of adhesion molecules. Excessive and inappropriate activation of leukocytes, particularly neutrophils, is thought to be a primary mechanism of organ dysfunction during sepsis.[105-107]

Table 2 Therapeutic Approaches to Increase Oxygen Delivery

1. Optimization of circulating blood volume
2. Selected treatment of brady or tachyarrhythmias
3. Increasing hemoglobin (10–12 g/dl)
4. Maintenance of adequate arterial oxygen saturation
5. Increasing cardiac contractility with β-agonists
6. Reducing afterload with vasodilators
7. Increasing mean arterial pressure with vasoconstrictors to improve tissue perfusion

IV. POTENTIAL THERAPIES

Central to the prevention and treatment of MOD from a microcirculation focus are therapies that minimize cellular injury by restoring tissue perfusion or controlling the host's systemic inflammatory response to the initial stimulus. Maintenance of optimal tissue perfusion is important to minimize ischemia-induced cellular injury and to decrease ischemia that results from the stress and inflammatory responses.[107,108] A critical concept to the prevention of MOD is the realization that an inadequate oxygen supply to tissues relative to cellular consumption results in an "oxygen debt" that impairs cellular function. Several studies demonstrate that an oxygen debt frequently exists after episodes of shock or critical illnesses in spite of clinical evidences of adequate central hemodynamic resuscitation.[22,109,110] Early optimization of oxygen delivery at the time of resuscitation is more effective in the prevention of cellular injury than after the microvascular events of MOD become clinically evident.

In general, clinical variables such as vital signs are not accurate indicators of the extent of oxygen delivery impairment due to compensatory central hemodynamic mechanisms. For this reason, patients with a significant risk of oxygen debt or MOD, such as the elderly, those with preexisting or acute cardiac or pulmonary dysfunction, or those with major traumatic injuries, should be monitored invasively with a pulmonary artery catheter. This permits an assessment of the adequacy of volume loading, a rapid measurement of cardiac function, and most importantly, determination of oxygen delivery and consumption. An aggressive treatment regimen that maintains a hyperdynamic state and an increased oxygen delivery to peripheral organs has been shown to decrease the incidence of primary MOD.[111-113] In spite of apparently adequate whole-body perfusion, certain visceral organs, particularly in the splanchnic circulation, may have persistent hypoperfusion.[20] Clinical indicators, including whole-body oxygen consumption, do not accurately reflect splanchnic perfusion,[114] and techniques such as gastric or colonic tonometry have been recommended in selected patients.[114,115] Standard therapies for the restoration and maintenance of oxygen delivery to vital organs are summarized in Table 2.

The second proposed therapeutic approach to MOD is the control of the systemic inflammatory response to the initial stimulus (e.g., hemorrhage, traumatic injury, infection, cardiac failure, etc.). Nonspecific therapies include adequate volume resuscitation, minimization of additional tissue trauma, debridement of nonviable tissue such as burn eschar, early fracture fixation, drainage of purulent collections, and appropriate systemic antimicrobials. Some of these have been demonstrated to decrease the occurrence of secondary MOD.[116] Attenuation of additional stress hormone release, particularly catecholamines,[117-119] may be effected by control of hypothermia or pyrexia, paralysis to stop shivering, and adequate control of pain and anxiety.[120,121]

Several additional systemic therapies that are directed toward specific mediators or enzyme systems involved in the inflammatory response have been studied in experimental models of hemorrhagic and septic shock, and in some human trials. These treatments

Table 3 Experimental Approaches to
Therapy of Shock

Cytokine Inhibition/Neutralization
    Anti-endotoxin antibodies
    Anti-TNF-α antibodies
    Recombinant soluble TNF receptor
    Interleukin 1 receptor antagonist
Antiinflammatory Agents
    Nonsteroidal antiinflammatory agents
    Leukotriene receptor antagonists
    Platelet activating factor antagonists
    Thromboxane synthesis antagonists
    Corticosteroids
    Aminosteroids (lazaroids)
Exogenous Antioxidants
    Xanthine oxidase inhibitors
    NADPH oxidase inhibitors
    Catalase
    Superoxide dismutase
    Iron chelators
    Free radical scavengers
Antineutrophil Agents
    CD11/CD18 monoclonal antibodies
Other
    ATP-MgCl$_2$
    Pentoxifylline
    Nitric oxide synthase agonists/antagonists

are summarized in Table 3; but for most of them, specific effects on the microcirculation have not been well characterized.

REFERENCES

1. **Tilney, N., Batley, G., and Morgan, A.,** Sequential system failure after rupture of abdominal aortic aneurysms: An unsolved problem in post-operative care, *Ann. Surg.*, 178, 117, 1973.
2. **Barton, R. and Cerra, F.,** The hypermetabolism multiple organ failure syndrome, *Chest*, 96, 1153, 1989.
3. **Crump, J., Duncan D., and Wears, R.,** Analysis of multiple organ system failure in trauma and non-trauma patients, *Ann. Surg.*, 54, 702, 1988.
4. **Pinsky, M. and Matuschak, G.,** A unifying hypothesis of multiple systems organ failure: Failure of host defense homeostasis, *J. Crit. Care*, 5, 108, 1990.
5. **Norton, L.,** Does drainage of intra-abdominal pus reverse multiple organ failure?, *Am. J. Surg.*, 199, 347, 1985.
6. **Fry, D., Pearlstein, L., Fulton, R., and Polk, H. C., Jr.,** Multiple system organ failure. The role of uncontrolled infection, *Arch. Surg.*, 115, 136, 1980.
7. **Carrico, C. J., Meakins, J. L., Marshall, J. C., Fry, D., and Maier R.,** Multiple-organ-failure syndrome, *Arch. Surg.*, 121, 196, 1986.
8. **Maship, L., McMillen, R., and Brown, J.,** The influence of sepsis and multi-system organ failure on mortality in the surgical intensive care unit, *Ann. Surg.*, 50, 94, 1984.
9. **DeCamp, M. and Demling, R.,** Post-traumatic multi-system organ failure, *JAMA*, 260, 530, 1988.
10. **Goris, R., Boekhorst T., Nuytinck, J., and Gimbrère, J.,** Multiple organ failure: Generalized autodestructive inflammation?, *Arch. Surg.*, 120, 1109, 1985.
11. **Demling, R., LaLonde, C., Saldinger, P., and Knox, J.,** Multiple-organ dysfunction in the surgical patient: Pathophysiology, prevention, treatment, *Curr. Prob. Surg.*, 30, 345, 1993.

12. **Goris, R. J. A.,** Shock, sepsis, and multiple organ failure: The result of whole body inflammation, in *Pathophysiology of Shock, Sepsis, and Organ Failure*, Schlag, G., and Redl, H., Eds., Springer-Verlag, Berlin, 1993.

13. **Garrison, R. N. and Cryer, H. M.,** Role of the microcirculation to skeletal muscle during shock, in *Perspectives in Shock Research: Metabolism, Immunology, Mediators and Models*, Passmore, J. C., Reichard, S. M., Reynolds, D. G., and Traber, D. L., Eds., Liss, New York, 1989.

14. **Mohsenifar, S., Amin, D., Jasper, A. C., Shah, P. K., and Koerner, S. K.,** Dependence of oxygen consumption on oxygen delivery in patients with chronic congestive heart failure, *Chest*, 92, 447, 1987.

15. **Chappell, T. R., Rubin, L. J., Markham, R. V., and Firth, B. G.,** Independence of oxygen consumption and systemic oxygen transport in patients with either stable pulmonary hypertension or refractory left ventricular failure, *Am. Rev. Respir. Dis.*, 128, 30, 1983.

16. **Rackow, E.,** Cellular oxygen metabolism during sepsis and shock: Relationship of oxygen consumption to oxygen delivery, *JAMA*, 259, 1989, 1988.

17. **Wang, P., Hauptman, J., and Chaudry, I.,** Hepatocellular dysfunction occurs early after hemorrhage and persists despite fluid resuscitation, *J. Surg. Res.*, 48, 464, 1990.

18. **Van der Kleij, A. J., de Koning, J., Beerthuizen, G., Goris, R. J. A., Kreuzer, F., and Kimmich, H. P.,** Early detection of hemorrhagic hypovolemia by muscle oxygen pressure assessment: Preliminary report, *Surgery*, 93, 518, 1983.

19. **Blum, H., Schnall, M., Renshaw, P., and Buzby, G. P.,** Metabolic and ionic changes in muscle during hemorrhagic shock, *Circ. Shock*, 26, 341, 1988.

20. **Flynn, W. J., Cryer, H. G., and Garrison, R. N.,** Pentoxifylline restores intestinal microvascular blood flow during resuscitated hemorrhagic shock, *Surgery*, 110, 350, 1991.

21. **Scalia, S., Burton, H., Van Wylen, D., Steinberg, S., Hoffman, A., Roche, F., and Flint, L.,** Persistent arteriolar constriction in microcirculation of the terminal ileum following moderate hemorrhagic hypovolemia and volume restoration, *J. Trauma*, 30, 713, 1990.

22. **Townsend, M., Schirmer, W., Schirmer, J., and Fry, D.,** Low dose dopamine improves effective hepatic blood flow in murine peritonitis, *Circ. Shock*, 21, 149, 1987.

23. **Deitch, E.,** Intestinal permeability is increased in burn patients shortly after injury, *Surgery*, 107, 411, 1990.

24. **Ozawa, K., Aoyama, H., Yasuda, K., Shimahara, Y., Nakatani, T., Tanaka, J., Yamamoto, M., Kamiyama, Y., and Tobe, T.,** Metabolic abnormalities associated with post-operative organ failure, *Arch. Surg.*, 118, 1245, 1983.

25. **Green, H. D., Bond, R. F., Rapela, C. E., Schmid, H. E., Manley, E., and Farrar, D. J.,** Competition between intrinsic and extrinsic controls of resistance vessels of major vascular beds during hemorrhagic hypotension and shock, *Adv. Shock Res.*, 3, 77, 1985.

26. **Adiseshiak, M. and Baird, J. R.,** Correlation of the changes in diastolic tissue pressure and regional coronary blood flow in hemorrhagic and endotoxin shock, *J. Surg. Res.*, 24, 20, 1978.

27. **Bohlen, H. G, Hutchins, P. M., Rapela, C. E., and Green, H.,** Microvascular control in the intestinal mucosa of normal and hemorrhaged rats, *Am. J. Physiol.*, 299, 1159, 1975.

28. **Bond, R. F., Bond, C. H., and Johnson, G., III,** Intrinsic versus extrinsic regional vascular control during hemorrhagic hypotension and shock, *Circ. Shock*, 18, 115, 1986.

29. **Flynn, W. J., Gosche, J. R., and Garrison, R. N.,** Intestinal blood flow is restored with glutamine or glucose suffusion after hemorrhage, *J. Surg. Res.*, 52, 499, 1992.

30. **Gosche, J. R. and Garrison, R. N.,** Prostaglandins mediate the compensatory responses to hemorrhage in the small intestine of the rat, *J. Surg. Res.*, 50, 584, 1991.

31. **Myers, S., Parks, L., Smith, G., and Miller, T.,** Elevated PGI$_2$ and PGE$_2$ in the rat ileum following mild hypotension, *J. Trauma*, 28, 1202, 1988.

32. **Myers, S. I., Taylor, B. J., and Stanislawska, M.,** Reperfusion inhibits elevated splanchnic prostanoid production following hemorrhagic shock, *Ann. Surg.*, 212, 688, 1991.

33. **Jodal, M. and Lundgren, O.,** Plasma skimming in the intestinal tract, *Acta Physiol Scand*, 80, 50, 1970.

34. **Jacobson, L. F. and Noer, R. F.,** The vascular pattern of the intestinal villi in various laboratory animals and man, *Anat. Rec.*, 114, 85, 1952.

35. **Lundgren, O.,** Studies on blood flow distribution and countercurrent exchange in the small intestine, *Acta Physiol. Scand.*, 303, 1, 1967.

36. **Kampp, M., Lundgren, O., and Nilsson, N. J.,** Extravascular shunting of oxygen in the small intestine of the cat, *Acta Physiol. Scand.*, 72, 396, 1968.

70

37. **Lundgren, O. and Svanvik, J.,** Mucosal hemodynamics in the small intestine of the cat during reduced perfusion pressure, *Acta Physiol. Scand.*, 88, 551, 1973.
38. **Navar, L. G., Marsh, D. J., Blantz, R. C., Hall, J., Ploth, D. E., and Nasjlett, A.,** Intrinsic control of renal hemodynamics, *Fed. Proc.*, 41, 3022, 1982.
39. **Fleming, J. T., Zhang, C., Chen, J., and Porter, J. P.,** Selective preglomerular constriction to nerve stimulation in rat hydronephrotic kidneys, *Am. J. Physiol.*, 262, F348, 1992.
40. **Neiberger, R. E., Levin, J. I., and Passmore, J. C.,** Renal effects of dopamine during prolonged hemorrhagic hypotension in the dog, *Circ. Shock*, 7, 129, 1980.
41. **Passmore, J. C., Leffler, C. W., and Neiberger, R. E.,** A critical analysis of renal blood flow distribution during hemorrhage in dogs, *Circ. Shock*, 5, 327, 1978.
42. **Stein, J. H., Boonjarern, S., Mauk, R. C., and Ferris, T. F.,** Mechanism of the redistribution of renal cortical blood flow during hemorrhage in the dog, *J. Clin. Invest.*, 52, 39, 1973.
43. **Passmore, J. C. and Baker, C. H.,** Intrarenal blood flow distribution in irreversible hemorrhagic shock in dogs, *J. Trauma*, 13, 1066, 1973.
44. **Carriere, S., Thorburn, G. D., O'Morchoe, C. C. C., and Barger, A. C.,** Intrarenal distribution of blood flow in dogs during hemorrhagic hypotension, *Circ. Res.*, 19, 167, 1966.
45. **Hock, C. E., Passmore, J. C., Levin, J. I., and Neiberger, R. E.,** Angiotensin II and alpha adrenergic control of the intrarenal circulation in hemorrhage, *Circ. Shock*, 9, 81, 1982.
46. **Pomeranz, B. H., Birtch, A. G., and Barger, A. C.,** Neural control of intrarenal blood flow, *Am. J. Physiol.*, 215, 1067, 1968.
47. **Kolozsi, W. Z. and Passmore, J. C.,** Renal krypton-85 washout in sinoaortic denervated dogs, *J. Surg. Res.*, 22, 37, 1977.
48. **Grandchamp, A., Ayer, G., and Truniger, B.,** Pathogenesis of redistribution of intrarenal blood flow in hemorrhagic hypotension, *Eur. J. Clin. Invest.*, 1, 271, 1971.
49. **Carriere, S. and Daigneault, B.,** Effect of retransfusion after hemorrhagic hypotension on intrarenal distribution of blood flow in dogs, *J. Clin. Invest.*, 49, 2205, 1970.
50. **LaChance, J. G., Arnoux, E., Brunette, M. G., and Carriere, S.,** Factors responsible for the outer cortical ischemia observed during hemorrhagic hypotension in dogs, *Circ. Shock*, 1, 131, 1974.
51. **Leffler, C. W. and Passmore, J. C.,** Effects of indomethacin on hemodynamics of dogs in refractory hemorrhagic shock, *J. Surg. Res.*, 23, 393, 1977.
52. **Wang, P., Hauptman, J. G., and Chaudry, I. H.,** Hemorrhage produces depression in microvascular blood flow which persists despite fluid resuscitation, *Circ. Shock*, 32, 307, 1990.
53. **Wang, P., Zheng, F., Dean, R. E., and Chaudry, I. H.,** ATP-MgCl$_2$ restores the depressed hepatocellular function and hepatic blood flow following hemorrhage and resuscitation, *J. Surg. Res.*, 50, 368, 1991.
54. **Flynn, W. J., Cryer, H. G., and Garrison, R. N.,** Pentoxifylline but not saralasin restores hepatic blood flow after resuscitation from hemorrhagic shock, *J. Surg. Res.*, 50, 584, 1991.
55. **Clemens, M. G., McDonagh, P. F., Chaudry, I. H., and Baue, A. E.,** Hepatic microcirculatory failure after ischemia and reperfusion: Improvement with ATP-MgCl$_2$ treatment, *Am. J. Physiol.*, 248, H804, 1985.
56. **Marzi, I., Bauer, C., Hower, R., and Buhren, V.,** Leukocyte-endothelial cell interactions in the liver after hemorrhagic shock in the rat, *Circ. Shock*, 40, 105, 1993.
57. **Bauer, M., Marzi, I., Ziegenfub, T., Seeck, G., and Larsen, R.,** Impact of isotonic and hypertonic resuscitation on hepatic leukocyte adhesion after hemorrhagic hypotension, in *Cells of the Hepatic Sinusoid*, Vol. 4, Wisse, E. and Knook, D. L., Eds., The Kupffer Cell Foundation, Rijswijk, The Netherlands, 1993.
58. **Bagge, U., Amundson, B., and Lauritzen, C.,** White blood cell deformability and plugging of skeletal muscle capillaries in hemorrhagic shock, *Acta Physiol. Scand.*, 180, 159, 1980.
59. **Marotto, M. E., Thurman, R. G., and Lemasters, J. J.,** Early midzonal cell death during low-flow hypoxia in the isolated-perfused rat liver: Protection by allopurinol, *Hepatology*, 8, 585, 1988.
60. **Mellander, S. and Lewis, D. H.,** Effect of hemorrhagic shock on the reactivity of resistance and capacitance vessels and on capillary filtration transfer in cat skeletal muscle, *Circ. Res.*, 13, 105, 1963.
61. **Bond, R. F., Manley, E. S., and Green, H. D.,** Cutaneous and skeletal muscle vascular responses to hemorrhage and irreversible shock, *Am. J. Physiol.*, 212, 488, 1967.

62. Flint, L. M., Cryer, H. M., Simpson, C. J., and Harris, P. D., Microcirculatory norepinephrine constrictor response in hemorrhagic shock, *Surgery*, 96, 240, 1984.

63. Cryer, H. M., Kaebnick, H. W., Harris, P. D., and Flint, L. M., Effects of tissue acidosis on skeletal muscle microcirculatory responses to hemorrhagic shock in unanesthetized rats, *J. Surg. Res.*, 39, 59, 1985.

64. Myers, S. I. and Hernandez, R., Role of oxygen radicals on rat splanchnic eicosanoid production during hemorrhagic shock, *Prostglandins*, 44, 25, 1992.

65. Suzuki, M., Inauen, W., Kvietys, P. R., Grisham, M. B., Meininger, C., Schelling, M. E., Granger, H. J., and Granger, D. N., Superoxide mediates reperfusion-induced leukocyte-endothelial cell interactions, *Am. J. Physiol.*, 257, H1740, 1989.

66. Lehr, H. A., Guhlman, A., Nolte, D., Keppler, D., and Messmer, K., Leukotrienes as mediators in ischemia-reperfusion injury in a microcirculation model in the hamster, *J. Clin. Invest.*, 87, 2036, 1991.

67. Ogletree, M. L., Overview of physiological and pathophysiological effects of thromboxane A_2, *Fed. Proc.*, 46, 133, 1987.

68. Beutler, B. and Cerami, A., Cachectin: More than a tumor necrosis factor, *N. Engl. J. Med.*, 316, 379, 1987.

69. Okusawa, S., Gelfand, J. A., Ikejima, T., et al., Interleukin 1 induces a shock-like state in rabbits: Syndergism with tumor necrosis factor and the effect of cyclooxygenase inhibition, *J. Clin. Invest.*, 81, 1162, 1988.

70. Bond, R. F., Peripheral vascular adrenergic depression during hypotension induced by *E. coli* endotoxin, *Adv. Shock Res.*, 9, 157, 1983.

71. Cryer, H. M., Garrison, R. N., Harris, P. D., and Anderson, G. L., Microvascular responses during hyperdynamic and hypodynamic phases of bacteremia in decerebrate rats, *Circ. Shock*, 18, 369, 1986.

72. Cryer, H. M., Garrison, R. N., Kaebnick, H. W., Harris, P. D., and Flint, L. M., Skeletal microcirculatory responses in hyperdynamic *E. coli* sepsis in unanesthetized rats, *Arch. Surg.*, 122, 86, 1987.

73. Cryer, H. M., Garrison, R. N., Harris, P. D., Anderson, G. L., and Flint, L. M., Similarity in microvascular responses between hemorrhagic and bacteremic shock in decerebrate rats, *Congr. Intl. Union of Physiological Sci.*, July 13–18, 1986. Vancouver, Canada.

74. Luebbe, A. S., Garrison, R. N., and Harris, P. D., Endothelium-dependent microvascular responses to activated complement, *J. Surg. Res.*, 57, 654, 1994.

75. Cryer, H. M., Garrison, R. N., Harris, P. D., Greenwald, B. H., and Alsip, N. L., Prostaglandins mediate skeletal muscle arteriole dilation in hyperdynamic bacteremia, *Am. J. Physiol.*, 259, H728, 1990.

76. Cryer, H. M., Garrison, R. N., Harris, P. D., and Polk, H. C., Role of the muscle microvasculature during hyperdynamic and hypodynamic phases of endotoxin shock in decerebrate rats, *J. Trauma*, 28, 312, 1988.

77. Wang, P., Ba, Z. F., Ayala, A., and Chaudry, I. H., Hepatic extraction of indocyanine green is depressed during early sepsis despite increased hepatic blood flow and cardiac output, *Arch. Surg.*, 126, 219, 1991.

78. Wang, P., Ba, Z. F., Tait, S. M., Zhou, M., and Chaudry, I. H., Alterations in circulating blood volume during polymicrobial sepsis, *Circ. Shock*, 40, 92, 1993.

79. Wang, P., Zhou, M., Rana, M. W., Ba, Z. F., and Chaudry, I. H., Differential alterations in microvascular perfusion in various organs during early and late sepsis, *Am. J. Physiol.*, 263, G38, 1992.

80. Unger, L. S., Cryer, H. M., and Garrison, R. N., A differential response of the centrilobular microvessels in the liver during bacteremia, *Circ. Shock*, 29, 335, 1989.

81. McCuskey, R. S., Urbaschek, R., McCuskey, P. A., and Urbaschek, B., *In vivo* microscopic studies of the responses of the liver to endotoxin, *Klin. Wochenschr.*, 60, 749, 1982.

82. McCuskey, R. S., Urbaschek, R., McCuskey, P. A., and Urbaschek, B., *In vivo* microscopic observations of the response of Kupffer cells and the hepatic microcirculation to Mycobacterium bovis BCG alone and in combination with endotoxin, *Infec. Immunol.*, 42, 362, 1983.

83. Unger, L. S. and Reilly, F. D., Hepatic miccrovascular regulatory mechanisms. VII. Effects of endportally infused endotoxin on microcirculation and mast cells in rats, *Microcirc. Endothelium Lymphatics*, 3, 47, 1986.

72

84. **Ferguson, D., McDonagh, P. F., Biewer, J., Paidas, C. N., and Clemens, M. G.,** Spatial relationship between leukocyte accumulation and microvascular injury during reperfusion following hepatic ischemia, *Int. J. Microcirc. Clin. Exp.*, 12, 45, 1993.

85. **Whitworth, P. W., Cryer, H. M., Garrison, R. N., Baumgarten, T. E., and Harris, P. D.,** Hypoperfusion of the intestinal microcirculation without decreased cardiac output during live *Escherichia coli* sepsis in rats, *Circ. Shock*, 27, 111, 1989.

86. **Scalia, S., Sharma, P., Rodriguez, J., Roche, F., Luchette, F., Chambers, R., Flint, L. M., and Steinberg, S.,** Decreased mesenteric blood flow (MBF) in experimental multiple organ failure (MOF), *J. Surg. Res.*, 52, 1, 1992.

87. **Theuer, C. J., Wilson, M. A., Steeb, G. D., and Garrison, R. N.,** Microvascular vasoconstriction and mucosal hypoperfusion of the rat small intestine during bacteremia, *Circ. Shock*, 40, 61, 1993.

88. **Cohn, S. M., Kruithoff, K. L., Rothschild, H. R., Wang, H., Antonsson, J. B., and Fink, M. P.,** Beneficial effects of LY203647, a novel leukotriene C_4/D_4 antagonist, on pulmonary function and mesenteric perfusion in a porcine model of endotoxic shock and ARDS, *Circ. Shock*, 33, 7, 1991.

89. **Wilson, M. A., Steeb, G. D., and Garrison, R. N.,** Endothelins mediate intestinal hypoperfusion during bacteremia, *J. Surg. Res.*, 55, 168, 1993.

90. **Tracey, K. J., Beutler, B., Lowry, S. F., et al.,** Shock and tissue injury induced by recombinant human cachectin, *Science*, 234, 470, 1986.

91. **Cryer, H. M., Unger, L. S., Garrison, R. N., and Harris, P. D.,** Prostaglandins maintain renal microvascular blood flow during hyperdynamic bacteremia, *Circ. Shock*, 26, 71, 1988.

92. **Cryer, H. G., Bloom, I. T. M., Unger, L. S., and Garrison, R. N.,** Factors affecting renal microvascular blood flow in rat hyperdynamic bacteremia, *Am. J. Physiol.*, 264, H1988, 1993.

93. **Kon, V. and Badr, K. F.,** Biologic actions and pathophysiologic significance of endothelin in the kidney, editorial review, *Kidney Int.*, 40, 1, 1991.

94. **Badr, K. F., Kelley, V. E., Rennke, H. G., and Brenner, B. M.,** Roles for thromboxane A2 and leukotrienes in endotoxin-induced acute renal failure, *Kidney Int.*, 30, 474, 1986.

95. **Takabashi, K., Nammour T. M., and Fukunaga, M.,** Glomerular actions of a free radical-generated novel prostaglandin, 8-epi-$PGF_{2\alpha}$, in the rat: Evidence for interaction with thromboxane A2 receptors, *J. Clin. Invest.*, 90, 136, 1992.

96. **Young, J. S. and Passmore, J. C.,** Hemodynamic and renal advantages of dual cyclooxygenase and leukotriene blockade during canine endotoxic shock, *Circ. Shock*, 32, 243, 1990.

97. **Julou-Schaeffer, G., Gray, G. A., Fleming, I., Schott, C., Parratt, J. R., and Stoclet, J. C.,** Loss of vascular responsiveness induced by endotoxin involves L-arginine pathway, *Am. J. Physiol.*, 259, H1038, 1990.

98. **Martin, W., Furchgott, R. F., Villani, G. M., and Jothianandan, D.,** Depression of contractile responses in rat aorta by spontaneously released endothelium-derived relaxing factor (EDRF), *J. Pharmacol. Exp. Ther.*, 237, 529, 1989.

99. **Gray, G. A., Furman, B. L., and Parratt, J. R.,** Endotoxin-induced impairment of vascular reactivity in the pithed rat: Role of arachidonic acid metabolites, *Circ. Shock*, 31, 395, 1990.

100. **Wurster, S. H., Wang, P., Dean, R. E., and Chaudry, I. H.,** Vascular smooth muscle contractile function is impaired during early and late sepsis, *J. Surg. Res.*, 56, 556, 1994.

101. **Palmer, R. M. J.,** The discovery of nitric oxide in the vessel wall: A unifying concept in the pathogenesis of sepsis, *Arch. Surg.*, 120, 396, 1993.

102. **Jacobs, R. F. and Tabor, D. R.,** Immune cellular interactions during sepsis and septic injury, *Crit. Care Clin.*, 5, 9, 1989.

103. **McMillen, M. A., Huribal, M., and Sumpio, B.,** Common pathway of endothelial-leukocyte interaction in shock, ischemia, and reperfusion, *Am. J. Surg.*, 166, 557, 1993.

104. **Malech, H. L. and Gallin, J. I.,** Neutrophils in human diseases, *N. Engl. J. Med.*, 317, 687, 1987.

105. **Movat, H. Z., Cybulsky, M. I., Colditz, I. G., Chan, M. K. W., and Dinarello, C. A.,** Acute inflammation in gram-negative infection: Endotoxin, interleukin 1, tumor necrosis factors, and neutrophils, *Fed. Proc.*, 46, 97, 1987.

106. **Kavlovsky, R. A., Horgan, M. J., Lum, H., McCandless, B. K., Gilboa, N., Wright, S. D., and Malik, A. B.,** Pulmonary edema induced by phagocytosing neutrophils. Protective effects of monoclonal antibody against phagocyte CD 18 integrin, *Circ. Res.*, 67, 795, 1990.

107. **Kaufman, B. S., Rackow, E. C., and Falk, J. L.,** The relationship between oxygen delivery and consumption during fluid resuscitation of hypovolemic and septic shock, *Chest*, 85, 336, 1984.

108. **Carden, D. L., Smith, J. K., Zimmerman, B. J., et al.,** Reperfusion injury following circulatory collapse: The role of reactive oxygen metabolites, *J. Crit. Care*, 4, 294, 1989.

109. **Haupt, M., Gilbert, E., and Carlson, R.,** Fluid loading increases oxygen consumption in septic patients with lactic acidosis, *Am. Rev. Respir. Dis.*, 131, 912, 1985.

110. **Skootsky, S. and Abraham, E.,** Continuous oxygen consumption measurement during initial emergency department resuscitation of critically ill patients, *Crit. Care Med.*, 16, 706, 1988.

111. **Moore, F. A., Haenel, J. B., Moore, E. E., and Whitehall, T. A.,** Incommensurate oxygen consumption in response to maximal oxygen availability predicts post injury multiple organ failure, *J. Trauma*, 33, 58, 1992.

112. **Bishops, T. and Shoemaker, W.,** Prospective trial of supranormal values as goals of resuscitation in severe trauma, *Arch. Surg.*, 127(10), 1175, 1992.

113. **Scalea, T. M.,** Geriatric blunt multiple trauma: Improved survival with early invasive monitoring, *J. Trauma*, 30, 129, 1990.

114. **Gutierrez, G., Palizas, F., Doglio, G., Wainsztein, N., Gallesio, A., Pacin, J., Dubin, A., Schiavi, E., Jorge, M., Pusajo, J., Klein, F., San Roman, E., Dorfman, B., Shottlender, J., and Giniger, R.,** Gastric mucosal pH as a therapeutic index of tissue oxygenation in critically ill patients, *Lancet*, 399, 195, 1992.

115. **Guys, T., Hubens, A., Neels, H., Lauwers, L. F., and Peeters, R.,** Prognostic value of gastric intramural pH in surgical intensive care patients, *Crit. Care Med.*, 16, 1222, 1988.

116. **Border, J. and Bone, L.,** Multiple trauma, major extremity wounds, their immediate management and its consequences, *Adv. Surg.*, 21, 263, 1988.

117. **Heindorff, H., Schulze, S., Mogenson, T., Almdal T., Kehlet, H., and Vilstrup, H.,** Hormonal and neural blockade prevents the post-operative increase in amino acid clearance and urea synthesis, *Surgery*, 111, 543, 1992.

118. **Chernow, B., Kasinski, N., and Salem, M.,** Catecholamines in critical illness, in *Critical Care: State of the Art*, Vol. 11, Lumb, P. and Shoemaker, W., Eds., Society of Critical Care Medicine Publisher, Fullerton, CA, 1990, 75–130.

119. **Chiolera, R., Breitenstein, E., Thorin, D., Christin, L., De Tribolet, N., Freeman, J., Jequier, E., and Schutz, Y.,** Effect of propranolol on resting metabolic rate after severe head injury, *Crit. Care Med.*, 17, 328, 1989.

120. **Figge, H., Huang, V., Kaul, A., et al.,** The pharmacotherapy of the behavioral manifestations of the ICU syndrome, *J. Crit. Care Med.*, 2, 199, 1987.

121. **Bouckoms, A.,** Pain relief in the intensive care unit, *J. Intens. Care Med.*, 3, 32, 1988.

Chapter 6

Leukocyte/Endothelial Cell Adhesion and Ischemia/Reperfusion Injury

Gary D. Dunn, D. Neil Granger, and Ronald J. Korthuis

CONTENTS

I. INTRODUCTION

The early restitution of blood flow to ischemic tissues is essential to halt the progression of cellular injury associated with decreased delivery of oxygen and metabolic substrates, and for removal of potentially harmful metabolic byproducts. However, it is now apparent that reperfusion also initiates a complex series of pathologic events that paradoxically injure tissues.[1-8] Moreover, a growing body of evidence indicates that ischemia/reperfusion (I/R) injury is initiated by events that occur within the microcirculation. For example, neutrophils must adhere to microvascular endothelium to induce the increases in microvascular permeability and transcapillary fluid filtration that occur in reperfused tissues.[6,9-14] In addition, neutrophil adhesion appears to play an essential role in the development of postischemic capillary no-reflow and has been implicated in the reduced arteriolar sensitivity to vasoactive substances induced by I/R.[6,7,15-19] These neutrophil-mediated microvascular changes may contribute to tissue injury and dysfunction by impairing cellular nutrition during reperfusion. In addition, the infiltrating leukocytes are able to direct a focused attack on the cells to which they become adherent, thereby exacerbating cell dysfunction and tissue injury during reperfusion. The aim of this review is to summarize the rapidly accumulating evidence implicating leukocyte/endothelial cell adhesive interactions in the pathogenesis of I/R.

II. MICROVASCULAR MANIFESTATIONS
OF ISCHEMIA/REPERFUSION

The microcirculation appears to be particularly vulnerable to the deleterious effects of reperfusion in that microvascular dysfunction precedes the development of parenchymal

0-8493-4870-6/95/$0.00+$.50

cell injury. The cumulative toll of the pathologic events associated with I/R is manifested as neutrophil adherence to microvascular endothelium and emigration of these inflammatory phagocytic cells into the interstitium, leukocyte capillary plugging, formation of intravascular thrombi, disruption of the endothelial cell glycocalyx, basement membrane, and interstitial matrix, endothelial cell swelling and denudation, reduced vascular sensitivity to vasoactive substances, and activation (and inactivation) of various enzymes and membrane receptors.[6,7,9-24] As a consequence of these I/R-induced changes in the microvasculature, vascular permeability and transcapillary fluid filtration are increased and capillary no-reflow becomes apparent. The severity of this postischemic microvascular pathology varies with the magnitude and duration of the ischemic period.[20]

The aforementioned microvascular alterations contribute to postischemic cellular dysfunction through several mechanisms. For example, the marked accumulation of fluid in the interstitial spaces induced by the loss of endothelial barrier function, coupled with the incomplete and maldistributed blood flow associated with capillary no-reflow, increases the functional diffusion path length for nutrients during reperfusion.[6,20,22] As a consequence, cellular nutrition can be severely limited during reperfusion despite successful therapeutic resolution (e.g., thrombolysis, embolectomy) of the pathologic event that initiated tissue ischemia. In the small intestine, accumulation of excessive interstitial fluid has an important pathologic consequence in addition to increasing diffusion distance. That is, edema formation may contribute to postischemic intestinal injury by increasing interstitial fluid pressure to a level sufficient to induce epithelial barrier disruption (filtration-secretion).[25] Provision of cellular nutrients during reperfusion may also be compromised by I/R-induced alterations in microcirculatory vasoregulatory function. For example, reduced arteriolar sensitivity to vasoactive substances associated with shock states may contribute to the difficulty in restoring arterial blood pressure to levels sufficient to maintain perfusion of vital organs when patients are resuscitated ("whole body ischemia/reperfusion").[26-28] Regional (i.e., organ) ischemia impairs endothelium-dependent vasodilatory responses and may contribute to postischemic vasospasm.[17-19]

A second important functional consequence of the microvascular pathology induced by I/R relates to the ability of neutrophils to accumulate specifically in ischemic foci and produce damage to host tissue.[29,30] The site specificity of neutrophil infiltration is dependent upon the expression of adhesive molecules on the surface of the microvascular endothelium within the ischemic regions. This enhances the destructive potential of the neutrophil by allowing its cytotoxic arsenal to be focused at specific sites within the ischemic tissue. Indeed, granulocyte adhesion enhances the oxidative burst and initiates the direct transfer of reactive oxygen metabolites from the neutrophil to the intracellular compartment of the cell to which they adhere.[31-34] Given the destructive potential of the infiltrating neutrophil, the participation of the microvascular endothelium in leukocyte trafficking to ischemic regions of a tissue underscores the importance of the microcirculation as an active participant in the pathogenesis of I/R.

It should be obvious from the foregoing discussion that postischemic alterations in the microcirculatory function play a critical role in the development of I/R injury. Moreover, it is becoming increasingly apparent that the establishment of adhesive interactions between circulating leukocytes and postcapillary venular endothelium is the rate-limiting microvascular event in I/R. Recognition of this fact has led to a major research effort directed at evaluating the potential for inhibition of leukocyte adherence to postcapillary venular endothelium as a novel approach to the treatment of reperfusion injury. In the next section, we will summarize the rapidly evolving evidence that neutrophil/endothelial cell adhesion plays a critical role in disorders characterized by ischemia and reperfusion.

Table 1 Immunoneutralization of the Common β-Subunit CD18 or the α-Subunits CD11a or CD11b of the Neutrophil Membrane Glycoprotein Adherence Complex CD11/CD18 Reduces Ischemia/Reperfusion-Induced Leukocyte Sequestration and Tissue Dysfunction

	Ref.
CD18 Antibodies Attenuate Reperfusion-Induced:	
Neutrophil sequestration	6,9,13,30,58–60
Myocardial necrosis	17,61,62
Alterations in coronary endothelium-dependent vascular reactivity	17
Capillary no-reflow	6,16,85
Skeletal muscle and myocardial contractile dysfunction	61,63
Reexpansion edema in atelectatic lungs	64
Neurologic deficits related to spinal cord ischemia	65
Intestinal mucosal injury	58
Increased microvascular permeability and edema formation	6,9–14,57
Pulmonary injury after hindlimb ischemia/reperfusion	90
Necrosis of frostbitten tissue	148
Burn wound extension	151
Antibodies Against CD11a or CD11b Reduce Postischemic:	
Neutrophil sequestration	62,66,69
Liver injury and necrosis	69
Myocardial necrosis	62,66
Hepatic and pulmonary injury induced by intestinal ischemia/reperfusion	86

From Korthuis, R. J., Carden, D. L., and Granger, D. N., Role of neutrophil-endothelial cell adhesion in inflammatory disorder, *J. Crit. Care*, 9, 1, 1994.

III. LEUKOCYTE/ENDOTHELIAL CELL ADHESION AND THE PATHOGENESIS OF POSTISCHEMIC TISSUE INJURY

A. ISCHEMIA/REPERFUSION

The observation that neutrophils accumulate in postischemic tissues in proportion to the severity of the ischemic insult, when coupled with the recognition that inflammatory granulocytes can damage host tissue, provides indirect support for the notion that neutrophils contribute to cellular injury in I/R.[20-22,29,30] More compelling support for this concept was provided by studies in which the potential participation of neutrophils in I/R was eliminated by either administration of compounds that interfere with granulocyte function[45-55] or by removal of circulating leukocytes from the blood during reperfusion.[6,9,10,35-44] The reduction in postischemic tissue injury noted in these studies indicates that neutrophils are a cause, and not an effect, of I/R injury.

The development of monoclonal antibodies directed against adhesive molecules expressed on the surface of leukocytes and endothelial cells has spurred an explosion of research directed at evaluating the potential therapeutic benefit of immunoneutralizing neutrophil/endothelial cell interactions in I/R. For example, a large number of studies have explored the potential contribution of adhesive interactions mediated by the leukocyte β2 integrin CD11/CD18 in the development of postischemic tissue injury (Table 1). This adhesive glycoprotein complex includes three structurally and functionally related heterodimers, each of which is comprised of an immunologically distinct α-subunit (CD11) that is linked with a common β-subunit (CD18).[138] Neutralizing antibodies directed against CD18 attenuate stationary leukocyte adhesion to postcapillary venular endothelium, but do not inhibit the weaker adhesive interaction associated with leukocyte rolling.[56,57] Administration of antibodies directed against the common β-chain of CD11/CD18 attenuate I/R-induced neutrophil accumulation,[6,9,13,30,58] granulocyte adherence and

Table 2 Neutralizing Antibodies Directed Against the Endothelial Cell Adhesion Molecules, Intercellular Adhesion Molecule-1 (ICAM-1) and P-Selectin, Reduces Ischemia/ Reperfusion-Induced Leukocyte Sequestration and Tissue Dysfunction

	Ref.
ICAM-1 Immunoneutralization Attenuates I/R-Induced:	
Neutrophil sequestration	12,18,62
Pulmonary permeability and edema	12
Myocardial necrosis	18,62
Coronary endothelial-dependent vasoregulatory dysfunction	18
Capillary no-reflow	15
Neurologic deficit associated with reversible spinal cord ischemia	71
P-Selectin Antibodies Reduce Postischemic:	
Myocardial necrosis	19
Alterations in coronary endothelium-dependent vascular reactivity	19
Capillary no-reflow	15
Pulmonary injury after intestinal I/R	81

From Korthuis, R. J., Carden, D. L., and Granger, D. N., Role of neutrophil-endothelial cell adhesion in inflammatory disorder, *J. Crit. Care*, 9, 1, 1994.

emigration in postcapillary venules,[59,60] microvascular dysfunction,[6,9-14,17,57,64] and parenchymal cell injury and necrosis.[17,58,61-63,65]

Although much of the work in this area has been directed at assessing the contribution of the common β-subunit of CD11/CD18 to the pathogenesis of I/R, an understanding of the role of the different α-subunits (CD11a, CD11b, and CD11c) is beginning to emerge (Table 1). For example, antibodies directed against CD11b decrease the release of hepatic-specific enzymes, attenuate granulocyte accumulation, and reduce the extent of necrosis noted in livers subjected to I/R.[69] It was suggested that a functional inactivation of the respiratory burst by inflammatory granulocytes may contribute to the protective effects induced by CD11b immunoneutralization inasmuch as antibody treatment reduced superoxide production.[69] Infarct size is also reduced by immunoneutralizing CD11a or CD11b in experimental models of myocardial I/R in which the ischemic period exceeds 30–45 minutes.[62,66] However, CD11b antibodies do not reduce the myocardial stunning induced by shorter periods of ischemia.[67] Since neutrophil depletion has also proven ineffective in preventing the myocardial dysfunction induced by short periods of ischemia, it does not appear that neutrophils play a role in myocardial stunning.[68]

The observation that postischemic neutrophil infiltration is confined primarily to regions of the tissue that were subjected to ischemia suggests that leukocyte trafficking must involve adhesive structures expressed on the surface of the endothelium in the affected area. Intercellular adhesion molecule-1 (ICAM-1) may fulfill this role since this adhesive molecule is a ligand for CD11/CD18.[20,21,24,70] Additional support for this notion is provided by the observation that many of the bioactive compounds that are involved in the pathogenesis of I/R upregulate ICAM-1 on the endothelial cell surface.[20,21,24,70] Indeed, ICAM-1 antibody treatment reduces I/R-induced neutrophil infiltration and edema in the lung,[12] decreases myocardial necrosis,[18,62] restores endothelial-dependent vasodilator responses in coronary arteries,[18] and attenuates the neurologic problems induced by spinal cord ischemia[71] (Table 2). ICAM-1-dependent leukocyte adherence to parenchymal cells may enhance targeted cellular destruction by emigrated cells. This notion is based on the observation that blocking antibodies to ICAM-1 prevent leukocyte adhesion to cardiac myocytes.[72] Furthermore, the establishment of CD18/ICAM-1-dependent adherence reactions initiates the direct transfer of oxidants from the adherent neutrophil to the intracellular compartment of the myocyte.[34]

A growing body of evidence indicates that the weak adhesive interaction associated with leukocyte rolling is mediated by the selectin family (P-selectin, L-selectin, and E-selectin) of adhesion molecules.[73-79] Since it appears that leukocytes that become firmly adherent are recruited almost exclusively from the rolling cell population,[80] inhibition of leukocyte rolling should be as effective as blockade of stationary adhesion in the prevention of postischemic tissue injury. Indeed, P-selectin antibody treatment reduces postischemic myocardial necrosis,[19] attenuates I/R-induced alterations in coronary endothelial-dependent vasodilatory responses,[19] prevents the development of capillary no-reflow,[15] and limits the pulmonary injury associated with intestinal I/R[81] (Table 2). Since P-selectin mediates the homotypic aggregation of platelets and platelet-leukocyte interactions,[76,82] it is possible that inhibition of these effects contributes to the protective actions of P-selectin antibody treatment.

The contributions of endothelial E-selectin and leukocyte L-selectin in the pathogenesis of postischemic cellular dysfunction have not been evaluated. However, a role for E-selectin in the recruitment of leukocytes during early reperfusion seems unlikely since the molecule is not normally present on the endothelial cell surface and requires 4–8 h to achieve full expression after exposure to proinflammatory mediators such as interleukin-1 or bacterial lipopolysaccharide.[83,84] It is possible that the formation of cytokines during early reperfusion upregulates the expression of E-selectin, which then contributes to the development of more delayed adherence reactions induced by I/R. Furthermore, since skin and skeletal muscle are very resistant to the short periods of ischemia that are so devastating to other organs such as the heart and brain, the duration of ischemia required to produce injury in the extremities (>4 h) may allow for changes that ultimately promote E-selectin expression during reperfusion. Indeed, a preliminary report indicates that E-selectin antibodies reduce microvascular dysfunction in a mouse dorsal skin fold model that involves exposure of the tissue to 4 h of ischemia.[85]

When a large mass of tissue is subjected to I/R, cellular injury is not confined to the tissue subjected to the ischemic insult, but also occurs in distant organs. For example, the remote consequences of I/R affecting large portions of the lower limbs or the small intestine include neutrophil sequestration in the liver and lungs and the development of hepatic injury and noncardiogenic pulmonary edema.[81,86-94] However, ischemia affecting a single muscle, a small group of muscles, or a small segment of the bowel is not associated with the development of systemic complications, at least in the short term. Since neutrophil depletion effectively eliminates the formation of pulmonary edema induced by lower torso ischemia, it appears that granulocytes play an important role in the production of remote tissue injury.[89] Additional support for this concept is provided by the observation that antibodies directed against CD11b or CD18 prevent the increase in pulmonary microvascular permeability and attenuate the release of liver enzymes induced by hindlimb or intestinal I/R (Table 1).[86,90] P-selectin antibody treatment has been shown to reduce the extent of microvascular barrier disruption in the lung after intestinal ischemia and reperfusion (Table 2).[81]

Although granulocyte infiltration occurs in many organs following reperfusion of a large tissue mass, pulmonary neutrophil accumulation is particularly impressive in these models.[87,91-94] Despite the reduction in lung injury associated with CD11/CD18 and P-selectin immunoneutralization after remote I/R, antibody treatment failed to prevent leukocyte sequestration in the lungs of these animals.[81,86,90] This suggests that leukocyte accumulation in the lungs of animals subject to intestinal I/R may involve other adhesive ligands or results from physical trapping of activated, and thus less deformable, leukocytes in pulmonary capillaries. Whatever the mechanism, the fact that antibody treatment prevented pulmonary microvascular injury but did not attenuate leukocyte sequestration in the lung after intestinal I/R suggests that these events may not be causally related. Since superoxide production can be inhibited by antibody binding to CD11b, it is possible that the protective action associated with immunoneutralization of this alpha subunit is due to a functional inactivation of neutrophils.[69] A similar argument may apply to the effect of P-selectin antibodies since it has been suggested that endothelial P-selectin may influence leukocyte or platelet activation or the ability of these cells to aggregate.[76,82,95-98] Thus, the protective effects of P-selectin antibody treatment may relate to reducing the propensity to form cell aggregates or prevention of the release of platelet-derived products. Finally, it is possible that by reducing injury in the tissue subjected to I/R, CD11b/CD18 and P-selectin immunoneutralization may prevent the release of bioactive compounds from the ischemic tissue into the bloodstream that, when delivered to the lungs, would induce endothelial barrier disruption.

B. POSTISCHEMIC CAPILLARY NO-REFLOW

When blood flow to certain organs (e.g., the heart, brain, liver, kidney, and skeletal muscle) is reinstituted after ischemia, a large proportion of capillaries fail to reperfuse, a phenomenon referred to as capillary no-reflow.[6,7,14-16,48,99-119,124] Despite being recognized for over 50 years, the mechanisms underlying the development of the no-reflow phenomenon remain unclear. Although it has been suggested that I/R-induced microvascular thrombus formation may contribute to this capillary perfusion deficit,[107] heparin treatment is not effective in restoring capillary perfusion after I/R[106] and microvessel thrombosis is rarely observed in postischemic tissues.[106,108,109] A better supported hypothesis is that activated neutrophils are significant contributors to the development of postischemic capillary no-reflow.[6,15,16,100-104,110,119,124] Not only is there a strong correlation between the percent of capillaries exhibiting no-reflow and the number of leukocytes present in these capillaries in postischemic tissues,[101-104] neutrophil depletion virtually abolishes no-reflow in reperfused myocardium, brain, and skeletal muscle.[6,15,100] Inasmuch as allopurinol and superoxide dismutase prevent leukocyte/endothelial cell adhesion and restore capillary perfusion, it appears that oxidant generation contributes to the enhanced neutrophil adhesion and the development of no-reflow in postischemic tissues.[111,120] Additional support for the concept that leukocytes are involved in the development of capillary no-reflow is provided by the observation that treatment with antibodies directed against CD18, ICAM-1, or P-selectin restores capillary perfusion in postischemic skeletal muscle (Tables 1 and 2).[6,15,85] CD18 immunoneutralization also prevents the development of no-reflow in the brain after I/R (Table 1).[16]

Inasmuch as CD11/CD18, ICAM-1, and P-selectin-dependent adherence reactions are almost exclusively confined to the venular segment of the microcirculation in postischemic tissues,[21] the results discussed above suggest that leukocyte adherence to postcapillary venules plays an important role in the development of capillary no-reflow. However, the mechanism whereby leukocyte adhesion to postcapillary venules causes capillary no-reflow is uncertain (see Figure 1). One explanation relates to the possibility that the adherent leukocytes reduce the effective lumenal diameter of postcapillary venules to which they adhere, thereby altering microhemodynamics such that flow in upstream vessels (i.e., capillaries) ceases.[111,116]

Leukocyte/capillary plugging has also been suggested to underlie the development of capillary no-reflow in postischemic tissues.[102-104] While this may contribute to the reduction in capillary perfusion during ischemia, physical impaction of leukocytes within the capillaries does not appear to play a role in the pathogenesis of no-reflow in skeletal muscle when normal perfusion pressures are established at reperfusion.[111,122] It is also possible that the mechanisms involved in the regulation of endothelial cell volume are disrupted by the release of oxidants or hydrolytic enzymes by adherent leukocytes (Figure 1). As a consequence, endothelial cells swell and reduce capillary diameter.[112-115] Endothelial cell swelling occur has been shown to occur during ischemia but is exacerbated by reperfusion.[113] Support for the endothelial cell swelling hypothesis is provided by the observation that treatment with a hypertonic, hyperosmotic saline dextran solution pre-

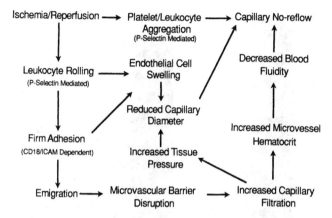

Figure 1 Mechanisms whereby leukocyte-endothelial cell adhesive interactions may contribute to the development of postischemic capillary no-reflow. See text for details. (From Akimitsu, T., Jerome, S. N., Gute, D., and Korthuis, R. J., Reactive oxygen species, neutrophil infiltration, and postischemic microvascular dysfunction, in *Reoxygenation Injury in Skeletal Muscle*, Fantini, G. O., Ed., Landis Publications, Austin, TX, 1994, 5–32.)

vents the reduction in capillary lumenal diameter induced by I/R[114,115] and reduces the extent of postischemic no-reflow.[123,124] Although postischemic endothelial cell swelling appears to result from altered sodium-hydrogen exchange,[115] the effect of oxidants or neutrophil activation on cell swelling and the regulation of intracellular pH by the endothelium has not been evaluated.

It is also possible that leukocyte adhesion to postcapillary venules contributes to the genesis of no-reflow by a mechanism that involves the ability of activated neutrophils to induce microvascular barrier disruption (Figure 1).[110,125] That is, as granulocytes adhere to the postcapillary venular endothelium and emigrate into the tissue spaces, microvascular permeability is increased. As a consequence of these events, transcapillary fluid filtration rate is enhanced such that excessive volumes of interstitial fluid accumulate. The rate of edema formation may be further enhanced by an increase in capillary pressure that results as a consequence of the physical reduction in the diameter of postcapillary venules induced by leukocytes adhering to the endothelium in these vessels.[116] Because many tissues cannot readily expand due to enclosure by restrictive boundaries, I/R-induced, neutrophil-mediated edema formation can be accompanied by a rise in interstitial fluid pressure sufficient to produce significant extravascular compression. For example, swelling of the brain is prevented by the cranial vault, while expansion of the kidney is limited by its capsular investment. Similarly, many muscles are surrounded by a tight fascial sheath that limits swelling.

Microhemodynamic alterations induced by neutrophil-mediated microvascular barrier disruption and altered membrane ion fluxes may also contribute to the development of no-reflow (Figure 1). That is, the enhanced transcapillary fluid filtration induced by increased capillary permeability can increase microvessel hematocrit.[117] As a consequence, the viscosity of blood in the capillaries increases, which in turn raises vascular resistance and thereby limits perfusion. Support for this notion is derived from studies in which prophylactic isovolemic hemodilution was used to restore hematocrit to preischemic levels and capillary no-reflow did not develop.[118]

C. SHOCK AND RESUSCITATION — WHOLE-BODY ISCHEMIA/REPERFUSION

Resuscitation after circulatory collapse is widely regarded as an event that results in whole-body I/R.[126] In view of the demonstrated role for neutrophils in the tissue injury

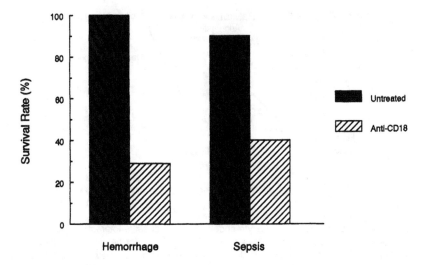

Figure 2 Treatment with antibodies directed against the common β-subunit of the leukocyte glycoprotein adherence complex CD11/CD18 (Anti-CD18) increase survival rates in septic animals and rats subjected to hemorrhagic hypotension and resuscitation relative to untreated controls. (Figure modified from data presented in References 128 and 141.)

induced by regional (i.e., organ) I/R, it is not surprising that granulocyte depletion reduces tissue injury and increases survival rates in animals resuscitated after the development of hemorrhagic shock.[44,100] Leukocyte adhesion to vascular endothelium appears to be required for the production of cellular dysfunction induced by circulatory collapse since prophylactic immunoneutralization of the common β chain of CD11/CD18 increases survival rates in rabbits subjected to hypovolemic hypotension and resuscitation (Figure 2), an effect presumably related to attenuated neutrophil infiltration, endothelial barrier disruption, edema formation, and hemorrhagic necrosis in the liver and intestinal mucosa noted with this treatment.[126-128] A similar protective effect was achieved when CD18 antibody treatment was initiated at the time of resuscitation.[126-128] This latter observation indicates that a major proportion of cellular injury induced by circulatory collapse and resuscitation occurs after the hypotensive episode. The effectiveness of CD18 antibody treatment at the time of resuscitation has important therapeutic implications since the need for prophylactic therapy cannot be anticipated.

In contrast to the protective effect of CD18 antibody administration noted in splanchnic organs, the pulmonary injury induced by hemorrhagic shock was not reduced.[126,128] This observation suggests either that neutrophils do not contribute to the pulmonary complications induced by circulatory collapse or that hemorrhage-induced neutrophil adherence and emigration is not dependent on CD11/CD18. Moreover, the ineffectiveness of CD18 antibody therapy in preventing the development of acute respiratory distress induced hemorrhagic shock and resuscitation is in direct contrast to the observation that immunoneutralization of CD18 ameliorates the pulmonary injury induced by lower torso ischemia/reperfusion.[88,90] This dichotomy suggests that fundamental differences exist with regard to the regulation of neutrophil adherence reactions in these conditions.

Septic shock results from an acute invasion of the bloodstream by microbial organisms or their products. This form of shock is particularly devastating in that it afflicts 300,000 to 500,000 people per year and is associated with a mortality rate of approximately 50%. The fact that neutrophil activation is a key component of host defense against invading pathogens strongly suggests that granulocytes contribute to the pathogenesis of septicemia. Indeed, the tissue injury induced by endotoxin or tumor necrosis factor (TNF) is attenuated by prior neutrophil depletion in many, but not all, septic models.[129-131] Moreover, the development of shock induced by injection of lethal doses of *E. coli* is prevented by administration of antibodies to these mediator.[132-136]

A role for neutrophil adhesion in the pathogenesis of sepsis is suggested by the results of *in vivo* and *in vitro* experiments that indicate that TNF and endotoxin upregulate the expression of CD11/CD18 on neutrophils and induce the appearance of ELAM-1 on the surface of endothelial cells.[83,84,137,138] In addition, neutrophils obtained from septic patients or naive granulocytes exposed to plasma from septic patients demonstrate increased adhesivity *in vitro*.[139] Increased neutrophil adhesiveness in septic patients would induce neutrophil margination and extravasation, thereby accounting for the neutropenia associated with this shock state. This latter idea is supported by the observation that CD18-specific antibodies attenuate the neutropenia associated with Gram-negative sepsis.[140]

More compelling support for the notion that neutrophil/endothelial cell adhesion is a prerequisite for the genesis of cellular injury in septic animals is provided by the observations that CD18 antibody treatment attenuates alveolar capillary membrane injury and protects the systemic circulation from the deleterious effects of septicemia.[141,142] Similarly, administration of neutralizing antibodies directed against CD11b or CD18 reduces the hepatic injury, extracellular oxidant production, and neutrophil accumulation associated with the development of endotoxin shock.[69] CD18 immunoneutralization has also been shown to improve survival rates in several models of experimental sepsis (LPS or TNF administration and appendiceal ligation) (Figure 2).[141,143]

Although the aforementioned observations have provided important insight regarding the role of neutrophil/endothelial cell adhesion in the pathogenesis of septic shock, it is not clear whether such an approach would be useful as a clinical treatment because of the potential risk for uncontrolled bacterial invasion.[126] In fact, granulocyte depletion has been shown to result in higher mortality rates in one model of septic shock, while CD18 antibody treatment increases the incidence and severity of subcutaneous abscesses in rabbits inoculated with *Staphylococcus aureus*.[144,145] Presumably, these effects were due to inhibition of neutrophil-dependent bacterial cytolysis. However, it has been suggested that *transient* inhibition of granulocyte adherence in conjunction with antibiotic therapy may represent a viable therapeutic avenue in sepsis. Support for this notion is provided by the observation that concomitant treatment with CD18 antibodies and cefazolin improved survival rates in septic animals when compared to rats receiving either the antibiotic or the antibody alone.[146] Since CD18-dependent adherence reactions were only inhibited during the first hours following induction of septicemia in these experiments, it appears that transient inhibition of neutrophil adherence may represent a useful adjunct to conventional antibiotic therapy in sepsis.

D. THERMAL TRAUMA, NEUTROPHIL ADHESION, AND ISCHEMIA/REPERFUSION

Cellular injury induced by exposure to extremes in temperature is also thought to involve I/R. One example is frostbite. Ice crystal formation in tissues exposed to intense cold induces microvascular barrier disruption, progressive vascular occlusion, and cellular injury.[147] When the frostbitten tissue is rewarmed, blood flow is initially restored but interstitial edema worsens and leukocyte activation becomes apparent. As rewarming continues, a progressive reduction in tissue perfusion occurs secondary to thromboxane-induced vasoconstriction and microvessel occlusion by leukocyte/platelet aggregates.[147] Administration of antibodies directed against functional epitopes on CD18 at the onset or following completion of rewarming prevented microvascular occlusion and reduced the tissue edema and necrosis noted in frostbitten rabbit extremities.[148] These observations suggest that inhibition of leukocyte adherence prevented the reduction in blood flow that normally accompanies rewarming of frozen tissues, thereby preventing ischemia-induced necrosis in frostbitten tissue.

The progression or extension of tissue loss into areas adjacent to a cutaneous burn appears to result from ischemia inasmuch as blood flow is markedly reduced in this marginal zone.[151] A role for neutrophils in burn wound progression has also been suggested because granulocytes are activated on exposure to burn blister fluid.[149] In addition, circulating leukocytes also demonstrate increased surface expression of CD11b/CD18 following burn injury.[150] Pre- or postburn administration of CD18 or ICAM antibodies restores blood flow and reduces tissue injury in areas adjacent to cutaneous burns.[151] The fact that postburn antibody administration was as effective as prophylactic treatment suggests that a therapeutic window may exist in the early postburn period that will allow for salvage of marginal zone tissue after production of burn injury. However, the possibility that inhibition of leukocyte adherence may increase the susceptibility to infection at burn sites must be addressed before the clinical relevance of this therapeutic approach can be assessed.

E. REPERFUSION INJURY IN TRANSPLANTATION

Only 30 years ago, successful clinical transplantation of solid organs was considered to be an unobtainable goal. However, the recent discovery of potent immunosuppressive agents has allowed transplantation to become a viable option for the treatment of end-stage disease involving the heart, liver, and kidneys. Despite these advances, the mechanisms underlying problems induced when transplanted organs are reperfused remain enigmatic and still contribute to acute rejection. The large body of evidence implicating a role for neutrophils in postischemic tissue injury, when coupled with the observation that acute rejection is associated with massive polymorphonuclear leukocyte and lymphocyte infiltration, suggests that leukocytes may contribute to tissue dysfunction when transplanted organs are reperfused. The influx of inflammatory leukocytes may be enhanced by rejection-induced endothelial cell activation, which appears to cause capillaries to undergo a postcapillary venule-like transformation.[152] More compelling support for the notion that granulocytes contribute to the myocardial injury associated with transplantation of human hearts is provided by the observation that neutropenic perfusion after implantation reduces ultrastructural evidence of reperfusion injury.[153] This observation suggests that the inflammatory infiltrate is a cause, rather than an effect, of allograft rejection.

A role for leukocyte adhesion has been postulated based on the fact that endothelial ICAM-1 expression is upregulated during cellular rejection in cardiac, renal, hepatic, and corneal allografts.[154-162] This finding is of particular relevance to the notion that leukocyte/endothelial cell adhesion may contribute to allograft rejection since endothelial cells of the transplanted organ form the major interface or boundary between the allograft and the recipient's immune defenses and as such represent the principal target in hyperacute and acute rejection. In addition, since the molecular determinants of neutrophil/endothelial cell adhesion are upregulated in acute rejection, quantitation of adhesion molecule expression may represent an important diagnostic tool for prediction of impending allograft rejection.

Inasmuch as inflammatory cell infiltration and increased expression of the molecular determinants of neutrophil/endothelial cell adhesion are characteristic pathologic features of acute graft rejection, it is reasonable to suggest that the infiltrated cells play an important role in transplantation-induced tissue injury. This notion is supported by studies that demonstrated that monoclonal antibodies against ICAM-1 prolong the survival of cardiac and renal allografts.[163,164] Similarly, immunoneutralization of either ICAM-1 or CD18 reduces myocardial inflammation and improves perfusion and ventricular function in transplanted hearts.[165] CD11a does not appear to act as a ligand for ICAM-1 in acute

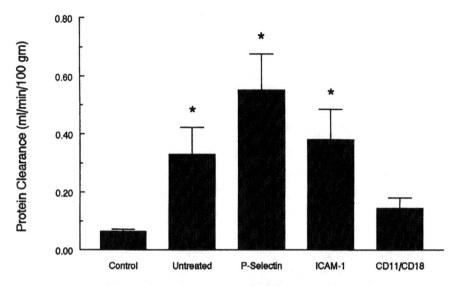

Figure 3 Administration of antibodies directed against CD11/CD18, but not intercellular adhesion molecule-1 (ICAM-1) or P-selectin, attenuates microvasular barrier disruption in intestinal allografts exposed to 6 h of hypothermic ischemia. Control refers to values obtained in intestinal preparations that were subjected to all surgical procedures but were not subjected to ischemia and reperfusion. (Modified from data presented in Reference 168.)

rejection of transplanted kidneys since monoclonal antibodies directed against this alpha subunit do not improve renal function.[166] Nevertheless, the observation that CD18 or ICAM-1 antibody treatment improves graft survival suggests that modulation of leukocyte adhesion may represent a novel mechanism of action for drugs presently used in the prevention of organ rejection following transplantation. Indeed, such an explanation may partially explain the beneficial effects of cyclosporine and FK-506 to enhance graft survival in that both immunosuppressive agents significantly attenuate leukocyte/endothelial cell adhesion.[167]

In contrast to the beneficial effects noted in transplanted hearts and kidneys, antibodies directed against ICAM-1 do not prevent microvascular and mucosal dysfunction in small intestinal allografts (Figure 3).[168] Although immunoneutralization of P-selectin was also ineffective, treatment with a CD18 antibody prevented the microvascular (but not mucosal) barrier disruption associated with small intestinal transplantation (Figure 3).[168] The reasons for the discrepant results regarding the role of ICAM-1 in cardiac and renal transplants vs. intestinal allografts are not clear, but may relate to tissue differences or the fact that intestinal mucosal disruption may allow for uncontrolled bacterial invasion. Whatever the explanation, these observations indicate that results obtained in one organ should not be extrapolated to another without proper validation.

F. HYDRODYNAMIC DISPERSAL FORCES, LEUKOCYTE ADHESION, AND ISCHEMIA/REPERFUSION

The large body of evidence summarized above clearly indicates that the proadhesive force generated on the surface of activated leukocytes and endothelial cells plays an important role in the pathogenesis of disorders characterized by I/R. However, other factors act to modulate neutrophil adhesion within the microcirculation. For example, hydrodynamic dispersal forces (shear stress) act to dislodge leukocytes from the vessel wall.[20,21,23] Thus, one might predict that reductions in blood flow and shear rate would tend to promote

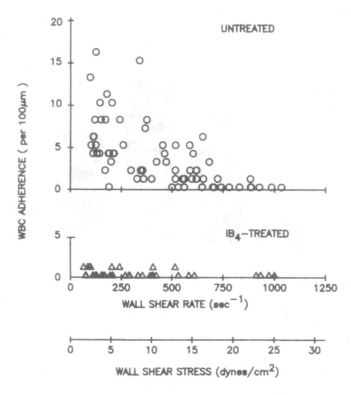

Figure 4 Relation between wall shear rate and leukocyte adhesion to postcapillary venules in the rat mesentery in the presence and absence of a monoclonal antibody directed against CD11/CD18. (From Reference 57.)

leukocyte adhesion to the endothelium, while just the opposite would occur with increased wall shear rate. Quantitative examine of these relationships under conditions of both high and low blood flow rates is particularly relevant to the understanding of the kinetics of leukocyte adhesion and emigration during ischemia and following reperfusion because of the wide range of blood flows associated with these conditions.

The influence of shear rate on leukocyte adherence to endothelium has been evaluated using intravital microscopic approaches.[23,57,78,169] The results of these studies indicate that as shear stress is reduced from its normal value, there is a progressive increase in the number of adherent leukocytes (Figure 4). Indeed, at the very low shear rates that are encountered in severely ischemic tissues, the number of adherent leukocytes increases even more dramatically (Figure 4).[57] The shear rate dependence of leukocyte adherence was localized primarily to postcapillary venules and was abolished by immunoneutralization of the CD11/CD18 glycoprotein adhesion complex.[57]

The mechanisms underlying leukocyte adhesion at low shear rates *in vivo* are not clear. One explanation for this behavior is that there is a low level of CD11/CD18 expression in normal circulating leukocytes. When tissue blood flow is normal, the proadhesive force generated by these adhesion molecules is not sufficient to overcome the anti-adhesive force generated by shear. However, as shear rate is reduced during ischemia, the balance between proadhesive and hydrodynamic dispersal forces changes such that adhesive bonds can be created between leukocytes and endothelial cells. An alternative explanation for the recruitment of adherent leukocytes at low shear rates is that there may be minimal or no expression of CD11/CD18 on circulating leukocytes; but as venular blood flow is reduced, there is a concomitant reduction in the washout of proinflammatory agents normally produced by endothelial and/or parenchymal cells. This accumulation of a chemotactic stimulus would elicit the expression of CD11/CD18 on rolling leukocytes and ultimately lead to firm adherence. The lower the shear rate, the greater the number of adherent leukocytes. Support for this proposal is provided by the observation that shear rate-dependent leukocyte adherence in cat mesenteric venules is enhanced when the mesenteric surface is superfused at a lower rate, thereby further promoting the accumulation of inflammatory mediators.[169]

G. ENDOTHELIAL CELL CYTOSKELETAL ALTERATIONS AND POSTISCHEMIC NEUTROPHIL EMIGRATION

The accumulation of neutrophils in postischemic tissues is well-documented and it is assumed that these extravasated leukocytes are responsible for the production of parenchymal cell injury. Recent studies indicate that alterations in the endothelial cell cytoskeleton play an important role in neutrophil accumulation in inflamed tissues. For example, microfilament-rich endothelial cell lamellopodia extend luminally and envelope leukocytes as they emigrate.[170] In addition, stabilization of F-actin in endothelial cells with phalloidin prevents the alterations in cytoskeletal architecture and leukocyte emigration that occurs in response to a variety of proinflammatory agents both *in vitro* and *in vivo*.[171,172] Recent studies indicate that postischemic microvascular dysfunction and neutrophil sequestration can be attenuated by stabilization of microfilamentous cytoskeletal elements in the endothelium.[46] Intravital microscopic studies indicate that phalloidin does not alter the increased leukocyte adherence to venular endothelium induced by I/R or venular exposure to PAF, LTB$_4$, and FMLP.[124,173] However, this agent completely prevented leukocyte emigration induced by these interventions.[173] These studies suggest that prevention of leukocyte emigration by use of compounds that stabilize the architecture of the endothelial cell cytoskeleton may represent a useful new therapeutic approach to ameliorate neutrophil-dependent I/R injury.

IV. SUMMARY

A growing body of evidence indicates that the molecular determinants of neutrophil/ endothelial cell adhesion play a critical role in modulating granulocyte-dependent cellular dysfunction in pathologic disorders that are characterized by ischemia and reperfusion. Given the destructive potential of the infiltrating neutrophil, the participation of the microvascular endothelium in leukocyte trafficking to ischemic regions of a tissue underscores the importance of the microcirculation as an active participant in the pathogenesis of I/R.

Since inhibition of leukocyte-endothelial cell adhesive interactions at the onset of reperfusion is as effective as prophylactic treatment, it appears that neutrophil-mediated tissue injury induced by I/R occurs primarily during reperfusion. The importance of this observation lies with the fact that therapy can rarely be instituted prior to the development of ischemia. However, administration of therapeutic agents that inhibit leukocyte/endothelial cell interactions at the time the defect that produced ischemia is repaired may significantly reduce tissue injury. Thus, elucidation of the mechanisms involved in the modulation of neutrophil adherence to postcapillary venular endothelium in different pathophysiologic conditions may lead to the development of novel therapeutic agents that prevent granulocyte-mediated tissue injury.

The information presented in this review is consistent with the following model of leukocyte recruitment to postischemic tissues.[20,21,174,175] The initial adhesive interaction between neutrophils and the endothelium involves upregulation of adhesion molecules

(ICAM-1, E-selectin, and P-selectin) on the surface of endothelium in ischemic regions of a tissue. L-selectin may mediate the initial adhesion (leukocyte rolling and reversible sticking) between nonactivated neutrophils and the stimulated endothelium by interacting with P-selectin and/or E-selectin. The transiently bound neutrophils are exposed to low concentrations of chemoattractants that are elaborated by the ischemic tissues, thus allowing for engagement of CD11/CD18 and downregulation (shedding) of L-selectin. Subsequent steps involve strengthening of the adhesive interaction and transendothelial migration. Thus, this model suggests that the selectins (L-selectin, P-selectin, and E-selectin) modulate neutrophil margination (rolling) in postischemic tissues, while the leukocyte integrins (CD11a/CD18 and CD11b/CD18) and ICAM-1 mediate firm adhesion and extravasation.

REFERENCES

1. **Hearse, D. J.,** Reperfusion of ischemic myocardium, *J. Mol. Cell. Cardiol.*, 9, 605, 1977.
2. **Parks, D. A. and Granger, D. N.,** Contributions of ischemia and reperfusion to mucosal lesion formation, *Am. J. Physiol.*, 250, G749, 1986.
3. **Korthuis, R. J., Smith, J. K., and Carden, D. L.,** Hypoxic reperfusion attenuates postischemic microvascular injury, *Am. J. Physiol.*, 256, H315, 1989.
4. **Perry, M. A. and Wadhwa, S. S.,** Gradual reintroduction of oxygen reduces reperfusion injury in cat stomach, *Am. J. Physiol.*, 254, G366–G372, 1988.
5. **Dahlback, L. O. and Rais, O.,** Morphological changes in striated muscle following ischemia: Immediate postischemic phase, *Acta Chir. Scand.*, 131, 430, 1966.
6. **Carden, D. L., Smith, J. K., and Korthuis, R. J.,** Neutrophil-mediated microvascular dysfunction in postischemic canine skeletal muscle: Role of granulocyte adherence, *Circ. Res.*, 66, 1436, 1990.
7. **Jerome, S. N., Smith, C. W., and Korthuis, R. J.,** CD18-dependent adherence reactions play an important role in the development of the no-reflow phenomenon, *Am. J. Physiol.*, 264, H479, 1993.
8. **Morris, J. B., Haglund, U., and Bulkley, G. B.,** The protection from postischemic injury by xanthine oxidase inhibition: Blockade of free radical generation or purine salvage, *Gastroenterology*, 92, 1542, 1987.
9. **Hernandez, L. A., Grisham, M. B., Twohig, B., Arfors, K.-E., Harlan, J. M., and Granger, D. N.,** Role of neutrophils in ischemia/reperfusion-induced microvascular injury, *Am. J. Physiol.*, 253, H699, 1987.
10. **Adkins, W. K. and Taylor, A. E.,** Role of xanthine oxidase and neutrophils in ischemia-reperfusion injury in rabbit lung, *J. Appl. Physiol.*, 69, 2012, 1990.
11. **Bishop, M. J., Kowalski, S. M., Guidotti, S. M., and Harlan, J. M.,** Antibody against neutrophil adhesion improves reperfusion and limits alveolar infiltrate following unilateral pulmonary artery occlusion, *J. Surg. Res.*, 52, 199, 1992.
12. **Horgan, M. J., Ge, M., Gu, J., Rothlein, R., and Malik, A. B.,** Role of ICAM-1 in neutrophil-mediated lung vascular injury after occlusion and reperfusion, *Am. J. Physiol.*, 261, H1578, 1991.
13. **Horgan, M. J., Wright, S. D., and Malik, A. B.,** Antibody against leukocyte integrin (CD18) prevents reperfusion-induced lung vascular injury, *Am. J. Physiol.*, 259, L315, 1990.
14. **Vedder, N. B., Winn, R. K., Rice, C. L., Chi, E. Y., Arfors, K. E., and Harlan, J. M.,** Inhibition of leukocyte adherence by anti-CD18 monoclonal antibody attenuates reperfusion injury in the rabbit ear, *Proc. Natl. Acad. Sci. U.S.A.*, 87, 2543, 1990.
15. **Jerome, S. N., Dore, M., Paulson, J. C., Smith, C. W., and Korthuis, R. J.,** P-selectin and ICAM-1 dependent adherence reactions: Role in the genesis of postischemic no-reflow, *Am. J. Physiol.*, 266, H1316, 1994.
16. **Mori, E., del Zoppo, G. J., Chambers, J. D., Copeland, B. R., and Arfors, K. E.,** Inhibition of polymorphonuclear leukocyte adherence suppresses no-reflow after focal cerebral ischemia in baboons, *Stroke*, 23, 712, 1992.
17. **Ma, X.-L., Tsao, P. S., and Lefer, A. M.,** Antibody to CD-18 exerts endothelial and cardiac protective effects in myocardial ischemia and reperfusion, *J. Clin. Invest.*, 88, 1237, 1991.
18. **Ma, X.-L., Lefer, D. J., Lefer, A. M., and Rothlein, R.,** Coronary endothelial and cardiac protective effects of a monoclonal antibody to intercellular adhesion molecule-1 in myocardial ischemia and reperfusion, *Circulation*, 86, 937, 1992.

19. **Weyrich, A. S., Ma, X., Lefer, D. J., Albertine, K. H., and Lefer, A. M.,** *In vivo* neutralization of P-selectin protects feline heart and endothelium in myocardial ischemia and reperfusion injury, *J. Clin. Invest.*, 91, 2620, 1993.

20. **Korthuis, R. J. and Granger, D. N.,** Pathogenesis of ischemia/reperfusion: Role of neutrophil-endothelial cell adhesion, in *Handbook of Immunopharmacology: Adhesion Molecules*, Wagner, C. J., Ed., Academic Press, London, 1994, 163–190.

21. **Korthuis, R. J., Anderson, D. C., and Granger, D. N.,** Role of neutrophil-endothelial cell adhesion in inflammatory disorders, *J. Crit. Care*, 9, 1, 1994.

22. **Gute, D. and Korthuis, R. J.,** Role of leukocyte adherence in reperfusion-induced microvascular dysfunction and tissue injury, in *Physiology and Pathophysiology of Leukocyte Adhesion*, Granger, D. N. and Schmid-Schonbein, G. W., Eds., New York, Oxford, 1995, 359–380.

23. **Granger, D. N., Kvietys, P. R., and Perry, M. A.,** Leukocyte-endothelial cell adhesion induced by ischemia and reperfusion, *Can. J. Physiol. Pharmacol.*, 71, 67, 1993.

24. **Korthuis, R. J., Carden, D. L., and Granger, D. N.,** Mechanisms of postischemic tissue injury: Role of reactive oxygen metabolites and neutrophils, in *Biological Consequences of Oxidative Stress: Implications for Cardiovascular Disease and Carcinogenesis*, Spatz, L. and Bloom, A., Eds., Oxford University Press, chap. 3, 50–77, 1992.

25. **Granger, D. N., Kvietys, P. R., Korthuis, R. J., and Premen, A. J.,** Microcirculation and intestinal mucosal function, in *Handbook of Physiology: The Gastrointestinal System., Vol. I, Part 2. Motility and the Circulation,* chap. 39, American Physiological Society, Williams & Wilkins, Bethesda, MD, 1405–1474, 1989.

26. **Gao, H., Korthuis, R. J., and Benoit, J. N.,** Effects of reactive oxygen metabolites on norepinephrine-induced vasoconstriction, *Free Rad. Biol. Med.*, 16, 839, 1994.

27. **Bond, R. F. and Johnson, G.,** Vascular adrenergic interactions during hemorrhagic shock, *Fed. Proc.*, 44, 281, 1985.

28. **Bond, R.F.,** A review of the skin and skeletal muscle hemodynamics during hemorrhagic hypotension and shock, *Adv. Shock Res.*, 8, 53, 1982.

29. **Go, L. O., Murray, C. E., Richard, V. J., Weischedel, G. R., Jennings, R. B., and Reimer, K. A.,** Myocardial neutrophil accumulation during reversible or irreversible ischemic injury, *Am. J. Physiol.*, 255, H1188, 1988.

30. **Dreyer, W. J., Michael, L. H., West, M. S., Smith, C. W., Rothlein, R., Rossen, R. D., Anderson, D. C., and Entman, M. L.,** Neutrophil accumulation in ischemic myocardium: Insights into time course, distribution, and mechanism of localization during early reperfusion, *Circulation,* 84, 400, 1992.

31. **Entman, M. L., Youker, K., Shappell, S. B., Seigel, C., Rothlein, R., Dreyer, W. J., Schmalstieg, F. C., and Smith, C. W.,** Neutrophil adherence to isolated adult canine myocytes: Evidence for a CD18-dependent mechanism, *J. Clin. Invest.,* 85, 1497, 1990.

32. **Nathan, C. F.,** Neutrophil activation on biological surfaces: Massive secretion of hydrogen peroxide in response to products of macrophages and lymphocytes, *J. Clin. Invest.*, 80, 1550, 1987.

33. **Nathan, C. F.,** Respiratory burst in adherent human neutrophils: Triggering by colony stimulating factors CSF-GM and CSF-G, *Blood*, 73, 301, 1989.

34. **Entman, M. L., Youker, K., Shoji, T., Kukielka, G. K., Shappel, S. B., Taylor, A. A., and Smith, C. W.,** Neutrophil-induced oxidative injury of cardiac myocytes: A compartmented system requiring CD11b/CD18-ICAM-1 adherence, *J. Clin. Invest.,* 90, 1335, 1992.

35. **Hellberg, P. O. A., Kallskog, O., Wolgast, M., and Ojteg, G.,** Effects of neutrophil granulocytes on the inulin barrier of renal tubular epithelium after ischaemic damage, *Acta Physiol. Scand.,* 134, 313, 1988.

36. **Jaeschke, H., Farhood, A., and Smith, C. W.,** Neutrophils contribute to ischemia/reperfusion injury in rat liver *in vivo*, *FASEB J.*, 4, 3355, 1990.

37. **Kochanek, P. M. and Hallenbeck, J. M.,** Polymorphonuclear leukocytes and monocytes/macrophages in the pathogenesis of cerebral ischemia and stroke, *Stroke*, 23, 1367, 1992.

38. **Kofsky, E. R., Julia, P. L., Buckberg, G. D., Quillen, J. E., and Acar, C.,** Studies of controlled reperfusion after ischemia. XXII. Reperfusate composition: Effects of leukocyte depletion and blood cardioplegic reperfusates after acute coronary occlusion, *J. Thorac. Cardiovasc. Surg.*, 101, 350, 1991.

39. **Lucchesi, B. R., Mickelson, J. K., Homeister, J. W., and Jackson, C. V.,** Interaction of formed elements of blood with the coronary vasculature *in vivo*, *Fed. Proc.*, 46, 63, 1987.

40. **Mullane, K. M., Read, N., Salmon, J. A., and Moncada, S.,** Role of leukocytes in acute myocardial infarction in anesthetized dogs: Relationship to myocardial salvage by anti-inflammatory drugs, *J. Pharmacol. Exp. Ther.,* 228, 510, 1984.

41. **Olof, P., Hellberg, A., Kallskog, O. T., Ojteg, G., and Wolgast, M.,** Peritubular capillary permeability and intravascular RBC aggregation after ischemia: Effects of neutrophils, *Am. J. Physiol.,* 258, F1018, 1990.

42. **Romson, J. L., Hook, B. G., Kunkel, S. L., Abrams, G. D., Schork, M. A., and Lucchesi, B. R.,** Reduction of the extent of ischemic myocardial injury by neutrophil depletion in the dog, *Circulation,* 67, 1016, 1983.

43. **Shiga, Y., Onodera, H., Kogure, K., Yamasaki, Y., Yashima, Y., Syozuharae, H., and Sendo, F.,** Neutrophil as a mediator of ischemic edema formation in the brain, *Neurosci. Lett.,* 125, 110, 1991.

44. **Smith, S. M., Rutili, L. H., Perry, M. A., Grisham, M. B. Arfors, K. E., Granger, D. N., Kvietys, P. R., and Russel, J. M.,** Role of neutrophils in hemorrhagic shock-induced gastric mucosal injury in the rat, *Gastroenterology,* 93, 466, 1987.

45. **Grisham, M. B., Hernandez, L. A., and Granger, D. N.,** Adenosine inhibits ischemia/reperfusion-induced leukocyte adherence and extravasation, *Am. J. Physiol.,* 257, H1334, 1989.

46. **Korthuis, R. J., Carden, D. L., Kvietys, P. R., Shepro, D., and Fuseler, J.,** Phalloidin attenuates postischemic neutrophil infiltration and increased microvascular permeability, *J. Appl. Physiol.,* 71, 1261, 1991.

47. **Korthuis, R. J., Grisham, M. B., Zimmerman, B. J., Granger, D. N., and Taylor A. E.,** Vascular injury in dogs during ischemia/reperfusion: Improvement with ATP-MgCl$_2$ pretreatment, *Am. J. Physiol.,* 254, H702, 1988.

48. **Lehr, H. A., Guhlmann, A., Nolte, D., Keppler, D., and Messmer, K.,** Leukotrienes as mediators in ischemia-reperfusion injury in a microcirculation model in the hamster, *J. Clin. Invest.,* 87, 2036, 1991.

49. **Lehr, H. A., Hubner, C., Nolte, D., Kohlschutter, A., and Messmer, K.,** Dietary fish oil blocks the microcirculatory manifestations of ischemia-reperfusion injury in striated muscle in hamsters, *Proc. Natl. Acad. Sci. U.S.A.,* 88, 6726, 1991.

50. **Mullane, K.,** Neutrophil and endothelial changes in reperfusion injury, *TCM,* 1, 282, 1991.

51. **Nolte, D., Lehr, H. A., and Messmer, K.,** Adenosine inhibits postischemic leukocyte-endothelium interaction in postcapillary venules of the hamster, *Am. J. Physiol.,* 261, H651, 1991.

52. **Nolte, D., Lehr, H. A., Sack, F. U., and Messmer, K.,** Reduction of postischemic reperfusion injury by the vasoactive drug buflomedil, *Blood Vessels,* 28, 8, 1991.

53. **Romson, J. L., Hook, B. G., Rigot, V. H., Schork, M. A., Swanson, D. P., and Lucchesi, B. R.,** The effect of ibuprofen on accumulation of 111 Indium labelled platelets and leukocytes in experimental myocardial infarction, *Circulation,* 66, 1002, 1982.

54. **Simpson, P. J., Mickelson, J., Fantone, J. C., Gallagher, K. P., and Lucchesi, B. R.,** Iloprost inhibits neutrophil function *in vitro* and *in vivo* and limits experimental infarct size in canine heart, *Circ. Res.,* 60, 666, 1987.

55. **Simpson, P. J., Mitsos, S. E., Ventura, A., Gallagher, K. P., Fantone, J. C., Abrams, G. D., Schork, M. A., and Lucchesi, B. R.,** Prostacyclin protects ischemic reperfused myocardium in the dog by inhibition of neutrophil activation, *Am. Heart J.,* 113, 129, 1987.

56. **Arfors, K. E., Lundberg, C., Lindholm, L., et al.,** A monoclonal antibody to the membrane glycoprotein complex CD18 inhibits polymorphonuclear leukocyte accumulation and plasma leakage *in vivo, Blood,* 69, 338, 1987.

57. **Perry, M. A. and Granger, D. N.,** Role of CD11/CD18 in shear rate-dependent leukocyte-endothelial cell interactions in cat mesenteric venules, *J. Clin. Invest.,* 87, 1798, 1991.

58. **Schoenberg, M. H., Poch, B., Younes, M., Schwarz, A., Baczako, K., Lundberg, C., Haglund, U., and Berger, H.G.,** Involvement of neutrophils in postischaemic damage to the small intestine, *Gut,* 32, 905, 1991.

59. **Oliver, M. G., Specian, R. D., Perry, M. A., and Granger, D. N.,** Morphologic assessment of leukocyte-endothelial cell interactions in mesenteric venules subjected to ischemia and reperfusion, *Inflammation,* 15, 331, 1991.

60. **Suzuki, M., Inauen, W., Kvietys, P. R., Grisham, M. B., Meininger, C., Schalling, M. E., Granger, H. J., and Granger, D. N.,** Superoxide mediates reperfusion-induced leukocyte-endothelial cell interactions, *Am. J. Physiol.,* 257, H1740, 1989.

61. **Gomoll, A. W., Lekich, R. F., and Grove, R. I.,** Efficacy of a monoclonal antibody (MoAb 60.3) in reducing myocardial injury resulting from ischemia/reperfusion in the ferret, *J. Cardiovasc. Pharmacol.*, 17, 873, 1991.

62. **Seewaldt-Becker, E., Rothlein, R., and Dammgen, J. W.,** In *Leukocyte Adhesion Molecules,* Springer, T., Anderson, D. C., Rosenthal, A., and Rothlein, R., Eds., Springer-Verlag, New York, 1989, 138–148.

63. **Weselcouch, E. O., Grove, R.I., Demusz, C. D., and Baird, A. J.,** Effect of *in vivo* inhibition of neutrophil adherence on skeletal muscle function during ischemia in ferrets, *Am. J. Physiol.*, 258, G185, 1991.

64. **Goldman, G., Welbourn, R., Rothlein, R., Wiles, M., Kobzik, L., Valeri, C. R., Shepro, D., and Hechtman, H. B.,** Adherent neutrophils mediate permeability after atelectasis, *Ann. Surg.*, 216, 372, 1992.

65. **Clark, W. M., Madden, K. P., Rothlein, R., and Zivin, J. A.,** Reduction of central nervous system ischemic injury in rabbits using leukocyte adhesion antibody treatment, *Stroke,* 22, 877, 1991.

66. **Simpson, P. J., Todd, P. J., III, Fantone, J. C., Mickelson, J. K., Griffen, J. D., and Griffen, B. R.,** Reduction of experimental canine myocardial reperfusion injury by a monoclonal antibody (anti-Mo1, anti-CD11b) that inhibits leukocyte adhesion, *J. Clin. Invest.*, 81, 624, 1988.

67. **Schott, R. J., Nao, B. S., McClanahan, T. B., Simpson, P. J., Stirling, M.C., Todd, R. F., III, and Gallagher, K. P.,** (F(ab′)2 fragments of anti-Mo1 (904) monoclonal antibodies do not prevent myocardial stunning, *Circ. Res.,* 65, 1112, 1989.

68. **O'Neill, P. G., Charlat, M. L., Harley, C. J., Michael, L. H., Roberts, R., and Bolli, R.,** Neutrophil depletion fails to attenuate post ischemic myocardial dysfunction (abstract), *Circulation,* 74, II–349, 1986.

69. **Jaeschke, H., Farhood, A., Bautista, A. P., Spolarics, Z., Spitzer, J. J., and Smith, C. W.,** Functional inactivation of neutrophils with a Mac-1 (CD11b/CD18) monoclonal antibody protects against ischemia-reperfusion injury in rat liver, *Hepatology,* 17, 915, 1993.

70. **Rothlein, R., Barton, R. W., and Winquist, R.,** The role of intercellular adhesion molecule-1 (ICAM-1) in the inflammatory response, in *Cellular and Molecular Mechanisms of Inflammation,* Vol. 2, Vascular Adhesion Molecules, Academic Press, San Diego, 1991, 171–180.

71. **Clark, W. M., Madden, K. P., Rothlein, R., and Zivin, J. A.,** Reduction of central nervous system ischemic injury by monoclonal antibody to intercellular adhesion molecule, *J. Neurosurg.*, 75, 623, 1991.

72. **Smith, C. W., Entman, M. L., Lane, C. L., Beaudet, A. L., Ty, T. I., Youker, K., Hawkins, H. K., and Anderson, D. C.,** Adherence of neutrophils to canine cardiac myocytes *in vitro* is dependent on intercellular adhesion molecule-1, *J. Clin. Invest.,* 88, 1216, 1991.

73. **Ley, K., Gaehtgens, P., Fennie, C., Singer, M. S., Lasky, L. A., and Rosen, S. D.,** Lectin-like adhesion molecule-1 mediates leukocyte rolling in mesenteric venules *in vivo, Blood,* 77, 2553, 1991.

74. **Tozeren, A. and Ley, K.,** How do selectins mediate leukocyte rolling in venules, *Biophys. J.,* 63, 700, 1992.

75. **Bevilacqua, M. P., Corless, C., and Lo, S. K,** Endothelial-leukocyte adhesion molecule-1 (ELAM-1): A vascular selectin that regulates inflammation, in *Cellular and Molecular Mechanisms of Inflammation, Vol. 2: Vascular Adhesion Molecules,* Cochrane, C. G. and Gimbrone, M. G., Eds., Academic Press, San Diego, 1991, 1–14.

76. **McEver, R. P.,** Selectins: Novel adhesion receptors that mediate leukocyte adhesion during inflammation, *Thromb. Haem.,* 65, 223, 1991.

77. **Lawrence, M. B. and Springer, T. A.,** Leukocytes roll on a selectin at physiologic flow rates: Distinction from and prerequisite for adhesion through integrins, *Cell,* 65, 859, 1991.

78. **Bienvenu, K. and Granger, D. N.,** Molecular determinants of shear rate-dependent leukocyte adhesion in postcapillary venules, *Am. J. Physiol.,* 264, H1504, 1993.

79. **Dore, M., Korthuis, R. J., Granger, D. N., et al.,** P-selectin mediates spontaneous leukocyte rolling *in vivo, Blood,* 82, 1308, 1993.

80. **Lindbom, L., Xie, X., Raud, J., et al.,** Chemoattractant-induced leukocyte adhesion to vascular endothelium *in vivo* is critically dependent on initial leukocyte rolling, *Acta Physiol. Scand.* 146, 415, 1992.

81. **Carden, D. L., Young, J. A., and Granger, D. N.,** Pulmonary microvascular injury following intestinal ischemia/reperfusion: Role of P-selectin, *J. Appl. Physiol.,* 75, 2529, 1993.

82. **McEver, R. P.,** Leukocyte interactions mediated by GMP-140, in *Cellular and Molecular Mechanisms of Inflammation, Vol. 2: Vascular Adhesion Molecules,* Cochrane, C. G. and Gimbrone, M. G., Eds., Academic Press, San Diego, 1991, 15–30.

83. **Bevilacqua, M. P., Corless, C., and Lo, S. K.,** *Cellular and Molecular Mechanisms of Inflammation, Vol. 2: Vascular Adhesion Molecules,* Academic Press, San Diego, 1991, 1–14.

84. **Bevilacqua, M.P., Strengelin, S., Gimbrone, M. A., and Seed, B.,** Endothelial leukcoyte adhesion molecule 1: An inducible receptor for neutrophils related to complement regulatory proteins and lectins, *Science,* 243, 1160, 1989.

85. **Nolte, D., Hecht, R., Botzlar, A., Menger, M. D., Sinowatz, F., Messmer, K., and Vestweber, D.,** Role of adhesion proteins during postischemic reperfusion of mouse striated muscle, *Eur. Surg. Res.,* 25, 414, 1992.

86. **Hill, J., Lindsay, T., Rusche, J., Valeri, C. R., Shepro, D., and Hechtman, H. B.,** A Mac-1 antibody reduces liver and lung injury but not neutrophil sequestration after intestinal ischemia-reperfusion, *Surgery,* 112, 166, 1992.

87. **Pogetti, R. S., Moore, E. E., Moore, F. A., Koike, K., and Banerjee, A.,** Gut ischemia/reperfusion-induced liver dysfunction occurs despite sustained oxygen consumption, *J. Surg. Res.,* 52, 436, 1992.

88. **Welbourn, R., Goldman, G., Paterson, I. S., Shepro, D., and Hechtman, H. B.,** Pathophysiology of ischaemia reperfusion injury, central role of the neutrophil, *Br. J. Surg.,* 78, 651, 1991.

89. **Klausner, J. M., Anner, H., Paterson, I. S., Shepro, D., and Hechtman, H. B.,** Lower torso ischemia-induced lung injury is leukocyte dependent, *Ann. Surg.,* 209, 231, 1988.

90. **Welbourn, R., Goldman, G., Hill, J., Lindsay, T., Shepro, D., and Hechtman, H. B.,** Role of neutrophil adherence receptors (CD18) in lung permeability following lower torso ischemia, *Circ. Res.,* 71, 82, 1992.

91. **Horton, J. W. and White, D. J.,** Cardiac contractile injury after intestinal ischemia-reperfusion, *Am. J. Physiol.,* 261, H1164, 1991.

92. **Pogetti, R. S., Moore, E. E., Moore, F. A., and Banerjee, A.,** Liver injury is a reversible neutrophil-mediated event following gut ischemia, *Arch. Surg.,* 127, 175, 1992.

93. **Schmeling, D. J., Caty, M. G., Oldham, K. T., Guice, K. S., and Hinshaw, D. B.,** Evidence for neutrophil-related acute lung injury after intestinal ischemia-reperfusion, *Surgery,* 106, 195, 1989.

94. **Turnage, R. H., Bagnasco, J., Berger, J., Guice, K. S., Oldham, K. T., and Hinshaw, D. B.,** Hepatocellular oxidant stress following intestinal ischemia-reperfusion injury, *J. Surg. Res.,* 51, 467, 1991.

95. **Lasky, L. A.,** Selectins: Interpreters of cell-specific carbohydrate information during inflammation, *Science,* 258, 964, 1992.

96. **Lorant, D. E., Topham, M. K., Whatley, R. E., McEver, R. P., McIntyre, T. M., Prescott, S. M., and Zimmerman, G. M.,** Inflammatory roles of P-selectin, *J. Clin. Invest.,* 92, 559, 1993.

97. **Nagata, K., Tsuji, T., Todoroki, N., Katagiri, Y., Tanoue, K., Yamazaki, H., Hanai, N., and Irimura, T.,** Activated platelets induce superoxide anion release by monocytes and neutrophils through P-selectin (CD62), *J. Immunol.,* 151, 3267, 1993.

98. **Palabrica, T., Lobb, R., Furie, B. C., Aronovitz, M., Benjamin, C., Hsu, Y. M., Sajer, S. A., and Furie, D.,** Leukocyte accumulation promoting fibrin deposition is mediated *in vivo* by P-selectin on adherent platelets, *Nature,* 359, 848, 1992.

99. **Ames, A., Wright, L. W., Kowada, J. M., Thurston, J. M., and Majno, G. M.,** Cerebral ischemia. II. The no-reflow phenomenon, *Am. J. Pathol.,* 52, 437, 1968.

100. **Barrosa-Arranda, J., Schmid-Schonbein, G. W., Zweifach, B. W., and Engler, R. L.,** Granulocytes and the no-reflow phenomenon in irreversible hemorrhagic shock, *Circ. Res.,* 63, 437, 1988.

101. **del Zoppo, G. J., Schmid-Schonbein, G. W., Mori, E., Copeland, B. R., and Chang, C. M.,** Polymorphonuclear leukocytes occlude capillaries following middle cerebral artery occlusion and reperfusion in baboons, *Stroke,* 22, 1276, 1991.

102. **Engler, R. L., Dahlgren, M. D., Morris, D. D., Peterson, M. A., and Schmid-Schonbein, G. W.,** Role of leukocytes in response to acute myocardial ischemia and reflow in dogs, *Am. J. Physiol.,* 251, H314, 1986.

103. **Engler, R. L., Dahlgren, M. D., Peterson, M. A., Dobbs, A., and Schmid-Schonbein, G. W.,** Accumulation of polymorphonuclear leukocytes during 3-h experimental myocardial ischemia, *Am. J. Physiol.,* 251, H93, 1986.

104. **Engler, R. L., Schmid-Schonbein, G. W., and Pavelec, R. S.,** Leukocyte capillary plugging in myocardial ischemia and reperfusion in the dog, *Am. J. Pathol.*, 111, 98, 1983.

105. **Grogaard, B., Schurer, L., Gerdin, B., and Arfors, K. E.,** Delayed hypoperfusion after incomplete forebrain ischemia in the rat: The role of polymorphonuclear leukocytes, *J. Cereb. Blood Flow Metab.*, 9, 500, 1989.

106. **Strock, P. E. and Majno, G. M.,** Vascular responses to experimental tourniquet ischemia, *Surg. Gynecol. Obstet.*, 129, 309, 1969.

107a. **Quinones-Baldrich, W. J., Chervu, A., Hernandez, J. J., et al.,** Skeletal muscle function after ischemia: "No-reflow" versus reperfusion injury, *J. Surg. Res.*, 51, 5, 1991.

107b. **Messina, L. M.,** *In vivo* assessment of acute microvascular injury after reperfusion of ischemic tibialis anterior muscle of hamster, *J. Surg. Res.*, 48, 615, 1990.

108. **Harmon, J. W.,** The significance of local vascular phenomenon in production of ischemic necrosis in skeletal muscle, *Am. J. Pathol.*, 24, 625, 1941.

109. **Bagge, U., Amundson, B., and Lauritzen, C.,** White blood cell deformability and plugging of skeletal muscle capillaries in hemorrhagic shock, *Acta Physiol. Scand.*, 108, 159, 1980.

110. **Jerome, S. N., Akimitsu, T., and Korthuis, R. J.,** Leukocyte adhesion, edema, and the development of postischemic capillary no-reflow, *Am. J. Physiol.*, 267, H1329, 1994.

111. **Menger, M. D., Steiner, D., and Messmer, K.,** Microvascular ischemia-reperfusion injury in striated muscle: Significance of "no-reflow", *Am. J. Physiol.*, 263, H1892, 1992.

112. **Mazzoni, M. C., Borgstrom, P., Intaglietta, M., et al.,** Lumenal narrowing and endothelial cell swelling in skeletal muscle capillaries during hemorrhagic shock, *Circ. Shock*, 29, 27, 1989.

113. **Gidlof, A., Lewis, D. H., and Hammersen, F.,** The effect of prolonged total ischemia on the ultrastructure of human skeletal muscle capillaries: A morphometric analysis, *Int. J. Microcirc. Clin. Exp.*, 7, 67, 1987.

114. **Mazzoni, M. C., Borgstrom, P., Intaglietta, M., et al.,** Capillary narrowing in hemorrhagic shock is reduced by hyperosmotic saline-dextran reinfusion, *Circ. Shock*, 31, 407, 1990.

115. **Mazzoni, M. C., Intaglietta, M., Crogue, Jr., et al.,** Amiloride sensitive Na^+ pathways in capillary endothelial cell swelling during hemorrhagic shock, *J. Appl. Physiol.*, 73, 1467, 1992.

116. **House, S. D. and Lipowshy, H. H.,** Leukocyte-endothelium adhesion: Microhemodynamics in messentery of the cat, *Microvasc. Res.*, 34, 363, 1987.

117. **Hammersen, F., Barker, J. H., Gidlof, A., et al.,** The ultrastructure of the microvessels and their contents following ischemia and reperfusion, *Prog. Appl. Microcirc.*, 13, 1, 1989.

118. **Menger, M. D., Sack, F. U., Barker, J. H., et al.,** Quantitative analysis of microcirculatory disorders after prolonged ischemia in skeletal muscle. Therapeutic effects of prophylactic isovolemic hemodilution, *Res. Exp. Med.*, 188, 151, 1988.

119. **Schmid-Schonbein, G. W.,** Capillary plugging by granulocytes and the no-reflow phenomenon in the microcirculation, *Fed. Proc.*, 46, 2397, 1987.

120. **Menger, M. D., Pelikan, S., Steiner, D., et al.,** Microvascular ischemia-reperfusion injury in striated muscle: Significance of "reflow paradox", *Am. J. Physiol.*, 263, H1901, 1992.

121. **Granger, D. N., Benoit, J. N., Suzuki, M., et al.,** Leukocyte adherence to venular endothelium during ischemia-reperfusion, *Am. J. Physiol.*, 257, G683, 1989.

122. **Hansell, P., Borgstrom, P., and Arfors, K. E.,** Pressure-related capillary leukostasis following ischemia-reperfusion and hemorrhagic shock, *Am. J. Physiol.*, 265, H381, 1993.

123. **Nolte, D., Bayer, M., Lehr, H. A., Becker, M., Krombach, F., Kreimeier, U., and Messmer, K.,** Attenuation of postischemic microvascular disturbances in striated muscle by hyperosmolar saline dextran, *Am. J. Physiol.*, 263, H1411, 1992.

124. **Jerome, S. N., Akimitsu, T., Gute, D. C., and Korthuis, R. J.,** Ischemic preconditioning attenuates capillary no-reflow induced by prolonged ischemia and reperfusion, *Am. J. Physiol.*, 268, H2063, 1995.

125. **Akimitsu, T., Jerome, S. N., Gute, D. C., and Korthuis, R. J.,** Reactive oxygen species, neutrophil infiltration, and postischemic microvascular dysfunction, in *Reoxygenation Injury in Skeletal Muscle*, Fantini, G. O., Ed., Landis Publications, Austin, TX, 1994, 5–32.

126. **Vedder, N. B., Winn, R. K., Rice, C. L., and Harlan, J. M.,** *Perspectives in Shock Research: Metabolism, Immunology, Mediators, and Models*, Alan R. Liss, New York, 1987, 181–191.

127. **Mileski, W. J., Winn, R. K., Vedder, N. B., Pohlman, T. H., Harlan, J. M., and Rice, C. L.,** Inhibition of CD18-dependent neutrophil adherence reduces organ injury after hemorrhagic shock in primates, *Surgery*, 108, 206, 1990.

128. **Vedder, N. B., Winn, R. K., Rice, C. L., Chi, E., Arfors, K.-E., and Harlan, J. M.,** A monoclonal antibody to the adherence promoting leukocyte glycoprotein CD18 reduces organ injury and improves survival from hemorrhagic shock and resuscitation in rabbits, *J. Clin. Invest.*, 81, 939, 1988.

129. **Heflin, A. C. and Brigham, K. L.,** Prevention by granulocyte depletion of increased vascular permeability of sheep lung following endotoxemia, *J. Clin. Invest.*, 68, 1253, 1981.

130. **Matsuda, T., Rubinstein, I., Robbins, R. A., Koyama, S., Joyner, W. L., and Rennard, S. I.,** Role of neutrophils in endotoxin-mediated microvascular injury in hamsters, *J. Appl. Physiol.*, 71, 307, 1991.

131. **Winn, R., Maunder, R., Chi, E., and Harlan, J.,** Neutrophil depletion does not prevent lung edema after endotoxin infusion in goats, *J. Appl. Physiol.*, 62, 116, 1987.

132. **Baumgartner, J., Glauser, M. P., McCutchen, J. A., Van Melle, G., Ziegler, E. J., Klauber, R., Vogt, M., Muehlen, E., Leuthy, R., Chioler, R., and Geroulanos, S.,** Prevention of gram-negative shock and death in surgical patients by antibody to endotoxincore glycolipid, *Lancet*, II, 59, 1985.

133. **Calandra, T., Glauser, M. P., Schellekens, J., and Verhoef, J.,** Swiss-Dutch J5 Immunoglobulin Study Group. Treatment of gram-negative septic shock with human IgG antibody to *Escherichia coli* J5. A prospective, double-blind, randomized trial, *J. Infect. Dis.*, 158, 312, 1988.

134. **Dal Nogare, A. R.,** Southwestern internal medicine conference: Septic shock, *Am. J. Med. Sci.*, 302, 50, 1991.

135. **Sheppard, B. C., Fraker, D. L., and Norton, J. A.,** Prevention and treatment of endotoxin and sepsis lethality with recombinant human tumor necrosis factor, *Surgery*, 106, 156, 1989.

136. **Shiga, Y., Onodera, H., Kogure, K., Yamasaki, Y., Yashima, Y., Syozuharae, H., and Sendo, H.,** Neutrophil as a mediator of ischemic edema formation in the brain, *Neuroscience Lett.*, 125, 110, 1991.

137. **Nathan, C. and Sporn, M.,** Cytokines in context, *J. Cell. Biol.*, 113, 981, 1991.

138. **Tonnenson, M. G.,** Neutrophil-endothelial cell interactions: Mechanisms of neutrophil adherence to vascular endothelium, *J. Invest. Dermatol.*, 93, 53S, 1989.

139. **Venezio, F. R., Westenfelder, G. O., and Phair, J. P.,** The adherence of polymorphonuclear leukocytes in patients with sepsis, *J. Infect. Dis.*, 145, 351, 1982.

140. **Walsh, C. J., Leeper-Woodford, S. K., Carey, P. D., Cook, D. J., Bechard, D. E., Fowler, A. A., and Sugarman, H. J.,** CD18 adhesion receptors, tumor necrosis factor, and neutropenia during septic lung injury, *J. Surg. Res.*, 50, 323, 1991.

141. **Thomas, J. R., Harlan, J. M., Rice, C. L., and Winn, R. K.,** Role of leukocyte CD11/CD18 complex in endotoxic and septic shock in rabbits, *J. Appl. Physiol.*, 73, 1510, 1992.

142. **Walsh, C. J., Carey, P. D., Cook, D. J., Bechard, D. E., Fowler, A. A., and Sugerman, H. J.,** Anti-CD18 antibody attenuates neutropenia and alveolar-capillary membrane injury during gram-negative sepsis, *Surgery*, 110, 205, 1991.

143. **Jaeschke, H., Farhood, A., and Smith, C. W.,** Neutrophil-induced liver cell injury in endotoxin shock is CD11b/CD18-dependent mechanism, *Am. J. Physiol.*, 261, G1051, 1991.

144. **Crowley, J. P., Dennis, R. C., Pivacek, L., Metzger, J., Carvalho, A., and Valeri, C. R.,** Effects of granulocytopenia on the hemodynamic responses of dogs during *E. coli* bacteremia, *Circ. Shock*, 22, 91, 1987.

145. **Sharar, S. R., Winn, R. K., Murray, C. E., Harlan, J. M., and Rice, C. L.,** A CD18 monoclonal antibody increases the severity of subcutaneous abscess formation after high-dose Staphylococcus aureus injection in rabbits, *Surgery*, 110, 213, 1991.

146. **Mileski, W. J., Winn, R. K., Harlan, J. M., and Rice, C. L.,** Transient inhibition of neutrophil adherence with the anti-CD18 monoclonal antibody 60.3 does not increase mortality rates in abdominal sepsis, *Surgery*, 109, 497, 1991.

147. **Britt, L. D., Dascombe, W. H., and Rodriguez, A.,** New horizons in management of hypothermia and frostbite injury, *Surg. Clin. N. Am.*, 71, 345, 1991.

148. **Mileski, W. J., Raymond, J. F., Winn, R. K., Harlan, J. M., and Rice, C. R.,** Inhibition of leukocyte adherence and aggregation for treatment of severe cold injury in rabbits, *J. Appl. Physiol.*, 74, 1432, 1993.

149. **Deitch, E. A., Lu, Q., Da-Zhong, X., and Special, R. D.,** Effect of local and systemic burn microenvironment on neutrophil activation as assessed by complement receptor expression and morphology, *J. Trauma*, 30, 259, 1990.

150. **Nelson, R., Hasslen, S., Ahrenholz, D., Haus, E., and Solem, L.,** Influence of minor thermal injury on expression of complement receptor CF3 on human neutrophils, *Am. J. Pathol.*, 125, 563, 1986.

151. **Mileski, W., Borgstrom, D., Lightfoot, E., Rothlein, R., Fautnes, R., Lipsky, P., and Baxter, C.,** Inhibition of leukocyte-endothelial adherence following thermal injury, *J. Surg. Res.*, 52, 334, 1992.

152. **Ianyi, B., Hansen, H. E., and Olsen, T. S.,** Postcapillary venule-like transformation of peritubular capillaries in acute renal allograft rejection: An ultrastructural study, *Arch. Pathol. Lab. Med.*, 116, 1062, 1992.

153. **Pearl, J. M., Drinkwater, D. C., Laks, H., Stein, D. G., Capouya, E. R., and Bhuta, S.,** Leukocyte-depleted reperfusion of transplanted human hearts prevents ultrastructural evidence of reperfusion injury, *J. Surg. Res.*, 52, 298, 1992.

154. **Adams, D. H., Hubscher, S. G., Shaw, J., Rothlein, R., and Neuberger, J. M.,** Intercellular adhesion molecule 1 on liver allografts during rejection, *Lancet*, ii, 1122, 1989.

155. **Adams, D. H., Wang, L. F., Burnett, D., Stockley, R. A., and Neuberger, J. M.,** Neutrophil activation — An important cause of tissue damage during liver allograft rejection?, *Transplantation*, 50, 86, 1990.

156. **Briscoe, D. M., Schoen, F. J., Rice, G. E., Bevilaqua, M. P., and Pober, J. S.,** Induced expression of endothelial-leukocyte adhesion molecules in human cardiac allografts, *Transplantation*, 51, 537, 1991.

157. **Elner, V. M., Elner, S. G., Pavilack, M. A., Todd, R. F., III, Yue, B. Y., and Huber, A. R.,** Intercellular adhesion molecule-1 in human corneal endothelium, *Am. J. Pathol.* 138, 525, 1991.

158. **Hubscher, S. G. and Adams, D. H.,** ICAM-1 expression in normal liver, *J. Clin. Pathol.*, 44, 438, 1990.

159. **Matsuno, T., Sakagami, K., and Orita, K.,** Expression of intercellular adhesion molecule-1 and perforin on kidney allograft rejection, *Transplant. Proc.*, 24, 1306, 1992.

160. **Omura, T., Ishikura, H., Nakajima, Y., Kimura, J., Ito, K., Isai, H., Tamatani, T., Miyasaka, M., Yoshiki, T., and Uchino, J.,** The expression of LFA-1/ICAM-1 in liver transplantation in rats, *Transplant. Proc.*, 24, 1618, 1992.

161. **Sedmak, D. D. and Orosz, C. G.,** The role of vascular endothelial cells in transplantation, *Arch. Pathol. Lab. Med.*, 115, 260, 1991.

162. **Takei, Y., Marzi, I., Gao, W., Gores, G. J., Lemasters, J. J., and Thurman, R. G.,** Leukocyte adhesion and cell death following orthotopic liver transplantation in the rat, *Transplantation*, 51, 959, 1991.

163. **Flavin, T., Ivens, K., Rothlein, R., et al.,** Monoclonal antibodies against intercellular adhesion molecule 1 prolong cardiac allograft survival in cynomolgus monkeys, *Transplant. Proc.*, 23, 533, 1991.

164. **Wee, S. L., Cosimi, A. B., Preffer, F. I., Raanes, R., Conti, D., and Colvin, R. B.,** Functional consequences of anti-ICAM-1 (CD54) in cynomolgus monkeys with renal allografts, *Transplant. Proc.*, 23, 279, 1991.

165. **Byrne, J. G., Smith, W. J., Murphy W. J., Couper, G. S., Appleyard, R. F., and Cohn, L. J.,** Complete prevention of myocardial stunning, contracture, low-reflow, and edema after heart transplantation by blocking neutrophil adhesion molecules during reperfusion, *J. Thoracic Cardiovasc. Surg.*, 104, 1589, 1992.

166. **Le Mauff, B., Hourmant, M., Rougier, J. P., Hirn, M., Dantal, J., Baatard, R., Cantarovich, D., Jacques, Y., and Soulillou, J. P.,** Effect of anti-LFA1 (CD11a) monoclonal antibodies in acute rejection in human kidney transplantation, *Transplantation*, 52, 291, 1991.

167. **Asako, H., Kubes, P., Baethge, B,A., Wolf, R. E., and Granger, D. N.,** Reduction of leukocyte adherence and emigration by cyclosporine and L683,590 (FK506) in postcapillary venules, *Transplantation*, 54, 686, 1992.

168. **Slocum, M. M. and Granger, D. N.,** Early mucosal and microvascular changes in feline intestinal transplants, *Gastroenterology*, 105, 1761, 1993.

169. **Bienvenu, K., Russell, J., and Granger, D. N.,** Leukotriene B_4 mediates shear rate-dependent leukocyte adhesion in mesenteric venules, *Circ. Res.*, 71, 906, 1992.

170. **Lewis, R. E. and Granger, H. J.,** Diapedesis and the permeability of venous microvessels to protein macromolecules: The impact of leukotriene B_4, *Microvasc. Res.*, 35, 27, 1988.

171. **Doukas, J., Shepro, D., and Hechtman, H. B.,** Vasoactive amines directly modify endothelial cells to affect polymorphonuclear leukocyte diapedesis *in vitro, Blood,* 69, 1563, 1987.

172. **Paterson, I. S., Klausner, J. M., Goldman, G., Welbourn, R., Alexander, J. S., Shepro, D., and Hechtman, H. B.,** The endothelial cell cytoskeleton modulates extravascular polymorphonuclear leukocyte accumulations *in vivo, Microvasc. Res.,* 38, 49, 1989.

173. **Asako, H., Wolf, R., Granger, D. N., and Korthuis, R. J.,** Phalloidin reduces leukocyte emigration and vascular permeability in postcapillary venules, *Am. J. Physiol.,* 263, H1637, 1992.

174. **Kishimoto, T. K.,** A dynamic model for neutrophil localization to inflammatory sites, *J. NIH Res.,* 3, 75, 1991.

175. **Kishimoto, T. K., Jutila, M. A., Berg, E. L., et al.,** Neutrophil Mac-1 and MEL-14 adhesion proteins are inversely regulated by chemotactic factors, *Science,* 245, 1238, 1991.

Chapter 7

The Adult Respiratory Distress Syndrome and the Microcirculation

Michael A. Matthay

CONTENTS

I. INTRODUCTION

The adult respiratory distress syndrome (ARDS) is a common clinical syndrome of acute respiratory failure that is associated with a high mortality (about 60%).[1-3] This syndrome of acute respiratory failure is an excellent example of how injury to the microcirculation of the lung results in a serious clinical disorder.

The primary purpose of this chapter is to discuss the pathogenesis of ARDS as an example of a pathologic condition that occurs primarily because of injury to the pulmonary microcirculation. The chapter will be divided into three sections. The first section describes the clinical manifestations of ARDS including the clinical disorders that predispose the development of ARDS. The second section will consider the pathologic basis for ARDS with an emphasis on mechanisms of injury as they relate to the pulmonary microcirculation. The third section discusses the physiologic basis of current treatment modalities. This latter section also considers future therapeutic options that may be useful in minimizing injury to the pulmonary microcirculation and thereby preventing the development of ARDS.

II. CLINICAL FEATURES OF ARDS

ARDS is a syndrome of acute respiratory failure that is characterized by severe arterial hypoxemia that is associated with bilateral infiltrates on the chest radiograph (Figure 1).[4,5] A recent North American-European consensus conference has agreed on the following definition for ARDS: $PaO_2/FiO_2 < 200$ and the presence of bilateral pulmonary infiltrates.[6] Left heart failure should be excluded by clinical criteria or with the measurement of a pulmonary arterial wedge pressure <18 mmHg. The majority of patients who meet these criteria will need positive pressure ventilation in order to treat the severe arterial hypoxemia as well as the high work of breathing that is associated with ARDS.[7] The primary etiology of the arterial hypoxemia is related to the development of noncardiogenic pulmonary edema that is also associated with atelectasis. Consequently, the lungs are edematous and have a marked decrease in their normal compliance. Thus, higher than normal airway pressures are required to inflate the lungs.[8]

The clinical disorders that are associated with ARDS have been carefully identified in several studies.[4,9,10] The most common clinical disorder is sepsis syndrome, either from a pulmonary or nonpulmonary source.[2,8,9] By definition, sepsis syndrome requires that the

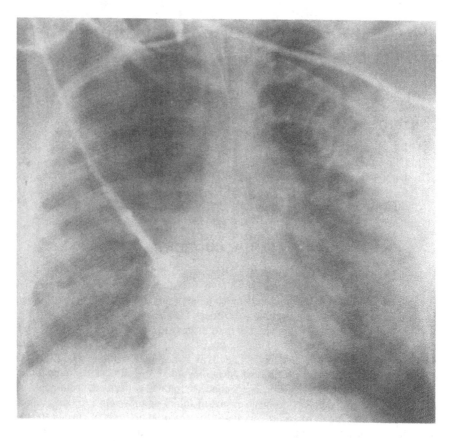

Figure 1 Typical appearance of increased permeability edema in a 22-year-old woman with adult respiratory distress syndrome and a high protein ratio. The cardiac size and vascular pedicle width (5.8 cm) are normal. The distribution of edema is peripheral, with prominent air bronchograms. There are no interstitial changes. Radiographic diagnosis was increased permeability edema.

patient have hyperthermia (T > 38.3°C) or hypothermia (T < 35.0°C) in association with systemic hypotension (systolic BP < 100 mmHg) or clinical evidence of sepsis as manifested by metabolic acidosis, decreased mental status, and/or oliguria with renal failure.[10-12] The second most common cause of ARDS is aspiration of gastric contents.[4,9,10] Perhaps the third most common cause, depending on the patient population that has been studied, are those individuals who have suffered major trauma requiring emergency surgery and multiple transfusions of blood products.[9] Other clinical disorders associated with ARDS include patients with a severe viral or opportunistic pneumonia, victims of near-drowning, patients who have taken an overdose of hypnotic or sedative drugs, and some patients following major cardiac or vascular surgery.

Prognosis for recovery in ARDS depends on multiple factors. Patients who develop ARDS in association with sepsis have a significantly higher mortality than those who develop ARDS from aspiration of gastric contents, following major trauma, or from a primary pneumonia that is not associated with sepsis syndrome.[2,10,11] There are several other factors that adversely affect the prognosis for survival including age over 60, the presence of nonpulmonary organ failure (such as renal failure, liver failure, hematologic failure, neurologic failure), metabolic acidosis at the onset of ARDS, and an underlying unfavorable medical diagnosis such as the presence of a hematologic malignancy or metastatic carcinoma.[1-3,10,12] As will be discussed in the section under treatment, therapeutic maneuvers for patients with ARDS must be directed both at treatment of the underlying cause of ARDS (such as sepsis) as well as providing supportive therapy for the respiratory failure and any other nonpulmonary organ failure, such as dialysis for renal failure. Prognosis may also be related to the severity of acute lung injury itself. For example, there is good evidence from our own clinical studies that some patients who develop ARDS have a more limited degree of acute lung injury with a greater capacity to resolve some of the pulmonary edema during the early phase of the syndrome. These patients may have less severe endothelial as well as less severe epithelial injury to the lung.[13]

III. PATHOGENESIS AND MECHANISMS OF ARDS

For over 25 years, there has been an intensive effort to understand the basic mechanisms that lead to ARDS in both clinical as well as in experimental studies. The experimental work has focused on models of acute lung injury that have been designed to reproduce many of the features of the clinical syndrome. Of course, the experimental models have been limited because they do not reproduce the entire clinical condition that leads to the development of ARDS. Nevertheless, the information that has been generated from the experimental work has provided a sound pathophysiologic understanding of the basic mechanisms of acute lung injury.

The physiologic basis for filtration of liquid and protein across any semipermeable barrier was proposed by Starling in 1986.[14] Starling's equation has been used extensively in the last 25 years for both experimental and clinical purposes to understand the pathophysiologic basis for the pulmonary edema that occurs in ARDS. The Starling equation predicts that the net flow of liquid across a semipermeable barrier is the product of the driving pressure (both hydrostatic and osmotic pressures) and the conductance, or permeability, of the barrier. The equation is:

$$Q_f = K[(P_{mv} - P_{pmv}) - \sigma \, (pmv - ppmv)] \tag{1}$$

In this equation, Q_f identifies the net liquid filtration rate and K is the conductance or the filtration coefficient across the barrier. The hydrostatic pressures are described by P_{mv} for the microvascular hydrostatic pressure and P_{pmv} for hydrostatic pressure in the perimicrovascular or lung interstitial space. The protein osmotic pressure is described by p. The term pmv designates the osmotic pressure within the circulation, and ppmv indicates the protein osmotic pressure in the perimicrovascular or lung interstitial space. In the setting of acute lung injury, the primary abnormality that leads to the development of pulmonary edema is an increase in the permeability of the barrier, which is indicated by the reflection coefficient (σ).[15-18]

The normal value for σ is estimated to be approximately 0.9 for the lung endothelium. In experimental acute lung injury and in clinical ARDS, the reflection coefficient is abnormally low, resulting in the movement of greater quantities of liquid and protein into the interstitium of the lung. Thus, the basic mechanism of edema fluid formation in the lung is related to an alteration in the normal barrier properties or permeability of the lung endothelial barrier. Consequently, the concentration of edema fluid in the lung in cases of increased permeability is between 80 and 100% of plasma protein concentration.[13,15,18] Several experimental and clinical studies have also emphasized, of course, that a simultaneous increase in the hydrostatic pressure in the microcirculation of the lung (P_{mv}) will markedly increase the degree of pulmonary edema that will form in the lung if there is an alteration in the normal barrier properties of the pulmonary endothelium.[19-21]

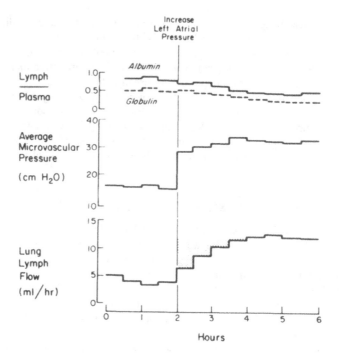

Figure 2 Time course of the effect of increased pulmonary microvascular pressure on lung lymph flow and the lymph-to-plasma protein concentration ratios in unanesthetized sheep. After 2 h of baseline study, left atrial pressure was elevated by inflating a chronically implanted balloon. Note the rise in lymph flow is more than double baseline values, and the lymph-to-plasma protein concentrations falls. (From Staub, N. C., *Circ. Res.*, 37, 271–284, 1975.)

In the lung, edema fluid first accumulates in the interstitium, where it can be removed by either lung lymphatics or directly across the visceral pleura of the lung into the pleural space. If the volume of fluid exceeds 500 ml in both lungs in man, then some of the edema fluid will usually move through the normally tight alveolar epithelium with flooding of the distal airspaces of the lung with protein-rich edema fluid that will then result in a severe decrease in gas exchange with marked arterial hypoxemia.[18,22,23] This sequence of events leads to clinical acute respiratory failure. In addition, the protein-rich pulmonary edema fluid in the airspaces of ARDS patients may be inactive surfactant, an important constituent of the normal alveolar space that prevents alveolar collapse by reducing surface tension.[24] Thus, the development of protein-rich pulmonary edema can lead to inactivation of surfactant, which will result in atelectasis or collapse of alveoli.[25]

Investigators at our institution as well as other medical centers have used a variety of animal models to examine the mechanisms of acute lung injury. One of the most useful models has been to study sheep and goats because it is possible to measure nearly pure lung lymph flow from these animals. Measurement of the volume of lung lymph flow as well as the protein concentration in the lymph makes it possible to measure the quantity and protein concentration of fluid filtration across the microcirculation of the lung. If the cause of increased transvascular fluid flow in the lung is elevated left atrial pressure, as in clinical left heart failure or volume overload, then the lung lymph flow will increase, but the ratio of protein in the lymph compared to plasma will decline (Figure 2).[14] Lymph flow increases because of the rise in P_{mv}, as predicted by Starling (Equation 1). The concentration of protein in the lung lymph declines because the endothelial barrier or the reflection coefficient(s) of the lung microcirculation is normal, thus the increase in transvascular fluid flux primarily

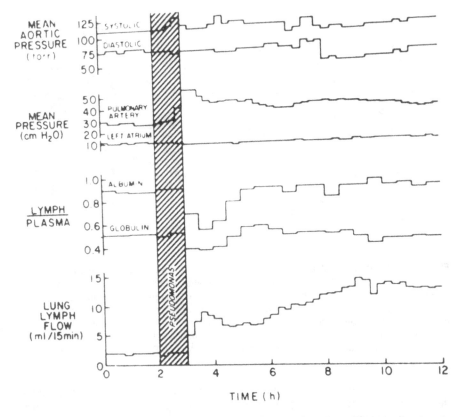

MEAN AORTIC PRESSURE (torr)

125 SYSTOLIC
100 DIASTOLIC
75
50

MEAN PRESSURE (cm H₂O)

50
40 PULMONARY ARTERY
30
20 LEFT ATRIUM
10

LYMPH PLASMA

1.0 ALBUMIN
0.8
0.6 GLOBULIN
0.4

LUNG LYMPH FLOW (ml/15min)

15
10
5
0

PSEUDOMONAS

TIME (h)

0   2   4   6   8   10   12

Figure 3 Effects of infusion of *Pseudomonas aeruginosa* on lung vascular pressures, lymph flow, and lymph-to-plasma protein concentration in unanesthetized sheep. Note that there is an initial rise in lymph flow associated with a fall in the lymph-to-plasma protein concentration ratio when pulmonary artery pressure had doubled. Then, there is a later, more dramatic increase in lung lymph flow with a return of the lymph-to-plasma protein concentration ratios to baseline levels when the pulmonary artery pressure has returned toward baseline levels. This is the late phase of increased lung vascular permeability with protein-rich lymph. A similar response occurs with *E. coli* endotoxin. (From Brigham, K. L., *J. Clin. Invest.*, 54, 792–804, 1974.)

consists of water and solutes, not protein. Therefore, clinically, the pulmonary edema fluid protein concentration from patients with left heart failure has a relatively low protein concentration (40–60%) compared to the plasma protein concentration.[13,16]

In order to simulate some of the clinical syndromes that lead to acute respiratory failure, several studies have been carried out in sheep and goats in which live bacteria or endotoxin, an important product of bacteria, have been given intravenously. The results of these studies demonstrate that following these clinically relevant insults, there is a marked increase in protein-rich lung lymph flow, indicating that there has been injury to the endothelial barrier of the microcirculation (Figure 3).[14] If there is injury to the lung microcirculation, as in endotoxemia, sepsis, or aspiration of gastric contents, then the lung lymph flow will markedly increase and the concentration of protein in the lymph compared to plasma will stay the same or increase, thus demonstrating that there is increased permeability to protein of the lung microcirculation with a decrease in σ or the reflection coefficient of the lung endothelial barrier (Figure 3).[14,16] Sometimes, injury to the alveolar epithelial barrier occurs in the experimental setting, although the normally tight epithelial barrier is more resistant to injury than the lung endothelial barrier.[26-28]

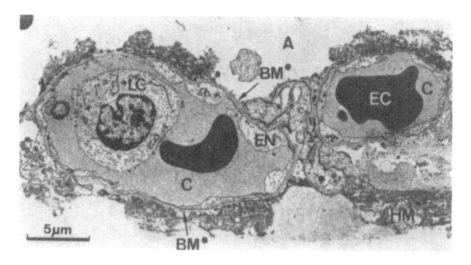

Figure 4 Ultrastructure of a lung specimen, showing the alveolar septum with extensive epithelial destruction in a 19-year-old woman who died after 4 days of fulminant capillary leakage as a result of septicemia. Note the irregularly swollen and damaged endothelium. Also note that there is a loss of the epithelial cell lining in some areas where the basement membrane is exposed to the alveolar space. A = alveolar space; BM = denuded basement membrane; C = capillary; EC = intravascular erythrocyte; EN = swollen endothelial cell; HM = hyaline membrane; LC = intravascular leukocyte. (From Bachofen, M. and Weibel, R. R., *Clin. Chest Med.*, 3, 35–46, 1982.)

The basic mechanisms responsible for the injury to the endothelial barrier depend on the associated cause of acute lung injury. For example, in the presence of primary bacterial pneumonia, work from our own research group indicates that products of the bacteria probably play an important role in causing the initial lung injury.[29] However, in the presence of bacterial sepsis with systemic hypotension, several studies suggest that some of the injury may depend on the release of toxic to oxygen products from neutrophils that adhere to the pulmonary microcirculation in the presence of sepsis.[30] Also, in aspiration of gastric contents, some of the injury may be neutrophil dependent, although there is a component of direct injury that also depends on the low pH content of the aspirated material as well as lung injury that may occur from a bacterial pneumonia that complicates the aspiration of gastric and oral pharyngeal contents. Regardless of the exact mechanism of acute lung injury, ultrastructural pathological studies of the lungs from patients who have died from ARDS always demonstrate widespread lung endothelial injury (Figure 4).[31,32] The list of possible mediators of lung injury can be broken down into effects from circulating cells, resident lung cells, as well as from circulating mediators (Table 1). The interaction of these mechanisms in causing injury to lung endothelial barrier may be complex. For example, intravascular bacteremia with septicemia will cause the release of cytokines, such as tumor necrosis factors, from circulating monocytes, which can upregulate integrin adhesion molecules on neutrophils (like the CD18,11 complex) and also upregulate selection binding molecules on the endothelium (such as E-selectin and P-selectin).[33-35] Neutrophils will then adhere in the lung and systemic microcirculation. These activated neutrophils can then cause endothelial injury through both release of their own intracellular enzymes as well as through generation of toxic oxygen radicals. Also, the bacterial products of the infecting organism causing the septicemia may cause direct lung endothelial injury. As will be discussed in the next section, the ideal treatment would be one that prevented, reduced, or reversed the injury to the lung microcirculation.

Table 1 Cellular and Humoral Factors That Have Been Implicated in Mediating Injury to the Lung Microcirculation in Acute Lung Injury

Circulating Cells:	Neutrophils
	Platelets
	Monocytes
Resident Lung Cells:	Alveolar macrophages
	Fibroblasts
Possible Mediators:	Complement system
	Prostaglandins
	Oxygen radicals
	Proteases
	Cytokines
	Bacterial products

IV. CURRENT AND FUTURE TREATMENT OF ARDS

Initial treatment for patients with ARDS is directed toward improving gas exchange. In order to accomplish this objective, most patients require mechanical ventilation with positive pressure ventilation. Standard therapy has been to provide tidal volumes in the range of 12–15 ml/kg, with positive end expiratory pressure (PEEP) between 5 and 15 cm H_2O.[7,8,36] With this approach, most patients will have an improvement in their arterial oxygenation and it will be possible to lower the fraction of inspired oxygen from 1.0 to a lower level. This is regarded as an important objective because high fractions of oxygen for an extended period of time may cause additional lung injury.[37,38] However, the guidelines for what levels of oxygen delivery are safe have never been clearly defined. Interestingly, oxygen toxicity experimentally first affects the endothelial barrier of the lung and then results in injury to the epithelial barrier along with evidence of interstitial fibrosis. These findings are characteristic of many patients with ARDS, so it is difficult to distinguish oxygen toxicity from the primary lung injury itself.

Additional therapy is directed to managing the patient's hemodynamics and fluid requirements. In general, if possible, it is advisable to maintain the pulmonary arterial wedge pressure in the normal range so as not to further increase the quantity of pulmonary edema that forms in the lung in the presence of increased lung endothelial permeability.[36,39] This objective may be difficult to achieve because some patients, particularly those with septicemia, may need a higher filling pressure in order to maintain systemic arterial pressure and cardiac output to perfuse the kidneys and other vital systemic organs.[36]

Therapy is also directed at attempts to treat the primary cause of the lung injury. If the patient has a primary pneumonia, antibiotic therapy should be given to treat this problem. Sometimes, it is difficult to make the exact diagnosis of the etiology of the pneumonia, particularly if the patient is immunocompromised. Diagnostic evaluations with bronchoscopy and bronchoalveolar lavage may help reveal specific pathogens that can be treated directly. In other patients, the cause of lung injury may be related to bacterial sepsis. Broad spectrum antibiotics are given to treat the septicemia. In some cases, surgical therapy is needed to treat the primary source of infection, such as a perforated viscus in the abdomen or a collection of intraabdominal pus from a ruptured appendix.

The limitation of current treatment is that there is no specific therapy that can be given to reduce or minimize the severity of lung injury. For example, because of their global antiinflammatory effects, high doses of glucocorticoids have been evaluated. However, in several well-controlled studies, high doses of glucocorticoids did not alter the severity of ARDS or the mortality associated with ARDS.[40,41] New therapies are being evaluated currently, most of which are designed to reduce the severity of injury to the pulmonary microcirculation. For instance, as already discussed, neutrophils have been implicated as an important cellular factor in mediating injury to the lung endothelium in some causes of ARDS, such as sepsis or aspiration-induced lung injury.[30] Therefore, new treatments are being developed that reduce or prevent neutrophil adhesion to the lung endothelium by blocking either one of the integrin or binding sites on the neutrophil or the selection binding sites on the endothelium in order to prevent neutrophil-dependent injury to the pulmonary microcirculation.[36] Another approach is to inhibit release of interleukin-8, the major chemotactic peptide that drives transendothelial migration of neutrophils in the lung.[42] However, these treatments may have unfavorable effects clinically if they significantly reduce the patient's ability to recover from an extravascular source of infection (peritonitis, pneumonitis, cellulitis). Clinical trials will be needed to assess their potential therapeutic value.[43]

V. SUMMARY

ARDS is a complex clinical syndrome of hypoxemic acute respiratory failure that is associated with several disorders including sepsis, aspiration, drug overdose, and major trauma.[1,2,4,5,10] In most, if not all clinical cases of ARDS, the initial site of injury is the pulmonary microcirculation with a subsequent increase in lung endothelial permeability. This damage to pulmonary circulation leads to exudation of protein-rich edema fluid and inflammatory cells into the interstitium and eventually into the airspaces of the lung.[13,16,31] Current treatment is primarily supportive with supplemental oxygen, positive pressure ventilation, fluids, and vasoactive agents as needed to treat systemic hypotension, particularly in patients with sepsis syndrome.[36,39,44] Mortality is high (60%), partly because ARDS is often complicated by nonpulmonary organ failure and recurrent infections.[2,12,45] Although no specific antiinflammatory therapy has yet been proven to be effective clinically, some promising new therapeutic strategies are being tested.[33,42,46] These and other new treatment modalities are designed to reduce the initial injury to the lung microcirculation and the alveolar epithelium early in the course of ARDS.

Another strategy to increase survival in ARDS is to design treatment modalities that will enhance recovery from ARDS, both in terms of recovery of the endothelium and the epithelium following acute lung injury. This concept includes remodeling of the lung since acute lung injury often involves the loss of the microcirculation as well as the normal alveolar epithelium.[31,32] Growth factors and cytokines undoubtedly play an important role in this process.[28] More basic and clinical research is needed to better understand both the mechanisms of injury and recovery to the lung microcirculation in acute lung injury syndromes.[47]

ACKNOWLEDGMENTS

The author appreciates the assistance of Jill Richardson and Barbara Walker in the preparation of this manuscript.

REFERENCES

1. **Fowler, A. A., Hamman, R. F., Zerbe, G. O., Benson, K. N., and Hyers, T. M.,** Adult respiratory distress syndrome: Prognosis after onset, *Am. Rev. Resp. Dis.*, 132, 472–478, 1985.
2. **Montgomery, A. B., Stager, M. A., Carrico, C. J., and Hudson, L. D.,** Causes of mortality in patients with the adult respiratory distress syndrome, *Am. Rev. Respir. Dis.*, 132, 485–489, 1985.
3. **Gee, M. H., Gottlieb, J. E., Albertone, K. H., et al.,** Physiology of aging related to outcome of the adult respiratory distress syndrome, *J. Appl. Physiol.*, 69, 822–829, 1990.

4. **Fowler, A. A., Hamman, R. F., Good, J. T., Petty, T. L., and Hyers, T.,** Adult respiratory distress syndrome: Risks with common predispositions, *Ann. Int. Med.*, 98, 593–597, 1983.

5. **Murray, J. F., Matthay, M. A., Luce, J. M., and Flick, M. R.,** An expanded definition of the adult respiratory distress syndrome, *Am. Rev. Respir. Dis.*, 138, 720–723, 1988.

6. **Bernard, G. R. and Artigas, A.,** European-American consensus conference on ARDS, *Am. Rev. Respir. Dis.*, in press, 1995.

7. **Ralph, D. D., Robertson, H. T., Weaver, L. J., and Hudson, L. D.,** Distribution of ventilation and perfusion during positive end-expiratory pressure in adult respiratory distress syndrome, *Am. Rev. Respir. Dis.*, 131, 54–60, 1985.

8. **Tantucci, C., Corbeil, C., Chasse, M., Robatto, F. M., Nava, S., Braidy, J., Matar, N., and Milic-Emili, J.,** Flow and volume dependence of respiratory system flow resistance in patients with adult respiratory distress syndrome, *Am. Rev. Respir. Dis.*, 145, 355–360, 1992.

9. **Pepe, P. E., Potkin, R. T., Reus, D. H., et al.,** Clinical predictors of the adult respiratory distress syndrome, *Am. J. Surg.*, 144, 124–129, 1982.

10. **Doyle, R. L., Szaflarski, N., Medin, G., Wiener-Kronish, J. P., and Matthay, M. A.,** Identification of patients with acute lung injury: Predictors of mortality, *Am. J. Respir. Crit. Care Med.*, in press, 1995.

11. **Bone, R. C., Balk, R., Slotman, G., et al.,** Adult respiratory distress syndrome: Sequences and importance of development of multiple-organ failure, *Chest*, 101, 320–326, 1992.

12. **Rubin, D. B., Wiener-Kronish, J. P., Murray, J. F., et al.,** Elevated von Willebrand actor-antigen is an early plasma predictor of impending of acute lung injury and death in non-pulmonary sepsis syndrome, *J. Clin. Invest.*, 86, 474–480, 1990.

13. **Matthay, M. A. and Wiener-Kronish, J. P.,** Intact epithelial barrier function is critical for the resolution of alveolar edema in humans, *Am. Rev. Respir. Dis.*, 142, 1250–1257, 1990.

14. **Matthay, M. A.,** Pathophysiology of pulmonary edema, *Clin. Chest Med.*, 6, 301–314, 1985.

15. **Staub, N. C.,** Pulmonary edema, *Physiol. Rev.*, 54, 678–811, 1974.

16. **Fein, A., Grossmann, R. F., Jones, J. G., et al.,** The value of edema fluid protein measurements in patients with pulmonary edema, *Am. J. Med.*, 67, 32–39, 1979.

17. **Ohkuda, K., Nakahara, K., Binder, A., and Staub, N. C.,** Venous air emboli in sheep: Reversible increase in lung microvascular permeability, *J. Appl. Physiol.*, 51, 887–894, 1981.

18. **Vreim, C. F., Snashall, P. D., Demling, R. H., et al.,** Lung lymph and free interstitial fluid protein composition in sheep with edema, *J. Appl. Physiol.*, 230, 1650–1653, 1976.

19. **Vreim, C. F. and Staub, N. C.,** Protein composition of lung fluids in acute alloxan edema in dogs, *Am. J. Physiol.*, 230, 376–379, 1976.

20. **Huchon, G. J., Hopewell, P. C., and Murray, J. F.,** Interactions between permeability and hydrostatic pressure in perfused dogs' lung, *J. Appl. Physiol.*, 51, 905–911, 1981.

21. **Unger, K. M., Shibel, E. M., and Moser, K. M.,** Detection of left ventricular failure in patients with the adult respiratory distress syndrome, *Chest*, 67, 8–13, 1975.

22. **Prewitt, R. M., McCarthy, J., and Wood, L. D. H.,** Treatment of acute low pressure pulmonary edema in dogs, *J. Clin. Invest.*, 67, 409–418, 1988.

23. **Staub, N. C.,** The pathogenesis of pulmonary edema, *Prog. Cardiovasc. Dis.*, 23, 53–80, 1980.

24. **Clements, J.,** Pulmonary edema and permeability of alveolar membranes, *Arch. Environ. Health*, 2, 280–283, 1961.

25. **Gregory, T. J., Longmore, W. J., Moxley, M. A., Whitsett, J. A., Reed, C. R., Fowler, A. A., III, Hudson, L. D., Maunder, R. J., Crim, C., and Hyers, T. M.,** Surfactant chemical composition and biophysical activity in acute respiratory distress syndrome, *J. Clin. Invest.*, 88, 1976–1981, 1991.

26. **Wiener-Kronish, J. P., Albertine, K. H., and Matthay, M. A.,** Differential effects of *E. coli* endotoxin on the lung endothelial and epithelial barriers of the lung, *J. Clin. Invest.*, 88, 864-875, 1991.

27. **Wiener-Kronish, J. P., Broaddus, V. C., Albertine, K. H., Gropper, M., Matthay, M. A., and Staub, N. C.,** Pleural effusions are associated with increased permeability pulmonary edema in anesthetized sheep, *J. Clin. Invest.*, 82, 1422–1429, 1988.

28. **Matthay, M. A., Folkesson, G., Campagna, A., and Kheradmand, F.,** Alveolar epithelial barrier and acute lung injury, *N. Horizons*, 1, 613–622, 1993.

29. **Wiener-Kronish, J. P., Sakuma, T., Kudoh, I., Pittet, J. F., Frank, D., Dobbs, L. G., Vasil, M. L., and Matthay, M. A.,** Alveolar epithelial injury and pleural empyema in acute *P. aeruginosa* pneumonia in anesthetized rabbits, *J. Appl. Physiol.*, 75, 1661–1669, 1993.

30. **Tate, R. M. and Repine, J. E.,** Neutrophils and the adult respiratory distress syndrome, *Am. Rev. Respir. Dis.*, 144, 251–252, 1991.
31. **Bachofen, M. and Weibel, E. R.,** Alterations of the gas exchange apparatus in adult respiratory insufficiency associated with septicemia, *Am. Rev. Respir. Dis.*, 116, 589–615, 1977.
32. **Tomashefski, J. F.,** Pulmonary pathology of the adult respiratory distress syndrome, *Clin. Chest Med.*, 11, 593–620, 1990.
33. **Windsor, C. J. W., Walsh, C. J., Mullen, P. G., Cook, D. J., Fisher, B. J., Blocher, C. R., Leeper-Woodford, S. K., Sugerman, H. J., and Fowler, A. A., III,** Tumor necrosis factor — a blockade prevents neutrophil oxygen radical generation, *J. Clin. Invest.*, 1459–1468, 1993.
34. **Newman, W., Beall, L. D., Carson, C. W., Hunder, G. G., Graber, N., Randhawa, Z. I., Gopal, T. V., Wiener-Kronish, J. P., and Matthay, M. A.,** Soluble E-selectin is found in supernatants of activated endothelial cells and is elevated in the serum of patients with septic shock, *J. Immunol.*, 150, 644–655, 1993.
35. **Wortel, C. H. and Doerschuk, C. M.,** Neutrophils and neutrophil-endothelial cell adhesion in adult respiratory distress syndrome, *N. Horizons*, 1, 631–637, 1993.
36. **Matthay, M. A. and Broaddus, V. C.,** Fluid and hemodynamic management in acute lung injury, *Sem. Respir. Med.*, 15, 271–288, 1994.
37. **Witchi, H. R., Haschek, W. M., Klein-Szanto, A. J. P., and Hakkinen, P. J.,** Potentiation of diffuse lung damage by oxygen: Determining variables, *Am. Rev. Respir. Dis.*, 123, 98–103, 1981.
38. **Cheny, F. W., Huang, T. W., and Graonka, R.,** The effects of 50% oxygen on the resolution of pulmonary injury, *Am. Rev. Respir. Dis.*, 122, 373–379, 1980.
39. **Schuster, D. P.,** The case for and against fluid restriction and occlusion pressure reduction in adult respiratory distress syndrome, *N. Horizons*, 1, 478–488, 1993.
40. **Bernard, G. R., Luce, J. M., Sprung, C. L., et al.,** High-dose corticosteroids in patients with the adult respiratory distress syndrome, *N. Engl. J. Med.*, 317, 1565–1570, 1987.
41. **Luce, J. M, Montgomery, A. B., Marks, J. D., Turner, J., Metz, C. A., and Murray, J. F.,** Ineffectiveness of high-dose methylprenisolone in preventing parenchymal lung injury and improving mortality in patients with septic shock, *Am. Rev. Respir. Dis.*, 138, 62–68, 1988.
42. **Folkesson, H. G., Matthay, M. A., Hebert, C. A., and Broaddus, V. C.,** Acid aspiration induced lung injury in rabbits is mediated by interleukin-8 dependent mechanisms, *J. Clin. Invest.*, in press, 1995.
43. **Dellinger, R. P.,** Clinical trials in the adult respiratory distress syndrome, *N. Horizons*, 1, 584–592, 1993.
44. **Matthay, M. A.,** Editorial — New modes of mechanical ventilation for ARDS: How should they be evaluated?, *Chest*, 95, 1175–1177, 1989.
45. **Hyers, T. M.,** Prediction of survival and mortality in patients with adult respiratory distress syndrome, *N. Horizons*, 1, 466–470, 1993.
46. **Zapol, W. M. and Hurford, W. E.,** Inhaled nitric oxide in the adult respiratory distress syndrome and other lung diseases, *N. Horizons*, 1, 638–650, 1993.
47. **Matthay, M. A.,** Fibrosing adhesives in the adult respiratory distress syndrome, *Ann. Int. Med.*, 122, 65–66, 1995.

Chapter 8

Malignant Tumors and the Microcirculation

Bernhard Endrich and Peter Vaupel

CONTENTS

I. INTRODUCTION

Cancer is a disease characterized by the insidious progressive growth of cells. These cells ultimately destroy tissue after invading it and will metastasize to organs away from the primary site. However, the inherent loss of proliferative control will allow the cell mass to reach a volume of only about 1 mm^3 (ca. 10^6 cells) without "nutritive deficiency".[1-4] Beyond this "preclinical growth stage", diffusional supply is inadequate. Further growth and tumor progression depend on a nutrient supply via a network of microvessels.[5-11] In fact, the vascularization of solid tumors is a prerequisite if a *clinically relevant size* is to be reached, and for hematogenic metastases of malignant cells. It is the aim of this review to: (1) summarize today's understanding of the microanatomy and pathophysiology of microvessels in tumors, and (2) address the possible relevance of these findings for diagnosis and treatment.

We will distinguish between new, sprouting blood vessels and the "mature" tumor microcirculation. On the basis of the data presented, a possible impact of various factors on clinical oncology will be discussed after each section.

II. VASCULAR ANATOMY OF TUMORS DURING EARLY GROWTH

A. PREEXISTING VESSELS

Blood and nutrients are supplied to a malignant tumor via preexisting ("parasitized" or recruited normal vessels) and newly formed vessels. A neoplasm incorporates arterial vessels of all categories because the wall of arteries exhibits a striking "immunity" for neoplastic invasion and retains its normal wall structure and function.[7,12-16] When the blood supply to small tumors is traced from its inception (possible in transparent observation chambers), a great number of channels are seen that have developed from capillary sprouts, eventually forming a chaotic microvascular network (for reviews, see References 5–11, 15, and 17).

B. NEOVASCULARIZATION

To allow the enlargement of a tumor mass, host tissue must provide the building blocks for vascular stroma. This was basically stated in the last century, when Paget[18] presented his "seed and soil" hypothesis of metastatic growth. The nonrandom pattern of visceral metastases suggested to Paget a special affinity that tumor cells possess for the "milieu" of specific organs. In an attempt to verify this notion, Gullino and Grantham[19] found 30 years ago that a hepatoma cell culture was unable to form collagen. However, when transplanted into a host, tumors developed with a collagen content equal to that obtained by implanting small fragments of whole hepatoma tissue.

The presence of an angiogenic stimulus, as first suggested in the early 1970s,[20,21] can promote the generation of new tumor blood vessels, which in turn were found to be critical for tumor expansion. Subsequently, a number of angiogenesis factors were identified.[22] As a specific feature of malignant growth, many tumors impose modifications on the microvascular bed that are different from angiogenesis induced by non-malignant cells.[23] For instance, a histologic cross-section of a capillary in the normal brain reveals one or two endothelial cells per lumen; in brain tumors such as the glioblastoma, however, 5 to 10 endothelial cells may occupy one lumen. Most tumor microvessels are dilated and they sometimes contain tumor cells within the endothelial lining.[24-34] Although microvessels in tumors are usually pericyte-poor and do not regain their normal density of pericytes until after capillary growth has ceased, capillaries in some tumors contain excessive numbers of pericytes. It is not clear why such enormous differences exist, nor whether they are of clinical significance.[35,36] In recent years, biochemical events during angiogenesis have received increasing attention among clinicians, particularly because of the capacity of endothelial cells to respond in a characteristic way to a specific stimulus.

III. DIAGNOSTIC AND THERAPEUTIC IMPLICATIONS OF ANGIOGENESIS IN MALIGNANT TUMORS

The angiogenic capacity of excretions and transcellular fluid that do not have such a capacity in benign tissue, might be of *diagnostic* value. The search for such diagnostic tools revealed media that became angiogenic on contact with growing tumors *in vivo*. Examples are urine for bladder carcinomas, cerebrospinal fluid for glioblastomas and meningiomas, and aqueous humor for ocular tumors. In fact, the release of an angiogenic stimulus into the extracellular compartment could be of use in early diagnosis. Such angiogenesis tests, however, cannot be applied easily in clinical practice.[4,37-40]

In clinical *pharmacology*, much attention was focused on the development of so-called angiogenesis inhibitors for anticancer therapy. Many of these compounds, however, were found to prevent neovascularization in chronic inflammatory diseases such as arthritis or psoriasis only. A summary of the most recent information in this field has been provided by Folkman and Brem.[23] They addressed some promising approaches related to clinical oncology as follows:

(1) Steroid-heparin combinations were found to dissolve the basement membrane of growing capillaries.[41] One application presently under discussion among clinicians is the treatment of corneal neovascularization, which is refractory to conventional therapy. It also seems possible to suppress neovascularization in mast cell-rich inflammatory lesions or hemangiomas by corticosteroids alone, because of the high levels of endogenous heparin.

(2) A number of studies suggest that components of the basal lamina such as fibronectin, collagen type IV, and laminin undergo a more rapid turnover in growing capillaries. Consequently, agents that interfere with the synthesis of these components or accelerate their degradation favor a dissolution of the basement membrane, thus inhibiting angiogenesis. In particular, interferon-alpha has received marked attention during recent years. This agent was used to successfully treat at least 20 children suffering from pulmonary capillary hemangiomatosis as well as systemic hemangiomatosis where steroid therapy had already failed.[42] Beyond this rare disease with its excessive growth of capillaries, however, interferon-alpha has not been established as a potent agent in medical oncology.[43]

This illustrates that the effectiveness of all antiangiogenic agents may be restricted to specific capillary beds since some tumors are more angiogenic than others.[44] Other medical subspecialties such as rheumatology have already introduced the "antiangiogenetic treatment approach" successfully; for instance, gold thiomalate and penicillamine are known to inhibit neovascularization in rheumatoid arthritis.[45,46]

Quite recently, angiogenesis was proposed for use as a *prognostic tool*. A prospective, blind study of 165 consecutive patients helped to identify the microvessels within primary invasive breast carcinoma as a potential indicator for the identification of high-risk groups. Immunocytochemical staining was used to detect factor VIII-related antigen. Weidner et al.[47] found microvessel density as the only statistically significant predictor of overall survival among node-negative women. It was concluded that counting capillary density would be useful in selecting those node-negative patients with breast cancer who are at high risk for having occult metastases. These patients could receive adjuvant chemotherapy earlier. Using the JC70 antibody to the platelet/endothelial cell adhesion molecule, Horak et al.[48] published a study on 103 primary breast cancer patients. Again, angiogenesis was closely linked to metastasis. A microvascular density above a "critical value" was also found as tumors enlarge or become poorly differentiated. They also concluded that counting of newly formed microvessels that were stained with endothelium specific antibodies could be a useful tool in the early detection of metastatic potential of breast cancer. The great clinical potential of angiohistogenesis, as well as these new microvascular techniques, recently have been addressed.[49]

Microvascular techniques were also chosen by Wakui et al.[50] and Bigler et al.[51] in prostatic carcinomas with the aim of predicting tumor progression and bone marrow metastasis in patients. Moreover, Brem et al.[52] found fibroblast growth factor predominantly present in surgical specimens from 52 human brain tumors. This suggests a cellular depot for this potent growth factor that mediates angiogenesis and tumorigenesis. Based on these findings, Brem et al. concluded that fibroblast growth factor may not only play a role in the transition from the benign to the malignant phenotype, but identified microvascular proliferation as a possible target for anti-cancer therapy.[52] Special attention should be given to the work of Gagliardi and Collins;[53] their novel findings showed that anti-estrogens are effective inhibitors of angiogenesis in breast cancer. Moreover, the fact that angiostatic activity is not altered in the presence of excess estrogens suggests that this activity is exerted via mechanisms other than through their inhibition of estrogen action. They also suggested that this angiostatic activity may contribute to the therapeutic effect

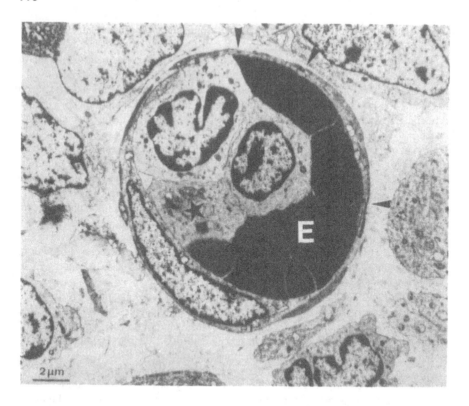

Figure 1A. Cross-sectioned capillary sprout from a BA 1112 Rhabdomyosarcoma grown for 2 weeks in a dorsal skinfold chamber in the rat. The vessel lumen is completely packed with erythrocytes (E) while the proliferating endothelium displays a high number of various organelles such as mitochondria and cisternae of the rough ER. There is a great structural similarity between some endothelial cells (★) and the adjacent tumor cells. Note the attenuated endothelial junctions (◄) with poorly differentiated adhesive devices. (Magnification 5500×.)

of anti-estrogens in estrogen receptor-negative tumors. Even though the microscopic counting was very time consuming (despite modern computer technology), it is expected to be a valuable prognostic index in the future. Not only medical oncology, but ophthalmology in particular could benefit from these new microvascular techniques.[54]

IV. PATHOPHYSIOLOGY OF THE MATURE ("ESTABLISHED") TUMOR MICROCIRCULATION

As a tumor grows, "tumorous" blood channels form a chaotic network of microvessels ("established" tumor microcirculation[55]). Such vessels are characterized by a lack of smooth muscle cells and nervous components, exhibit tortuosity, arteriovenous anastomoses, irregular vessel branching pattern and vessels with little or no endothelial lining (Figures 1 and 2). In addition to such structural abnormalities of microvessels,[24] a functioning lymphatic system is absent in most solid tumors. Thus, interstitial fluid drainage is limited even though the number of venous vessels is often much larger in tumor tissue than in its normal counterpart. Therefore, it is not surprising that interstitial pressures as high as 45 mmHg have been reported for human tumors.[56,57] Such hydrostatic pressures were identical to arteriolar pressures reported for tumors in the rat and in the hamster.[8,58,59] Quite recently, simultaneous measurements of interstitial and venular pressure on the surface of a mammary adenocarcinoma in the rat also showed more or less

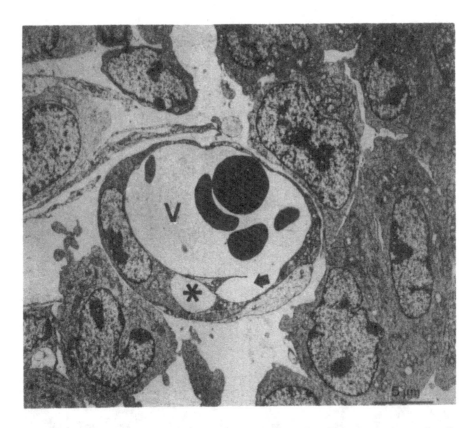

Figure 1B. Larger capillary with a wall of extremely varying thickness from a melanotic melanoma (MOHR) grown in the hamster. The development of intracytoplasmic cisternae (*) and their secondary access (♦) to the vessel lumen (V) lead to its enlargement with concomitant attenuation of the endothelium. Note that size, structure, and number of cellular organelles within the endothelium very much resembles that of the adjacent tumor cells. (Magnification 2300×.)

identical values.[59] However, local changes in pressure and diameter might also be elicited by swelling and destruction of endothelial cells, adhesion of leukocytes, platelets, or even cancer cells. It is evident that all of the factors mentioned above may contribute to making the blood flow through any malignant tumor more chaotic, sluggish, heterogeneous, and ultimately, inadequate.[8-10]

For many years, the disorganization of the microvascular network of tumors associated with a poor delivery of blood, oxygen (Figure 3), nutrients or anticancer agents has been considered a major drawback for obtaining a substantial improvement in radiation and chemotherapy regimens.[60-62] To precisely define that segment where the therapeutic problems arise in the microcirculation, it is useful to consider separately the "transport" and "exchange" functions in malignant tumors.

A. "TRANSPORT" FUNCTION IN TUMOR MICROVESSELS

As in the normal microcirculation, blood flow through the microvascular network of a tumor is assumed to be proportional to the pressure difference between arterial and venous vessels, and inversely proportional to the viscous and geometric resistances.[62] Arteriolar pressures in tumors are almost identical for both tumor and normal microcirculation.[8,58] Venular pressures, however, are significantly lower in a tumor, a fact that can be explained by a much higher number of outflow vessels.[8,58]

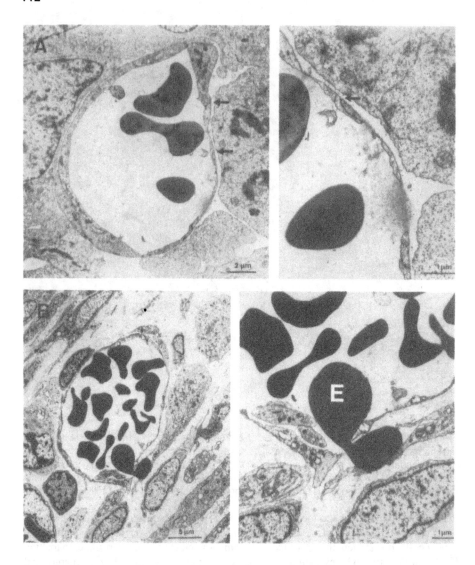

Figure 2 **A:** Oblique section of a capillary of the amelanotic melanoma A-Mel-3. In the endothelium, there is a defect of more than 1 μm in diameter still retaining some electron-dense material. Near this defect, there are closed intercellular endothelial junctions (arrows). Furthermore, a basal lamina cannot be identified. **B:** Capillary with extremely attenuated and partly disintegrated (right side) endothelium from a BA 1112 Rhabdomyosarcoma of the rat. One erythrocyte (E) is passing through a large endothelial defect while being deformed by contact with another cellular structure that closely resembles a tumor cell.

The *viscous resistance* (apparent viscosity) of blood is affected by the number and flow behavior of blood cells and to a much smaller extent by the plasma viscosity. Therefore, the possibility of purposely inducing changes in erythrocyte fluidity has received great attention in recent years. In animal experiments, red blood cell rigidity could be increased by hypoxia, lowering the pH, elevating the temperature or raising the plasma glucose concentration. It should be noted that because of their larger capillary diameter, tumors may already reveal a less pronounced Fahraeus and Fahraeus-Lindqvist effect, which in turn could lead to an increased number of microvessels with low or no

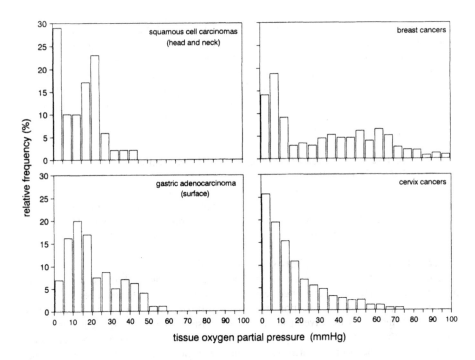

Figure 3 Frequency distributions of pO$_2$-values (pO$_2$-histograms) for squamous cell carcinomas of the head and neck, for breast cancers, a gastric carcinoma (surface-pO$_2$) and cervix cancers as summarized from the literature. The data indicate tumor tissue hypoxia in all malignomas studied. (For further details, see References 7, 10, 136, and 143).

perfusion as long as red blood cells are less flexible than normal. Therefore, information on geometric resistance, which is limited at present, should include the number of vessels (capillary density), their length and diameter, as well as the branching pattern.[62]

For unknown reasons, malignant cells rarely invade vessels of the arterial tree. As a result of the well-maintained contractile and nervous apparatus, one would assume that these vessels might respond to physical, pharmacological, and chemical stimuli, and may reveal the phenomenon of vasomotion.

Even though the earliest studies of "normal" microcirculation referred to the presence of rhythmic diameter changes of arterioles associated with a modulation of capillary flow, vasomotion in tumors as well as its impact on tumor microvessels have widely been neglected. One possible explanation might be that vasomotion has been seen only rarely in tumors.[8,12,13,15]

The clinical significance of this phenomenon becomes apparent in one example from angiology. The periodic activity of vasomotion shows pronounced alterations when arterial stenosis of the lower extremity associated with ischemic disease is treated by transluminal angioplasty. Using laser Doppler flowmetry in a clinical situation, it was shown that normal microcirculatory function is highly nonlinear. Tissue perfusion, exchange of materials, fluid balance, and peripheral vascular resistance are fundamentally different if the diameter of the vessel is oscillatory instead of steady, even though the mean diameter might be the same.[63]

Apparently, a different situation is found in tumors in which vasomotion is nearly eliminated even though tumor arteries and arterioles, with their original morphological features, are incorporated into tumor tissue. Tumor arterioles in particular might experience a condition where a presumed constrictor stimulus from a local pacemaker is inadequate in producing oscillatory behavior.[64-67] A significant effect of vasomotion on homeostasis was further substantiated by calculations from Tsai and Intaglietta.[68] They demonstrated in a mathematical model that under flowmotion (cyclic time varying fluctuations of capillary blood flow), tissue — which under steady-state conditions would remain anoxic — becomes oxygenated. Thus, experimental and clinical evidence[63-67] indicate that slow wave flowmotion constitutes a physiological mechanism to improve tissue oxygenation in situations where the oxygen supply is reduced; this mechanism is lacking in tumors to an unknown extent.[15]

B. EXCHANGE OF FLUID AND SOLUTES IN THE TUMOR MICROVASCULATURE

Considering the lack of vasomotion as one important difference between the normal and the tumor microcirculation, it is not surprising that a number of exchange parameters show differences when compared to the normal tissue "microenvironment". These alterations are summarized in a number of comprehensive reports.[69-77]

1. Transport Across the Microvascular Wall

As a rule, transport of anticancer agents over long distances within the body is accomplished by convection. On reaching exchange vessels, substances extravasate and meet their target through the interstitium by two primary modes, diffusion and convection. *Diffusion* is defined as transport of dissolved particles on the basis of their thermokinetic energy. A prerequisite for the movement of particles is the existence of a concentration gradient. Diffusion will depend on the diffusion medium, the molecular weight of the diffusing particles and on the temperature. In general, transport of low molecular weight substances is diffusion dominated, while convective transport in the microcirculation becomes important at higher molecular weights. For larger molecules, and particularly for those with polar groups, the microvascular wall can be a considerable obstacle to diffusion.

In malignant tumors, however, where most of the exchange vessels arise from the expansion of the vascular network by angiogenesis, the vessels have wide (water-filled) interendothelial gaps with discontinuous or absent basement membranes.[24-30,78] This feature alone suggests that there should be a much higher diffusive exchange rate compared to vessels in most normal tissues. On the other hand, the average microvascular surface area decreases with tumor growth: hence, one would expect reduced diffusive exchange in bulky tumors compared to smaller ones.

Convective fluid flow through the microvascular wall is defined as *filtration*. Morphologic characteristics of tumor microvessels suggest that the filtration coefficient should be higher than in most normal tissues. Extravasation of macromolecules, however, is poor in tumors. This is due to high interstitial fluid pressures which limit fluid extravasation.[72] Recent investigations of intratumor pressure gradients show that although the interstitial pressure is elevated throughout the tumor, it drops precipitously to normal levels in the tumor's periphery.[76] As the tumor grows, the interstitial fluid pressure rises, presumably due to proliferation of tumor cells in a confined space, high vascular permeability, and the absence of lymphatic vessels.[76]

In normal tissue, the oncotic pressure difference between vascular and interstitial space is approximately 5 to 20 mmHg. Oncotic pressure in the tumor interstitium is most likely higher than that in normal tissues based on high vascular permeability and thus higher concentrations of plasma proteins in the tumor interstitium than in the interstitial compartment of normal tissue.

2. Transport Within the Interstitial Space

Once an agent has passed the endothelium, its interstitial transport occurs by *diffusion and convection*. In general, the interstitial space in tumors is large compared with that in host normal tissue, hyaluronate and proteoglycan are present in lower concentrations, and the relative volume of free fluid in tumors is high.[71,78] These features suggest a relatively high diffusion coefficient in malignant tumors. Diffusion coefficients for macromolecules are an order of magnitude higher in tumors than for several normal tissues,[78] and this should favor diffusion of large-sized molecules. The opposite, however, is true! Since diffusion distances are significantly increased in many malignant tumors, agents need more time to traverse these longer distances to reach their targets. For instance, the time required for the diffusion of IgG in tumors is of the order of 0.5 h for a distance of 100 μm; for its Fab fragment, it would take about 0.2 h to move the same distance in the tumor's interstitium.[74]

Based on the characteristics of the interstitial space in tumors (high relative volume of free water, interstitial hypertension, low levels of glycosaminoglycan, increase in fractional volume of interstitial compartment), convective transport is of significance in tumors, especially for substances of larger molecular size. Bulk flow of free fluid in the interstitial compartment is a typical pattern for malignant tumors. Whereas, in normal tissues, convective currents in the interstitial space are estimated to be 0.5 to 1.0% of plasma flow; in tumors, bulk flow of free fluid can reach 14% of the plasma flow rate, provoking a significant hemoconcentration during the passage of blood through the tumor.[79] Since interstitial fluid pressure is high in the center of the tumor and decreases toward the invasion frontier at the tumor's periphery, interstitial fluid motion is from the center toward its periphery, from where it will ooze out into the surrounding tissue, contributing to the formation of a peri-tumor edema. This fluid leakage leads to an interstitial fluid velocity of 0.1 to 25 μm/s directed radially outward.[80,81] This outward convection has to be overcome by macromolecules diffusing from peripheral to central areas.

To sum up the pros and cons of tumor characteristics for the delivery of anti-cancer agents (especially macromolecules), the physiological "benefits" include high values for vascular permeability, diffusion coefficient, and hydraulic conductivity, whereas the problems arise from a heterogeneous microcirculation, elevated interstitial pressures and the enlarged volume of the interstitial space, larger intercapillary distances and a radially directed bulk flow of free water toward the tumor periphery. This aspect, which is of great clinical relevance in chemotherapy, is often neglected. It might still limit this approach to a great extent.

V. DIAGNOSTIC AND PROGNOSTIC TOOLS IN THE CLINICAL SETTING

A. DIAGNOSTIC PROCEDURES

New possibilities of monitoring a tumor's response to therapy performed using imaging modalities have received increased attention during recent years. Tumor size is still the main criterion, although a reduction in tumor size after therapy will only become evident after several weeks. NMR spectroscopy could quickly define the effects of therapy in quantitative terms, so that one could optimize tumor therapy sooner.[82-86] Recently, blood flow related data were obtained using dynamic CT and dynamic magnetic resonance imaging.[87,88] In pelvic tumors, Feldmann et al.[89] were able to differentiate between areas of low and high perfusion. Encouraged by the possibility of having an additional tool for the prediction of tumor response to thermoradiotherapy and radiation, they have started to evaluate changes in tumor perfusion by positron emission tomography. Lammertsma et al.[90] also reported some of their experience in women suffering from breast carcinomas while utilizing positron emission tomography for *in vivo* measurements of tumor perfusion. Positron emission tomography might have great possibilities in oncology for the staging and follow-up of proliferation of tumors as well as for the evaluation of the distribution of labeled chemical agents in tumor metastases. It should, however, be noted that due to perfusion heterogeneities, a quantitative estimate of oxygen utilization is still not possible with this technique.

In contrast, "metabolic imaging" in cryosections of tissue using quantitative biolumi-nescence renders feasible data on the relation between the tumor's histology and the spatial distribution of compounds such as ATP, glucose, and lactate.[60,91] This novel technique and its clinical potential has been evaluated directly in specimens of human tumors such as the cervix carcinoma.[11]

B. PROGNOSTIC PARAMETERS

As discussed in Section III, there seems to be some clinical evidence of a relation between tumor cell proliferation and vascularity. However, experimental data on the relationship between cell proliferation and vascularization in transplantable animal tumors and human xenografts do not always support this notion.[92-96]

In some experimental studies, the percentage of labeled cells as well as the mitotic index were high in the vicinity of microvessels (or at high oxygen tensions in the tissue) and decreased with increasing distance from blood vessels. According to the radial O_2 tension gradient from the vessel into the tissue, these results merely confirm the role of oxygen as a limiting substrate for tumor cell proliferation. In addition, there is an intravascular O_2 tension gradient from the arterial to the venous end. This implies that there should be substantial differences in the proliferative indices, not only as a function of distance from microvessels but also as a function of the position with respect to the arterial and venous ends of the microvessels. This difference has not yet been evaluated experimentally and needs further evaluation.

The question, whether the above-mentioned correlation between proliferation indices and distance from blood vessels applies to all tumors irrespective of their degree of differentiation, has been addressed by Gabbert et al.[97] They reported experiments dealing with cell proliferation in chemically induced colon carcinomas in the rat. These tumors were characterized by different degrees of differentiation but had an equally developed vascularization. Since significant differences in proliferation patterns were found, the authors concluded that the proliferation behavior of a tumor may depend primarily on inherent properties of the tumor cell proliferation, while vascularization merely provides the conditioning for tumor enlargement.

In human tumors, similar studies are scarce. Using six different human melanoma xenograft lines, Lyng et al.[96] concluded that blood supply (number of vessels) per viable tumor cell was likely to be the key to proliferative activity of tumor cells. Studying cell proliferation and vascularization in human breast carcinomas, Monschke et al.[98] found that highly vascularized tumors exhibited a greater proliferative activity than tumor specimens with a lower vascular density. Much work, however, still needs to be done to solve the discrepancy between clinical and experimental data that presently exists.

VI. THERAPEUTIC MEASURES RELATED TO THE MICROCIRCULATION IN TUMORS

A. REVERSIBLE ALTERATIONS OF TUMOR BLOOD FLOW INDUCED BY DRUGS

Despite the problems in the tumor microcirculation discussed earlier, a great number of studies on blood flow in human and experimental tumors are reported (Figure 4). In addition, a reasonable number of drugs has been tested for their effect on blood flow in experimental tumors.[99] The compound most extensively evaluated is angiotensin II,[100-106] which is known to be a potent vasoconstrictor that induces hypertension upon adminis-tration. This agent was found to restore flow in regions within the tumor whose interstitial pressure was higher than the intravascular pressure. From the clinical point of view, a

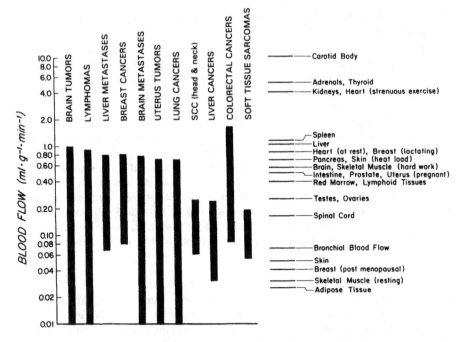

Figure 4 Variability of blood flow in human malignancies as compared to mean flow values of nonmalignant tissues. In the left part of the picture, data are given for various tumors; on the right side, values are listed for normal tissue. Note that colorectal cancers have a rather high perfusion rate. For further details, see Reference 10.

short-term infusion of angiotensin could be beneficial when used during radiation or chemotherapy.[106] Even though this drug has been shown to improve the efficiency of chemotherapy, it is not used to a great extent in medical oncology. The same is true for diagnostic imaging although blood vessel visualization is greatly improved. One reason for its very limited use might be extensive variations in the dose-response relationship between individuals as well as between different organs.

The use of another group of drugs might be of more clinical significance. To improve the cytotoxicity of antineoplastic drugs, *calcium antagonists* have been tested under *in vitro* and *in vivo* conditions. Moreover, these agents may have the capability to inhibit the respiration of malignant cells *in vitro*.[15] There is also some experimental evidence that verapamil and nifedipine inhibit spontaneous and experimental tumor metastasis. At the microcirculatory level, calcium antagonists can lead to an increase of peripheral blood flow at a constant perfusion pressure via arteriolar dilation. Vaupel and Menke[15] have recently summarized their findings in the rat DS-carcinosarcoma and have found that, of the drugs tested, only flunarizine caused a 20% increase in tumor flow that lasted for more than 30 min. It should again be mentioned that they observed rhythmic oscillations of red blood cell flux in about 15% of the subepidermal tumors. The average time for these oscillations was nearly 3 min, with about 21 cycles per hour.[16] Upon application of all calcium antagonists tested, these rhythmic variations slowed down significantly to a mean of more than 5 min with 11 cycles per hour. Comparing these data with results from the literature,[15] the flow increase seems to be a rather consistent finding. Presently, however, one can only speculate on the clinical usefulness of these agents as adjuvants in diagnosis and anticancer treatment as they might modulate pharmacokinetics and pharmacodynamics of cytostatic agents, increase radiosensitivity or improve the delivery of monoclonal antibodies and biological response modifiers.

B. SIDE EFFECTS OF TUMOR THERAPY AS RELATED TO THE MICROVASCULATURE

Very recently, Gerl et al.[107] reviewed acute and late vascular complications following chemotherapy of germ cell tumors. Among "central" and life-threatening side effects such as myocardial infarction, cerebral insults, or pulmonary embolism, they focused in particular on Raynaud's phenomenon because this occurs in a considerable number of patients. As a consequence to use with vinblastine and bleomycin, it was first described in 1977.[108] Subsequently, a number of studies report Raynaud's phenomenon upon chemotherapy in 2.6 to 41% of the patients treated; the combination of bleomycin and cisplatin seems to bear a rather high risk for developing this complication.[109-114] The onset of clinical symptoms of Raynaud's phenomenon is about 10 months after starting chemotherapy.[113] Therapeutic trials with topical application of nitroglycerin did not prove to be beneficial in this group of patients; a gradual resolution of symptoms was seen in about 50% of the patients.[114] Apparently, chemotherapy can be associated with both systemic and peripheral vascular toxicity, the latter affecting the microcirculation directly. Much more interest, however, was focused on the effects of physical measures on the microvasculature of tumors.

C. HYPERTHERMIA — A CLINICAL REALITY?

As an important addition to conventional treatment of cancer, hyperthermia has been more and more introduced into clinical oncology over the last decade. The great interest in this modality focused in particular on the pathophysiology of the tumor microcirculation. In this respect, hyperthermia is rather well understood, although great problems are still present with the uniform heating of deep-seated tumors. Today, it seems established that malignant tumors can be destroyed by a thermal dose undamaging to normal tissues. Moreover, small changes of flow at the microcirculatory level could have major effects on the microenvironment in tumors that in turn can modify the response to therapeutic modalities added to hyperthermia. It should, however, be noted that the question of whether normal and malignant cells have a different thermosensitivity is still being discussed controversially.

Dealing with hyperthermia, there are a number of reviews and books available.[115-125] In a recent review,[60] a diagram (Figure 5), showing the normal vascular response to heat and the effect of hyperthermia on tumor tissue vasculature, was designed on the basis of a literature search of clinical and experimental blood flow studies upon heating. Due to its low perfusion, a tumor creates its own heat reservoir with the convective heat dissipation being poorer in "low-flow" tumors. As a result, the tumor temperature will be higher than in normal tissue. On the other hand, the microcirculation of malignant tumors appears to have little tolerance to elevated tissue temperatures. The mechanisms of this vascular shut-down that permits, at least experimentally, a selective treatment of tumors, are rather complex (they are discussed in References 7, 60, 126, and 127). The hyperthermia-induced dysfunction of the microcirculation will not only be advantageous for a selective heating of the tumor as a whole, but can sensitize tumor cells to (subsequent) hyperthermic treatment by changing the "milieu interne" of the tumor. However, since these phenomena are established only experimentally in rapidly growing animal tumors, clinical relevance is likely but needs to be verified during clinical application of hyperthermia. Particularly for isolated extremity perfusion of melanomas and soft tissue sarcomas, a fair number of clinical studies are available.[7,128-131] Some clinicians have also begun to realize the tremendous impact of changes in tumor microcirculation upon regional hyperthermia, which affects the response of the cytostatic agents added and thus subsequent tumor growth.[130,131]

It should also be mentioned that comparable microvascular damage has been reported upon photodynamic and shock-wave therapy.[8,132,133] Based on encouraging experimental data, photodynamic therapy has also been used clinically.[132]

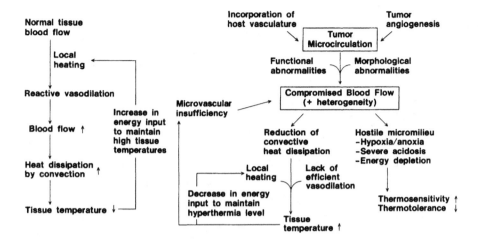

Figure 5 Diagram showing the normal vascular response to heat (left) and the impact of hyperthermia on the microvasculature of tumor tissue (right). If the temperature is elevated in normal tissue, vasodilation occurs and is associated with an increase in heat dissipation by convection. Due to low flow, an efficient heat transfer is not present in most malignant tumors. Vascular destruction leads to a further temperature rise rather than a temperature drop, as it would be expected in normal tissue. (From Vaupel, P., *Biological Basis of Oncologic Thermotherapy*, Gautherie, M., Ed., Springer, Berlin, 1990, 73.)

D. MICROVASCULAR CHANGES AFTER RADIATION: IMPLICATIONS FOR THERAPY

As early as 1927, changes in the tumor microvasculature upon radiation were discussed. Mervin and Algire[134] were the first to report a pronounced microvessel narrowing upon application of doses of 20 to 50 Gy in a single fraction. They also observed, as an effect of radiation, that tumor blood flow was variable, even for the same tumor and an identical dose of radiation. From a number of clinical and experimental studies, it appeared that unfractionated therapy employing a large dose would destroy the microvasculature and lead to parenchymal cell death, while fractionated radiation in a clinically relevant dose range could temporarily improve the oxygenation of experimental tumors, thus facilitating further radiation treatment.[135] The relative radiosensitvity as a function of pO_2 is graphically illustrated in Figure 6.

Beyond evaluating directly the response of the microvasculature to radiation, many factors have been considered as potentially useful *predictors* of tumor response to radiotherapy.[136] Besides clonogenic and growth assays and the evaluation of repair capacity to predict intrinsic radiosensitivity, proliferative indices, ploidy, tissue oxygenation, and vascularity have received attention as valid predictors. Vascular density and intercapillary distances have been correlated with the outcome of radiotherapy in carcinomas of the cervix,[137-142] the larynx, and nasopharynx.[143] In these studies, small intercapillary distances and/or high vascular density were associated with better local control of the disease or even a longer survival. In contrast, in a small series of 26 oral squamous cell carcinomas, a better local control was observed in poorly vascularized tumors.[144] An explanation for this striking difference cannot be provided at the present time.

Basically, these studies highlight the role of *tumor oxygenation* in determining the response to radiotherapy, particularly in cervical carcinomas. Since measurements of vascularity are laborious and not always descriptive of the functional status of microvessels (not all microvessels detected and counted by morphometric techniques are perfused at a given time), the results obtained indicate again that alternative, more rapid and *direct*

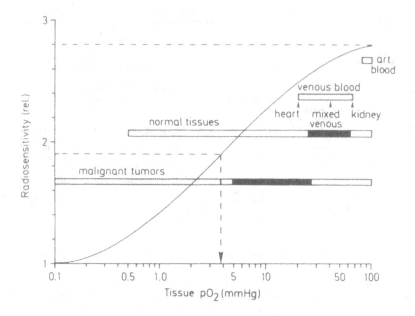

Figure 6 Schematic representation of relative radiosensitivity as a function of pO_2 at the cellular level. The usual range of pO_2 values for blood, normal as well as malignant tissue is graphically illustrated; in addition, the pO_2 value at which the sensitizing effect is half-maximal, is indicated by the arrow. (From Vaupel, P., Kallinowski, F., and Okunieff, P., Cancer Res., 49, 6449, 1989.)

methods for evaluation of tumor oxygenation could have a significant impact for individual radiotherapy.[144] In a recent study on cervical cancers treated with radiotherapy, this has been explicitly stated because tumor oxygenation was a predictor for both local control and overall survival.[145]

VII. FUTURE PERSPECTIVES

Tumor therapy depends on being able to remove the neoplasm as a whole or destroy the clonogenic activity of tumor cells still in place while keeping the normal tissue damage low. As for the latter, a variety of factors are needed to explain why chemical or physical treatment quite frequently fails. It becomes increasingly clear that physiological parameters are of utmost importance for a sufficient outcome in cases where surgery needs to be supplemented. As a result of the nonuniform vascular network and its inadequate function, blood flow and microcirculation, transcapillary and interstitial transport, tissue oxygen and nutrient supply, as well as the bioenergetic status will markedly change any therapeutic response beyond a genetically determined resistance.

Knowledge of microcirculatory and microenviromental parameters will be relevant to clinical oncology in two ways: (1) as a diagnostic aid when new methods such as NMR, positron emission tomography, and quantitative bioluminescence are utilized to evaluate tumor pathophysiology in clinical oncology. With wider use of these novel techniques, a new generation of clinical trials might be initiated using the increasing amount of preclinical data as a guideline for designing clinical protocols; (2) as a prognostic index derived from a surgical specimen. Some data on vascular density, obtained primarily in mammary carcinomas at the time of surgery, seem to open a new horizon in prognosis and patient selection.[146] The first encouraging results, however, need to be confirmed in a much larger number of patients.

REFERENCES

1. **Ausprunk, D. H. and Folkman, J.,** Migration and proliferation of endothelial cells in preformed and newly formed blood vessels during tumor angiogenesis, *Microvasc. Res.,* 14, 53, 1977.

2. **Folkman, J.,** How is blood vessel growth regulated in normal and neoplastic tissue?, *Cancer Res.,* 46, 467, 1986.

3. **Folkman, J., Merler, E., Abernathy, C., and Williams, G.,** Isolation of a tumor factor responsible for angiogenesis, *J. Exp. Med.,* 133, 275, 1971.

4. **Gullino, P. M.,** Tumor angiogenesis 1990: Comments on the state of the art, in *Tumor Blood Supply and Metabolic Microenvironment,* Vaupel, P. and Jain, R. K., Eds., Akademie der Wissenschaften und der Literatur, Mainz, Gustav Fischer Verlag, Stuttgart, 1991, 11.

5. **Denekamp, J.,** Angiogenesis, neovascular proliferation and vascular pathophysiology as targets for cancer therapy, *Br. J. Radiol.,* 66, 181, 1993.

6. **Denekamp, J., Hill, S.A., and Hobson, B.,** Vascular occlusion and tumor cell death, *Eur. J. Cancer,* 19, 271, 1983.

7. **Endrich, B.,** Hyperthermie und Tumormikrozirkulation — Eine kritische Wertung experimenteller und klinischer Befunde, in *Contributions to Oncology,* Vol. 31, Karger, Basel, 1988.

8. **Endrich, B. and Götz, A.,** Tumor microcirculation: Scope and clinical applicability, in *Tumor Blood Supply and Metabolic Microenvironment,* Vaupel, P. and Jain, R. K., Eds., Akademie der Wissenschaften, Mainz, Gustav Fischer Verlag, Stuttgart, 1991, 37.

9. **Jain, R. K.,** Determinants of tumor blood flow: A review, *Cancer Res.,* 48, 2641, 1988.

10. **Vaupel, P., Kallinowski, F., and Okunieff, P.,** Blood flow, oxygen and nutrient supply, and metabolic microenvironment of human tumors: A review, *Cancer Res.,* 49, 6449, 1989.

11. **Vaupel, P.,** Physiological properties of malignant tumors, *NMR in Biomed.,* 5, 220, 1992.

12. **Intaglietta, M., Myers, R. R., Gross, J. F., and Reinhold, H. S.,** Dynamics of microvascular flow in implanted mouse mammary tumours, *Bibl. Anat.,* 15, 273, 1977.

13. **Reinhold, H. S., Blachewiecz, B., and Blok, A.,** Oxygenation and reoxygenation in "sandwich" tumours, *Bibl. Anat.,* 15, 270, 1977.

14. **Reinhold, H. S.,** *In vivo* observations of tumor blood flow, in *Tumor Blood Circulation,* Peterson, H.-I., Ed., CRC Press, Boca Raton, FL, 1979, 115.

15. **Vaupel, P. and Menke, H.,** Effect of various calcium antagonists on blood flow and red blood cell flux in malignant tumors, *Progr. Appl. Microcirc.,* 14, 88, 1989.

16. **Vaupel, P., Kluge, M., and Ambroz, M. C.,** Laser Doppler flowmetry in subepidermal tumours and in normal skin of rats during localized ultrasound hyperthermia, *Int. J. Hyperthermia,* 4, 307, 1988.

17. **Skinner, S. A., Tutton, P. J. M., and O'Brien, P. E.,** Microvascular architecture of experimental colon tumors in the rat, *Cancer Res.,* 50, 2411, 1990.

18. **Paget, S.,** The distribution of secondary growths in cancer of the breast, *Lancet,* 1, 571, 1889.

19. **Gullino, P. M. and Grantham, F. H.,** Studies on the exchange of fluids between host and tumor. II. The blood flow of hepatomas and other tumors in rats and mice, *J. Natl. Cancer Inst.,* 27, 1465, 1961.

20. **Folkman, J.,** Tumor angiogenesis: Therapeutic implications. *N. Engl. J. Med.,* 285, 1182, 1971.

21. **Folkman, J. and Klagsburn, M.,** Angiogenic factors, *Science,* 235, 442, 1987.

22. **Folkman, J. and Brem, H.,** Angiogenesis and inflammation, in *Inflammation — Basic Principles and Clinical Correlates,* Gallin, J. I., Goldstein, I. M., and Snyderman, R., Eds., Raven Press, New York, 1992, 821.

23. **Brem, S., Cotran, R., and Folkman, J.,** Tumor angiogenesis: A quantitative method for histological grading, *J. Natl. Cancer Inst.,* 4, 347, 1972.

24. **Hammersen, F., Endrich, B., and Osterkamp-Baust, U.,** The fine structure of tumor blood vessels. I. Participation of non-endothelial cells in tumor angiogenesis, *Int. J. Microcirc. Clin. Exp.,* 4, 31, 1985.

25. **Hoeckel, M., Schlenger, K., Doctrow, S., Kissel, T., and Vaupel, P.,** Therapeutic angiogenesis, *Arch. Surg.,* 128, 423, 1993.

26. **Yamaura, H. and Sato, H.,** Quantitative studies on the developing system of rat hepatoma, *J. Natl. Cancer Inst.,* 53, 1229, 1974.

27. **Konerding, M. A., Steinberg, F., and Budach, V.,** The vascular system of xenotransplanted tumors — Scanning electron and light microscopic studies, *Scanning Microsc.,* 3, 327, 1989.

28. **Konerding, M. A., Steinberg, F., and Streffer, C.,** The vasculature of xenotransplanted human melanomas and sarcomas on nude mice. I. Vascular corrosion casting studies, *Acta Anat.*, 136, 21, 1989.

29. **Konerding, M.A., Steinberg, F., and Streffer, C.,** The vasculature of xenotransplanted human melanomas and sarcomas on nude mice. II. Scanning and transmission electron microscopic studies, *Acta Anat.*, 136, 27, 1989.

30. **Steinberg, F., Konerding, M. A., and Streffer, C.,** The vascular architecture of human xenotransplanted tumors: Histological, morphometrical, and ultrastructural studies, *J. Cancer Res. Clin. Oncol.*, 116, 517, 1990.

31. **Blood, C. H. and Zetter, B. R.,** Tumor interactions with the vasculature: Angiogenesis and tumor metastasis, *Biochim. Biophys. Acta*, 1032, 89, 1990.

32. **Folkman, J.,** What is the evidence that tumors are angiogenesis dependent?, *J. Natl. Cancer Inst.*, 82, 1, 1990.

33. **Klagsbrun, M. and D'Amore, P. A.,** Regulators of angiogenesis, *Annu. Rev. Physiol.*, 53, 217, 1991.

34. **Yamaura, H. K., Yamada, K., and Matsuzawa, T.,** Radiation effect on the proliferating capillaries in rat transparent chambers, *Int. J. Radiat. Biol.*, 30, 179, 1976.

35. **Wurschmidt, F., Beck-Bornholdt, H. P., and Vogler, H.,** Radiobiology of the rhabdomyosarcoma R1H of the rat: Influence of the size of irradiation field on tumor response, tumor bed effect, and neovascularization kinetics, *Int. J. Radiat. Oncol. Biol. Phys.*, 18, 879, 1990.

36. **Verhoeven, D. and Buyssens, N.,** Desmin-positive stellate cells associated with angiogenesis in a tumour and non-tumour system, *Arch. Biol. Cell Pathol.*, 54, 263, 1988.

37. **Chodak, G. W., Scheiner, C. J., and Zetter, B. R.,** Urine from patients with transitional cell carcinoma stimulates migration of capillary endothelial cells, *N. Engl. J. Med.*, 305, 869, 1981.

38. **López-Pousa, S., Ferrier, I., Vich, J. M., and Domenech-Mateu, J.,** Angiogenic activity of CSF in human malignancies, *Experientia*, 37, 413, 1981.

39. **Glaser, B. M., D'Amore, P. A., Lutty, G. A., Fenselau, A. H., Michels, R. G., and Patz, A.,** Chemical mediators of intraocular neovascularization, *Trans. Ophthal. Soc.*, 100, 369, 1980.

40. **Tapper, D., Scheiner, C., Frissora, H., and Zetter, B.,** The stimulation of capillary endothelial cell migration by aqueous humor, *J. Surg. Res.*, 30, 262, 1981.

41. **Ingber, D. E., Madri, J. A., and Folkman, J.,** A possible mechanism for the inhibition of angiogenesis, *Endocrinology*, 119, 1768, 1986.

42. **White, C. M., Sondheimer, H. M., Crouch, E. C., Wilson, H., and Fan, L. L.,** Treatment of pulmonary hemangiomatosis with recombinant interferon alfa-2a, *N. Engl. J. Med.*, 320, 1197, 1989.

43. **Folkman, J.,** Successful treatment of an angiogenic disease, *N. Engl. J. Med.*, 320, 1211, 1989.

44. **Takamiya, Y., Friedlander, R. M., Brem, H., Malick, A., and Martuza, R. L.,** Inhibition of angiogenesis and growth of human nerve-sheath tumors by AGM-1470, *J. Neurosurg.*, 78, 470, 1993.

45. **Matsubara, T., Saura, R., Hirohata, K., and Ziff, M.,** Inhibition of human endothelial cell proliferation *in vitro* and neovascularization *in vivo* by D-penicillamine, *J. Clin. Invest.*, 83, 158, 1989.

46. **Matsubara, T. and Ziff, M.,** Inhibition of human endothelial cell proliferation by gold compounds, *J. Clin. Invest.*, 79, 1440, 1987.

47. **Weidner, N., Folkman, J., Pozza, F., Bevilacqua, P., Allred, E. N., Moore, D. H., Meli, S., and Gasparini, G.,** Tumor angiogenesis — A new significant and independent prognostic indicator in early-stage breast carcinoma, *J. Natl. Cancer Inst.*, 84, 1875, 1992.

48. **Horak, E. R., Leek, R., Klenk, N., Lejeune, S., Smith, K., Stuart, N., Grenall, M., Stepniewska, K., and Harris, A. L.,** Angiogenesis, assessed by platelet endothelial cell adhesion molecule antibodies, as indicator of node metastases and survival in breast cancer, *Lancet*, 340, 1120, 1992.

49. **Page, D. L. and Dupont, W. D.,** Breast cancer angiohistogenesis — Through a narrow window, *J. Natl. Cancer Inst.*, 84, 1850, 1992.

50. **Wakui, S., Furusato, M., Itoh, T., Sasaki, H., Akiyama, A., Kinoshita, I., Asano, K., Tokuda, T., Aizawa, S., and Ushigome, S.,** Tumor angiogenesis in prostatic carcinoma with and without bone marrow metastasis — A morphometric study, *J. Pathol.*, 168, 257, 1992.

51. **Bigler, S. A., Deering, R. E., and Brawer, M. K.,** Comparison of microscopic vascularity in benign and malignant prostate tissue, *Hum. Pathol.*, 24, 220, 1993.

52. **Brem, S., Tsanaclis, A. M. C., Gately, S., Gross, J. L., and Herblin, W. F.,** Immunolocalization of basic fibroblast growth factor to the microvasculature of human brain tumors, *Cancer,* 70, 2673, 1992.

53. **Gagliardi, A. and Collins, D. C.,** Inhibition of angiogenesis by antiestrogens, *Cancer Res.,* 53, 533, 1993.

54. **Folberg, R., Peer, J., Gruman, L. M., Woolson, R. F., Jeng, G., Montaque, P. R., Moninger, T. O., Yi, H., and Moore, K. C.,** The morphologic characteristics of tumor blood vessels as a marker of tumor progression in primary human uveal melanoma — A matched case-control study, *Hum. Pathol.,* 23, 1298, 1992.

55. **Endrich, B., Reinhold, H. S., Gross, J. F., and Intaglietta, M.,** Tissue perfusion inhomogeneity during early tumor growth in rats, *J. Natl. Cancer Inst.,* 62, 387, 1979.

56. **Boucher, Y., Baxter, L. T., and Jain, R. K.,** Interstitial pressure gradients in tissue-isolated and subcutaneous tumors: Implications for therapy, *Cancer Res.,* 50, 4478, 1990.

57. **Less, J. R., Posner, M. C., Boucher, Y., Borochovitz, D., Wolmark, N., and Jain, R. K.,** Interstitial hypertension in human tumors. 4. Interstitial hypertension in human breast and colorectal tumors, *Cancer Res.,* 52, 6371, 1992.

58. **Peters, W., Teixeira, M., Intaglietta, M., and Gross, J. F.,** Microcirculatory studies in rat mammary carcinoma. I. Transparent chamber method, development of microvasculature, and pressures in tumor vessels, *J. Natl. Cancer Inst.,* 65, 631, 1980.

59. **Boucher, Y. and Jain, R. K.,** Microvascular pressure is the principal driving force for interstitial hypertension in solid tumors: Implications for vascular collapse, *Cancer Res.,* 52, 5110, 1992.

60. **Vaupel, P.,** Pathophysiological mechanisms of hyperthermia in cancer therapy, in *Biological Basis of Oncologic Thermotherapy,* Gautherie, M., Ed., Springer, Berlin, 1990, 73.

61. **Vaupel, P., Schlenger, K., and Höckel, M.,** Blood flow and oxygenation of human tumors, in *Tumor Blood Supply and Metabolic Microenvironment,* Vaupel, P. and Jain, R. K., Eds., Akademie der Wissenschaften, Mainz, Gustav Fischer Verlag, Stuttgart, 1991, 165.

62. **Jain, R. K.,** Parameters governing tumor blood flow, in *Tumor Blood Supply and Metabolic Microenvironment,* Vaupel, P. and Jain, R. K., Eds., Akademie der Wissenschaften, Mainz, Gustav Fischer Verlag, Stuttgart, 1991, 27.

63. **Intaglietta, M.,** Reactivation of the microcirculation in ischemia, *Progr. Appl. Microcirc.,* 13, 27, 1989.

64. **Slaaf, D. W., Oude Vrielink, H. H. E., Tangelder, G.-J., and Reneman, R. S.,** Vasomotion under altered perfusion conditions, *Progr. Appl. Microcirc.,* 15, 75, 1989.

65. **Intaglietta, M.,** Vasomotion as normal microvascular activity and a reaction to impaired homeostasis, *Progr. Appl. Microcirc.,* 15, 1, 1989.

66. **Meyer, J.-U., Borgström, P., Lindbom, L., and Intaglietta, M.,** Vasomotion patterns in skeletal muscle arterioles during changes in arterial pressure, *Microvasc. Res.,* 35, 193, 1988.

67. **Meyer, J.-U., Lindbom, L., and Intaglietta, M.,** Coordinated diameter oscillations at arteriolar bifurcations in sceletal muscle, *Am. J. Physiol.,* 253, H568, 1987.

68. **Tsai, A. G. and Intaglietta, M.,** Evidence of flow motion induced changes in local tissue oxygenation, *Int. J. Microcirc. Clin. Exp.,* 12, 75, 1993.

69. **Baxter, L. T. and Jain, R. K.,** Transport of fluid and macromolecules in tumors. I. Role of interstitial pressure and convection, *Microvasc. Res.,* 37, 77, 1989.

70. **Curti, B. D., Urba, W. J., Alvord, W. G., Janik, J. E., Smith, J. W., Madara, K., and Longo, D. L.,** Interstitial pressure of subcutaneous nodules in melanoma and lymphoma patients: Changes during treatment, *Cancer Res.,* 53, 2204, 1993.

71. **Gullino, P. M.,** Extracellular compartments of solid tumors, in *Cancer,* Vol. 3, Becker, F. F., Ed., Plenum Press, New York, 1975, 327.

72. **Jain, R. K.,** Transport of molecules in the tumor interstitium: A review, *Cancer Res.,* 47, 3039, 1987.

73. **Jain, R. K.,** Transport of molecules across tumor vasculature, *Cancer Metastasis Rev.,* 6, 559, 1987.

74. **Jain, R. K.,** Delivery of novel therapeutic agents in tumors: Physiological barriers and strategies, *J. Natl. Cancer Inst.,* 81, 570, 1989.

75. **Jain, R. K.,** Vascular and interstitial barriers to delivery of therapeutic agents in tumors, *Cancer Metastasis Rev.,* 9, 253, 1990.

76. **Jain, R. K.,** Haemodynamic and transport barriers to the treatment of solid tumors, *Int. J. Radiat. Biol.,* 60, 85, 1991.

77. **Reinhold, H. S.,** Improved microcirculation in irradiated tumours, *Eur. J. Cancer,* 7, 273, 1971.

78. **Vaupel, P. and Müller-Klieser, W.,** Interstitieller Raum und Mikromilieu in malignen Tumoren, *Mikrozirk. Forsch. Klin.,* 2, 78, 1983.

79. **Vaupel, P. and Kallinowski, F.,** Hemoconcentration of blood flowing through human tumor xenografts, *Int. J. Microcirc. Clin. Exp.,* 6, 72, 1987.

80. **Young, J. S., Lumsden, C. E., and Stalker, A. L.,** The significance of the "tissue pressure" of normal testicular and of neoplastic (Brown-Pearce carcinoma) tissue in the rabbit, *J. Path. Bact.,* 62, 313, 1950.

81. **Butler, T. P., Grantham, F. H., and Gullino, P. M.,** Bulk transfer of fluid in the interstitial compartment of mammary tumors, *Cancer Res.,* 35, 3084, 1979.

82. **Molls, M. and Feldmann, H. J.,** Clinical investigations of blood flow in malignant tumors of the pelvis and the abdomen in patients undergoing thermoradiotherapy, in *Tumor Blood Supply and Metabolic Microenvironment,* Vaupel, P. and Jain, R. K., Eds., Gustav Fischer Verlag, Stuttgart, 1991, 143.

83. **Semmler, W., Bachert, P., and van Kaick, G.,** Human tumor response to therapy monitored by magnetic resonance spectroscopy, in *Tumor Blood Supply and Metabolic Microenvironment,* Vaupel, P. and Jain, R. K., Eds., Gustav Fischer Verlag, Stuttgart, 1991, 257.

84. **Okunieff, P., Singer, S., and Vaupel, P.,** Magnetization transfer 31P-NMR to measure metabolic states, dynamic changes, and enzyme kinetics, in *Tumor Blood Supply and Metabolic Microenvironment,* Vaupel, P. and Jain, R. K., Eds., Gustav Fischer Verlag, Stuttgart, 1991, 267.

85. **Okunieff, P., Vaupel, P., Sedlacek, R., and Neuringer, L. J.,** Evaluation of tumor energy metabolism and microvascular blood flow after glucose or mannitol administration using 31P nuclear magnetic resonance spectroscopy and laser Doppler flowmetry, *Int. J. Radiat. Oncol. Biol. Phys.,* 16, 1493, 1989.

86. **Vaupel, P., Okunieff, P., Kallinowski, F., and Neuringer, L. J.,** Correlations between ^{31}P-NMR spectroscopy and tissue O_2 tension measurements in a murine fibrosarcoma, *Radiat. Res.,* 120, 477, 1989.

87. **Adler, L. P., Crowe, J. P., Alkaisi, N. K., and Sunshine, J. L.,** Evaluation of breast masses and axillary lymph nodes with (F-18)-2-Deoxy-2-fluoro-D-glucose PET, *Radiology,* 187, 743, 1993.

88. **Evelhoch, J. L., Larcombe-McDouall, J. B., McCoy, C. L., Mattiello, J., Simpson, N. E., and Sayedsadr, M.,** Deuterium NMR imaging of regional tumor blood flow: Effect of size in RIF-1 murine tumors, in *Tumor Blood Supply and Metabolic Microenvironment,* Vaupel, P. and Jain, R. K., Eds. Gustav Fischer Verlag, Stuttgart, 1991, 293.

89. **Feldmann, H. J., Sievers, K., Fuller, J., Molls, M., and Lohr, E.,** Evaluation of tumor blood perfusion by dynamic MRI and CT in patients undergoing thermoradiotherapy, *Eur. J. Radiol.,* 16, 224, 1993.

90. **Lammertsma, A. A., Wilson, C. B., and Jones, T.,** *In vivo* physiological studies in human tumors using positron emission tomography, in *Tumor Blood Supply and Metabolic Microenvironment,* Vaupel, P. and Jain, R. K., Eds., Gustav Fischer Verlag, Stuttgart, 1991, 319.

91. **Kroeger, M., Walenta, S., Rofstad, E. K., and Müller-Klieser, W.,** Imaging of structure and function in human tumor xenografts, in *Tumor Blood Supply and Metabolic Microenvironment,* Vaupel, P. and Jain, R. K., Eds., Gustav Fischer Verlag, Stuttgart, 1991, 305.

92. **Thomlinson, R. H. and Gray, L. H.,** The histological structure of some human lung cancers and the possible implications for radiotherapy, *Br. J. Cancer,* 9, 539, 1955.

93. **Tannock, I. F.,** The relation between cell proliferation and the vascular system in a transplanted mouse mammary tumour, *Br. J. Cancer,* 22, 258, 1968.

94. **Brammer, I., Zywietz, F., and Jung, H.,** Changes of histological and proliferative indices in the Walker carcinoma with tumour size and distance from blood vessel, *Eur. J. Cancer,* 15, 1329, 1979.

95. **Hirst, D. G. and Denekamp, J.,** Tumour cell proliferation in relation to the vasculature, *Cell Tissue Kinet.,* 12, 31, 1979.

96. **Lyng, H., Skretting, A., and Rofstad, E. K.,** Blood flow in six human melanoma xenograft lines with different growth characteristics, *Cancer Res.,* 52, 584, 1992.

97. **Gabbert, H., Wagner, R., and Höhn, P.,** The relation between tumor cell proliferation and vascularization in differentiated and undifferentiated colon carcinomas in the rat, *Virchows Arch. Cell Pathol.,* 41, 119, 1982.

98. **Monschke, F., Müller, W.-U., Winkler, U., and Streffer, C.,** Cell proliferation and vascularization in human breast carcinomas, *Int. J. Cancer,* 49, 812, 1991.

99. **Chaplin, D. J. and Trotter, M. J.,** Chemical modifiers of tumor blood flow, in *Tumor Blood Supply and Metabolic Microenvironment,* Vaupel, P. and Jain, R. K., Eds., Gustav Fischer Verlag, Stuttgart, 1991, 65.

100. **Jirtle, R. L.,** Chemical modification of tumour blood flow, *Int. J. Hyperthermia,* 4, 355, 1988.

101. **Burton, M. A., Gray, B. N., and Coletti, A.,** Effect of angiotensin II on blood flow in the transplanted sheep squamous cell carcinoma, *Eur. J. Cancer,* 45, 54, 1988.

102. **Burton, M. A., Gray, B. N., Self, G. W., Heggie, J. C., and Townsend, P. S.,** Manipulation of experimental rat and rabbit liver tumor blood flow with angiotensin II, *Cancer Res.,* 45, 5390, 1985.

103. **Suzuki, M., Hori, K., Abe, I., Saito, S., and Sato, H.,** A new approach to cancer chemotherapy: selective enhancement of tumor blood flow with angiotensin II, *J. Natl. Cancer Inst.,* 67, 663, 1981.

104. **Kuroiwa, T., Aoki, K., Taniguchi, S., Hasuda, K., and Baba, T.,** Efficacy of two route chemotherapy using *cis*-diamminedichloroplatinum (II) and its antidote sodium thiosulphate in combination with angiotensin II in a rat limb tumor, *Cancer Res.,* 47, 3618, 1987.

105. **Takematsu, H., Tomita, Y., and Kato, T.,** Angiotensin-induced hypertension and chemotherapy for multiple lesions of malignant melanoma, *Br. J. Dermatol.,* 113, 463, 1985.

106. **Ekelund, L. and Lunderquist, A.,** Pharmacoangiography with angiotensin, *Radiology,* 110, 533, 1974.

107. **Gerl, A., Clemm, C., and Wilmanns, W.,** Acute and late vascular complications following chemotherapy for germ cell tumors, *Onkologie,* 16, 88, 1993.

108. **Teutsch, C., Lipton, A., and Harvey, H. A.,** Raynaud's phenomenon as a side effect of chemotherapy with vinblastine and bleomycin for testicular carcinoma, *Cancer Treat. Rep.,* 61, 925, 1977.

109. **Vogelzang, N. J., Bosl, G. J., Johnson, K., and Kennedy, B. J.,** Raynaud's phenomenon: A common toxicity after combination chemotherapy for testicular cancer, *Ann. Intern. Med.,* 95, 288, 1981.

110. **Hansen, S. W. and Olsen, N.,** Raynaud's phenomenon in patients treated with cisplatin, vinblastine, and bleomycin for germ cell cancer: Measurement of vasoconstrictor response to cold, *J. Clin. Oncol.,* 7, 940, 1989.

111. **Aass, N., Kaasa, S., Lund, E., Kaalhus, O., Heier, M. S., and Fossa, S. D.,** Long-term somatic side effects and morbidity in testicular cancer patients, *Br. J. Cancer,* 61, 151, 1990.

112. **Bissett, D., Kunkeler, L., Zwanenburg, L., Paul, J., Gray, C., Swan, I. R. C., Kerr, D. J., and Kaye, S. B.,** Long-term sequelae of treatment for testicular germ cell tumours, *Br. J. Cancer,* 62, 655, 1990.

113. **Scheulen, M. E. and Schmidt, C. G.,** Raynaud-Syndrom nach kombinierter zytostatischer Behandlung von Patienten mit malignen Hodentumoren, *Dtsch. Med. Wschr.,* 107, 1640, 1982.

114. **Heier, M. S., Nilsen, T., Graver, V., Aass, N., and Fossa, S. D.,** Raynaud's phenomenon after combination chemotherapy of testicular cancer, measured by laser Doppler flowmetry. A pilot study, *Br. J. Cancer,* 63, 550, 1991.

115. **Streffer, C.,** Hyperthermia and the therapy of malignant tumors, *Recent Results in Cancer Research,* Vol. 104, Springer, Berlin, 1987.

116. **Hinkelbein, W., Bruggmoser, G., Engelhardt, R., and Wannenmacher, M.,** Preclinical hyperthermia. *Recent Results in Cancer Research,* Vol. 109, Springer, Berlin, 1988.

117. **Issels, R. D. and Wilmanns, W.,** Application of hyperthermia in the treatment of cancer. *Recent Results in Cancer Research,* Vol. 107, Springer, Berlin, 1988.

118. **Anghileri, L. J. and Robert, J.,** *Hyperthermia in Cancer Treatment,* Vols. I–III, CRC Press, Boca Raton, FL, 1986.

119. **Reinhold, H. S. and Endrich, B.,** Tumour microcirculation as a target for hyperthermia, *Int. J. Hyperthermia,* 2, 111, 1986.

120. **Endrich, B. and Hammersen, F.,** Morphologic and hemodynamic alterations in capillaries during hyperthermia, in *Hyperthermia in Cancer Treatment,* Vol. II, Anghileri, L. J. and Robert, J., Eds., CRC Press, Boca Raton, FL, 1986, 17.

121. **Mayer, W.-K., Stohrer, M., Krüger, W., and Vaupel, P.,** Laser Doppler flux and tissue oxygenation of experimental tumours upon local hyperthermia and/or hyperglycemia, *J. Cancer Res. Clin. Oncol.,* 118, 523, 1992.

122. **Kalmus, J., Okunieff, P., and Vaupel, P.,** Dose-dependent effects of hydralazine on microcirculatory function and hyperthermic response of murine FSall tumors, *Cancer Res.,* 50, 14, 1990.

123. **Vaupel, P., Okunieff, P., and Kluge M.,** Response of tumour red blood cell flux to hyperthermia and/or hyperglycemia, *Int. J. Hyperthermia,* 5, 199, 1989.

124. **Waterman, F. M., Tupchong, L., Nerlinger, R. E., and Matthews, J.,** Blood flow in human tumors during local hyperthermia, *Int. J. Radiat. Oncol. Biol. Phys.*, 20, 1255, 1991.

125. **Acker, J. C., Dewhirst, M. W., Honoré, G. M., Samulski, T. V., Tucker, J. A., and Oleson, J. R.,** Blood perfusion measurements in human tumours: Evaluation of laser Doppler methods, *Int. J. Hyperthermia*, 6, 287, 1990.

126. **Seegenschmiedt, M. H., Sauer, R., Miyamoto, C., Chalal, J. A., and Brady, L. W.,** Clinical experience with interstitial thermoradiotherapy for localized implantable pelvic tumors, *Am. J. Clin. Oncol.*, 16, 210, 1993.

127. **Lyng, H., Monge, O. R., Sager, E. M., and Rofstad, E. K.,** Prediction of treatment temperatures in clinical hyperthermia of locally advanced breast carcinoma — The use of contrast enhanced computed tomography, *Int. J. Radiat. Oncol. Biol. Phys.*, 26, 451, 1993.

128. **Gilly, F. N., Carry, P. Y., Sayag, A. C., Panteix, G. G., Bienvenu, J., Brachet, A., Salle, B., and Braillon, G.,** Gastric cancer with peritoneal carcinomatosis — Does hyperthermia constitute a new therapeutic approach? *Ann. Chir.*, 47, 414, 1993.

129. **Henneking, K., Binder, J., Weyers, W., and Schwemmle, K.,** Chirurgische Behandlung und regionale Chemotherapie beim Extremitätenmelanom, *Chirurg*, 64, 134, 1993.

130. **Schlag, P. M. and Kettelhack, Ch.,** Weichteilsarkome: Die isolierte Extremitätenperfusion, *Chirurg*, 64, 455, 1993.

131. **Issels, R. D., Bosse, D., Starck, M., Abdel-Rahman, S., Jauch, K. W., Schildberg, F. W., and Wilmanns, W.,** Weichteiltumoren: Indikation und Ergebnisse der Hyperthermie, *Chirurg*, 64, 461, 1993.

132. **Lowdell, C. P., Ash, D. V., Driver, I., and Brown, S. B.,** Interstitial photodynamic therapy. Clinical experience with diffusing fibres in the treatment of cutaneous and subcutaneous tumours, *Br. J. Cancer*, 67, 1398, 1993.

133. **Gamarra, F., Spelsberg, F., Kuhnle, G. E. H. and Goetz, A. E.,** High-energy shock waves induce blood flow reduction in tumors, *Cancer Res.*, 53, 1590, 1993.

134. **Merwin, R. and Algire, G. H.,** Transparent-chamber observations of the response of a transplantable mouse mammary tumor to local roentgen irradiation, *J. Natl. Cancer Inst.*, 10, 593, 1950.

135. **Dewhirst, M. W.,** Microvascular changes induced by radiation exposure: Implications for therapy, in *Tumor Blood Supply and Metabolic Microenvironment*, Vaupel, P. and Jain, R. K., Eds, Gustav Fischer Verlag, Stuttgart, 1991, 109.

136. **West, C. M. L.,** Predictive assays in radiation therapy, *Adv. Radiat. Biol.*, 18, 149, 1994.

137. **Kolstadt, P.,** Intercapillary distance, oxygen tension and local recurrence in cervix cancer, *Scand. J. Clin. Lab. Invest.*, 106, 145, 1968.

138. **Siracka, E., Siracky, J., Pappova, N., and Révész, L.,** Vascularization and radiocurability in cancer of the uterine cervix. A retrospective study, *Neoplasma*, 29, 183, 1982.

139. **Siracka, E., Révész, L., Kovac, R., and Siracky, J.,** Vascular density in carcinoma of the uterine cervix and its predictive value for radiotherapy, *Int. J. Cancer*, 41, 819, 1988.

140. **Siracky, J., Siracka, E., Kovac, R., and Révész, L.,** Prognostic significance of vascular density and a malignancy grading in radiation treated uterine cervix carcinoma, *Neoplasma*, 35, 289, 1988.

141. **Révész, L., Siracka, E., Siracky, J., Delides, G., and Pavlaki, K.,** Variation of vascular density within and between tumors of the uterine cervix and its predictive value for radiotherapy, *Int. J. Radiat. Oncol. Biol. Phys.*, 16, 1161, 1989.

142. **Awwad, H. K., Naggar, M., Mocktar, N., and Barsoum, M.,** Intercapillary distance measurement as an indicator of hypoxia in carcinoma of the cervix uteri, *Int. J. Radiat. Oncol. Biol. Phys.*, 12, 1329, 1986.

143. **Delides, G. S., Venizelos, J., and Révész, L.,** Vascularization and curability of stage III and IV nasopharyngeal tumours, *J. Cancer Res. Clin. Oncol.*, 114, 321, 1988.

144. **Lauk, S., Skates, S., Goodman, M., and Suit, H. D.,** A morphometric study of the vascularity of oral squamous cell carcinomas and its relation to outcome of radiation therapy, *Eur. J. Cancer Clin. Oncol.*, 25, 1431, 1989.

145. **Höckel, M., Knoop, C., Schlenger, K., Vorndran, B., Baußmann, E., Mitze, M., Knapstein, P. G., and Vaupel, P.,** Intratumoral pO_2 predicts survival in advanced cancer of the uterine cervix, *Radiother. Oncol.*, 26, 45, 1993.

146. **VanHoef, M., Knox, W. F., Dhesis, S. S., Howell, A., Schor, A. M.,** Assessment of tumor vascularity as a prognostic factor in lymph node negative invasive breast cancer, *Eur. J. Cancer*, 29A, 1141, 1993.

Section III

Development of Microcirculation Research

Chapter 9

Historical Aspects of Microcirculation Research

Benjamin W. Zweifach

CONTENTS

I. GENERAL BACKGROUND

The roots of the field of microcirculation can be traced back several hundred years to the observations of Malpighi[1] and Leuwenhoek[2] who were able with the aid of crude microscopes to describe for the first time the unceasing flow of blood through the tiny tubes that were referred to as capillaries. These microscopic-sized blood vessels were envisaged originally as being analogous to a set of irrigation ditches. In fact, for a time there was some uncertainty as to whether they were indeed vascular conduits or merely tissue spaces. The recognition of these peripheral ramifications of the vascular tree as an independent functional entity emerged only gradually as an outcome of work on the tissue response to local injury or inflammation.

The usage of the term "microcirculation" in an organic context is of comparatively recent vintage, first appearing consistently in the literature during the 1950s. Claude Bérnard[3] had recognized as far back as 1880 that paramount for the physiological organization of multicellular organisms is the maintenance of a stable environment, the "milieu interieur" in which the parenchymal cells carry out their functional activities. Walter B. Cannon, in *The Wisdom of the Body*,[4] which was concerned with the basic integrative issue for which the autonomic nervous system is responsible, advanced the term "homeostasis" to focus on the overriding necessity to safeguard the integrity of the tissue milieu. The terminal vascular bed was the obvious modus operandi for this seminal function. In this context, a local feedback of some kind was necessary not only to ensure a stable tissue milieu, but set into motion mechanisms for readjusting tissue perfusion of blood in response to the fluctuating metabolic activities of the body. Intravital microscopy in humans has provided provocative evidence over the years that the terminal vascular bed is intimately involved at a primary, as well as a secondary, level in major disease processes and indeed in the aging process per se.

Quantitative concepts dealing with the exchange of fluid between the blood and tissue compartments had been advanced by Ludwig in 1861[5] and later elaborated by Starling.[6] The behavior of the terminal vascular bed attracted at that time primarily pathologists so that details of the control of blood flow within the tissues and its selective distribution remained largely inferential. The data on the behavior of individual components of the terminal vascular network continued to be descriptive in nature until the classical work

0-8493-4870-6/95/$0.00+$.50
© 1995 by CRC Press, Inc.

of August Krogh in the 1920s and 1930s[7] brought to our attention the cardinal aspects of tissue perfusion that had to be addressed.

Much of the change in the direction and emphasis in microvascular research has evolved through the application of the tools and principles from related basic disciplines, such as engineering, physics, and chemistry. However, until dynamic measurements of microvascular behavior became available, there was only a superficial interaction with these disciplines in terms of early manifestations of disease.

Two methodological departures were major factors in setting the stage for substantial advances in our understanding of microcirculatory dynamics — the introduction of electron microscopy[8,9] in the 1970s and 1980s brought the intracellular organization of the minute vessels and their associated organellae into clearer focus. More recently, the advancements in cell culture techniques, together with the development of specific immunological probes, have uncovered an immense vista of biochemical and biophysical relationships concerned with the multicellular organization and selective modification of living structures.

A survey of the historical sequence of attempts in this direction provides a useful framework for the evaluation of the particular milestones that were key determinants in laying the foundations for the currently accepted directions of microcirculatory research. It is important at the outset to keep in perspective the primary physiological function performed by this segment of the cardiovascular system — the maintenance of the exchange of materials between the blood and the interstitial compartment at a level that is commensurate with the changing metabolic needs of a given tissue.

As researchers continued to delve more deeply into the organizational fabric of living systems, the information became increasingly focused on cellular and subcellular phenomena that are far removed from the level of information used to describe the behavior of organ systems that have been the signposts of physiology.

A trend has appeared to replace the term "physiology" with the term "biology" as an indication that the core of current investigation is concerned with the physicochemical attributes of living materials. Just how a molecular database can be meaningfully integrated into the functional activities of the various organ systems is not readily apparent since what appeared to be discreet reactions have been found to be complex cascades that encompassed alternative, overlapping pathways. Local cell-to-cell communication appears to be a dominant factor in the modulation of tissue functions. The diversity that has been encountered has been handled in the past by the formulation of theoretical models[10] for which individual variables could be tested singly or in combination. The diverse source of the data from the very start, by itself, creates a great deal of uncertainty in the extrapolation from *in vitro* to *in situ* situations. Because of this, many different ways to categorize microvascular information have been tried and are shown in Table 1.

Despite its shortcomings, intravital microscopy has served as a practical approach for the study of the components of human microcirculation in a clinical setting for well over 75 years.[11] The information is in many ways self-limiting since it is confined to more accessible tissues, such as the skin or the eye. The nailfold region of the digits, because of its thinness and relative transparency, has been an especially attractive site for the study of the circulation within individual capillary loops in which flow could be followed and documented at repeated intervals. As data accumulated on changes associated with tissue injury and local inflammation, an appreciation began to develop for the importance of factors affecting the physicochemical characteristics of the bloodstream.

The observations of Thomas Lewis[12] dealing with the responsiveness of the skin vessels to local injury led him to recognize the need to distinguish between several subsets of microvessels. He preferred the term "minute blood vessels" when referring to the active adjustments of the flow through the microscopic-sized vessels. It was clear that

Table 1 Functional Behavior of the Microvascular Network

I. Vasomotor Modulation
- Redistribution of flow via in-series vs. in-parallel offshoots of arterioles
- Sphincter control of precapillary side-arm offshoots
- Active contractility of endothelium vs. Rouget Cell [pericyte]
- Geometric constraints vs. selective modulation

II. Regional Differences
- Design of network relative to the range of tissue metabolic activity

III. Functional Modulation
- Endothelial cell shape changes (cytoskeleton)
- Match exchange area with volumetric flow
- Local endothelial vs. systemic or neurogenic origin
- Shifting formation and release of cytokines

---

within the tissue proper, the volumetric flow, as well as its distribution, were selectively modulated by changes at different segmental branchings.

In view of the highly specialized nature of the skin or eye circulation, an overriding difficulty with respect to the significance of data in humans to specific aspects of disease has been the question of its relevance to the status of other microcirculatory beds throughout the body. Repeated observations that major systemic diseases are associated with perturbations in blood rheology, evidence of microthrombosis, red cell aggregation, and macromolecular leakage have, however, led investigators to consider the relevance of such phenomena to the circulation in general, as well as serving as predisposing factors to organ damage. Considerable support in this regard has been forthcoming for diabetes[13] and hypertension.[14] Attempts at quantification have utilized direct photography and indirect estimates of blood flow through the use of laser Doppler recording.

The expanding literature base dealing with intravital microscopy in disease contains references to the increased incidence of microangiopathies.[14] Microvascular abnormalities in conditions such as hypertension include micro-aneurysms, vessel tortuosity, wall thickening, intravascular aggregation, and stasis. Evidence has been presented[10] that the hypertensive syndrome was associated with a striking ischemia of the capillary-sized vessels, presumably due to a bypassing of whole groups of capillaries.

II. CONCEPTUAL FRAMEWORK

Early concepts of the organization of the microcirculation depicted the network as the end result of a repeated dichotomous subdivision of the feed arteries within the tissue in which the successive branchings taper down to capillary dimensions (about the size of the red blood cells for that species) to form a seemingly nondescript meshwork.

A variety of approaches have been used to explore the possibility of a representative modular design as a frame of reference for dealing with the microcirculatory behavior in the various organs of the body.[15] In essence, such studies have demonstrated a spectrum of branching configurations in different tissues that depend upon the architectural peculiarities of the constituent parenchymal cells, as well as the range of biochemical activities encountered in each tissue. Thus, in tissues where parenchymal cell metabolism remains relatively stable, the terminal vascular bed was found to be deployed as a seemingly random, dichotomous branching network that is in contrast to the modular design exhibited by skeletal muscle preparations, where perfusion requirements vary widely at rest and during mechanical work (exercise). Differences between tissues are especially striking on the precapillary side of the network reinforcing the idea that the precapillary arterioles represent the principal sites for selective adjustment of capillary perfusion.

Specialized organs, such as the liver,[16] show extensive departures from the ideal dichotomous branching, in line with their unique functions.

III. SHIFTING FOCUS OF MICROCIRCULATORY RESEARCH

If one examines the database covering microvascular behavior over the past 60 to 70 years, it can be seen that there has been a series of shifts in focus to more fundamental organizational levels.

Organ physiology — Descriptive
Tissue physiology — *In vitro* biochemistry
Cell physiology — Micromanipulative intervention
Molecular biology — Tissue culture of cell lines
Extracellular domain — Macromolecule properties

With the application of the tools and principles from related basic disciplines, such as mathematics, physics, and chemistry, the field has shifted from a largely phenomenological database to a more analytical approach. The earliest application of engineering principles and tools to microvascular dynamics is to be found mainly in the analysis of the rheological properties of the blood. Until dynamic measurements of microvascular behavior became available, there was only a cosmetic interaction with this discipline.

The application of electron microscopy in particular has brought to the fore the contribution of extracellular macromolecules in conjunction with intracellular organellae.[17] More recently, information derived from *in vitro* cultures of selected cell lines has revealed adaptive controls at increasingly more basic organizational levels. As an example, it was shown that endothelial cell surfaces were covered with unique glycoprotein materials that could be visualized and analyzed with a series of monoclonal probes.

A. ENDOTHELIUM

Physiological studies have in the past come to grips with the exchange process mainly by measuring the A-V extraction of selected materials across whole organs or tissues. Although permeability studies at the organ level are informative, such phenomenological data by themselves do not address many of the essential features of the problem, such as the selective distribution of the volume of blood coursing through the terminal vascular bed so as to provide for a surface area commensurate with optimal exchange.

It has been estimated that there are some 60,000 miles of blood vessels in the human body — all of which are lined by endothelial cells — so that the population of endothelial cells makes up one of the largest organs of the body that enters into almost every conceivable facet of tissue homeostasis.

Prior to 1950, the endothelium was looked upon as an inert tile-like lining that was designed to minimize the frictional interaction with the moving bloodstream and the suppression of intravascular coagulation. Alterations in the lumenal surface properties were known to serve as the nidus for the injury cascade involving platelets and leukocytes. It was speculated that the adsorption of a precursor protein, such as fibrinogen, was a key factor in this regard. However, the shift in focus to the outer cell glycocalyx has shown that a family of glycoproteins serve as a dynamic interface between the intra- and the extracellular compartments.[18]

In view of the graded perviousness of the blood vascular exchange barrier to a range of different-sized water-soluble molecules, it was originally suggested that the unique permeability of the endothelial cell could be ascribed to its thinness and undifferentiated cellular organization. With time, it has become clear, however, that endothelial cells contained characteristic cytoplasmic organellae.

Some of the ultrastructural features of endothelium are given in Table 2.

Table 2 Ultrastructural Organization — Electron Microscopy of Capillary Bed

- Cell to cell junctional complexes
- Cytoplasmic organellae
- Interlocking cellular and extracellular features
- Microvascular changes in humans vs. experimental models of disease

When cultured *in vitro* on a suitable physical scaffold, endothelial cells formed sheets that exhibited properties not unlike those exhibited by the endothelium *in situ*. Recent studies have shown that endothelial cells not only participate in a broad array of local tissue reactions through the formation and secretion of selective cytokines, but that the endothelial lining of blood vessels responds to changes in intravascular pressure as well as fluctuations in shear rate so as to modulate vascular smooth muscle cell tone and reactivity.

Macromolecular complexes contribute to the permselectivity of the barrier in several contexts — either by way of a physicochemical modification in the functional attributes of different adhesive ligands or by way of an effect on special groupings in these macromolecular complexes that can lead to reactions with particular ligands or with related surface materials of other cells such as leukocytes or platelets. For example, a family of macromolecules, the integrins or selectins, are believed to serve as the electro-mechanical transducers for responses that may even include interstitial tissue pressure.[19]

Histological and electron microscopy studies show that the endothelium lining of the vascular system varies from continuous multicellular sheets to discontinuous structures. The discontinuous type is seen in tissues such as the intestinal mucosa on the postcapillary or venous side of the vascular network, or in the glomerular capillaries of the kidney. The work of Rous, Gilding, and Smith[20] in the 1930s demonstrated in skeletal muscle a gradient in the permeability of the microvessels to macromolecules, with a more pronounced extravasation of macromolecular markers occurring in the venules despite the fact that in skeletal muscle the postcapillary vessels do not have a demonstrably discontinuous endothelium. When considered as a whole, the observations in the literature suggest not only that the substantial differences in the endothelial barrier lining these vessels are intrinsic in nature, but that they can be induced by particular agents. Evidence has been advanced that adaptation along these lines may be associated with the expression of different phenotypes, but the functional basis for these striking cellular differences remains largely speculative. (For detailed information on endothelial cells, see Chapter 30 in this volume.)

B. DESIGN OF THE TERMINAL VASCULAR BED

It has long been appreciated from work on embryological preparations that the terminal vascular bed in the adult arises out a primitive meshwork of endothelial tubes that become differentiated as the heart delivers an increasing volumetric flow through the network so as to stimulate the formation of larger, heavier walled vessels with an outer investment of smooth muscle cells. This progressive remodeling process is closely dependent upon the physical path taken by the bloodstream. Essentially, the array of true capillaries in the adult tissue represents those vessels that were least affected by the progressive increase in volumetric flow and remain as endothelial tubes whose properties are determinants of the physicochemical characteristics of the blood-tissue barrier.

A basic feature relative to the deployment of terminal vascular networks that has been largely overlooked in dealing with the dynamics of the peripheral circulation is the extensive head-on interconnections between comparatively large arterioles (100–125 μm) and between analogous venular vessels so as to form arcades.[11] The majority of offshoots leading into the microvascular network proper originate as sidearm branches from such arteriole-to-arteriole interconnections, a feature that in effect provides a series of in-parallel pathways with respect to the parent trunk. (For further details on microvascular networks, refer to Chapter 33 of this volume.)

C. INTRINSIC CONTROL OF MICROVASCULAR SMOOTH MUSCLE

The blood ejected by the heart into the arterial system is distributed along regional lines through adjustments of vascular caliber of 100 to 150 µm arteries, a segmental hierarchy in which the prevailing *tone* is dominated by the autonomic nervous system. It then became necessary to explain how an adjustment that is geared to buffer systemic blood pressure within a prescribed range was integrated with changes in the small arterioles that are designed to meet shifting local metabolic needs.[21]

A large body of evidence indicates that the local modulation of pressure-flow relationships is achieved by a shift in the response characteristics of vascular smooth muscle.[22] Spontaneous adjustments in the diameter of the terminal arterioles and precapillaries have been observed in situations where the prevailing transmural pressure is increased or decreased. The magnitude of this response is strongly influenced by local environmental factors such as oxygen or carbon dioxide tensions, metabolites, and specific vasoactive mediators.

D. SYSTEMIC MODULATION OF MICROVASCULAR BEHAVIOR

It has long been recognized that the reactive state of the arteriolar vessels is influenced by blood-borne vasoactive materials. Most studies of this kind have been concerned with the nature of the response to specific mediators, especially when examined in the context of a disease such as hypertension. A large body of such investigations have dealt with comparisons of the microvascular perturbations associated with two extreme types of circulatory imbalance — hypotensive as opposed to hypertensive conditions. The database for these diametrically opposite perturbations demonstrates that they are characterized by shifts in either a compensatory or decompensatory direction that, in final analysis, is related to changes induced in the state of responsiveness of vascular smooth muscle. The development of a hyperresponsive state has been found to be more evident in the arterioles than in the parent feed arteries. Under chronic conditions where an induced shift in the functional status of the smooth muscle cells persists, a substantial remodeling of the affected small blood vessels develops including changes in length, diameter, wall thickness, and number of vessels.[22]

At the other extreme are various forms of peripheral circulatory insufficiency or shock that are associated with an imbalance of systemic as well as peripheral control mechanisms. Under conditions of hypovolemia and hypotension, tissue perfusion falls below critical levels. The entire vascular array within the microcirculation proper is involved initially in an attempt to counter the failing systemic driving force. Such mechanisms serve only as a temporary expedient since the resulting underperfusion of the tissue can be tolerated for only short periods. Local factors arise that interfere with the response of the smooth muscle cells and thereby undermine local homeostatic readjustments. The ensuing hyporesponsive state was found[23] to be associated with the appearance of materials that blunt the capacity of the smooth muscle to contract, as for example, SH compounds, various peptides, organic iron complexes, free radicals, etc. More recently, the endothelial cell via nitrous oxide mechanisms has been shown to act as a chemical transducer for the modulation of constrictor vs. dilator responses to agonists, a feature that introduces another pathway through which smooth muscle tone or reactivity can be adjusted.[24,25]

IV. MICROCIRCULATORY STUDIES IN MAN

The range of clinical indices listed in Table 3 illustrates the far-reaching implications of microvascular pathophysiology to organ survival and the course of different disease states.

Table 3 Microvascular Abnormalities in Patients

RBC aggregation — sludging, blood rheology, stasis
Intravascular thrombosis
Increased permeability (macromolecules)
Micro-aneurysms (material failure)
Capillary fragility (basement membrane)
Vasospasm
Venular enlargement
Tortuosity of capillaries and venules
Atypical reactivity to agonists
Maldistribution within network
Inflammatory sequelae
Angiogenesis

Note: Hypertension, diabetes mellitus, aging, sepsis.

There has been an increasing interest in the status of the microcirculation during chronic disorders such as arteriosclerosis, different forms of diabetes, and hypertension, among others. Although the use of vital microscopy in man is confronted with a number of limitations, it has been possible, nevertheless, to establish an extensive information base in accessible organs, such as the bulbar conjunctiva of the eye or the nailfold skin vessels. Despite the fact that the conjunctiva is not an organic structure in which vascular deterioration is life-threatening, its symptomology may reflect comparable changes in other key organs. Furthermore, the ubiquitous involvement of the microvasculature in most diseases has raised the possibility that vascular beds in general may be undermined to varying extents in chronic disease, with regional differences reflecting only a matter of the degree of change.

Advances in data acquisition techniques and electronic analysis of recorded images, as well as newly developed scanning techniques should enable investigators to quantify the *in vivo* information obtained in patients so as to be in a position to evaluate better their significance with respect to primary and/or secondary aspects of diabetes, hypertension, immune reactions, and predisposition of individuals to given complications.

The use of morphometric techniques as a yardstick to evaluate the status of the microvasculature has a number of unique advantages. The continuous shifting in nutritive exchange needs are met at the microcirculatory level by modulation of the caliber of particular segmental vessels. Under conditions where the microvasculature is confronted with a persistent imbalance of the physicochemical environment, a readjustment of volumetric flow rate by itself is no longer adequate to ensure local homeostasis so that the microvasculature begins to undergo various degrees of remodeling, which includes structural changes in individual segments as well as in the deployment of the network hierarchical constituents.

V. OVERVIEW

It is apparent that the microcirculation is a labile organic entity with a significant capacity to undergo remodeling in a positive as well as a negative direction. Morphometric adaptation is more readily quantified by recording segmental changes in microcirculatory topology. As commonly used, the term "disease" implies either a structural abnormality and/or a functional imbalance. Adaptive changes in arteriolar length and dimensions serve to meet flow requirements; increased capillarization provides an increased surface area for exchange; venular widening or tortuosity appears to be secondary to changes in transmural pressure, and apparent blood viscosity. Some of these anatomical changes persist. Others are patchy and reversible.

Until recently, dynamic manifestations of abnormality have been documented in general terms; e.g., ischemic trends vs. a hyperemic trend, hyperplastic vs. atrophic networks on the assumption that a comparable set of changes exists throughout the vascular system. More current data clearly indicate that network remodeling is not uniform, but develops initially in focal portions of the bed and then spreads to other portions until more and more of the network is involved. The reason for the predilection of certain vessels to change is not clear, but may be purely random.

There still remains considerable ambiguity concerning the operational properties of the cellular building blocks of the microcirculation. Vital microscopy of this delicately poised functional unit provides a sensitive index not only for the effectiveness of local homeostasis, but for systemic homeostatic adjustments. Hopefully, a blending of *in vivo* and *in vitro* experimental data will allow for a further expansion of what is currently in man a laboratory tool to supplement and to strengthen our clinical base of information — in a prospective context as well as a guide for therapeutic intervention.

REFERENCES

1. **Malpighi, M.,** De pulmonibus: observationes anatomical Bologna, 1661, in *Selected Readings in the History of Physiology,* Fulton, J., Ed., Charles C Thomas, Springfield, IL, 1956.
2. **Leuwenhoek, A. von,** Den Waaragtigen Omloop des Bloeds, als mede dat de Arterien en Venae gecontinueerde Bloed — Vatem zijn Kloor veor de Ooegen gestelt. Verhandelt in een Brief geschreven aan de Koninglijke. Societeit tot London, 65th Missive, Sept. 7, 1688, *Opuscula selecta Neerlandicorum de Arte medica,* Fasc. 1, 45, 1907.
3. **Bérnard, C. L.,** *Lecons de Pathologie experimentale,* J. B. Bailbiare et Fils, Paris, 1880.
4. **Cannon, W. B.,** *The Wisdom of The Body,* W. W. Norton, New York, 1932.
5. **Ludwig, C.,** *Lehrbuch der Physiologie des Menschen,* C. F. Winter, Leipzig, 1861.
6. **Starling, E. H.,** On the absorption of fluids from the connective tissue spaces, *J. Physiol. (London),* 19, 312, 1896.
7. **Krogh, A.,** *The Anatomy and Physiology of Capillaries,* Yale University Press, New Haven, CT, 1922.
8. **Rhodin, J. A. G.,** The ultrastructure of mammalian arterioles and precapillary sphincters, *J. Ultrastruct. Res.,* 18, 181, 1967.
9. **Hammersen, F., Hammersen, E., and Osterkamp-Banst, U.,** Structure and function of the endothelial cell, *Prog. Appl. Microcirc.,* 1, 1, 1983.
10. **Lipowsky, H. H. and Zweifach, B. W.,** Network analysis of microcirculation of cat mesentery, *Microvasc. Res.,* 7, 73, 1974.
11. **Davis, E.,** Clinical vasomicroscopy in *Microcirculation,* Vol. III, Chap. 11, Kaley G. and Altura, B. M., Eds., University Park Press, Baltimore, 1980, 223.
12. **Lewis, T.,** The vascular reactions of the skin to injury. I. Reactions to stroking, *Heart,* 11, 119, 1924.
13. **Ruderman, N. B., Williamson, J. R., and Brownlee, M.,** Glucose and diabetic vascular disease, *FASEB J.,* 6, 2905, 1992.
14. **Zweifach, B. W.,** Microcirculation in health and disease, in *Circulatory Disorders,* Niimi, H. and Messmer, K., Eds., Springer-Verlag, Tokyo, 1988, 3.
15. **Zweifach, B. W.,** *Functional Behavior of the Microcirculation,* C. C. Thomas, Springfield, 1961.
16. **Oda, M., Tsukada, N., Honda, K., Komatsu, H., Kaneko, K., Azuma, T., Nishizaki, N., and Tsuchiya, M.,** Hepatic sinusoidal endothelium — its functional implications in the regulation of sinusoidal blood flow, in *Microcirculation — An Update, 2.,* Elsevier, Amsterdam, 1987, 317.
17. **Simionescu, S., Simionescu, M., and Palade, G. E.,** Structural basis of permeability in sequential segments of the microvasculature of the diaphragm. II. Pathways followed by microperoxidase across the endothelium, *Microvasc. Res.,* 15, 17, 1978.
18. **Hardingham, T. F. and Fosang, A. J.,** Proteoglycans: Many forms and many functions, *FASEB J.,* 6, 861, 1992.
19. **Ingber, D. E.,** Fibronectin controls capillary endothelial cell growth by modulating cell shape, *Proc. Natl. Acad. Sci. U.S.A.,* 87, 3579, 1990.

20. **Rous, P., Gilding, H. P., and Smith, F.,** The gradient of vascular permeability, *J. Exp. Med.,* 51, 807, 1930.
21. **Johnson, P. C.,** Autoregulation of blood flow, *Circ. Res.,* 59, 483, 1986.
22. **Zweifach, B. W. and Lipowsky, H. H.,** Pressure-flow relations in blood and lymph microcirculation, in *Handbook of Physiology — The Cardiovascular System. IV. The Microcirculation,* Renkin E. M. and Michel, C. C., Eds., Am. Physiological Society, Washington, D.C., Chap. 7, 1984, 251.
23. **Furchgott, R. F. and Vanhoutte, P. M.,** Endothelium-derived relaxing and contracting factors, *FASEB J.,* 3, 2007, 1989.
24. **Koller, A. and Kaley, G.,** Prostaglandins mediate arteriolar dilation to increased blood flow in skeletal muscle microcirculation, *Circ. Res.,* 67, 529, 1990.
25. **Ryan, U. S.,** The endothelial surface and response to injury, *Fed. Proc.,* 45, 101, 1986.

Chapter 10

Technological Developments in the Study of the Microcirculation

Marcos Intaglietta and Konrad Messmer

CONTENTS

I. HISTORICAL PERSPECTIVE

The analysis of events that occur in the microcirculation began with the development of the microscope and was circumscribed to primarily descriptive approaches that focused on morphological features and the observation of events in the flowing blood. This was consequent to the lack of methods for recording the dynamics of the microscopic image, and techniques for measuring mechanical phenomena at the cellular level. Roy and Brown[30] and Landis,[31] in a period spanning from 1880 to 1930, were the first investigators that developed the ingenious concept of comparing visually detected signals from unknown microscopic parameters to macroscopic counterparts, thus measuring microvascular pressures. From this time up to the 1960s, there were advances in recording of microscopic images by photography and film, which allowed researchers to document microvascular flow and to quantify capillary fluid exchange.[51] The decade of 1960–1970, coinciding with the rapid advances in electronic instrumentation, led Wiederhielm, Baez, and Wayland and Johnson to the development of quantitative methods for the measurement of pressure,[33] diameter,[5] and flow velocity.[13] Progress in television and introduction of video equipment for consumer use in 1970s allowed Intaglietta and co-workers to introduce the electronic techniques for obtaining dynamic information directly from the microvascular video image.[6,15] From the beginning of the 1980s, the advances in fluorescence microscopy used in conjunction with low light level video cameras has expanded the range of phenomena accessible to *in vivo* microscopy to include tissue injury, tissue metabolism, and biochemistry.

As history reveals, advances in our understanding of the structure and function of the microcirculation are a direct consequence of the development of quantitative techniques for the measurement of microvascular parameters mostly encoded in and generated by the intravital microscope. The techniques use optical and electronic signal processing and provide dynamic data on microvascular diameter, hematocrit, microvessel blood flow velocity, tissue perfusion, hemoglobin oxygen saturation, and plasma oxygen tension. By contrast, micromanipulative techniques dependent on the construction of fine glass needles and electrodes, although important and fully developed, are few and restricted to the measurement of pressure, fluid filtration, and oxygen tension.

Although direct quantitative techniques are difficult to implement in the clinical setting, they provide advantages over indirect methods such as plethysmography because the microcirculation does not respond uniformly to either physiological and pharmacological interventions. The direct techniques allow one to correctly identify the compartment under scrutiny, as well as the type of microvascular vessel or cellular component within that compartment.

II. IMAGE ENHANCEMENT

The images of the microcirculation often have a complex background, and lack contrast and resolution, complicating the process of quantifying dimensions and dynamic events visualized through the optical microscope. Optical techniques are used to circumvent this situation, where the most frequently used technique is the enhancement of the column of blood by selective optical filtering, where light from a mercury or xenon arc is passed through a blue filter, illuminating the tissue at a wavelength where hemoglobin maximally absorbs, thus increasing the contrast of the blood vessels. The plasma can be made phosphorescent through the use of sodium-fluorescein, fluorescein-dextran, and indocyanine green, which remain in the circulation for varying periods.[1] The images obtained outline the inner vessel wall of the microvessels. These techniques require visualization by means of low-light video cameras; and once the image is in video format, it can be further enhanced by electronic processing.

Video gray-scale stretching increases contrast by selectively amplifying a portion of the image that is the encoded by a greater range of gray levels.[2] An instrument that accomplishes this is manufactured by IPM Inc., San Diego, CA. This instrument does not require a computer imaging board, and operates directly with the video signal on-line. On-line, real-time analog gray-scale stretching and compression prior to other forms of data processing are highly recommended in processing video images of the microcirculation, since it processes the signals in conditions of infinite resolution and allows to maximize the range of levels that encode the information of interest. By contrast, when this procedure is carried out by computer where the image is first digitized and then processed, gray-scale stretching and compression is made on the limited portion of the gray-scale range of the low contrast features causing the appearance of digitization image noise.

III. DIAMETER MEASUREMENTS

Diameter measuring techniques are mostly based on the conversion of the microscope optical image into a video signal where the necessary information can be obtained by image shearing and the use of electronic calipers. Image shearing is based on the ability of the eye to recognize alignment[3,4] according to the scheme developed by Baez.[5] In this procedure, a portion of the image of the blood is translated in a direction perpendicular to its axis (sheared) until the opposite edges align. One may manually align the edge of the blood column, or align the inner or outer vessel wall utilizing the pattern recognition ability of the observer.[6] A practiced operator can reproduce variations of vessel diameter with a frequency response sufficient to encode all vasomotion-related activity, which rarely exceeds the frequency of 30 cycles per minute.[7]

Electronic calipers consist of generating two vertical lines within the video screen that are electronically controlled and manually superposed to opposite sides of the blood column, or to the opposite inner or outer walls via manually operated controls. The separation is obtained directly from the circuitry that generates the lines. Since the lines are fixed relative to the video frame, this technique requires continuous adjustment for tissue movements with two independent controls as well as the adjustment of any change in dimension. By contrast, with image shearing, tissue motion is essentially ignored and thus requires the operation of only one control, and has the advantage that the features of the blood vessel used for identifying the diameter can be directly superposed and compared.

A continuous tracking method has been reported for image shearing.[8] An automated edge tracking technique[9] is available commercially (IPM, San Diego, CA) and is based on the independent detection of the change of light level due to the optical contrast of the vessel wall in two independent windows superposed to each opposing wall of the blood vessels. This technique is operator independent and provides temporal resolution for diameter variations up to the limit of the frequency response of the video system (in the range of 20 cps, where greater frequency response can be achieved by decreasing the number of scanned horizontal lines). This technique, as is the image shearing method, is insensitive to the motion of the preparation.

A continuous signal proportional to vessel diameter can be obtained from microvessels where there is a continuous column of blood by measuring the light absorbed by the lumen. This procedure measures the width of the column of blood[10] and can be implemented with a photometer and an appropriate calibration. Other techniques that have been implemented to obtain continuous diameter records depend on the traversal scanning of the microvessel image by means of a flying spot detector[11] or sweeping the image past a fixed detector.[12] These techniques are usually dependent on setting a threshold gray level that identifies a feature of the vessel that is used to begin and terminate the measurement.

IV. FLOW MEASUREMENTS

Blood flow in microscopic vessels cannot be measured directly due to the small size of the conduits. This parameter is derived from red blood velocity and diameter measurements obtained optically.

The direct measurement of blood flow velocity is mostly centered on the dual slit approach developed by Wayland and Johnson,[13] where the delay between upstream and downstream photosignals is measured by a cross-correlation calculation between the two signals. The time resolution of this methodology is dependent on the quality of signals generated by the photowindows, namely their degree of similarity. The dual slit method is relatively insensitive to microscope focus, and gives the same result regardless of which part of the image of the flowing blood is in focus. The measured centerline velocity is smaller than the actual value and must be multiplied by a correction factor[14] that has the numerical value of 1.6 for vessels in the 15 to 80 μm diameter range, and decreases gradually to the value of 1.0 for narrow capillaries, where cells move single file.

The dual sensor method has been implemented by Intaglietta et al.[15] in a video configuration, which allows a recording of the dynamic images of the microvessels in real time and measurement of diameter and velocity in playback, allowing one to obtain data from several vessels in temporal registration. This technique is primarily applicable to capillaries, which are the vessels where the optoelectronic signatures caused by the passage of red blood cells are well differentiated from the noise. The video framing rate limits the frequency content of the signals, which in turn sets a limit to the maximum interwindow delay that can be measured, and therefore the flow velocity. This problem is circumvented by increasing the framing rate of the video system, which allows for an increase in the frequency response of the system in direct relation to the decrease in video image height. Conversely, flows that are too slow for automated measurements are conveniently quantified by the flying spot technique.[16]

The principal problem of red blood cell velocimetry is the method for conversion of the optical signature of the passing red blood cells into an electronic signal. Originally,[13] this was accomplished by photomultipliers, which to date provide the maximum sensitivity and signal-to-noise ratio. Television cameras, even the cooled image intensified CCD types, do not approach the performance of these devices.

The use of a nonideal signal transductor, as well as the complexity of the microvascular image, limits velocity measurements in the microcirculation — a problem that can in part be overcome by either optimally utilizing or increasing the amount of information derived from the available images. The interdetector optical signature transit time is optimally measured by the variable time base tracking cross-correlation method (IMP Inc., San Diego, CA). This technique yields a virtually infinite temporal resolution in the measurement of time delay, and utilizes all the information available from the detectors. The cross-correlation has also been implemented in a PC-based digital computer configuration for clinical use (Capiflow® AB, Stockholm, Sweden); but due to the nature of the digital instrumentation, the computation is made at discrete intervals, with finite data records, leading to a significant reduction in the amount of data used relative to the data available. Furthermore, PC-based digital batch correlation is significantly less efficient at computing the cross-correlation than the available analog systems. Since the usable signals are marginal and at the verge of being buried in the noise, the reduction of usable data due to digital implementation as well as its nonoptimal treatment often prevents obtaining valid velocity measurements that otherwise can be readily obtained with analog instrumentation. Furthermore, PC-based digital systems such as Capiflow rely solely on video sources of data, at the standard framing rate, and therefore are unable to provide flow velocity measurement beyond those obtainable from capillaries.

Several other approaches have been taken to maximize the utilization of the available data. One of these uses spatial correlation where optical scans are made along the axis of the blood vessels under investigation. When two of these signals are obtained in succession and transformed into electronic format, they can be cross-correlated to determine the displacement that has taken place in the period between scans.[17] A different approach is the direct frequency analysis of the photometric signals. This can be implemented by projecting the image of the moving red blood cells through a grating that has the effect of generating a frequency that is proportional to the velocity and the spacing in the grating.[18-22] The grating-photodetector configuration can be replaced by a linear array of photodetectors[18] or a sequence of four video windows photometers,[23] which allow one to obtain the difference between the photometric signals from two contiguous windows and to form two difference signals. This constitutes a spatial differentiation of the signals that significantly improves the cross-correlation measurement of transit time relative to the one obtainable from only two windows, has an improved frequency response, and is less sensitive to motion in the preparation.[23] Riva et al.[24] have successfully implemented a laser Doppler velocimeter for measurements in the human retina.

In many tissues, illumination can only be obtained by incident light, which poses an additional limitation on contrast and resolution of the moving red blood cells. This problem has been in part resolved by the use of fluorescent markers that stain either the red blood cells or the plasma and therefore enhance contrast and provide more distinct optical signatures for the passage of red blood cells. Epifluorescence microscopy is shown to underestimate the actual velocity by at most 20%.[25]

In recent years, there has been a tendency to incorporate the various components of data processing needed for video velocimetry in self-contained, preprogrammed, dedicated PC-based digital systems. In these systems, the number of variables that the operator has to deal with is decreased at the expense of flexibility and optimization of the utilization of the data. While digital and analog methods function properly in the presence of ideal signals, red blood cell velocimetry is usually at the limit of measurability, which requires the maximal flexibility in controls and data utilization that is provided by multiple window analog cross-correlation instrumentation.

V. HEMATOCRIT

Information on microvascular hematocrit is in principle contained within the signals used in flow velocity measurements. Two different hematocrits must be considered: namely, the tube hematocrit (the instantaneous value in the blood vessel) and the discharge hematocrit (measured by collecting the fluid that exits the blood vessel). These parameters are different because of the relative velocities of red blood cells and plasma.

Tube hematocrit can be measured by manual count in capillaries, and by labeling a small fraction of red blood cells with a fluorescent marker. Automated cell counting has been implemented[26] for conditions where red blood cells produce distinct optical signatures. In larger vessels, the measurements of optical density provides information that can be converted into hematocrit data, where the principal schemes have been reviewed by Lipowsky.[27] Densitometric methods are particularly sensitive to dynamic hematocrit fluctuations caused by vasomotion.[28] Hematocrit and flow velocity can be combined to calculate flux according the scheme of Intaglietta et al.[29]

VI. PRESSURE MEASUREMENTS

The measurement of blood pressure in the microscopic blood vessels constitutes a specialized methodology because of the minimal hydraulic energy present in the microvascular blood. This situation was recognized from the beginning of microvascular studies, leading to the concept of comparing the microvascular pressure with a known pressure source through some nonmechanical means, i.e., an optical or electric signal.

Such a method was first devised by Roy and Brown[30] in 1880; they installed on the front of the microscope objective (which was used to observe the microcirculation) a transparent and flexible cover forming a balloon that could be inflated against the tissue. In this configuration, they noted the balloon pressure that was needed to stop flow in the various blood vessels, thus using an optical signal to compare the known balloon pressure to the unknown blood vessel pressure. This technique is approximate since the mechanical properties of the tissue influence in an unknown way the pressure at which microvessels will collapse.

Landis[31] developed an active pressure-measuring system that utilized a glass micropipette that could be inserted directly into the microvessels, establishing direct hydraulic contact with blood. The pipettes where filled with saline that was hydraulically connected to a fluid reservoir whose pressure could be changed by varying its height relative to the tip of the pipette. A dye in the saline made it possible to observe through the microscope when the pipette fluid exited or plasma entered the pipette. The same principle is now used in commercial instruments, where the detection of the pressure balance point is made by an electrical measurement.

The electrical comparison of pressures between the outside of the tip of the glass micropipette and the fluid in its shank is made on the basis of the pressure sensitivity of the electrical resistance of electrolyte-filled glass pipettes.[32] This feature was incorporated into the servo-nulling pressure measuring system developed by Wiederhielm et al.[33] and Intaglietta et al.[34] In this system, 2 M NaCl solution fills the glass micropipette and the electrical resistance of the tip is measured when the micropipette is inserted in the blood vessel of interest. The electrical resistance is developed at the tip, which is of the order of 1 μm in diameter, and its measurement is made from anywhere in the tissue to any portion of the fluid in the shank of the microneedle. When the pressure of plasma is greater than that in the shank, it will enter the tip, causing the electrical resistance to increase. This change of resistance is detected and a pressure is servoed back to maintain the resistance constant. The required pressure is identical to that in the blood vessel.

The measurement of the resistance of the plasma-saline interface in the glass microcannulae is made via AC excitation to avoid DC null drift arising from the polarization of the electrodes. In the glass pipette, the hypertonic saline and the plasma, two conductive media, are separated by an insulator, which constitutes a capacitor generating an impedance in parallel to the resistance of the saline-plasma interface. The need for high frequency (520 Hz) bridge excitation, in order to operate in a frequency band removed from 60-Hz power line harmonics aggravates the problem. Intaglietta and Tompkins[35] introduced an operator-adjusted negative capacitance amplifier to cancel a major portion of this stray capacity.

A new system[36] obviates the need for manual capacitance balance, eliminates the possibility of negative capacitance loop oscillation, and allows of total compensation for signal loss due to the capacitance associated with the pipette, the pipette holder, and wiring. In this system, a miniature preamplifier and current source is used to electrically excite the pipette with an AC current that produces a voltage proportional to pipette electrical resistance. Following amplification, this voltage is compared by a differential amplifier to that from the balancing resistance in a Wheatstone bridge. After further amplification and in-phase synchronous detection, the difference signal actuates a pump that generates an opposing pressure, thus maintaining bridge balance. In this system, signal loss due to stray capacitance is corrected, not by cancellation by negative capacitance, but rather by automatically increasing the pipette AC current excitation with the proper amplitude and phase to precisely make up for the stray capacitance current loss.

The new system, with its automatic features, renders the electronic operational problems much less severe and the main remaining problems for the new user involve becoming adept at the fabrication, filling, and selection of the pipettes, as well as some precautions for reducing noise in the electrical operating environment.

VII. OXYGEN TENSION MEASUREMENTS

Intra- and extravascular measurements of pO_2 in the microcirculation have been obtained by means of spectrophotometry of the hemoglobin molecule and with microelectrodes that are a miniaturized version of the Clark oxygen electrodes. Microelectrodes have been used for the measurement of pO_2 in the vicinity of the blood vessels[37,38] where they are inserted into the tissue. This procedure requires anesthesia and exposure of the tissue to be examined, in such a fashion that it is isolated from the environmental oxygen.[39,40]

The multiwire electrode configuration[41] measures the oxygen distribution from the surface of tissues. It consists of eight platinum electrodes, each 15 µm in diameter, assembled in a glass rod of 5-mm diameter. The electrodes are present on the surface of the glass and sample a tissue volume of approximately 25-µm radius. The electrode surface contacts the tissue via a Cuprophan and a Teflon® membrane providing a continuous record from each sensor, which is used to create a histogram of oxygen tension. This technique measures oxygen near the surface, where the microcirculation may have special features not present in the depth of the tissue. Penetration to a greater depth can be implemented at the expense of spatial resolution. Different types of electrode configurations have been implemented, as reviewed by Fatt.[42]

Optical techniques are implemented in the light microscope and determine the oxygen saturation of red blood cells by spectrophotometric principles[43,44] where light absorption is measured at an isosbestic wavelength of the hemoglobin absorption spectrum, and at a wavelength where there is a maximum difference between oxy- and deoxyhemoglobin. This method can be implemented noninvasively and yields reliable measurements when the light from other portions of the tissue can be accounted for or effectively shielded. However, it is a concentration-dependent determination and the results are a function of the intensity of the light, absorption by the tissue, and hematocrit.

A new optical method for measuring pO_2 in normal tissues[45-47] is based on the injection of the die palladium-porphyrin bound to albumin, where the rate of decay of the phosphorescence excited by a brief light flash is independent of both the concentration of the compound and of the intensity of excitation light, but is a function of the amount of oxygen present. Thus, pO_2 information is only related to the time-dependent features of the phosphorescence signal and not to the intensity of emission, and the information of interest is neither concentration nor light intensity dependent. This method measures the intravascular pO_2 in single microvessels simultaneously with other microvascular parameters like diameter and blood flow.

The technique is implemented[48] by delivering an intravenous injection of palladium (Pd)-meso-tetra (4-carboxyphenyl)porphyrin (Porphyrin Products, Inc.) previously bound to albumin. The solution is prepared by dissolving the porphyrin in dimethylsulfoxide and then adding a mixture containing NaCl and bovine serum albumin in bidistilled water. The pH is kept at 7.4 and the final dosage used is 30 mg/kg body weight at a concentration of 15 mg/ml. The phosphorescence is excited with the light from a xenon strobe source arc passed through a narrow bandpass interference filter (420 ± 50 nm). The phosphorescence emission from the epi-illuminated area is passed through a bandpass light filter (630 nm) and measured by a photomultiplier that yields intensity vs. time information of the signal decay. The pO_2 of blood is determined by mathematically fitting the decay of phosphorescence to a single exponential using a conventional least squares method and measuring the time constant of the fitted exponential curve. This data is then used to determine pO_2 from the Stern-Volmer equation.[49]

VIII. CAPILLARY FLUID PERMEABILITY

The permeability of capillaries to fluid can be measured directly with a technique devised by Landis,[50] which consists in mechanically compressing a portion of the capillary with a glass micro-tool until flow stops and recording the motion of red blood cells trapped in the occluded capillary. Any post-occlusion motion is due to either changes of the capillary dimensions or the exchange of fluid between the blood and tissue. This technique was further developed by Intaglietta and Zweifach,[51] who tracked different types of relative red blood cell trajectories, and has also been implemented with a densitometric method whereby the exchange of fluid is tracked by noting the increase or decrease of intensity of a fluorescent die present in the plasma.[52,53] A more precise technique consists of placing an oil droplet in the capillary by microinjection methods, a procedure that seals the capillary lumen and more precisely delineates the motion of the fluid trapped between occluding droplets.[54]

IX. LEUKOCYTE ADHESION

Ischemia followed by reperfusion activates leukocytes, causing them to roll and adhere to the microvascular endothelium. The quantification of this phenomenon plays an important role in the analysis of pharmacological activity in inflammatory processes. Several techniques have been utilized for the determination of leukocyte velocity and mobility, mostly based on manual tracing of the leukocyte path on either film or video images.[55-57] The introduction of the system CAMAS[58] has notably simplified this time-consuming process, rendering the data acquisition automatic, computer-controlled, and therefore free of operator bias, and allowing one to obtain a greater amount of data in a systematic way.

The method is used in experimental investigations where the microcirculation can be observed by fluorescent intravital microscopy and the leukocytes are rendered visible by staining with a dye such as acridine orange. It is based on the acquisition of images through a video camera and digitizing and storing the images in a computer memory. The velocity of the cells is obtained by identifying each cell in a pair of video images separated by a preset time delay. The method is versatile to the extent that all the cells within the video image can be tracked and measured. Observer bias is reduced by making the choice of images independent from the observer.

An important feature of this system is the quantification of the leukocyte/endothelium interaction by means of an adhesion coefficient defined as the ratio between the difference of red blood cell velocity and the leukocyte velocity, divided by the red blood cell velocity.[59] The methodology is not restricted to leucocyte analysis: through image substraction, the system is able to quantify functional capillary density, and by optical intensity thresholding, the system can also be used as a planimeter to evaluate tissue phenomena such as injury and how materials diffuse.[60]

REFERENCES

1. **Bollinger A. and Fagrell, B.,** Clinical capillaroscopy, Hogrefe & Huber, Lewiston, NY, 1990.
2. **Intaglietta, M. and Tompkins, W. R.,** Contrast enhancement amplifier for television microscopy, *Int. J. Microcirc.: Clin. Exp.,* 7, 253, 1988.
3. **Barer, R. A.,** A new micrometer microscope, *Nature,* 188, 398, 1960.
4. **Dyson, J.,** Precise measurement by image splitting, *J. Opt. Soc. Am.,* 50, 754, 1960.
5. **Baez, S.,** Recording microvascular dimensions with an image splitter microscope, *J. Appl. Physiol.,* 211, 299, 1966.
6. **Intaglietta, M. and Tompkins, W. R.,** Microvascular measurements by video image shearing and splitting, *Microvasc. Res.,* 5, 309, 1973.
7. **Meyer, J.-U. and Intaglietta, M.,** Measurement of the dynamics of arteriolar diameter, *Ann. Biomed. Eng.,* 14, 109, 1986.
8. **Kaufman, A. G. and Intaglietta, M.,** Automated diameter measurement of vasomotion by cross-correlation, *Int. J. Microcirc.: Clin. Exp.,* 4, 45, 1985.
9. **Yin, F. C. P., Tompkins, W. R., Peterson, K. L., and Intaglietta, M.,** A video dimension analyzer, *IEEE Trans. Biomed.,* 19, 376, 1972.
10. **Auer, L. M. and Haydn, F.,** Multichannel videoangiometry for continuous measurement of pial microvessels, *Acta Neurol. Scand.,* 60(Suppl.72), 208, 1979.
11. **Johnson, P. C.,** Measurement of microvascular dimensions *in vivo, J. Appl. Physiol.,* 23, 593, 1967.
12. **Richardson, D. R.,** Measurement of microvascular diameter by sensor scan technique, *Microvasc. Res.,* 5, 100, 1973.
13. **Wayland, H. and Johnson, P. C.,** Erythrocyte velocity measurement in microvessels by a two slit method, *J. Appl. Physiol.,* 22, 333, 1967.
14. **Baker, M. and Wayland, H.,** On line volume flow rate and velocity profile measurement for blood in microvessels, *Microvasc. Res.,* 7, 131, 1974.
15. **Intaglietta, M., Silverman, N. R., and Tompkins, W. R.,** Capillary flow velocity measurements *in vivo* and *in situ* by television methods, *Microvasc. Res.,* 10, 165, 1975.
16. **Tyml, K. and Ellis, C. G.,** Evaluation of the flying spot technique as a television method for measuring cell velocity in microvessels, *Int. J. Microcirc.: Clin. Exp.,* 1, 145, 1982.
17. **Goodman, A. H., Guyton, A. C., Drake, R., and Laflin, J. H.,** A television method for measuring capillary red blood cell velocity, *J. Appl. Physiol.,* 37, 126, 1974.
18. **Borders, J. L. and Granger, H. J.,** An optical Doppler intravital velocimeter, *Microvasc. Res.,* 27, 117, 1984.
19. **Fleming, B. P., Klitzman, B., and Johnson, W. O.,** Measurement of erythrocyte velocity by use of a periodic differential detector, *Am. J. Physiol.,* 249, H899, 1985.
20. **Intaglietta, M. and Tompkins, W. R.,** Capillary video red blood cell velocimetry by cross correlation and spatial filtering, *Microvasc. Res.,* 34, 108, 1987.

21. **Nitta, J., Koyama, T., Kikuchi, Y., and Shinod, Y.,** Measurement of erythrocyte flow velocity by means of grating laser microscope, *Jpn. J. Physiol.,* 33, 377, 1983.

22. **Slaaf, D., Rood, J. P. S., Tangelder, G. J., Jeurens, T. J. M., Alewijnse, R., Reneman, R. S., and Arts, T.,** Bidirectional optical (BDO) three stage prism grating system for on-line measurement of red blood cell velocity in microvessels, *Microvasc. Res.,* 22, 110, 1981.

23. **Intaglietta, M., Breit, G. A., and Tompkins, W. R.,** Four window differential capillary velocimeter, *Microvasc. Res.,* 40, 46, 1990.

24. **Riva, C. E., Grunwald, J. E., Sinclair, S. H., and Petrig, B. L.,** Blood velocity and volumetric flow rate in human retinal vessels, *Invest. Opthal. Vis. Sci.,* 26, 1124, 1985.

25. **Seki, J. and Lipowsky, H. H.,** *In vivo* and *in vitro* measurements of red cell velocity under epifluorescence microscopy, *Microvasc. Res.,* 38, 110, 1989.

26. **Johnson, P. C., Blaschke, J., Burton, K. S., and Dial, J. H.,** Influence of flow variations on capillary hematocrit in mesentery, *Am. J. Physiol.,* 221, 105, 1971.

27. **Lipowsky, H. H.,** In situ measurement of microvascular hematocrit, in *Microcirculatory Technology,* Baker, C. H. and Nastuk, W. L., Eds., Academic Press, Orlando, FL, 1986, 161.

28. **Fagrell, B., Intaglietta, M., and Östergren, J.,** Relative hematocrit in human skin capillaries and its relation to capillary blood flow velocity, *Microvasc. Res.,* 20, 327, 1980.

29. **Intaglietta, M., Mirhashemi, S., and Tompkins, W. R.,** Capillary fluxmeter: The simultaneous measurement of hematocrit, velocity and flux, *Int. J. Microcirc.: Clin. Exp.,* 8, 313, 1989.

30. **Roy, C. S. and Brown, J. G.,** The blood pressure and its variation in arterioles, capillaries and smaller veins, *J. Physiol.,* 2, 323, 1880.

31. **Landis, E. M.,** The capillary pressure in frog mesentery as determined by microinjection methods, *Am. J. Physiol.,* 75, 548, 1926.

32. **Rubio, R. and Zubieta, G.,** The variation of electrical resistance of microelectrodes during the flow of current, *Acta Physiol. Lat. Am.,* 11, 211, 1961.

33. **Wiederhielm, C. A., Woodbury, J. W., Kirk, S., and Rushmer, R. F.,** Pulsatile pressure in the microcirculation of the frog's mesentery, *Am. J. Physiol.,* 207, 173, 1964.

34. **Intaglietta, M., Pawula, R. F., and Tompkins, W. R.,** Pressure measurements in the mammalian microvasculature, *Microvasc. Res.,* 2, 212, 1970.

35. **Intaglietta, M. and Tompkins, W. R.,** Micropressure measurement with 1 micron and smaller cannulae, *Microvasc. Res.,* 3, 211, 1971.

36. **Intaglietta, M. and Tompkins, W. R.,** Simplified micropressure measurements via bridge current feedback, *Microvasc. Res.,* 39, 386, 1990.

37. **Duling, B. R. and Berne, R. M.,** Longitudinal gradients in peri-arteriolar oxygen tension. A possible mechanism for the participation of oxygen in local regulation of blood flow, *Circ. Res.,* 27, 669, 1970.

38. **Whalen, W. J., Riley, J., and Nair, P.,** A microelectrode for measuring intracellular pO_2, *J. Appl. Physiol.,* 23, 798, 1967.

39. **Kessler, M. and Lübers, D. W.,** Aufbau und Anwendungsmöglichkeiten Verschiedener pO_2-Elektroden, *Pflügers Arch.,* 291, 82, 1966.

40. **Pittman, R. N.,** Microvessel blood oxygen measurement techniques, in *Microcirculatory Technology,* Baker, C. H. and Nastuk, W. L., Eds., Academic Press, Orlando, FL, 1986, 367.

41. **Kessler, M., Harrison, D. K., and Hoper, J.,** Tissue oxygen measurement techniques, in *Microcirculatory Technology,* Baker, C. H. and Nastuk, W. L., Eds., Academic Press, Orlando, FL, 1986, 391.

42. **Fatt, I.,** *Polarographic Oxygen Sensors,* CRC Press, Cleveland, OH, 1976.

43. **Ellis, C. G., Ellsworth, M. L., and Pittman, R. N.,** Determination of red blood cell oxygenation *in vivo* by dual video densitometric image analysis, *Am. J. Physiol.,* 258, H1216, 1990.

44. **Ellsworth, M. L., Pittman, R. N., and Ellis, C. G.,** Measurement of hemoglobin oxygen saturation in capillaries, *Am. J. Physiol.,* 252, H1031, 1987.

45. **Rumsey, W. L., Vanderkooi, J. M., and Wilson, D. F.,** Imaging of phosphorescence: A novel method for measuring oxygen distribution in perfused tissue, *Science,* 241, 1649, 1988.

46. **Shonat, R. D., Wilson, D. F., Riva, C. E., and Pawlowski, M.,** Oxygen distribution in the retinal and choroidal vessels of the cat as measured by a new phosphorescence imaging method, *Appl. Optics,* 31, 3711, 1992.

47. **Wilson, D. F., Pastuszko, A., DiGiacomo, J. E., Pawlowski, M., Schneiderman, R., and Delivoria-Papadopoulos, M.,** Effect of hyperventilation on oxygenation of the brain cortex of newborn piglets, *J. Appl. Physiol.,* 70, 2691, 1991.

48. **Torres Filho, I. P. and Intaglietta, M.,** Microvessel pO_2 measurements by phosphorescence decay method, *Am. J. Physiol.,* 265, 1434, 1993.

49. **Vanderkooi, J. M., Maniara, G., Green, T. J., and Wilson, D. F.,** An optical method for measurement of dioxygen concentration based upon quenching of phosphorescence, *J. Biol. Chem.,* 262, 5476, 1987.

50. **Landis, E. M.,** Micro-injection studies of capillary permeability. II. The relation between capillary pressure and the rate at which fluid passes through the walls of single capillaries, *Am. J. Physiol.,* 82, 217, 1927.

51. **Intaglietta, M. and Zweifach, B. W.,** Indirect method for measurement of pressure in blood capillaries, *Circ. Res.,* 19, 199, 1966.

52. **Levick, J. R. and Michel, C. C.,** A densitometric method for determining the filtration coefficient of single capillaries in the frog mesentery, *Microvasc. Res.,* 13, 141, 1977.

53. **Curry, F.-R. E.,** The measurement of hydraulic conductivity, in *Microcirculatory Technology,* Baker, C. H. and Nastuk, W. L., Eds., Academic Press, Orlando, FL, 1986, 429.

54. **Baldwin, A. L. and Gore, R. B.,** Simultaneous measurement of capillary distensibility and hydraulic conductance, *Microvasc. Res.,* 38, 1, 1989.

55. **Braide, M., Amundson, B., Chien, S., and Bagge, U.,** Qualitative studies on the influence of leukocytes on the vascular resistance in skeletal muscle preparations, *Microvasc. Res.,* 27, 331, 1984.

56. **Gruler, H. and Bueltman, B. D.,** Analysis of cell movement, *Blood Cells,* 10, 61, 1984.

57. **Burton, J. L., Law, P., and Bank, H. L.,** Video analysis of chemotactic locomotion of stored human polymorphonuclear leukocytes, *Cell Motil. Cytoskeleton,* 6, 485, 1986.

58. **Zeintl, H., Tompkins, W. R., Messmer, K., and Intaglietta, M.,** Static and dynamic microcirculatory video image analysis applied to clinical investigations, *Prog. Appl. Microcirc.,* 11, 1, 1986.

59. **Zeintl, H., Sack, F.-U., Intaglietta, M., and Messmer, K.,** Computer assisted leukocyte adhesion measurement in intravital microscopy, *Int. J. Microcirc.: Clin. Exp.,* 8, 293, 1989.

60. **Zeintl, H., Seltsam, A., Funk, W., Enrich, B., and Messmer, K.,** Computer assisted measurement of capillary density, *Int. J. Microcirc.: Clin. Exp.,* 3, 536, 1984.

Chapter 11

Application of Microcirculation Research to Clinical Disease

Bengt Fagrell and Alfred Bollinger

CONTENTS

I. INTRODUCTION

The morphology of microcirculation can only be studied by direct techniques such as vital capillaroscopy. This technique has been used for studying skin capillaries in humans since the beginning of the 20th century. One of the most extensive publications is that by Otfried Müller in Tübingen, who published the book *Die Kapillaren der menschlichen Körperoberfläsche in gesunden und kranken Tagen* already in 1922.[1] This was a milestone in clinical capillaroscopy and was later followed by several publications. Eugene Landis measured nailfold capillary pressure in 1930, and Davis and Landau published an important atlas of microvascular findings in the late 1960s.[2] An overview of modern microvascular techniques and their application in research and practice has recently been presented by Bollinger and Fagrell.[3]

Microcirculation is involved in many diseases. Microvessels in any part of the body may be the essential target of a disease process resulting in primary microangiopathy. Well-known examples are microangiopathy in diabetes and progressive systemic sclerosis. Secondary involvement is typical in ischemia or in venous disorders. Occlusions or obstructions of major arteries are bridged by collateral pathways. With inadequate collateral circulation, postocclusion blood pressure drops into a critical range that may lead to decompensation at the microvascular level. Ultimately, tissue necrosis develops as the consequence of microvascular failure on the basis of severe large vessel disease. In chronic venous insufficiency, blocked or incompetent deep veins and/or insufficient perforating veins cause high ambulatory pressures in the microcirculation, damaging the microvessels that exhibit typical secondary microangiopathy.

The development of television techniques, and different forms of video processing, made it possible to study dynamic phenomena like blood cell velocity, not only in experimental animal preparations, but also in human skin.[4,5] Automation was achieved by videodensitometry, and computerized systems are now also available for automatic image analysis and data processing.[3,5] New techniques, like fluorescence videomicroscopy, open a way to visualize previously invisible microvascular and interstitial compartments (pericapillary halo, plasma skimming) and to analyze transcapillary diffusion of Na-fluoresceine.[6,7] Indocyanine green binding almost completely to plasma proteins depicts

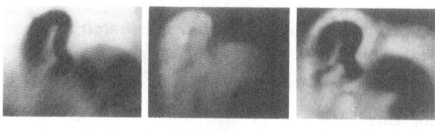

red cell column   indocyanine green   Na–fluorescein

Figure 1   Giant capillaries of the nailfold depicted by conventional capillaroscopy, where only the blood cell column provides enough contrast for visualization. After intravenous injection of indocyanine green, the whole capillary diameter is stained by the tracer fluorescing in the near-infrared portion of the spectrum. Na-fluoresceine diffuses through the capillary wall and visualizes the pericapillary halo, which is enlarged at the loop apex of the capillary on the right side. The images were taken in a patient with progressive systemic sclerosis.

the whole capillary diameter, including the plasma layer[8,9] and is used to detect capillary aneurysms filled by plasma alone.[8] Using servo-nulling micropressure systems, capillary pressure can be measured transcutaneously in controls and patients.[10-12]

Microlymphatics of human skin may be stained by FITC-labeled macromolecules in health and lymphatic diseases.[3,13] It is a prerequisite to determine microlymphatic pressure by the already-mentioned servo-nulling system.[14,15]

II. APPLICATION OF MICROVASCULAR TECHNIQUES IN CLINICAL MEDICINE

The techniques now available have been used in a considerable number of disease states like collagen vascular disease, diabetic microangiopathy, ischemia, chronic venous incompetence, and lymphedema. There are still many conditions affecting probably the microcirculation that have remained unexplored. Pathophysiology of vascular diseases is only understood in depth if microvascular studies are included. Moreover, methods for characterizing microvascular morphology and function contribute to diagnosis and classification of different disease states. Sequential examinations in a given patient allow one to follow the evolution of disease and to control treatment modalities. The application of microvascular techniques, especially capillary microscopy and microvascular flow velocity and pressure measurements, which require previous visualization of microvessels, has a large potential for better understanding and diagnosis of various pathologic conditions.

In the following subsections, some examples of disease states, where microvascular investigations play an important role, are briefly described.

A. PROGRESSIVE SYSTEMIC SCLEROSIS

Microangiopathy of blood capillaries is a well-known and diagnostically important condition in progressive systemic sclerosis or scleroderma.[16-19] In advanced cases, the capillaries are rarefied and enlarged (Figure 1). Na-fluoresceine applied by intravenous injection and diffusing through the capillary wall visualizes an enlarged pericapillary space called "halo".[16] The latter assumes a dwarf-hat aspect at the apex of the loop in scleroderma patients. Penetration of the dye into the more remote interstitial space is common since transcapillary diffusion across the capillary wall and the outer halo border is enhanced.[16] After intravenous bolus injection of indocyanine green, capillary aneu-

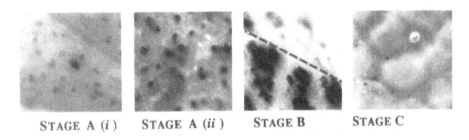

STAGE A (*i*)   STAGE A (*ii*)   STAGE B   STAGE C

Figure 2 Morphological structure of the capillaries of the dorsum of the feet in normal subjects and patients with a reduced arterial circulation to the area.
Stage A: i) Normal pattern with thin, point or comma-shaped capillaries. One dilated capillary, a "micro-pool," can be seen. ii) Most capillaries dilated. This is the first sign in an ischemic skin area, but still the risk of necrosis is minimal.
Stage B: Marked ischemia with edema, making the capillaries hazy (upper part of photo) and appearance of capillary hemorrages (lower part of photo).
Stage C: Complete ischemia where no blood-filled capillaries can be seen. The risk of necrosis is imminent.

rysms are often detected, even if they are only filled by plasma. In most instances, they are localized at the loop apex. Their prevalence is significantly increased in progressive systemic sclerosis and related disorders.[8]

The prevalence of microangiopathy in progressive systemic sclerosis reaches about 80% and may be still higher after the application of the fluorescent tracer Na-fluoresceine. Therefore, capillaropathy is an important component for the diagnosis of the disease, since immunological tests do not yield convincing results as in systemic lupus erythematodes. The combination of Raynaud's disease with typical capillaropathy predicts later development of the full clinical picture, including visceral involvement in a high proportion of patients.[17,19]

Tendency to vasospasms often accompanies microangiopathy in progressive systemic sclerosis. It may be objectively demonstrated by standardized cold provocation tests.[20] Like in primary Raynaud's disease, the blood cells stop for a longer or shorter period after blowing ice-cooled air or decompressed CO_2 on the finger nailfold. The same cold provocation does not provoke a complete stop in most normal subjects.

B. ARTERIAL ISCHEMIA

The capillaries of the dorsal skin of the foot and toes show significant changes of the nutritional skin capillaries in patients with severe peripheral arterial occlusive disease (PAOD). Capillaroscopy is one of the most sensitive methods for estimating the nutritional status of a given skin area and of predicting skin viability.[21] For studying feet and toes in skin ischemia, the patient should be in a sitting position in order to guarantee that the microvascular bed is filled with blood even in the presence of a marked decrease of arterial blood supply.[3]

The normal nutritional capillaries in the skin of the foot have a uniform appearance in healthy subjects, irrespective of age and sex (Figure 2). Most of the papillae are clearly outlined, and 1 to 3 capillaries are seen as dots or commas in each papilla. The capillary density of the forefoot varies from approximately 70/mm^3 on the dorsal skin of the toes to about 30 to 50/mm^3 on the foot. There is a normal tonicity in the capillary bed, that is, a permanent variation in the diameter of the visible capillaries, within the skin area studied. Age does not seem to influence significantly capillary morphology (Table 1), except for an apical dilatation of the capillaries, i.e., "micropools", which can be found in approximately 35% of elderly, but not in young or middle-aged subjects.[22]

Table 1 Capillary Structure in Patients with Peripheral Arterial Obliterative Disease

Stage A	is the normal stage where the skin capillaries are seen as small dot- or comma-shaped structures in the skin papillas. All of the capillaries are filled with blood, and sometimes in patients with mild PAOD a moderate or marked dilatation (= 'micropool') of the nutritional capillaries can be observed.
Stage B	represents indistinct capillaries where the capillaries cannot be sharply focused in the microscope. This is most often due to edema formation or structural changes in the skin papillae themselves, and is the earliest sign of an ischemic disturbance of the microvascular bed in the region. Capillary hemorrhages indicate a vast damage to the capillary wall, and these changes are seen in patients with more severe reduction of the arterial circulation to the region.
Stage C	represents a marked reduction or complete absence of the number of blood-filled capillaries, although the patients are in the sitting position during the investigation. These changes are seen in skin areas of patients with PAOD where the risk of tissue necrosis is imminent.

The majority of patients with PAOD have their ischemic symptoms in acral parts of the foot, and consequently it is in this region that the skin capillaries should most often be studied. Only patients with moderately or severely reduced arterial circulation, to the area show any marked capillary alterations. In patients with only a minor decrease of the arterial circulation the blood flow in the nutritional vascular bed is not reduced, and consequently no changes of the capillaries will be present.

In 1984, Fagrell and Lundberg[21] introduced a simplified classification system that has been shown to be very sensitive for evaluating the viability of the skin in patients with ischemia. In this system, the capillary changes have been gathered in three groups: Stage A, Stage B, and Stage C (Figure 2).

The correlation between the total arterial circulation of a leg, as evaluated by the systolic blood pressure (SBP) of the digit, and the capillary stages of the same foot, has been extensively studied in patients with PAOD.[3,22-24] In toes with an SBP of ≥ 30 mmHg, the whole spectrum of capillary morphology can be seen. Severe changes (Stage C) are almost exclusively seen in toes with a high risk of, or already present, skin ulcers. The prognosis for an ulcer in such an area to heal is almost zero; but if the capillaries can be filled with blood by some therapeutical procedure, the chances of healing is markedly improved.[3,22]

It has been shown by fluorescence videomicroscopy after Na-fluoresceine application that microvascular perfusion is inhomogeneous at the forefoot of patients with advanced ischemia.[3] After successful therapy by reconstructive vascular surgery or angioplasty, all the capillaries in a given field of observation fill within at least 40 seconds. Transcapillary diffusion of Na-fluoresceine is enhanced in severe skin ischemia (Figure 3). Single leaky capillaries exhibit a region of high fluorescent light intensity at their apex (candle light phenomenon).[3]

Not only the morphology, but also the capillary blood flow velocity (CBV) can be continuously studied in clinical practice by the use of microscopical techniques. The blood flow in the capillaries is recorded on videotape and analyses are performed on-line. During the past few years, a new computerized system has been developed for the whole process of analysis (CapiFlow® AB, Stockholm, Sweden).[3]

Up to now, the technique has been mostly used for studying capillary blood flow in the nailfold capillaries of patients with various degrees of peripheral arterial obliterans (PAOD) disease.[3] By combining the technique of capillaroscopy with the method of laser Doppler fluxmetry, it has been shown that the dynamics of the skin microcirculation is impaired in patients with PAOD.[25] Recently, it has also been shown that the reactivity of the microvascular bed in PAOD patients is quite different in those with diabetes than in those without diabetes (Figure 4).[26]

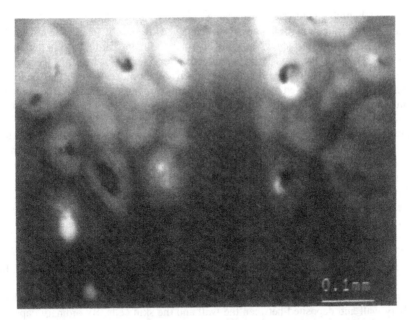

Figure 3 Capillaries at the foot dorsum of a patient with severe ischemia. The comma-shaped loops are embedded into the fluorescing halo. At the apex of some loops, brightly fluorescing spots are visualized because of increased permeability ("candle light phenomenon").

The technique of dynamic capillaroscopy has also been used for evaluating the effect of therapeutic procedures in PAOD patients. It has been shown that epidural spinal cord stimulation (ESCS) may improve the skin microcirculation in severely ischemic regions. Both capillary density and blood flow can be improved significantly in spite of the fact that the macrocirculation, as evaluated by ankle and toe pressure, does not change at all.[27]

C. CHRONIC VENOUS INSUFFICIENCY (CVI)

By 1949, Gilje had shown that the skin microcirculation of the lower leg was considerably affected in patients with different stages of peripheral venous insufficiency.[28] Later,

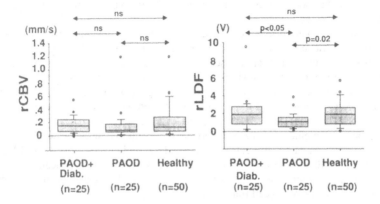

Figure 4 Skin microcirculation in ischemic feet of PAOD patients with and without diabetes. The resting subpapillary skin microcirculation (rLDF) was normal in the diabetic group but significantly reduced in the nondiabetics, while the capillary circulation (rCBV) was normal in both groups. This indicates a maldistribution of blood in the diabetic patients.

Ryan[29] and Fagrell[30] confirmed that the morphology of the skin capillaries changes dramatically in patients with venous insufficiency. However, it must be realized that microangiopathy from CVI shows a patchy distribution. In one particular skin region, for the most part close to the major insufficient perforators, severe changes may be present; whereas, not far away, only mild alterations or even normal skin capillaries may be found. The severe changes observed by clinical investigation are most often a reliable guide for the presence of microangiopathy, but sometimes it may be difficult to observe the pattern of capillary changes, for example, in areas with marked pigmentation or edema.[3]

Insufficiency of the deep venous system of the leg may cause severe disturbances of the skin nutritional circulation. When the venous valves are destroyed, which is most often caused by venous thrombosis, the pressure in the deep venous system increases markedly during walking.[31] This pressure increase is transmitted out through the ankle perforators into the superficial veins of the skin. The pressure during muscle contraction can reach 100 mmHg (13.3 kPa) above the hydrostatic pressure and may consequently approach that of the arteries. This also causes a marked pressure increase in the skin microcirculation, interfering with the normal nutritional circulation. However, during rest, the blood flow through the skin vessels is actually not increased in these patients.[31] The cause for skin ulceration is consequently not circulatory insufficiency in itself, but more a nutritional block between the capillaries and the skin cells.[30,32]

When the capillary pressure increases, blood components are pressed out through the capillary wall and deposited between the wall and the skin cells. By ordinary capillary microscopy, this can be seen as light areas around the capillaries (Figure 5a). The capillaries themselves become very tortuous (Figure 5b).[28,30] The number is decreased, but the capillaries may become so large that they can easily be seen also by the naked eye as small dots in the area.[3,32,33]

One of the most striking findings in the skin of the ankle region in patients with deep venous insufficiency and/or insufficient ankle perforators is the appearance of a "halo" formation around the nutritional skin capillaries.[3,34,35] This halo is caused by a specific microedema that can be easily demonstrated by ordinary capillaroscopy. In some patients, it has been possible to puncture the halo with an injection needle, and marked leakage of fluid can be seen concomitantly with a decrease in the halo size.[3,34] Recently, this microedema has been nicely demonstrated by fluorescence microangiography and microlymphography.[3,32] The edema fluid seems to contain high concentrations of fibrin,[36] other proteins, and neutral polysaccharides.[37] The development of the halo formation is most probably due not only to incompetence of the venous, but also of the lymphatic system of the affected leg.[38]

Additional information may be gained by fluorescence videomicroscopy. Since the dye stains the pericapillary halo and its outlines, the increased halo size is better documented than by conventional capillaroscopy and may be measured. In normals, mean halo diameter at the medial ankle is 81 ± 15 µm and 146 ± 47 µm in patients with severe disease ($p < 0.001$).[33] There is a direct relationship between the number of perfused capillaries in a given area and transcutaneous oxygen tension.[34,39] In atrophie blanche fields, transcutaneous oxygen tension drops to values close to zero that can be shown by special probes combining capillaroscopy and measurements of transcutaneous Po_2. Atrophie blanche is characterized by avascular fields. Na-fluoresceine needs long times like 30 to 60 minutes in fields with a mean diameter of 1 mm to reach its peak concentration in the center.[32] The destruction of capillaries is probably the result of microvascular thrombosis[3,33,35] or of white cell trapping.[40,41]

D. LYMPHEDEMA

Lymphatic microvessels are invisible with conventional capillaroscopy since they do not contain flowing blood cells. After subepidermal injection of minute amounts (0.01 ml) of

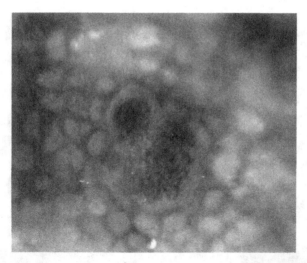

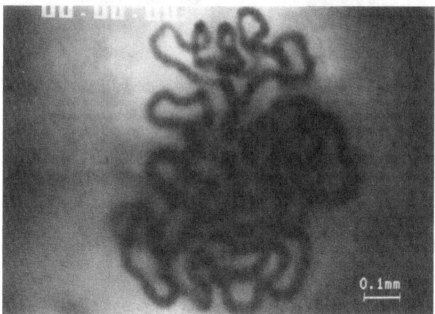

Figure 5 In patients with venous insufficiency, the capillary structure changes dramatically. A. Capillary changes in the skin of the medial part of the ankle in a patient with severe deep venous insufficiency. The photo is taken in an area over an insufficient ankle perforator. Marked dilatation of the capillaries with a 'halo' of micro-edema surrounding the capillaries. B. Glomerulus-like enlarged and tortuous capillaries convolute near the medial ankle in a patient with chronic venous insufficiency.

FITC-dextran 150'000 by microneedles, the superficial network of the skin may be delineated in the fluorescence microscope.[13] The technique is almost noninvasive and causes only minimal discomfort to the patient. No side effects other than rare local swelling and itching have been reported.[3]

The procedure called fluorescence microlymphography is useful for confirming the clinical diagnosis of lymphedema (Figure 6). In 85% of the patients with primary

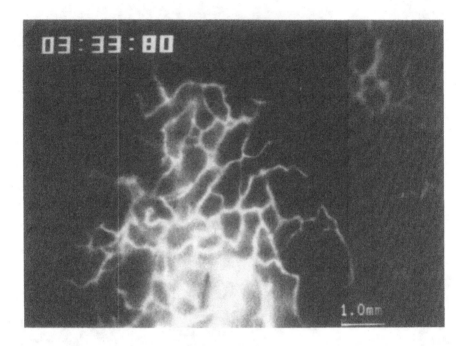

03:33:80

1.0mm

Figure 6 Fluorescence microlymphography (FITC-dextran 150'000) of a patient with primary lymphedema and onset after puberty. The depicted superficial network at the medial ankle has a large extension. In the right upper corner, another area of the network appears by cutaneous reflux of the fluorochrome from deeper channels.

lymphedema, the depicted network extends to more than 13 mm from the border of the dye deposit.[3] The dye transport into deeper precollectors is impeded, which leads to increased superficial propagation.

A distinction between primary and secondary lymphedema is not possible. However, the technique provides a means for classifying primary lymphedema into a form with normal superficial microlymphatics, aplasia and hyperplasia. Aplasia or hyperplasia are found in primary lymphedema manifesting at birth (Nonne-Milroy's disease), normal microlymphatics in primary lymphedema with onset after puberty.[3] Enlargement of lymphatic capillaries is detected in some patients with congenital lymphedema. These differences in microvascular morphology may have a prognostic and therapeutic impact in the future.

Visualization of lymphatic capillaries by FITC-dextran 150'000 is a prerequisite for insertion of glass micropipettes by a micromanipulator and measurement of intralymphatic pressure by servo-nulling systems.[14] In primary lymphedema, lymphatic capillary pressure is increased as has been published recently.[15] Mean lymphatic capillary pressure and standard deviations were 7.9 ± 3.4 mmHg in control subjects and 15.0 ± 5.1 mmHg in patients with primary lymphedema manifesting after puberty ($p < 0.001$). Site of measurement was the forefoot in recumbent position.[15] Microlymphatic hypertension seems to be an important feature for disease pathophysiology.

III. EVALUATION OF THERAPEUTIC PROCEDURES

To evaluate the effect of drugs in patients with critical limb ischemia is very difficult. Most macrociculatory methods are too insensitive for this purpose.[21-24] Very few tech-

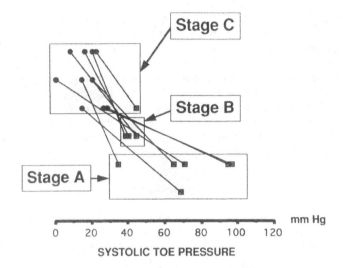

Figure 7 Capillary stages in 10 patients with critical limb ischemia (toe blood pressure ≤ 30 mmHg) before (●) and after (■) femoro-popliteal bypass operation. Concomitantly with an increase in the local toe pressure, the nutritional circulation (capillary stage C, to B or A) improved significantly in all but one patient.

niques for measuring the macrocirculation give any direct information on the nutritional status in an ischemic area.[21-24] The advantage of capillaroscopy is that it can be used in the whole ischemic region, and especially around the ischemic ulcer, where the effect of therapy should be studied. The technique has, for example, been used to evaluate the effect of prostaglandin (E1, I2) and other vasoactive substances.[3,42] The results of these studies have clearly shown that although the drugs may not influence the macrocirculation at all, the nutritional circulation can be significantly improved. This is most probably due to a redistribution of blood from the nonnutritional vascular beds into the nutritional capillaries of the ischemic areas.[42]

The effect of reconstructive vascular surgery has also been evaluated by the simple technique of capillaroscopy.[43] Improvement of the macrocirculation by the surgical procedures also improves the nutritinal circulation of the ischemic areas in most patients. Six weeks after arterial bypass operations in the leg, the nutritional circulation had improved dramatically, concomitantly with improvement of ischemic clinical signs (Figure 7). Like after reconstructive vascular surgery, microcirculation is improved after reopening of stenosed or occluded limb arteries by peripheral transluminal angioplasty.[3] Inhomogeneous microvascular perfusion is normalized after successful catheter therapy.

IV. CONCLUDING REMARKS

Our work has focused on skin microcirculation and specifically on the technique of vital capillaroscopy. Other methods, such as laser Doppler fluxmetry and transcutaneous oxygen tension measurements (for further details on these techniques, see Chapter 24 of this volume), are also used to measure the skin microcirculation, but capillaroscopy is the only method with which the circulation in the specific nutritional skin capillaries can be evaluated. As skin is one of the major targets in several major diseases (i.e., arterial and venous insufficiency, hypertension, scleroderma, and diabetes), extensive information on pathophysiology, prognosis, and effect of different treatments can be achieved. Moreover, attempts are made to introduce the techniques in other systems and organs as well. At present, efforts are made to evaluate microvascular flow of the gastrointestinal mucosa.[44] Preliminary results indicate that gastric ulcers are surrounded by a hyperemic zone and do not exhibit perfused microvessels at their center.

There is no question that more organs and systems will be accessible for microvascular studies in the future. Even in skin, the development is far from being accomplished. Many of the available techniques should be improved for easier practical application. In addition, there is a need for further methods capable of analyzing unknown structures and functions. For example, what do we know about convective and diffusive transport in the human interstitial compartment?

REFERENCES

1. **Müller, O.**, *Die Kapillaren der menschlichen Körperoberfläsche in gesunden und kranken Tagen*, Enke, Stuttgart, 1922.
2. **Davis, E. and Landau, J.**, *Clinical Capillary Microscopy*, Charles C. Thomas, Springfield, IL, 1966.
3. **Bollinger, A. and Fagrell, B.**, *Clinical Capillaroscopy — A Guide To Its Use in Clinical Research and Practice*, Hogrefe & Huber, Bern, 1990.
4. **Bollinger, A., Butti, P., Barras, J. P., Trachsler, H., and Siegenthaler, W.**, Red blood cell velocity in nailfold capillaries of man measured by a television microscopy technique, *Micrvasc. Res.*, 7, 61–72, 1974.
5. **Fagrell, B., Fronek, A., and Intaglietta, M.**, A microscope television system for studying flow velocity in human skin capillaries, *Am. J. Physiol.*, 233, H318–H 321, 1977.
6. **Bollinger, A., Frey, J., Jäger, K., Furrer, J., Seglias, J., and Siegenthaler, W.**, Patterns of diffusion through skin capillaries in patients with long-term diabetes, *N. Engl. J. Med.*, 307, 1305, 1982.
7. **Bollinger, A., Jäger, K., Roten, A., Timeus, Ch., and Mahler, F.**, Diffusion, pericapillary distribution and clearance of Na-fluorescein in the human nailfold, *Pflügers Arch.*, 382, 137, 1979.
8. **Bollinger, A., Saesseli, B., Hoffmann, U., and Franzeck, U. K.**, Intravital detection of skin capillary aneurysms by videomicroscopy with indocyanine green in patients with progressive systemic sclerosis and related disorders, *Circulation*, 83, 546, 1991.
9. **Moneta, G., Brülisauer, M., Jäger, K., and Bollinger, A.**, Infrared fluorescence videomicroscopy of skin capillaries with indocyanine green, *Int. J. Microcirc.: Clin. Exp.*, 6, 25, 1987.
10. **Mahler, F., Muheim, M. H., Intaglietta, M., Bollinger, A., and Anliker, M.**, Blood pressure fluctuations in human nailfold capillaries, *Am. J. Physiol.*, 236, H888, 1979.
11. **Sandeman, D. D., Shore, A. C., and Tooke, J. E.**, Relation of skin capillary pressure in patients with insulin-dependent diabetes mellitus to complications and metabolic control, *N. Engl. J. Med.*, 327, 760, 1992.
12. **Tooke, J. E.**, Microvascular physiology and its clinical relevance with special reference to diabetes, *Qu. J. Med.*, 83, 567, 1992.
13. **Bollinger, A., Jäger, K., Sgier, F., and Seglias, J.**, Fluorescence microlymphography, *Circulation*, 64, 1195, 1981.
14. **Spiegel, M., Vesti, B., Shore, A., Franzeck, U. K., Becker, F., and Bollinger, A.**, Pressure of lymphatic capillaries in human skin, *Am. J. Physiol.*, 262, H1208, 1992.
15. **Zaugg-Vesti, B., Dörffler-Melly, J., Spiegel, M., Wen, S., Franzeck, U. K., and Bollinger, A.**, Lymphatic capillary pressure in patients with primary lymphedema, *Microvasc. Res.*, 46, 128, 1993.
16. **Bollinger, A., Jäger, K., and Siegenthaler, W.**, Microangiopathy of progressive systemic sclerosis: Evaluation by dynamic fluorescence videomicroscopy, *Arch. Intern. Med.*, 146, 1541, 1986.
17. **Granier, F., Vayssairat, M., and Priollet, P.**, Nailfold capillary microscopy in mixed connective tissue disease, comparison with systemic sclerosis and systemic lupus erythematosus, *Arthritis Rheum.*, 29, 189, 1986.

18. **Jacobs, M. J. H. M., Breslau, P. D., Slaaf, D. W., Reneman, R. S., and Lemmens, J. A. J.,** Nomenclature of Raynaud's phenomenon: A capillary microscopic and hemorheologic study, *Surgery*, 101, 136, 1987.

19. **Maricq, H. R.,** Comparison of quantitative and semiquantitative estimates of nailfold capillary abnormalities in scleroderma spectrum disorders, *Microvasc. Res.*, 32, 271, 1986.

20. **Mahler, F., Saner, H., Boss, Ch., and Annaheim, M.,** Local cold exposure test for capillaroscopic examination of patients with Raynaud's syndrome, *Microvasc. Res.*, 33, 422, 1987.

21. **Fagrell, B. and Lundberg, G.,** A simplified evaluation of vital capillary microscopy for predicting skin viability in patients with severe arterial insufficiency, *Clin. Physiol.*, 4, 403, 1984.

22. **Fagrell, B.,** Vital capillary microscopy — A clinical method for studying changes of skin microcirculation in patients suffering from vascular disorders of the leg, *Scand. J. Clin. Lab. Invest.*, Suppl. 133, 1973.

23. **Fagrell, B.,** Vital capillaroscopy — A clinical method for studying changes of skin microcirculation in patients suffering from vascular disorders of the leg, *Angiology*, 23, 284–298, 1972.

24. **Fagrell, B.,** The use of capillaroscopy in the evaluation of skin viability, *Prog. Appl. Microcirc.*, 11, 40–46, 1986.

25. **Bongard, O. and Fagrell, B.,** Discrepancies between total and nutritional skin microcirculation in patients with peripheral arterial occlusive disease (PAOD), *VASA*, 8, 105–111, 1990.

26. **Jörneskog, G., Brismar, K., and Fagrell, B.,** Skin capillary circulation is more impaired in the toes of diabetic than non-diabetic patients with peripheral vascular disease, *Diabetic Med.*, 12, 36–41, 1995.

27. **Jacobs, M., Jörning, P., Joshi, S., Kitslaar, P., Slaaf, D., and Reneman, R.,** Epidural spinal cord electrical stimulation improves microvascular blood flow in severe limb ischemia, *Ann. Surg.*, 207, 179–183, 1988.

28. **Gilje, O.,** Ulcus cruris in venous circulatory disturbances, *Acta Derm.-Venereol.*,22 (Suppl.), 29, 1949.

29. **Ryan, T. J.,** The epidermis and its blood supply in venous disorders of the leg, *Trans. St. John's Hosp. Derm. Soc. (London)*, 55, 51, 1969.

30. **Fagrell, B.,** Local microcirculation in chronic venous incompetence and leg ulcers, *Vasc. Surg.*, 13, 217–225, 1979.

31. **Arnoldi, C. C. and Linderholm, H.,** On the pathogenesis of the venous leg ulcer, *Acta. Chir. Scand.*, 134, 427–440, 1968.

32. **Bollinger, A., Jäger, K., Geser, A., Sgier, F., and Seglias, J.,** Transcapillary and interstitial diffusion of Na-fluorescein in chronic venous insufficiency with white atrophy, *Int. J. Microcirc.: Clin. Exp.*, 1, 5, 1982.

33. **Leu, A. J., Yanar, A., Geiger, M., Pfister, G., Franzeck, U. K., and Bollinger, A.,** Mikoangiopathie bei chronischer venöser Insuffizienz, *Dtsch. Med. Wschr.*, 116, 447, 1991.

34. **Franzeck, U. K.,** *Transkutaner Sauerstoffdruck in der klinischen Mikrozirkulation*, Huber, Bern, 1992.

35. **Leu, H. J.,** Morphology of chronic venous insufficiency — light and electron microscopic examinations, *VASA*, 20, 330, 1991.

36. **Browse, N. L. and Burnand, K. G.,** The cause of venous ulceration, *Lancet*, 2, 243–245, 1982.

37. **Burnard, K. G., Whimster, I., Naido, A., and Browse, N. L.,** Pericapillary fibrin in the ulcer-bearing skin of the leg: The cause of lipodermatosclerosis and venous ulcerations, *Br. Med. J.*, 285, 1071–1072, 1982.

38. **Haselbach, P., Vollenweider, U., Moneta, G., and Bollinger, A.,** Microangiopathy in severe chronic venous insufficiency evaluated by fluorescence videomicroscopy, *Phlebology*, 1, 159, 1986.

39. **Franzeck, U. K., Bollinger, A., Huch, R., and Huch, A.,** Transcutaneous oxygen tension and capillary morphologic characteristics and density in patients with chronic venous incompetence (CVI), *Circulation*, 70, 806, 1984.

40. **Scott, H. J., Coleridge Smith, P. D., and Scurr, J. H.,** Histological study of white blood cells and their association with lipodermatosclerosis and venous ulceration, *Br. J. Surg.*, 78, 210, 1991.

41. **Thomas, P. R. S., Nash, G. B., and Dormandy, J. A.,** White cell accumulation in dependent legs of patients with venous hypertension: A possible mechanism for trophic changes in the skin, *Br. Med. J.*, 296 1693, 1988.

42. **Fagrell, B., Lundberg, G., Olsson, A. G., and Östergren, J.,** PGE_1 treatment of severe skin ischemia in patients with peripheral arterial insufficiency — the effect on skin microcirculation, *VASA,* 15, 56–60, 1986.

43. **Fagrell, B., Sonnenfeld, T., Cronestrand, R., and Lind, M.,** The microcirculatory response to reconstructive vascular surgery in patients with severe foot ischemia, *Bibl. Anat. (Karger, Basel),* 18, 385–388, 1979.

44. **Franzeck, U. K., Münch, R., Wächter, M., Vesti, B., Amman, R., and Bollinger, A.,** Gastrointestinal mucosal blood flow in humans by dynamic fluorescence video endoscopy, *Int. J. Microcirc.: Clin. Exp.,* 11, 58, 1992.

Section IV

Specific Application of Microcirculation Research

Chapter 12

Bone Microcirculation

Howard Winet and Harris Gellman

CONTENTS

I. ANATOMY AND FUNCTION

A. ANATOMY
1. General
Long bone has been the traditional model for circulation in the skeletal system. Redundancy characterizes the influx vasculature and collateral circulation. For example, the tibial diaphysis receives blood through (1) nutrient arteries (at least 67%),[83] (2) periosteal arteries (up to 33%), which are supplied by soft tissue (e.g., tendons), and geniculate arteries, and (3) metaphyseal arteries.

2. Influx Vasculature
General relationships of influx and efflux vasculature within the organ are illustrated in Figure 1. The nutrient artery enters a long bone through a diaphyseal perforation and does not branch until reaching the medullary canal. More than one nutrient artery/vein may perforate the diaphysis. Variations in number and location of nutrient arteries occur both within and between species. After branching in the medullary canal, there is a division into two main networks: marrow sinusoids and vessels radially penetrating the endosteum. Branching patterns vary between species. When applying nonprimate observations

0-8493-4870-6/95/$0.00+$.50
© 1995 by CRC Press, Inc.

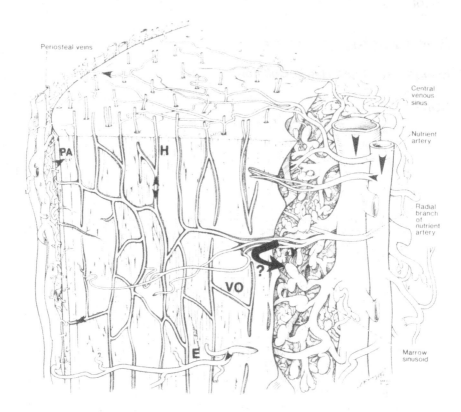

Periosteal veins

Central venous sinus

Nutrient artery

Radial branch of nutrient artery

PA   H

VO

E

Marrow sinusoid

Figure 1   Three-dimensional view of a cortical bone wedge in a representative diaphysis. Vessels in haversian canals (H) may flow in either direction and can reverse (Winet, unpublished), as indicated by two-headed arrow. Nutrient artery branches may split into endosteal (small arrow furthest right) and medullary (next small arrow to left) branches in a parallel arrangement or endosteal vessels may loop through sinusoids in a serial arrangement (largest arrow with "?"). Vessel in Volkmann's canals (VO) may be arteriolar or venular. Vessels emptying sinusoids and haversian canals supply emissary veins (E). Periosteal arteries (PA) provide blood from attached soft tissue. Pressure gradient is from right to left, but may reverse, and with it flow, as a result of trauma. (From Williams [1980],[106] with permission.)

to humans, the degree to which the branching pattern is in parallel or in series is of some significance.[63] In a parallel system, separate branches supply the medullary and endosteal microcirculation, while a series pattern has loops from the endosteum supplying bone marrow microcirculation. No clear demonstration of the dominant (exclusivity has not been determined) pattern in humans has been reported. In the medullary canal, branches from the nutrient artery form sinusoidal vessel networks that associate intimately with hematopoietic tissue before emptying into the central sinus.

Endosteal and periosteal vessels predominately follow a longitudinal path within haversian canals parallel with the long bone axis. Radial connections are maintained through side branches following Volkmann's canals as shown in Figure 1. Generally, a haversian canal is 25 to 175 μm wide[5] and contains one or two vessels of calibers ranging from 6 to 30 μm.[111] Volkmann's canals are generally smaller.

Metaphyseal circulation receives input from anastomoses with epiphyseal arteries, as well as through perforations in metaphyseal (trabecular) bone. The latter arteries arise through ligamentous attachments.[82] In the tibia, the epiphysis is supplied primarily by vessels from the genicular arteries, with some assistance from branches of the tibial artery. These arteries enter the epiphysis in its posterior portion from multiradial directions to form a spoke-like network.[70] Proximally, the epiphyseal network sends branches toward the articular surface, forming arcades in the subchondral bone as they regress distally.

3. Nutrient Vasculature

The anatomy of microvascular networks is unclear because identification of microvessels is inconsistent. Lumen sizes observed have been as small as 2 μm[23] and larger than 70 μm (H. Winet, unpublished data). They are commonly lined with one to two endothelial cells[107] and are occasionally surrounded with pericytes. Their basement membrane ranges from 40 to 60 nm. This large variability in caliber for apparently permeable vessels exceeds the standard limits of: about 5 μm, true capillary; 6 to 9 μm, precapillary; 10 to 20 μm terminal arteriole; 21 to 40 μm, arteriole, and more than 40 μm, artery[52]; as well as Diana's[24] restriction of true capillaries to the less than 15-μm range. The few vessels with smooth muscle are found near the endosteum where the microvasculature is most dense.[70] In general, the distance between parallel vessels in separate haversian canals remains within the 100 to 200 μm maximum proposed by Ham.[43]

4. Efflux Vasculature

Kelly[54] has estimated the capacity of veins draining bone to be six to eight times that of inflow arteries. Most of the drainage in long bone occurs at the epiphysis.[54] In general, venous output from the epiphysis and metaphysis is concomitant with arterial pathways. However, there are more arteries than veins in these networks.[70] The central sinus is assumed to empty into nutrient veins. Only about 10% of the venous drainage is through the nutrient veins, however, according to canine studies.[106] Blood not exiting these pathways follows the emissary veins, which collect from sinusoids and haversian vessels and course through enlarged Volkmann's canals to anastomose with periosteal and/or soft tissue veins.[106] Two separate efflux tributaries have been hypothesized by Oni,[71] who envisioned parallel efflux systems, one carrying blood to the haversian, emissary, and systemic vessels from nutrient arteries and sinusoids and the other the venous sinus to the nutrient veins (which are concomitant with the nutrient arteries).

5. Lymphatic Vessels

Lymphatic vessels have been detected only in the periosteal circulation.[106] There is physiological evidence for pathways to periosteal lymphatic capillaries, but no direct anatomic evidence.[70]

B. NORMAL PHYSIOLOGY OF BONE MICROCIRCULATION
1. Blood Supply

Long bones are contained within fascial compartments. The medullary canal forms an inner compartment with variations of intravascular hydrostatic pressure from 16 mm in the diaphysis to 27 mmHg in the metaphysis of the tibia, (± 7 mmHg for the heart pulse component).[30] Outside the bone compartment, the pressure drops to 19 mmHg in the nutrient vein, from an inflow nutrient artery value of 123 $\pm$ 15 mmHg.[104] High medullary canal pressures could result from contraction of muscles supplying vasculature to the periosteum or from increased compartment pressures outside the bone.

Dissociation of O_2 from hemoglobin is strongly influenced by P_{CO_2}, which is reflective of metabolic activity. In nonmedullary regions of bone, this may be viewed as a result of basic multicellular unit (BMU) operations. BMUs are the osteons that carry on remodeling and consist primarily of osteoblasts, osteoclasts and their matrix substrate, and usually two blood vessels. They are the initial form of haversian canals. Another inducer of O_2 release is H^+, which can be produced in large amounts by the osteoclasts as they resorb mineralized bone matrix. Hyperoxia as a stimulus for collagen synthesis has been established for other tissues.[20] In bone it has also been associated with collagen synthesis, while hypoxia, in contrast, stimulates osteogenesis.[13] There is thus an emerging picture that relates blood flow and bone remodeling.

Regulation of bone blood flow by O_2 has not been studied sufficiently to decide if its mechanism differs from that in other tissues. While the existence of paired veins and arteries is well established, the degree to which they extend to arterioles and venules that could exhibit counter-current diffusion of O_2 is not known for bone. In other tissues, smooth muscle cell hypoxia is accentuated in a counter-current environment, and mitochondrial support for contraction diminishes. As a result, the cell relaxes, allowing "reactive hyperemia" to develop.[40,45] In bone, one product of metabolism, adenosine diphosphate (ADP), has been shown to induce vasodilation.[42] Studies from other tissues suggest alternatives to this negative-feedback *metabolic* regulatory mechanism by which hypoxia stimulates arteriolar dilation.

Dilation may also be initiated by shear and/or hydrostatic pressure stimulation of arteriolar endothelium. As described by Kuo et al.,[59] shear stress activates endothelial K^+ channels that hyperpolarize the membrane and establish a gradient through which Ca^{2+} enters the endothelial cells and stimulates release of endothelial-derived relaxing factor (EDRF now known to be nitric oxide), Prostacyclin (PGI_2),[22] and/or other factors. Adjacent smooth muscle cells relax through the mediation of receptors for these dilating agents and appropriate second messengers. Humoral catecholamines may also initiate dilation of smooth muscle cells bearing β-receptors. This effect has been shown, however, to play a minor role in vasodilation.[91] Autonomic neuronal stimulation of muscarinic receptors probably does not occur in bone since no cholinergic nerve fibers have been identified.[22] Davis and Wood[22] have obtained indirect evidence that EDRF and PGI_2 (or PGE_2) are secreted by bone vascular endothelium. They measured an increase in vascular resistance after chemically blocking EDRF and prostaglandin production.

Vasoconstriction by adrenergic stimulation of α-receptors has been shown in non-bone tissues to occur in smooth muscle cells around both the capacitance (venular) and resistance (arteriolar) vessels. The ratio of response to stimulation at the two sites differs from organ to organ, but appears to have evolved so as to maintain a constant hydrostatic pressure in their associated capillaries.[91] Arteriole vasoconstriction decreases capillary pressure, allowing interstitial fluid to influx. Venule vasoconstriction increases capillary pressure, allowing plasma to extravasate.[66] In the Davis and Wood[22] study cited above, baseline values for resistance were obtained by perfusion with norepinephrine as well as by electrical stimulation of the "nutrient" nerve. They did not attempt to interpret the relative effects of the two vasoconstriction sites on their results. Yet, they assumed the response to the exogenous catecholamine and stimulation of the adrenergic sympathetic nerve differed only in the ability of the more diffusable agent (norepinephrine) to reach the endothelium. Endothelin (ET-1), a vasoconstrictive agent secreted by endothelial cells that has at least two receptors on vascular smooth muscle cells[47] has not been sufficiently investigated to clarify its normal role in bone vasoregulation. Direct injection into a nutrient artery in dogs generates an increase in artificial perfusion pressure,[16] as would be expected from vasoconstriction. One conclusion seems clear from the foregoing. Although smooth muscle cells do not appear to be present in large numbers in bone microvessels, their concentration near the endosteal surface[70] puts them on the arteriolar side of bone's microvascular system, where they can have their greatest influence.

Hormonal effects on bone blood flow have been poorly studied and appear to be of little significance. Parathormone (PTH) has a vasodilator effect on non-bone vascular smooth muscle that indirectly affects bone blood flow.[15] No direct effect on bone vascular smooth muscle has been demonstrated. Similarly, thyroxin increases blood flow to bone,[88] but no direct effect on bone vascular smooth muscle has been reported.

2. Nutrient Exchange

Among the ions in bone, Ca^{2+} is the most clinically important. Calcium does not have to reach the lymphatics (or alymphatics[70]) to be distributed outside the bone compartment. Its uptake by venular capillaries in more radial osteons allows its distribution to be related only to blood flow. One could conceive of this transfer as a counter-current arrangement. It has been suggested that the movement of Ca^{2+} and other ions between the mineralized and mobile phases is modulated by the intervening layer of osteoblasts. The organization of osteoblasts into a layer sufficiently continuous to be called a "barrier" implies that forces maintaining continuity (cell-to-cell adhesion) may compete with those attaching these cells to their mineralized matrix. At equilibrium, there could be an interstitial space between osteoblast layer and mineralized surface. Osteonal osteoblasts would thus be bounded by two interstitia. These cells must extract Ca^{2+} from one and expel it to the other. McCarthy and Hughes[64] found that blocking of osteoblast activity with KCN causes a decrease in the extraction of $^{85}Sr^{2+}$ into the mineralized phase. The notion of osteoblasts functioning as calcium pumps is well established in bone physiology.[96] Pump regulation by PTH[15] can be defined as two opposite ionic gradients.[4] Knowing the fraction of bone interstitial fluid trapped between osteoblasts and mineral phase would, accordingly, be necessary for determination of total transport in bone. The demonstration that osteoblasts form an effective syncytial blood-bone barrier would add bone to a small list of organs with similar boundaries, the most notable being the brain.

Movement of solvent and solutes through the vessel walls and matrix is by both diffusive and convective transport. The latter has been modeled in bone by both black-box/global relationships — e.g., Darcy's Law for filtration through sand[26] — and as the sum of local relationships — e.g., Piekarski and Munro's[78] stress-driven flow through the lacunar-canalicular network.

Levick,[61] evaluating the hydraulic conductivity of the interstitium as a porous matrix, concluded that glycosaminoglycan (GAG) concentration was the major determinant of interstitial convective transport. Since GAGs carry fixed negative charges, they interact directly with charged ions flowing through the interstitial matrix. In addition, other solutes with extensive hydration layers, along with macromolecules, interact more mechanically with the matrix. As a result, a more complex porous flow exists than would be predicted from a model based on dry bone. The magnitude of hydraulic conductivity is suggested by the extravasation and transport of ferritin, a 440-kDa protein with a Stokes-Einstein radius of 105 Å.[7] This molecule extravasates and moves through the bone matrix too fast to be merely diffusing. Moreover, the pattern of deposition of "halos" of this protein suggest that convective fluid flow follows the hydrostatic pressure gradient down from the medullary canal to the periosteum.[25,68] Emerging models for bone mineralization that replace piezoelectric with flow shear stress hypotheses attempt to incorporate these results into quantitative predictions.[102] One flow shear stress model for calcium exchange between mineralized matrix and osteocytes in canaliculi has been proposed by Weinbaum et al.[102]

II. PATHOPHYSIOLOGY OF BONE MICROCIRCULATION

A. DISEASES THOUGHT TO AFFECT OR BE AFFECTED BY BONE MICROCIRCULATION

1. Trauma

a. Fractures

The most common bone pathology is the fracture. Since it is the most rigid tissue in the body and the closest to a Hookean solid, bone cannot dissipate impact energy as well as other tissues. Yet, while its stiffness is relatively high and its porosity undermines the strength of its hydroxyapatite phase, bone's organic matrix and fluid phases raise the level of impact energy necessary for fracture.[17] Moreover, mechanical stress is *required* to maintain a balance between resorption and mineralization in normal bone. The development of disuse osteoporosis under microgravity conditions is well known. Mechanical stress in normal bone is not restricted to bending, compression, and/or tensile forces. Fluid shear has been shown to be sufficient to induce increased cAMP levels in osteoblasts.[80] Similar effects have also been observed in endothelial cells.[32]

The point at which mechanical stress becomes trauma was once thought to be marked by the "fracture" event. Studies on cadavers[97] and living bone from healthy subjects,[18] however, have indicated a progression of discontinuity:

molecular < ultrastructural < prefailure plane < frank cracks < complete fracture[31]

Below the "frank crack" level, the microdamage appears to stimulate remodeling.[18] Since fuchsin dye (used to detect prefailure planes) requires weeks to penetrate harvested samples,[18] it appears unlikely that extravascular convective flow is significantly enhanced by greater porosity. Where blood vessels are not damaged sufficiently, a wound healing response will be absent. Angiogenesis is, however, stimulated as part of the remodeling process.[99]

At some point between formation of prefailure planes and frank cracks, sufficient shear or tension is inflicted on vasculature to release platelets and clotting factors, which induces a clotting cascade. The fissure also provides additional pathways for macrophage migration. While trying to digest the clot by aiding in plasminogen activation, macrophages elaborate cytokines like basic fibroblast growth factor (bFGF), which stimulate fibroblast chemotaxis and collagen I and III secretion.[6]

Formation of type V collagen is associated with the invasion of endothelial cells soon after the fibroblasts. The former are responding to angiogenins like bFGF, primarily from macrophages.[58] They form tubes while secreting EDRF and PGI_2 to prevent further platelet aggregation and plasminogen activator[87] to assist the macrophages. A given venular capillary will grow about 0.2 mm/day.[50] Both fibroblasts and endothelial cells use the fibronectin remaining after clot digestion by macrophages as a scaffolding.[33] This glycoprotein and laminin mediate the adhesion of endothelial cells to type IV collagen,[51] which is produced during formation of vascular basement membrane.[72]

Healing long bone periosteum, which is bridging a nondisplaced fracture, is composed of fibrous tissue at day 3.[6] The periosteal fibrous bridge, located close to increasingly well-perfused soft tissue, is well vascularized, in contrast to the more endosteal callus. If the latter is thin enough to also be in contact with well-perfused soft tissue or healthy bone (perhaps as a result of early reduction and fixation), prechondrocytes (which require hypoxia for induction) do not develop and the periosteal layer eclipses the remaining callous to proceed to "intramembranous" healing. Because ossification takes place so quickly by this process where blood supply is adequate from outside the healing focus, intramembranous bone tends to be less perforated with vessel-bearing haversian canals.

If "micromotion" occurs at the fracture site, endochondral repair results. An example of such movement is that equivalent to 1-mm axial displacement by 360 Newtons force at 0.5 Hz for 500 cycles/day,[39] which will repeatedly tear the vasculature. Under these conditions, pluripotential mesenchymal cells that have migrated to help form the subperiosteal callus apparently respond to the resulting hypoxia by differentiating into chondroblasts.[6] These become chondrocytes that elaborate angiogenesis inhibitors[69] and collagen II. The resulting cartilage defines the avascular callus matrix. Chondrocytic antiangiogenic factors maintain the cartilage callus until the fracture gains sufficient stability to support mineralized struts that form in the callus along with the osteoblasts that make them. Such mineralization, along with chondrolysis, appears to take place at first in the absence of osteoblasts, which soon appear to accelerate the process. Vascu-

Table 1 Causes of Ischemic Necrosis
of Cartilage and Bone

Endocrine/metabolic
  Glucocorticoid therapy
  Cushing's disease
  Alcoholism
  Gout
  Osteomalacia
Storage diseases (e.g., Gaucher's disease)
Hemoglobinopathies (e.g., Sickle cell disease)
Trauma (e.g., dislocation, fracture)
Dysbaric conditions
Collagen vascular disorders
Irradiation
Pancreatitis
Renal transplantation idiopathic, familial

Note: See References 27 and 81.

lature also appears and is necessary to maintain the transformation. The cartilaginous callus ossification triumvirate — chondrolysis, angiogenesis, and mineralization — does not exhibit an obvious progression. Accordingly, their relationship is still a controversial subject.[38]

Revascularization of the periosteal surface is matched at the endosteal surface and is evident by 4 days post-trauma.[1] After penetrating the mineralizing cartilaginous callous, vessels reach a maximum density at 9 to 10 days.[74] Blood supply to the fracture site decreases slowly after this point, requiring more than 16 weeks to return to normal baseline values.[74] The lack of microcirculation in cartilaginous callus prior to day 4 results in a low P_{O_2}, starting at about 6.3 mm Hg in the hematoma,[13] which favors osteogenesis. The lack of committed osteoblasts at this point, however, frustrates any attempt at osteogenesis. There have been reports of a "primitive woven bone", occurring at this stage, which is transient.[2] As the day 10 peak is achieved and oxygen levels reach 22 to 40 mm Hg, macromolecular (presumably including collagens I and IV) synthesis becomes dominant.[13] Oxygen levels apparently fall faster than the blood supply after the hyperemic peak because osteoblasts, fibroblasts, and endothelial cells that are now in abundance are metabolizing.[46] Oxygen utilization increases to such an extent that P_{O_2} is zero in tissue 10 to 15 μm from the vessel.[13] It would seem that an increase in vascularity would be necessary to prevent a decrease of P_{O_2} to a level below that capable of supporting osteogenesis. Such an increase would result in a second hyperemic peak, which has not been reported except in bone chamber studies of healing defects.[108]

b. Traumatic Osteonecrosis
Bone dies when denied blood for as little as 6 hours.[86] The clinical entity designated "osteonecrosis" refers to a specific group of bone disorders some of which may occur in the absence of ischemia.[35]

"Ischemic bone disease"[103] (IBD) can be either "traumatic" or "atraumatic".[26] Clinical diagnosis of IBD requires only that both necrotic bone and compromised vasculature be found in the same biopsy. The etiology of IBD has yet to be defined because (1) it is initiated by a variety of apparently unrelated agents, and (2) no valid animal model has been developed for study.[63]

Whyte's[103] summary of the conditions presaging ischemic bone disease is presented in Table 1. Atraumatic IBD is linked to all the indications listed that are not a form of wounding. These appear to share the characteristic of altering vessels (e.g., corticosteroid therapy) or blood (e.g., sickle cell disease). Yet, a specific effect common to all is not obvious.

Pathophysiological approaches to the study of IBD have been dominated by radiological staging of the disease in the hip, its most common site by far. During the zero and first stages,[29] there is no radiological evidence of osteonecrosis and no symptomology. Accordingly, this interval has earned the name "silent hip".

It is during stage zero that osteonecrosis occurs. Whether osteocytes die directly[57] or following an ischemic event is not clear.[77] Those who accept an ischemic event as the etiological mechanism have been unable to find an experimental model that follows the clinical manifestation.[77] Meyers[67] has challenged all models proposing nonlocal causes on the basis that bone death is not evenly distributed over the pathologic region. Trauma that damages vessels critical for survival of the affected bone define traumatic IBD.[30,67,152]

The femoral head is the principal site for both forms of IBD and its principal at-risk vessels are the lateral epiphyseal and superior metaphyseal arteries, the main blood supply to the upper femoral epiphysis.[30] At a minimum, dislocation of the hip would affect only the medial epiphysial artery in the ligamentum teres. At a maximum, fracture of the femoral neck would sever all collaterals leading to the femoral head.

Alternatives to traumatic arterial injury could be capillary collapse during bone compression, an event unlikely without concomitant micro-damage/fracture, and venous injury that would block blood efflux from the bone. To test the viability of the latter prediction, Woodhouse[114] applied an intracapsular tamponade causing venous occlusion, leaving the medial epiphyseal artery as the only blood supply to the femoral head. Extensive osteonecrosis was produced and the resulting histological lesions were identical to those resulting from arterial occlusion.[30] Since the ratio of efflux to influx vessels in bone is about 6:1, any agent affecting efflux vessels would have to be more systemic than one resulting in arterial ischemia. Glimcher and Kenzora[37] have also argued against a venous stasis mechanism, but their reasoning that it would halt repair conflicts with the observations of Kelly.[54]

Malizos et al.[63] used liquid nitrogen to freeze canine femoral heads and induce osteonecrosis *in situ*. Histological examination 2 h post-insult confirmed the observations of Kenzora et al.[56] in osteotomized-femora rabbits: that osteocytes and osteoblasts appeared to be normal. This condition persisted up to 6 to 7 days in the latter study. *In vitro* evaluation of the cells determined that the osteocytes had lost the ability to synthesize collagen and were, in fact, functionally dead 12 to 24 h post-insult; the endothelial cells had suffered the same fate by 12 h. By 2 to 4 days post-insult, cells of the marrow vascular space along with endothelial cells showed histological signs of injury, while osteocytes still appeared to be normal.[56]

Death of osteocytes does not result in immediate resorption of their lacunar bone matrices. The ischemia that reduces migration of preosteoclast cells from the marrow is one explanation for the delay. Persistence of the mineralized matrix yields radiographs that are indistinguishable from healthy bone. In addition, absence of permeable vessels also restricts the paths for fluid transport to the extracellular matrix. The first stage of the disease is clinically detectable with a stress test, in which saline is injected into the medullary canal while its canal pressure is monitored. With disease, a much slower-than-normal return to baseline pressure occurs because of insufficient blood flow to carry away the excess fluid.

By 4 days post-trauma, mesenchymal cells and capillaries proliferate at the interface of necrotic and living bone. Revascularization of necrotic bone takes 8 to 12 weeks. According to Kenzora et al.,[56] no resorption is evident during this period, although the invading primitive mesenchymal cells continuously elaborate collagen matrix and proteoglycan. Malizos et al.[63] observed in the rabbit model that the invading mesenchymal cells are accompanied (probably preceded) by fibroblasts and macrophages, and the latter resorb necrotic trabeculae. This observation is supported by the clinical findings of Johnson and Crothers[51] and the "osteoporosis" reported in stage I by others.[30] In any case, the revascularization process is not uniform over the entire involved structure[67] and supports the contention that traumatic IBD is caused by local rather than systemic factors. Femoral head collapse usually occurs 1 to 2 years post-trauma.[51] This collapse creates a second traumatic condition that results in ischemia of the newly revascularized tissue.

2. Atraumatic Osteonecrosis

There are distinct differences in the pathologic courses between traumatically and atraumatically-induced IBD. The most dramatic difference is the tendency for all atraumatic cases to go on to collapse.[36] Each atraumatic etiological factor listed in Table 1 has a known deleterious effect on microcirculation. Sickle cell disease increases viscosity because the Fahraeus effect is retarded and small vessels are clogged with RBCs that cannot deform. In each of the other cases, an ischemic factor can be postulated based upon observed circulatory effects in other organs. Unfortunately, none of the non-human animal models developed to date have been able to clarify the early pathological events.[63] Four major pathological models appear to be popular at present:

1. Embolism (fat, nitrogen, etc.) usually blocking the venous microcirculation[53]
2. Edema or normal joint load crushing compliant vessels in the rigid Starling resistor-like medullary canal[104]
3. Osteocyte death from cytotoxic agents[101]
4. "Multifactorial" agents that cause cumulative stress on "bone cells"[55]

With the exception of the fourth, which is difficult to test, there is contradictory evidence for all the suggested factors.[67] An intriguing model combines mechanisms 1 and 2 by proposing that marrow fat is forced into arterial microvasculature by pressure from loaded joints.[89]

3. Compartment Syndrome (CS)

Compartment syndromes result from edema in a limb fascial compartment. Edema, under these circumstances, is caused by blockage of a vessel in the compartment so as to create increased transmural pressure in vessels with resultant hydraulic conductivity into the interstitium. Compartmental pressures, which are normally 4 to 8 mmHg in the leg,[44] may increase to more than 30 mmHg, a pressure sufficient to compress compliant tissue, including veins. As a consequence, ischemia spreads due to vascular compromise increasing hypoxia, and threatening tissue viability if maintained more than 6 h.[44] Sequelae range from the mild "shin splints"[1] to massive necrosis sufficient to require amputation. The leg is the most common site of CS, where etiological agents identified thus far include traumatic conditions such as fractures of the tibia, crush injuries, compression bandaging, and atraumatic conditions such as arteriolar embolism.[1] Similarities between CS etiology and the Wilkes and Visscher[104] model for atraumatic IBD become apparent when the medullary canal is modeled as a compartment.[49,101]

B. CLINICAL APPLICATIONS OF MICROCIRCULATORY STUDIES
1. Hyperbaric Oxygenation (HBO)

The need for oxygen to ensure transition from repair to the regenerative phase of bone healing has led to the proposal that enhancement of O_2 delivery by high pressure increases plasma O_2 concentration, which would enhance fracture healing.[21] High O_2 permeability and potential for saturating the interstitium have been the basis for the use of HBO to control anaerobes causing osteomyelitis.[90] Potential for reducing edema has been the basis of its use for the treatment of CS.[92] Hyperbaric oxygenation raises plasma O_2 concentration at 37°C from 0.236 ml_{O_2}/ml_{blood} at 10 mm Hg to 35.8 ml_{O_2}/ml_{blood} at 2 atmospheres absolute pressure. Patients are enclosed in a monoplace chamber for a minimum of 1 hour each day. Pressure and O_2 combine to: (1) enhance interstitial O_2 concentration by converting its vascular delivery from flow dependence (in RBCs) to permeability dependence (O_2 and pressure); (2) reduce edema by causing flow-decreasing constriction of vascular smooth muscle (O_2); and (3) decrease gas emboli (pressure).[94] Use of HBO for treatment of orthopedic conditions has been controversial.[34] Robin[85] has asserted that even if the proposed physiological effects occurred, it does not follow that HBO elicits cures for any of the proposed indications. In no case has a statistically valid randomized, double-blinded study been conducted that demonstrates clinical efficacy of HBO.[34] Non-human animal models for application of HBO have been successfully developed for treatment of acute fractures,[76] compartment syndrome,[93] and osteomyelitis.[28] While statistically significant positive effects were demonstrated in the former two, results from the latter were inconclusive.

2. Electrical Stimulation

Direct current delivered through implanted electrodes has been shown to have a beneficial effect on bone healing.[75] Noninvasive alternatives currently in use are pulsed electromagnetic fields (PEMFs)[41] and coupled capacitance (CC).[12] The former, delivered through a Helmholtz coil, maintains a strength of about 1.5 mV/cm in various pulse configurations from intermittent bursts to AC-form currents. CC delivers a calculated 16.5 V/cm through two signal generators placed on opposite sides of the appendage.[14]

Study of the influence of electrical stimulation on bone vascular phenomena has almost been ignored in comparison with that on osteogenesis. Yen-Patton et al.[115] studied PEMF effects and found enhancement of endothelial cell proliferation *in vitro*. Rinsky et al.[84] found that PEMFs stimulated blood supply to traumatically devascularized femoral heads, and Braun and Lemons[11] found an increase in vascularity, as measured by India-ink injected into traumatically devascularized femoral heads. In the latter study, an advantage over control specimens after 2 weeks of healing disappeared by the fourth week.[11] In some preliminary tests, neither PEMF nor ultrasound showed any marked effect on local blood flow (Winet, unpublished data). There are, however, preliminary data that suggest an effect on vascular permeability.[112]

III. QUANTITATION OF BONE MICROCIRCULATION

A. RESEARCH-LIMITED MEASURES

Of the global measurement techniques limited to non-human research, the most useful for blood flow has been arteriolar entrapment of 15 μm (usually) radioisotope-bearing microspheres.[98,105] A source of error in this technique is a significant incidence of A-V shunts that would cause flow to be underestimated.[107] Permeability is indicated by extraction of isotopes[48] with low reflection coefficient (δ) values. The most useful tracers for bone (where they accumulate) are ^{45}Ca, ^{18}F, and ^{85}Sr. Precise values for isotope extraction depend on δ being zero (assuming no other impediments to clearance). Unfortunately, most evidence suggests there is less than 100% clearance for all tracers tested.[107]

Dependence of local microcirculation models on intravital microscopy has presented a challenge to those seeking to discern the degree to which bone mimics other tissues. Brånemark[10] was the first to determine that blood flow in the endosteum was not "sluggish", as previous investigators had assumed. Brånemark developed an implantable window that allowed chronic observations following "osseointegration".[9] McCuskey et al.[65] and Brånemark's student Albrektsson[3] refined this optical bone chamber window implant (BCI) to a point where it could be used to obtain dynamic information from haversian vessels.[107]

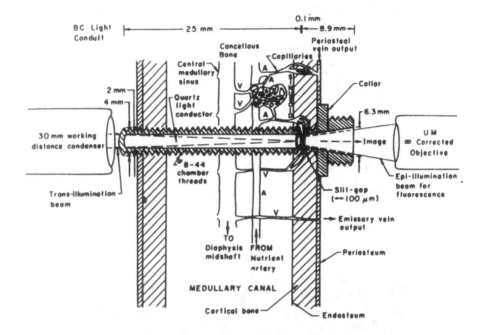

Figure 2 *In situ* niche of optical bone chamber. The tissue observed must heal from healthy haversian cortical bone across layers of necrotic bone (created by implantation surgery) and hematoma that must be resorbed. Fibrovascular ("repair") tissue and apposing trabeculae enter the field-of-view compartment through a 100 μm separation ("slit") of the quartz windows. Repair tissue is well established by W4 when trabeculae first appear at the distal and proximal entrances to the field-of-view cell/chamber. Bone covers the 2 mm diameter circle ("gap") by W8. (From Winet [1989],[107] with permission.)

The most recent version of the optical BCI is diagrammed *in situ* in Figure 2. Intravital microscopic observations commence 3 weeks after implantation (W3), 1 day before which, the BCI ends are exposed permanently. Daily lavage is required to prevent pin-tract infections. Weekly observations utilize fluorescein isothiocyanate-conjugated dex-trans (20 and 70 kDa) and fluorescent microspheres (1–1.75 μm in diameter), which are injected intravenously. Recorded intravital microscopic images are analyzed with video frame-grabber-based image processing software to determine vascularity (perfused vasculature) and microsphere velocity. Typically, the field-of-view for intravital microscopy is a 2-mm diameter circle 100 μm thick. Thus, the tissue volume observed is about 3.14×10^{-4} cm^3.

Vascularity is expressed as vessel length per unit tissue volume (L/V).[116] Weekly changes in L/V indicate *net* angiogenesis. Representative photographs of analyzed fields-of-view are shown in Figure 3. In this model, normal values of L/V were of the order 10^8 μm/cm^3. This may appear a large value, but it represented newly healed bone and *maximum* vasculature was perfused (as with other tissues, vessels are not all perfused simultaneously in bone so the total L/V obtained over the 2+ minutes of observation performed is a sum rather than a snapshot). During the first 2 weeks of cortical bone defect healing in the BCI, L/V peaked, reflecting post-traumatic inflammatory hyperemia. The tail end of this peak was observed at week 3, after which a minimum L/V of about 3×10^7 μm/cm^3 appeared. The next L/V peak at week 7.5 was 1.2×10^8 μm/cm^3, which

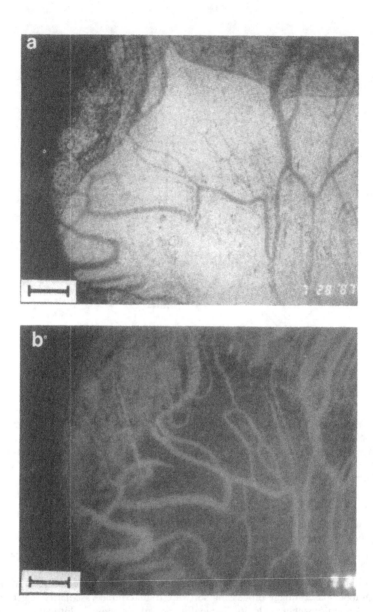

Figure 3 Typical field-of-view during intravital microscopy of the bone chamber. Usually, an 8-mm objective is used and the entire 2-mm circle of slit-gap is visible. Scale bar is 200 μm. Both panels show the same tissue sample. (a) Brightfield illumination. Bone trabeculae (B) are best resolved under this lighting. (b) Epifluorescence illumination. Vasculature carrying FITC-Dextran 70 kDa is shown fluorescing. Vessel caliber rarely exceeds 50 μm. (From Winet [1989],[107] with permission.)

was followed by a dip to the normal value cited above. Net angiogenesis between week 4 and week 7 was of the order 6×10^6 μm/cm^3/day.

Calculation of Q utilized $Q = Q_{in} = \sum \pi c^2 u_{in}/8$, with c = each vessel caliber (which averaged about 25 μm) and u_{in} = microsphere velocity in each influx vessel. Values of blood flow were as high as 370 ml/min/100 g, with normal bone closer to 100 ml/min/100 g. The pattern during healing paralleled that of L/V with minima near 10 and maxima near 200 ml/min/100 g. Values for bone blood flow during fracture healing obtained with global techniques were markedly different from BCI values in at least two ways: (1) local values were markedly higher and (2) global values indicated a steady decrease in blood flow following post-traumatic inflammatory hyperemia. While it probably has little effect on blood flow values, flow reversal, which has been observed in the local model (Winet, unpublished observations), would not be detectable in global models.

Vascular investigations utilizing the optical BCI have uncovered flaws in some of the assumptions about bone microcirculation. From Brånemark's[10] revelation that blood in bone is not "slow" (confirmed by data presented above) to Albrektsson's[2] detection of perfusion failures by vascularity markers, the need for intravital microscopic follow-up to nonphysiological or macroscopic techniques has become clear. Thus, BCI intravital microscopy has shown that:

1. Allogeneic bone grafts are easily penetrated by host vasculature, but will not form a continuous interface with host bone.[113]
2. Bone under pulsed electromagnetic fields, at least in the presence of metal implants, may alter vessel permeability. This was concluded after observing that under PEMF, bone apposition increased with increasing blood flow.[112] Normally, the reverse is true because permeability and osteogenesis are enhanced by decreased blood flow (when instituted by venous blockage).[74]
3. Hyperbaric oxygenation does not affect vascularization during acute fracture healing.[95]
4. In the presence of a bio-eroding polymer implant, which is not under bone stress (i.e., the polymer is in the BCI rather than press-fit into bone), healing tissue angiogenesis is both delayed and diminished, and blood flow is reduced.[109]

While these observations increase insight into local components of the process being investigated, they do not yield conclusive evidence with regard to mechanisms. What is actually taking place at the molecular level? The link that connects microvasculature with this level is the primary function of microcirculation — nutrient exchange. Accordingly, it is necessary to extend BCI observations to vessel permeability. Preliminary local data on bone vessel permeability at various time points during healing in the BCI have been obtained for large pores (sites of macromolecular filtration).[110] A count of the number of leak points per unit tissue volume (LP/V) yielded a positive correlation between bone apposition and LP/V, which agrees with results obtained by global techniques. In contrast, the relationship between blood flow and LP/V is less clear. The major trend of the data supports an inverse relationship, which agrees with global observations. At higher blood flow values, however, the trend appears to reverse.

B. CLINICAL MEASURES

Two techniques that have been used to quantitate blood flow clinically are laser Doppler velocimetry[60] (LDF) and clearance of radioisotopic tracers.[48,79] Since Doppler-based technology does not give a velocity value for blood flow, attempts have been made to correlate the values obtained with those from more direct techniques. Lausten et al.[60] found a correlation between LDF and microsphere measurements, but concluded that the LDF values had so much variation between sample sites in close proximity that the technique was suitable only for monitoring changes at one location. Of the radioisotopic tracers, ^{18}F has been the most useful for clinical determination of an "effective", rather than absolute blood flow because uptake of the tracer was determined from biopsies.[79] New techniques that show some promise for clinical determination of vascular transport are ultrasound Doppler velocimetry,[8] NMR/MRI,[19,100] and an alternative for the stress test of IBD, "hydraulic resistance", whereby a fluid is injected slowly and less painfully while outflow resistance is evaluated.[26]

176

REFERENCES

1. **Abramson, D. L. and Miller, D. S.**, *Vascular Problems in Musculoskeletal Disorders of the Limbs*, Springer-Verlag, New York, 1981.
2. **Albrektsson, T.**, A comparison between microangiography and vital microscopic in evaluation of bone vascularization, in *Bone Circulation*, Williams and Wilkins, 162–166, 1984.
3. **Albrektsson, T. and Albrektsson, B.**, Microcirculation in grafted bone, *Acta Orthop. Scand.*, 49, 1–7, 1978.
4. **Albright, J. A. and Skinner, H. C. W.**, Bone: Structural organization and remodeling dynamics, in *The Scientific Basis of Orthopaedics*, Albright, J. A. and Brand, R. A., Eds., Appleton & Lange, Los Altos, CA, 1987, 161–198.
5. **Arsenault, A. L.**, Vascular canals in bovine cortical bone studied by corrosion casting, *Calcif. Tiss. Int.*, 47, 320–325, 1990.
6. **Ashhurst, D. E.**, Macromolecular synthesis and mechanical stability during fracture repair, in *Bone*, Hall, B. K., Ed., CRC Press, Boca Raton, FL, 1992, 61–121.
7. **Bent-Hansen, L. and Svendsen, J. H.**, Tissue to plasma capillary permeability of 131Albumin in the perfused rabbit ear, *Microvasc. Res.*, 41, 141–148, 1991.
8. **Blair, W. F., Brown, T. D., and Greene, E. R.**, Pulsed ultrasound doppler velocimetry in the assessment of microvascular hemodynamics, *J. Orthop. Res.*, 6, 300–309, 1988.
9. **Brånemark, P.-I., Breine, U., Johansson, B., Roylance, P. J., Rökert, H., and Yoffey, J. M.**, Regneration of bone marrow, *Acta Anat. (Basel)*, 59, 1–46, 1964.
10. **Brånemark, P. I.**, Vital microscopy of bone marrow in rabbit, *Scand. J. Clin. Lab. Invest.*, 11, 1–82, 1959.
11. **Braun, K. A. and Lemons, J. E.**, Effects of electromagnetic fields on the recovery of circulation in mature rabbit femoral heads, *Trans. Orthop. Res. Soc. 28th Mtng.*, 7, 313, 1982.
12. **Brighton, C. T. and Pollack, S. R.**, Treatment of recalcitrant non-union with a capacitively coupled electrical field, *J. Bone Jt. Surg.*, 67A, 577–585, 1985.
13. **Brighton, C. T., Schaffer, J. L., Shapiro, D. B., Tana, J. J. S., and Clark, C. C.**, Proliferation and macromolecular synthesis by rat calvarial bone cells grown in various oxygen tensions, *J. Orthop. Res.*, 9, 847–854, 1991.
14. **Brighton, C. T., Tadduni, G. T., Goll, S. R., and Pollack, S. R.**, Treatment of denervation/disuse osteoporosis in the rat with a capacitively coupled electrical signal: Effects on bone formation and bone resorption, *J. Orthop. Res.*, 6, 676–684, 1988.
15. **Brindley, G. W., Williams, E. A., Bronk, J. T., Meadows, T. H., Montgomery, R. J., Smith, S. R., and Kelly, P. J.**, Parathyroid hormone effects on skeletal exchangeable calcium and bone blood flow, *Am. J. Physiol.*, 255, H94–H100, 1988.
16. **Brinker, M. R., Lippton, H. L., Cook, S. D., and Hyman, A. L.**, Pharmacological regulation of the circulation of bone, *J. Bone Jt. Surg.*, 72A, 964–975, 1990.
17. **Burger, E. H. and Veldhuijzen, J. P.**, Influence of mechanical factors on bone formation, resorption and growth *in vitro*, in *Bone 7: Bone Growth-B*, Hall, B. K., Ed., CRC Press, Boca Raton, FL, 1993, 37–56.
18. **Burr, D. B., Martin, R. B., Schaffler, M. B., and Radin, E. L.**, Bone remodeling in response to *in vivo* fatigue microdamage, *J. Biomech.*, 18, 189–200, 1985.
19. **Burstein, D., Gray, M. L., Hartman, A. L., Gipe, R., and Foy, B. D.**, Diffusion of small solutes in cartilage as measured by nuclear magnetic resonance (NMR) spectroscopy and imaging, *J. Orthoped. Res.*, 11, 465–478, 1993.
20. **Chang, N., Goodson, W. H., III, Gottrup, F., and Hung, T. K.**, Direct measurement of wound and tissue oxygen tension in postoperative patients, *Ann. Surg.*, 197, 470–478, 1983.
21. **Coulson, D. B., Ferguson, A. B., Jr., and Diehl, R. C., Jr.**, Effect of hyperbaric oxygen on the healing femur of the rat, *Surg. For.*, 17, 449–450, 1966.
22. **Davis, T. R. C. and Wood, M. B.**, Endothelial control of long bone bascular resistance, *J. Orthop. Res.*, 10, 344–349, 1992.
23. **De Bruyn, P. P. H., Breen, P. C., and Thomas, T. B.**, The microcirculation of the bone marrow, *Anat. Rec.*, 168, 55–68, 1970.
24. **Diana, J. E.**, Transcapillary water flux, *The Physiol.*, 25, 365–375, 1982.
25. **Dillaman, R. M., Roer, R. D., and Gay, D. M.**, Fluid movement in bone: Theoretical and empirical, *J. Biomech.*, 24, 163–177, 1991.

26. **Downey, D. J., Simkin, P. A., Lanzer, W. L., and Matsen, F. A. I.,** Hydraulic resistance: A measure of vascular outflow obstruction in osteonecrosis, *J. Orthop. Res.*, 6, 272–278, 1988.

27. **Eideiken, J., Dalinka, M., and Karasick, D.,** *Edeiken's Roentgen Diagnosis of Disease of Bone, 4th Ed.,* Williams and Wilkins, Baltimore, 1990.

28. **Esterhai, J. L., Jr., Clark, J. M., Morton, H. E., Smith, D. W., Steinbach, A., and Richter, S. D.,** Effect of hyperbaric oxygen exposure on oxygen tension within the medullary canal in the rabbit tibial osteomyelitis model, *J. Orthop. Res.*, 4, 330–336, 1986.

29. **Ficat, R. P.,** Idiopathic bone necrosis of the femoral head. Early diagnosis and treatment, *J. Bone Jt. Surg.*, 67B, 3–9, 1985.

30. **Ficat, R. P. and Arlet, J.,** *Ischemia and Necrosis of Bone,* Williams and Wilkins, Baltimore, 1980.

31. **Frost, H. M.,** Transient-steady state phenomena in microdamage physiology: A proposed algorithm for lamellar bone, *Calcif. Tiss. Int.*, 44, 367–381, 1989.

32. **Fry, D. L.,** Acute vascular endothelial changes associated with increased blood velocity gradients, *Circ. Res.*, 22, 165–197, 1968.

33. **Furcht, L. T.,** Critical factors controlling angiogenesis: Cell products, cell matrix and growth factors, *Lab. Invest.*, 55, 505–509, 1986.

34. **Gabb, G. and Robin, E. D.,** Hyperbaric oxygen. A therapy in search of disease, *Chest*, 92, 1074–1082, 1987.

35. **Glimcher, M. J. and Kenzora, J. E.,** The biology of osteonecrosis of the human femoral head and its clinical implications. I. Tissue biology, *Clin. Orthop. Rel. Res.*, 138, 284–309, 1979.

36. **Glimcher, M. J. and Kenzora, J. E.,** The biology of osteonecrosis of the human femoral head and its clinical implications. II. The pathological changes in the femoral head as an organ and in the hip joint, *Clin. Orthop. Rel. Res.*, 139, 283–312, 1979.

37. **Glimcher, M. J. and Kenzora, J. E.,** The biology of osteonecrosis of the human femoral head and its clinical implications. III. Discussion of the etiology and genesis of the pathological sequelae: Comments on treatment, *Clin. Orthop. Rel. Res.,* 140, 273–312, 1979.

38. **Glowacki, J.,** Influence of imflammation and vascularization on bone repair, in *Portland Bone Symposium*, Hollinger, J. O. and Seyfer, A., Eds., U. Oregon Health Sciences, Portland, 1993, 33–38.

39. **Goodship, A. E. and Kenwright, J.,** The influence of induced micromovement upon the healing of experimental tibial fractures, *J. Bone Jt. Surg.*, 67B, 650–655, 1985.

40. **Granger, H. J., Borders, J. L., Meininger, G. A., Goodman, A. H., and Barnes, G. E.,** Microcirculatory control systems, in *The Physiology and Pharmacology of the Microcirculation*, Mortillaro, N. A., Ed., Academic Press, San Francisco, 1983, 209–236.

41. **Greenough, C. G.,** The effects of pulsed electromagnetic fields on blood vessel growth in the rabbit ear chamber, *J. Orthop. Res.*, 10, 256–262, 1982.

42. **Gross, P. M., Heistad, D. D., and Marcus, M. L.,** Neurohumoral regulation of blood flow to bones and marrow, *Am. J. Physiol.*, 237, H440–H448, 1979.

43. **Ham, A. W.,** Some histophysiological problems peculiar to calcified tissues, *J. Bone Jt. Surg.*, 34A, 701–728, 1952.

44. **Hargens, A. R. and Akeson, W. H.,** Pathophysiology of the compartment syndrome, in *Compartment Syndromes and Volkmann's Contracture*, Mubarak, S. J. and Hargens, A. R., Eds., W. B. Saunders, Philadelphia, 1981, 47–70.

45. **Harris, P. D.,** Movement of oxygen in skeletal muscle, *NIPS*, 1, 147–153, 1986.

46. **Heppenstall, R. B.,** Fracture healing, in *Fracture Treatment and Healing*, Heppenstall, R. B., Ed., W. B. Saunders, Philadelphia, 1980, 35–64.

47. **Highsmith, R. F., Blackburn, K., and Schmidt, D. J.,** Endothelin and calcium dynamics in vascular smooth muscle, *Ann. Rev. Physiol.*, 54, 257–277, 1992.

48. **Hughes, S.,** Radionuclides in orthopaedic surgery, *J. Bone Jt. Surg.*, 62B, 141–150, 1980.

49. **Hungerford, D. S.,** Bone marrow pressure, venography, and core decompression in ischemic necrosis of the femoral head, in *The Hip: Proceedings of the Seventh Open Scientific Meeting of the Hip Society*, Sledge, C. B., Ed., C. V. Mosby, St. Louis, 1979, 218–237.

50. **Ingber, D. and Folkman, J.,** Inhibition of angiogenesis through modulation of collagen metabolism, *Lab. Invest.*, 59, 44–51, 1988.

51. **Ingber, D. and Folkman, J.,** How does extracellular matrix control capillary morphogenesis?, *Cell*, 58, 803–805, 1989.

52. **Johnson, J. T. H. and Crothers, O.,** Revascularization of the femoral head. A clinical and experimental study, *Clin. Orthop. Rel. Res.*, 114, 364–373, 1976.

53. **Jones, J. P. J.,** Fat embolism and osteonecrosis, *Orthop. Clin. N. Am.,* 16, 595–633, 1985.

54. **Kelly, P. J.,** Anatomy, physiology and pathology of the blood supply of bones, *J. Bone Jt. Surg.,* 50A, 766–783, 1968.

55. **Kenzora, J. E.,** The multifactorial etiology of idiopathic osteonecrosis associated with corticosteroid administration, *J. Rheumatol.,* 10, 48–58, 1983.

56. **Kenzora, J. E., Steele, R. E., Yosipovitch, Z. H., and Glimcher, M. J.,** Experimental osteonecrosis of the femoral head in adult rabbits, *Clin. Orthop. Rel. Res.,* 130, 8–46, 1978.

57. **Kenzora, J. E, Steele, R. E., Yosipovitch, Z. Y., and Glimcher, M. J.,** Experimental osteonecrosis of the femoral head in adult rabbits, *Clin. Orthop. Rel. Res.,* 130, 8-46, 1978.

58. **Klagsbrun, M. and D'Amore, P. A.,** Regulators of angiogenesis, *Ann. Rev. Physiol.,* 53, 217–239, 1991.

59. **Kuo, L., Davis, M. J., and Chilian, W. M.,** Endothelial modulation of arteriolar tone, *NIPS,* 7, 5–9, 1992.

60. **Lausten, G. S., Kiær, T., and Dahl, B.,** Laser doppler flowmetry for estimation of bone blood flow: Studies of reproducibility and correlation with microsphere technique, *J. Orthop. Res.,* 11, 573–580, 1993.

61. **Levick, J. R.,** Flow through interstitium and other fibrous matrices, *Q. J. Exp. Physiol.,* 72, 409–438, 1987.

62. **Lopez-Curto, J. A., Bassingthwaighte, J. B., and Kelly, P. J.,** Anatomy of the microvasculature of the tibial diaphysis of the adult dog, *J. Bone Jt. Surg.,* 62A, 1362–1369, 1980.

63. **Malizos, K. N., Quarles, L. D., Seaber, A. V., Rizk, W. S., and Urbaniak, J. R.,** An experimental canine model of osteonecrosis: Characterization of the repair process, *J. Orthop. Res.,* 11, 350–357, 1993.

64. **McCarthy, I. D. and Hughes, S. P. F.,** Is there a blood-bone barrier?, in *Bone Circulation and Bone Necrosis,* Arlet, J. and Maziéres, B., Eds., Springer-Verlag, New York, 1988, 30–33.

65. **McCuskey, R. S., McClugage, S. G., and Younker, W. J.,** Microscopy of living bone marrow *in situ, Blood,* 38, 87–95, 1971.

66. **Mellander, S. and Björnberg, J.,** Regulation of vascular smooth muscle tone and capillary pressure, *NIPS,* 7, 113–119, 1992.

67. **Meyers, M. H.,** Osteonecrosis of the femoral head, *Clin. Orthop. Rel. Res.,* 231, 51–61, 1988.

68. **Montgomery, R. J., Sutker, B. D., Bronk, J. T., Smith, S. R., and Kelly, P. J.,** Interstitial fluid flow in cortical bone, *Microvasc. Res.,* 35, 295–307, 1988.

69. **Moses, M. A., Sudhalter, J., and Langer, R.,** Identification of an inhibitor of neovascularization from cartilage, *Science,* 248, 1408–1410, 1990.

70. **Nelson, G. E., Kelly, P. J., Peterson, F. A., and Janes, J. M.,** Blood supply of the human tibia, *J. Bone Jt. Surg.,* 42A, 625–636, 1960.

71. **Oni, O. O. A., Stafford, H., and Gregg, P. J.,** An investigation of the routes of venous drainage from the bone marrow of the human tibial diaphysis, *Clin. Orthop. Rel. Res.,* 230, 237–244, 1988.

72. **Orlidge, A. and D'Amore, P. A.,** Cell specific effects of glycosaminoglycans on the attachment and proliferation of vascular wall components, *Microvasc. Res.,* 31, 41–53, 1986.

73. **Otter, M. W., Palmieri, V. R., and Cochran, G. V. B.,** Transcortical streaming potentials are gnerated by circulatory pressure gradients in living canine tibia, *J. Orthop. Res.,* 8, 119–126, 1990.

74. **Paradis, G. R. and Kelly, P. J.,** Blood flow and mineral deposition in canine tibial fractures, *J. Bone Jt. Surg.,* 57A, 220–226, 1975.

75. **Paterson, D. C., Lewis, G. N., and Cass, C. A.,** Treatment of delayed union and nonunion with an implanted direct current stimulator, *Clin. Orthop. Rel. Res.,* 148, 117–128, 1980.

76. **Penttinen, R., Niinikoski, J., and Kulonem, E.,** Hyperbaric oxygenation and fracture healing: A biochemical study with rats, *Acta Chir. Scand.,* 138, 39–44, 1972.

77. **Petty, W.,** Osteonecrosis, *J. Bone Jt. Surg.,* 68A, 1311–1312, 1986.

78. **Piekarski, K. and Munro, M.,** Transport mechanism operating between blood supply and osteocytes in long bones, *Nature,* 269, 80–82, 1977.

79. **Reeve, J., Arlot, M., Wooton, R., Edouard, C., Tellez, M., Hesp, R., Green, J. R., and Meunier, P. J.,** Skeletal blood flow, iliac histomorphometry, and strontium kinetics in osteoporosis: A relationship between blood flow and corrected apposition rate, *J. Clin. Endocrin. Metab.,* 66, 1124–1131, 1988.

80. **Reich, K. M., Gay, C. V., and Francos, J. A.,** Fluid shear stress as a mediator of osteoblast cyclic adenosine monophosphate production, *J. Cell. Physiol.,* 143, 100–104, 1990.

81. **Resnick, D. and Niwayama, G.,** *Diagnosis of Bone and Joint Disorders,* 2nd ed., W. B. Saunders, Philadelphia, 1988.
82. **Rhinelander, F. W.,** The normal microcirculation of diaphyseal cortex and its response to fracture, *J. Bone Jt. Surg.,* 50A, 784–800, 1968.
83. **Rhinelander, F.,** The blood supply of the limb bones, in *Scientific Foundations of Orthopaedics and Traumatology,* Owen, R., Goodfellow, J., and Bullough, P., Eds., William Heinemann, London, 1980, 126–151.
84. **Rinsky, L. A., Halpern, A., Schurman, D. B., and Bassett, C. A. L.,** Electrical stimulation of experimentally produced avascular necrosis of the femoral head, *Orthop. Trans.,* 4, 238, 1980.
85. **Robin, E. D.,** Differing opinions on hyperbaric oxygen therapy, *Chest,* 94, 667–674, 1988.
86. **Rösingh, G. E. and James, J.,** Early phases of avascular necrosis of the femoral head in rabbits, *J. Bone Jt. Surg.,* 51B, 165–174, 1969.
87. **Shih, G. C. and Hajjar, K. A.,** Plasminogen and plasminogen activator assembly on the human endothelial cell, *Proc. Soc. Exp. Biol. Med.,* 202, 258–264, 1993.
88. **Sim, F. H. and Kelly, P. J.,** Relationship of bone remodeling, oxygen consumption, and blood flow in bone, *J. Bone Jt. Surg.,* 52A, 1377–1389, 1970.
89. **Simkin, P. A. and Downey, D. J.,** Hypothesis: Retrograde embolization of fat marrow may cause osteonecrosis, *J. Rheumatol.,* 14, 870–872, 1987.
90. **Slack, W. K., Thomas, D. A., and Perrins, D.,** Hyperbaric oxygenation in chronic osteomyelitis, *Lancet,* 1, 1093–1094, 1965.
91. **Smith, J. J. and Kampine, J. P.,** *Circulatory Physiology,* Williams and Wilkins, Baltimore, 1990.
92. **Strauss, M. B.,** Role of hyperbaric oxygen therapy in acute ischemias and crush injuries — An orthopaedic perspective, *Hyperbar. Oxyg. Rev.,* 2, 87–106, 1981.
93. **Strauss, M. B., Hargens, A. R., Gershuni, D. H., Hart, G. B., and Akeson, W. H.,** Delayed used of hyperbaric oxygen for treatment of a model anterior compartment syndrome, *J. Orthop. Res.,* 4, 108–111, 1986.
94. **Strauss, M. B. and Hart, G. B.,** Hyperbaric oxygen and tissue viability, in *Tissue Nutrition and Viability,* Hargens, A. R., Ed., Springer-Verlag, New York, 1986, 285–300.
95. **Strauss, M. B., Winet, H., Bao, J. Y., Greenberg, D. A., Messina, V. A., and Hart, G. B.,** Reparative osteogenesis and neovascularization in a bone chamber: Effect of HBO, *Undersea Hyperbar. Med. Soc. Proc.,* 1989.
96. **Talmage, R. V.,** Calcium homeostasis — Calcium transport — Parathyroid action, *Clin. Orthop. Rel. Res.,* 67, 210–224, 1969.
97. **Todd, R. C., Freeman, A. R., and Pirie, C. J.,** Isolated trabecular fatigue fractures in the femoral head, *J. Bone Jt. Surg.,* 54B, 723–728, 1972.
98. **Tøndevold, E. and Eliasen, P.,** Blood flow rates in canine cortical and cancellous bone measured with ^{99}Tc^m-labelled human albumin microspheres, *Acta Orthop. Scand.,* 53, 7–11, 1982.
99. **Vaes, G. M.,** Cellular biology and biochemical mechanism of bone resorption, *Clin. Orthop. Rel. Res.,* 231, 239–271, 1988.
100. **Viegas, S. F. and Amparo, E.,** Magnetic resonance imaging in the assessment of revascularization in Kienbock's disease, *Orthopaed. Rev.,* 28, 1285–1288, 1989.
101. **Warner, J. J. P., Philip, J. H., Brodsky, G. L., and Thornhill, T. S.,** Studies of nontraumatic osteonecrosis. Manometric and histologic studies of the femoral head after chronic steroid treatment: An experimental study in rabbits, *Clin. Orthop. Rel. Res.,* 225, 128–140, 1987.
102. **Weinbaum, S., Cowin, S. C., and Zeng, Y.,** A model for the exitation of osteocytes by mechanical loading-induced bone fluid shear stresses, *J. Biomech.,* 27, 339–360, 1994.
103. **Whyte, M. P.,** Ischemic bone disease, in *Primer on the Metabolic Diseases and Disorders of Mineral Metabolism,* Favas, M. J., Ed., Raven Press, New York, 1993, 363–367.
104. **Wilkes, C. H. and Visscher, M. B.,** Some physiological aspects of bone marrow pressure, *J. Bone Jt. Surg.,* 57A, 49–57, 1975.
105. **Willans, S. M. and McCarthy, I. D.,** Heterogeneity of blood flow in tibial cortical bone. An experimental investigation using microspheres, *J. Orthop. Res.,* 9, 168–173, 1991.
106. **Williams, E. A., Fitzgerald, R. H. J., and Kelly, P. J.,** Microcirculation of bone, in *The Physiology and Pharmacology of the Microcirculation,* Mortillaro, N. A., Ed., Academic Press, San Francisco, 1984, 267–323.
107. **Winet, H.,** A horizontal intravital microscope bone chamber system for observing microcirculation, *Microvas. Res.,* 37, 105–114, 1989.

108. **Winet, H.,** Local microcirculatory changes in healing bone: A preliminary study in the rabbit tibial bone chamber, *Trans. Orthop. Res. Soc. 39th Mtng.,* 18, 253, 1993.

109. **Winet, H.,** Relationship of volume fraction, vascularity and blood supply in bone, *Proc. Microcir. Soc.,* 41, 1994.

110. **Winet, H. and Bao, J. Y.,** Microvascular leakage in apposing trabeculae of a healing cortical defect: A bone chamber study in the rabbit tibia, *Orthop. Trans.,* 15, 577–578, 1991.

111. **Winet, H., Bao, J. Y., and Moffat, R.,** A control model for tibial cortex neovascularization in the bone chamber, *J. Bone Min. Res.,* 5, 19–30, 1990.

112. **Winet, H., Bao, J. Y., Zmoelek, J., Gellman, H., and Lewonowski, K.,** PEMF effect on microvasculature and bone in healing tibial cortical defects in bone chambers: Preliminary results from the rabbit, *Orthop. Trans.,* 16, 544, 1993.

113. **Winet, H., Dossick, P., Bao, J. Y., Stetson, W., Anderson, S., Moore, T. M., and Menendex, L.,** Neovascularization of 2 mm allograft discs: A preliminary intravital microscope bone chamber study in the rabbit, in *Bone Circulation and Bone Necrosis,* Arlet, J. and Maziéres, B., Eds., Springer-Verlag, New York, 1988, 369–373.

114. **Woodhouse, C. F.,** Dynamic influences of vascular occlusion affecting the development of avascular necrosis of the femoral head, *Clin. Orthop. Rel. Res.,* 32, 119–129, 1964.

115. **Yen-Patton, A., Patton, W. F., Beer, D. M., and Jacobson, B. S.,** Endothelial cell response to pulsed electromagnetic fields: Stimulation of growth rate and angiogenesis *in vitro, J. Cell. Physiol.,* 134, 37–46, 1988.

116. **Zawicki, D. F., Jain, R. K., Schmid-Schoenbein, G. W., and Chien, S.,** Dynamics of neovascularization in normal tissue, *Microvasc. Res.,* 21, 27–47, 1981.

Chapter 13

Brain Microcirculation

William I. Rosenblum

CONTENTS

I. ANATOMY AND FUNCTION

A. VASCULAR ANATOMY OF THE BRAIN

The brains of most mammals, including man, have a similar vascular anatomy. The vertebral and internal carotid arteries supply the brain. Major anastomoses between these arteries are located at the Circle of Willis.[1] In some mammals, for example cats and goats, the carotid arteries supply a rete mirabile, which in turn supplies the brain.[2]

From the Circle of Willis, major arteries arise that supply the brain via branches on the surface of the brain.[1] These lie in the subarachnoid space and are covered by a membrane known as the pia-arachnoid. The arteries and arterioles in the subarachnoid space are commonly called "pial vessels". At the base of the brain, some arterial branches penetrate the brain rather directly, instead of arising as branches of vessels that have run for a significant distance in the subarachnoid space.

The arteries that branch from the pial arteries to penetrate the brain are generally less than 100 μm, even in very large mammals, including man.[3] Thus, virtually the entire parenchymal arterial system, plus much of the parenchymal venous system, and smaller pial vessels are all part of the microcirculation. The venules drain into pial veins, which drain into venous sinuses. The latter drain into the jugular veins.

Anastomoses between pial arteries or between pial veins are common.[1] However, anastomoses between parenchymal arterioles and venules are rare except at the precapillary level.[4] Precapillary anastomoses between penetrating arterioles are common, and the capillary network itself is rich and tortuous. There are numerous possibilities for shunting of oxygen between adjacent vessels, which precludes modeling based on a simple Krogh model that assumes a cylindrical vessel with a high and low O_2 end.

The pial vessels, both arteries and veins, are richly innervated by nerve nets in the adventitia. The axons lack synaptic contacts but releases transmitters from varicosities.[5] Adrenergic, cholinergic,[5] and peptidergic axons[6] are present, some containing more than one transmitter. The parenchymal arterioles are variably innervated, and frequently innervation ends at this point. Whether or not capillaries are innervated is still a matter of controversy.

The endothelium of cerebral vessels has several special adaptations that restrict or regulate permeability. These restrictions may be collectively called the "blood brain barrier".[7,8]

Myoendothelial junctions[9] are found in brain vessels of many species, including man. Their frequency in human brain increases in the microcirculation as compared with larger surface arterioles or small arteries.

B. FUNCTION OF BRAIN MICROCIRCULATION
1. Delivery Functions
The cerebral microcirculation distributes blood to its target organ. Aortic pressure is reduced in the carotid and vertebral circuits and again in the pial segment. The latter probably contributes 25% of the total cerebrovascular resistance.[10,11] This contribution can be increased or reduced depending upon the tone of the proximal or distal vessels and/ or pathologic reductions in the lumens of the proximal larger arteries. The parenchymal arterioles may also contribute 25% to total cerebrovascular resistance. Capillaries and venules may contribute another 25%. Pressure is more or less equalized over the cerebral surface by the anastomosing pial arteries and arterioles.

The adrenergic innervation of cerebral arteries and arterioles may act as a constricting pathway.[5,11] Its significance in man is unknown. In normal animals, cerebral vessels are generally less sensitive than other vessels to exogenous catechols, and to sympathetic (or cholinergic) nerve stimulation. However, in animals, the adrenergic stimulation has been shown to have greater importance during pathologic states, for example, limiting vascular distension in hypertension.[11]

Peptidergic innervation in animals has only recently been shown to serve as a dilating influence during a variety of pathologic states, acting apparently as part of an axon reflex.[12,13]

In normal conditions, the arterial and arteriolar tone of the cerebral circulation is controlled by three major mechanisms, not directly dependent upon neurogenic influences. These three are: pH at the vessel wall, which is greatly dependent upon CO_2; intraluminal pressure, which influences vascular tone by a myogenic mechanism; and metabolic factors that are in part dependent upon flow and hence on pressure, but which are largely determined by the metabolic activity of the brain itself. Diverse mediators play a role in this feedback between brain and vessels, which couples cerebral blood flow to metabolic demand.

2. Exchange Functions
The cerebral microcirculation acts as a barrier[7,8] to the entry of numerous substances that would otherwise enter the brain. Diverse mechanisms perform this function and, in major ways, the nature or importance of some mechanisms remain unsettled.

The barrier to protein is the classical "blood-brain barrier". This may reside in very tight junctions between endothelial cells. However, opening of these junctions may not be the way or the only way in which protein enters the brain in pathologic conditions. Normally, the endothelium of brain microvessels has only a scant number of vesicles.

However, in pathologic states, the number of vesicles may greatly increase and some evidence has been presented that vesicular transport is important.

Microvascular endothelium controls glucose and amino acid transport with a variety of specific transport systems that employ carrier molecules. Microvascular endothelium also contains a variety of enzymatic systems that metabolize small molecule substrates and prevent passage of the substrate through the vessel wall. The pial vessels do not share some of these enzyme mechanisms with the parenchymal vessels.

Contact with astrocytes and/or the presence of astrocytic processes very close to the vessels can induce a variety of enzymes regulating transport in one of the ways just mentioned.[14,16] However, the older idea that astrocytic foot processes are a physical barrier to transvascular transport is probably untenable.

II. PATHOLOGY

A. CEREBRAL EDEMA[17,18]

This complex condition is the lethal common denominator in virtually all destructive lesions of the brain. These lesions or conditions include cerebral infarction (due to obstruction of vessels), hypoxic encephalopathy, cerebral hemorrhage, trauma, and brain tumors. In all these conditions, the original lesion rarely destroys enough brain to cause death, and frequently would not, by itself, produce severe dysfunction. However, edema fluid, spreading from vessels within the lesion, diffuses widely and mostly within the extracellular space of the white matter, and greatly increases intracranial mass and hence intracranial pressure. The result is displacement of various brain structures, of which downward displacement of the brain stem is the most serious. This brain stem "herniation" may cause a secondary, lethal hemorrhage within the brain stem. In addition, severe elevation of intracranial pressure reduces cerebral perfusion pressure and can result in cessation of cerebral blood flow or reduction to a level incompatible with normal function and with cellular viability. Thus, the whole cerebrum may die as a result of cerebral edema. Finally, even if edema does not produce lethal or damaging increases of intracranial pressure, its presence may compromise nutrition of myelin, leaving areas of rarefaction in the deep white matter.[19,20] Since edema is a parenchymal phenomenon and since most parenchymal vessels are, in fact, microvessels, edema is a microvascular phenomenon.

Cerebral edema has been divided into at least three types: transependymal, cytotoxic, and vasogenic. Vasogenic edema results from a breakdown in transvascular barrier mechanisms. It is clinically the most important type of edema, accounting for the severe disturbances mentioned at the beginning of this section.

Vasogenic edema involves a breakdown of microvascular barriers to protein and possibly to water. The detection of abnormal amounts of protein in the brain has frequently been used to demarcate the onset of vasogenic edema; however, increases in water may precede the detection of protein entry, leading to the search for "idiogenic" osmols. The issue is confused by experimental findings indicating that the barrier to protein may open transiently at a much earlier time than previously thought, and that the delayed opening or "ripening" of vasogenic edema represents a second, now long-lasting disruption of the barrier to protein. In hypertension, there may be white matter edema.[21] However, experimental studies suggest that fluid enters the white matter from adjacent cortex, and that it is cortical arterioles rather than white matter arterioles or capillaries that leak.[22]

Hyperosmotic agents used to treat edema may act to pull edema fluid out of edematous brain via vessels with an intact barrier. These vessels could maintain the osmotic gradient essential for such action. However, evidence has also been presented for a different mode of action of hyperosmotic agents. These agents pull water from throughout the body into the blood, thereby causing hemodilution and decreased blood viscosity. Decreased viscosity is associated with vasoconstriction, as observed in studies of pial vessels, *in vivo*.[23]

The constriction reduces the volume of the vascular compartment within the closed skull and this will, in turn, reduce intracranial pressure.

Steroids are also used to treat edema. They may be more effective in edema produced by tumors than by ischemic lesions. In either case, the edema is vasogenic. The mechanism by which steroids work is not known, but may involve suppression of synthesis of one or more agents liberated by injured brain and then damage brain vessels.

B. HYPERTENSION

Brain arterioles are more susceptible than vessels elsewhere to the change that accompanies hypertension and is best described as fibrinoid arteritis.[24] The media undergoes degeneration accompanied by the passage of plasma proteins, like fibrin, into the vessel wall. The media then stains like fibrin. Fibrinoid necrosis may be the cause of vessel rupture, leading to cerebral hemorrhage in hypertension. Vessels throughout the body undergo fibrinoid necrosis during malignant or accelerated hypertension. However, brain arterioles undergo fibrinoid necrosis and lethal hemorrhage during otherwise benign hypertension. Prevention of this complication may be the most important reason for treating mild to moderate elevations of blood pressure. The reason for the selective vulnerability of brain arterioles to fibrinoid necrosis is not known.

C. AMYLOID[25]

Brain microvessels, including capillaries and arterioles, develop a type of amyloid known as beta amyloid, whose gene resides on chromosome 21. The reason for selective expression of this gene in brain vessels and in brain parenchyma is not known. The deposition of amyloid increases with age. Its presence in brain parenchyma is associated with and may be a causative factor in the development of Alzheimer's disease (senile dementia of the Alzheimer type). The presence of this amyloid in the vessels of the elderly (without dementia) appears to be the most important cause of cerebral hemorrhage in this age group.

D. VASCULAR "WICKWORKS"[26,27]

As we grow older, brain capillaries undergo a peculiar proliferation, with the proliferating branches wrapping around each other in the manner of strands in a candle wick. Such wicks must have a significant effect on cerebrovascular resistance, increasing resistance in proportion to the number and complexity of the wicks.

E. HYPERVISCOSITY

Studies of pial arterioles, *in vivo*, in mice have demonstrated that hyperviscous syndromes cannot be lumped into a single entity.[28] Diseases like polycythemia and macroglobulinemia certainly do affect the cerebral microcirculation of humans. However, macroglobulinemia is often accompanied by anemia. Reductions in hematocrit profoundly reduced blood viscosity and may nullify the effects of the elevated plasma viscosity that is caused by increased macroglobulin concentrations. The macroglobulin also increases blood viscosity by causing clumping of red blood cells (rouleaux), perhaps, in part, because the clumping of red cells increases the amount of plasma near the vessel wall. The overall effect of macroglobulinemia seems to be an increased plasma skimming so that plasma transit is slowed while red cell velocity is not impeded. Indeed, the anemia that accompanies the macroglobulinemia causes a significant increase in red cell velocity, perhaps aided by the central streaming of the rouleaux. This differential effect of hyperviscosity on plasma and red cell flow is not seen in polycythemia, where the increased viscosity is caused by an increased hematocrit rather than an increase in plasma viscosity. In polycythemia, only a slowing of plasma is observed. When increased whole blood viscosity is caused by an increase in the rigidity of erythrocytes, as in spherocytosis, the red cell velocity should be reduced; but again, the effect of accompanying anemia may nullify the adverse effects of the increased rigidity. Moreover, in the presence of the anemia accompanying spherocytosis, plasma velocity increases just as it does in simple anemia. The effect of the three important variables, hematocrit, red cell aggregation, and plasma viscosity, may also be observed by measuring red cell velocity[28] at the vessel wall and the vessel center. This gives a good impression of the velocity profile and demonstrates a relative blunting of the profile in hyperviscosity states as compared with anemia.

F. HUMAN BRAIN MICROCIRCULATION

Since the cerebral microcirculation of the brain can only directly be observed on the surface of that organ or in its most superficial millimeter (by confocal microscopy), and since a craniotomy is usually required, it is not feasible to directly study brain microcirculation in humans.

However, studies of cerebral blood flow, even in very small volumes of brain, are now possible. These are certainly studies of microcirculation. However, as an aid to our understanding of microvascular control mechanisms in brain, flow studies must be interpreted with great caution. Flow studies are still studies of a "black box" in which the behavior of individual elements remains unknown. Thus, at present, studies of surface microcirculation and *in vitro* studies of isolated vessels represent our best effort at understanding cerebral microcirculation.

The *in vitro* studies can be performed using human tissue. However, the presence of disease and the effects of aging may present serious barriers to our understanding of normal function. This is particularly obvious now that endothelium-dependent relaxation and constriction have been demonstrated in the cerebral microcirculation.[29-31] Atherosclerosis, hypertension, and diabetes can seriously disturb endothelium-dependent responses[32,33] and are common afflictions of humans, especially as they age. Hypertension, diabetes, and amyloid deposition may also directly alter the vessel wall. Therefore, sampling human vessels for *in vitro* studies may provide abnormal rather than normal data.

III. MODELS, TECHNIQUES, AND EQUIPMENT

A. MODELS

Animal models of atherosclerosis,[34] hypertension,[35,36] diabetes,[37,38] anemia,[28] malaria,[39] polycythemia,[28] macroglobulinemia,[28] and spherocytosis[28] all exist and can provide fruitful models for studying the effects of these respective disease states on the cerebral vessels, including the microcirculation.

B. TECHNIQUES

1. *In Vitro*

The *in vitro* study of cerebral microvessels requires that they be removed from the brain, cannulated,[40] and perfused or at least maintained at some preselected pressure where they develop spontaneous tone. Learning to isolate and cannulate microvessels, especially those under 50 μm in diameter, is a very time-consuming task with a learning curve of months.

2. *In Vivo*

The *in vivo* study of cerebral microcirculation generally requires performance of a craniotomy to enable one to view the cerebral surface. However, very young small mammals such as mice and gerbils have a very transparent, thin calvarium through which the pial vessels may be seen with *in vivo* microscopy.[41] Thus far, however, there have been virtually no studies[41,42] attempting to monitor changes in diameter through the intact skull. When, as is usually the case, a craniotomy is performed, the surface (pial) vasculature is exposed by stripping the dura.[41,43] The pial vessels lie beneath the dura in the subarachnoid space lying between the transparent arachnoid and the surface of the brain. The pial vessels are loosely tethered within the subarachnoid space by wisps of connective tissue bridging the space.

The craniotomy site may be bathed by a continuously flowing suffusate, or a chamber may be fixed to the skull around the craniotomy site.[44,45] The chamber may be continuously suffused. The chamber may be closed or open. However, because the tone of cerebral arteries and arterioles is very sensitive to change in local pH[11] and because the pH of stagnant bicarbonate buffered suffusates rapidly rises due to loss of CO_2 to the air, it is not advisable to use open, stagnant preparations unless pial arteriolar diameter is unimportant to the study. Closed chambers may be stagnant, provided they are impervious to CO_2 loss. A flowing suffusate may be used with an open preparation, provided the pH of the solution is adjusted along with the speed of suffusion to maintain a physiologic and constant pH over the craniotomy site. This is easy to do with small craniotomies such as those in mice, rats, and gerbils. I have found that flow rates of 1 to 2 ml/min are sufficient.

The suffusate is a mock cerebrospinal fluid.[35,46] Elliotts solution or a modification thereof is frequently used. Drugs may be topically applied via the suffusate. The pH of the mixture of drug and suffusate must be the same as that of the suffusate alone.

Some researchers prefer to apply drugs via micropipettes with which they puncture the arachnoid adjacent to the vessel.[47,48] The micropipette technique delivers drug to a single vessel rather than to many. The proponents of this technique frequently state that the application of minute amounts of drug in this manner avoids pitfalls inherent in suffusing the entire craniotomy site. However, I am unaware of major differences between results of the two methods. Where different results have been reported with one of the techniques as opposed to the other, subsequent studies have shown that the differences could not be ascribed to the use of suffusion instead of microapplication. If microapplication is used, care must be taken to distinguish the primary response directly under the pipette from possible propagated responses upstream and downstream.

C. EQUIPMENT

1. *In Vitro*

Measurements of *in vitro* dimensions of cerebral microvessels can be performed with a variety of devices.[52] These obviously involve using a microscope. This may be coupled to a TV camera and monitor. The diameter of the vessel on the monitor may be continuously or intermittently monitored with a video caliper, an image shearing device, or a variety of mechanoelectronic or electronic interfaces.

2. *In Vivo*

Similarly, the *in vivo* image of the pial surface is transmitted to a TV monitor for measurement by an image splitter, image shearing device, or video caliper. It should be noted that the original image splitter[53] used by Baez is no longer manufactured. A currently manufactured alternative is the image shearing monitor (Instrumentation Physiology and Medicine, La Mesa, CA).

Red blood cell velocity can be measured in pial microvessels using a two-slit velocimeter (IPM, La Mesa, CA) or similar instruments.[54,55] This gives on-line results. A different technique, ultra-high-speed cinematography, provides data only after the developing of motion picture film.[56,57] Transit time of a plasma label can be monitored by lower speed cine techniques[57] or by a variety of TV techniques.

Pial microvessels can be punctured by a micropipette and intraluminal pressure measured by the servo-null technique.[35,58]

Since the brain cannot be transilluminated, epillumination must be used. Care must be taken to avoid the heating effects of any light source. Heat filters usually are required because so called "cold" light guides transmit infrared light, even though they feel cool to the touch. The red wavelengths, if absorbed by the target, will heat the target.

Recent advances in confocal microscopy may conceivably result in marked improvements of our ability to monitor parenchymal vessels. Some conventional microscopes permit observations at depths 50 to 100 μm beneath the brain surface. However, image definition is poor. Confocal microscopy could, in theory, permit observation at much greater depths. In a small mammal like the mouse, this could be full cortical thickness. However, our trials of confocal microscopes thus far have not been fruitful, owing to the great loss of light inherent in confocal microscopy. This may be remedied by image-enhanced 3-dimensional reconstruction, but the usual timeframe for such computer-assisted observation is too long for practical on-line observations. The use of confocal microscopy with a fluorescent label for either red cells or plasma[59] may overcome the problem of limited light because a fluorescent image is so much brighter than a standard image. However, we are reluctant to employ fluorescent dyes because they can damage endothelium when excited by light.[29] We have shown that the effects of endothelial damage in both a fluorescent and a nonfluorescent "light/dye" model of endothelial injury may be restricted to functional rather than morphologically evident derangements.[29,30,60] Consequently, a healthy-looking preparation would not assure a functionally normal preparation. If we begin our investigations by assuming we know nothing of the functional characteristics of parenchymal vessels (e.g., their response to putative vasoactive agents), then we cannot compare their responses with those of pial vessels and conclude from the similarity that the parenchymal vessels are normal. The normal response might, in fact, differ from that of pial vessels. Conversely, if parenchymal vessels behave differently than pial vessels, we cannot conclude that the former have been damaged. The normal response may indeed be different from that of pial vessels. If, in the presence of a fluorescent marker, we cannot use the appearance of the vessels to assure ourselves that they are undamaged, then we have no way of assessing the influence of the fluorescent technique on the responses in question. Rather than pursue fluorescent confocal microscopy, we await further developments in confocal microscopy without fluorescence.

Microvascular flow within the upper layers of the brain, or through the full thickness of cortex in a small mammal, can be monitored using a laser Doppler flowmeter.[61,62] Laser Doppler flowmeters provide measurements that are highly correlated with flow measurements made by other techniques. However, they do not provide absolute flow values. Consequently, results of laser Doppler studies are best reported in terms of percent change in flow (e.g., flow increased 10%, or flow decreased 20%). Because of variability in values obtained by repeated measurements of the same tissue volume, it is difficult to use the technique to detect flow changes of less than 10%.[63]

REFERENCES

1. **Vander Eecken, H. M.,** *Anastomoses Between the Leptomeningeal Arteries of the Brain,* Charles C. Thomas, Springfield, 1959.
2. **Lluch, S., Dieguez, F., Garcia, A. L., and Gomez, B.,** Rete mirabile of goat: Its flow-damping effect on cerebral circulation, *Am. J. Physiol.,* 249, R482, 1985.
3. **Alexander, L. and Putnam, T. J.,** Pathological alterations of cerebral vascular patterns, in *The Circulation of the Brain and Spinal Cord,* Proc. Assoc. Res. Nervous Mental Dis., Vol. 18, Williams and Wilkens, Baltimore, 1938, 471.
4. **Ravens, J. R.,** Anastomoses in the vascular bed of the human cerebrum, in *The Cerebral Vessel Wall,* Cervos-Navarro, J., Betz, E., Matakos, F., and Wullenweber, R., Eds., Raven Press, New York, 1976, 175.

5. **Edvinsson, L. and MacKenzie, E. T.,** Amine mechanisms in the cerebral circulation, *Pharmacological. Rev.*, 28, 275, 1977.

6. **Owman, C. and Hardebo, J. E., Eds.,** *Neural Regulation of Brain Circulation*, Elsevier Science, Amsterdam, 1986, 302–418.

7. **Nagy, Z.,** Blood-brain barrier and the cerebral endothelium, in *Pathophysiology of the Blood Brain Barrier*, Johansson, B. B., Owman, Ch., and Widner, J., Eds., Elsevier Science, Amsterdam, 1990, 11.

8. **Rapoport, S. I.,** *Blood Brain Barrier in Physiology and Medicine*, Raven Press, New York, 1976.

9. **Aydin, F., Rosenblum, W. I., and Povlishock, J. T.,** Myoendothelial junctions in human brain arterioles, *Stroke*, 22, 1592, 1991.

10. **Rosenblum, W. I.,** Vascular resistance in the cerebral circulation: Location and potential consequences with respect to the effect of neurogenic stimuli on flow, in *Neurogenic Control of Brain Circulation*, Owman, Ch. and Edvinsson, L., Eds., Pergamon Press, New York, 1972, 221.

11. **Heistad, D. D. and Kontos, H. A.,** Cerebral circulation, in *Handbook of Physiology, Sect 2. The Cardiovascular System*, Vol. III. Peripheral Circulation and Organ Blood Flow, Part I, Shepherd, J. T. and Abboud, F. M., Eds., Am. Physiol. Soc., Bethesda, MD, 1983, 137.

12. **Moskowitz, M. A., Macfarlane, R., Tasdemiroglu, E., Wei, E. P., and Kontos, H. A.,** Neurogenic control of the cerebral circulation during global ischemia, *Stroke*, 21 (Suppl. III), 168, 1990.

13. **Macfarlane, R., Tasdemiroglu, E., Moskowitz, M. A., Uemura, Y., Wei, E. P., and Kontos, H. A.,** Chronic trigeminal ganglionectomy or topical capsaicin application to pial vessels attenuates postocclusive cortical hyperemia but does not influence postischemic hypoperfusion, *J. Cereb. Blood Flow Metab.*, 11, 261, 1991.

14. **Beck, D. W., Vintners, H. V., Hart, M. N., and Cancilla, P. A.,** Glial cells influence polarity of the blood brain barrier, *J. Neuropath. Exp. Neurol.*, 43, 219, 1984.

15. **Maxwell, K., Berliner, J. A., and Cancilla, P. A.,** Stimulation of glucose analogue uptake by cerebral microvessel endothelial cells by a product released by astrocytes, *J. Neuropath. Exp. Neurol.*, 48, 69, 1989.

16. **Cancilla, P. A., Berliner, J. A., and Bready, J. V.,** Astrocytes and the blood brain barrier: Kinetics of astrocyte activation after injury and inductive effects in endothelium, in *Pathophysiology of the Blood Brain Barrier*, Johansson, B. B., Owman, Ch., and Widner, J., Eds., Elsevier, Amsterdam, 1990, 31.

17. **Klatzo, I.,** Neuropathological aspects of brain edema, *J. Neuropath. Exp. Neurol.*, 26, 1, 1987.

18. **Garcia, J. H. and Lossinsky, A. S.,** in *Cerebrovascular Diseases*, Price, T. R. and Nelson, E., Eds., Raven Press, New York, 1979, 125.

19. **Feigin, I. and Popoff, N.,** Neuropathological changes late in cerebral edema: The relationship to trauma, hypertensive disease and Binswanger's encephalopathy, *J. Neuropath. Exp. Neurol.*, 22, 500, 1963.

20. **Feigin, I. and Budzilovich, G. N.,** The role of edema in diffuse sclerosis and other leukoencephalopathies, *J. Neuropath. Exp. Neurol.*, 37, 326, 1978.

21. **Adachi, M., Rosenblum, W. I., and Feigin, I.,** Hypertensive disease and cerebral edema, *J. Neurol. Neurosurg. Psychiat.*, 29, 69, 1966.

22. **Nag, S.,** Cerebral changes in chronic hypertension: Combined permeability and immunohistochemical studies, *Acta Neuropathol.*, 62, 178, 1984.

23. **Muizelaar, J. P., Wei, E. P., Kontos, H. A., and Becker, D. P.,** Mannitol causes compensatory cerebral vasoconstriction and vasodilation in response to blood viscosity changes, *J. Neurosurg.*, 59, 822, 1983.

24. **Rosenblum, W. I.,** Miliary aneurysms and fibrinoid degeneration of cerebral blood vessels, *Hum. Pathol.*, 8, 133, 1977.

25. **Yamaguichi, H., Yamazaki, T., Lemere, C. A., Frosch, M. P., and Selkoe, D. J.,** Beta amyloid is focally deposited within the outer basement membrane in the amyloid angiopathy of Alzheimer's disease, *Am. J. Pathol.*, 141, 249, 1992.

26. **Hassler, O.,** Vascular changes in senile brains, *Acta Neuropathol. (Berl.)*, 5, 40, 1965.

27. **Saunders, R. L. de Ch. and Bell, M. A.,** X-ray microscopy and histochemistry of the human cerebral blood vessels, *J. Neurosurg.*, 35, 128, 1971.

28. **Rosenblum, W. I.,** Complex microvascular effects involving plasma and red cell movement in brain following alterations of viscosity, in *Cerebral Ischemia and Hemorheology*, Hartman, A. and Kuschinsky, W., Eds., Springer, Berlin, 1987, 96.

29. **Rosenblum, W. I.,** Endothelial-dependent relaxation demonstrated *in vivo* in cerebral arterioles, *Stroke,* 17, 494, 1986.

30. **Rosenblum, W. I., Nelson, G. H., and Povlishock, J. T.,** Laser induced endothelial damage inhibits endothelium dependent relaxation in the cerebral microcirculation of the mouse, *Circ. Res.,* 60, 169, 1987.

31. **Rosenblum, W. I. and Nelson, G. H.,** Endothelium dependent constriction demonstrated *in vivo* in mouse cerebral arterioles, *Circ. Res.,* 62, 937, 1988.

32. **Forstermann, U., Mugge, A., Alheid, U., Haverick, A., and Frobich, J. C.,** Selective attenuation of endothelium mediated dilation in atherosclerotic human coronary arteries, *Circ. Res.,* 62, 185, 1988.

33. **Faraci, F. M. and Heistad, D. D.,** Regulation of cerebral blood vessels by humoral and endothelium dependent mechanisms, *Hypertension,* 17, 917, 1991.

34. **White, R. A., Ed.,** *Atherosclerosis and Arteriosclerosis: Human Pathology and Experimental Animal Methods and Models,* CRC Press, Boca Raton, FL, 1989.

35. **Baumbach, G. L., Dobrin, P. B., Hart, M. N., and Heistad, D. D.,** Mechanics of cerebral arterioles in hypertensive rats, *Circ. Res.,* 62, 56, 1988.

36. **Meininger, G. A., Harris, P. D., and Joshua, I. G.,** Distribution of microvascular pressure in skeletal muscle of one-kidney one clip, two-kidney one clip and deoxycorticosterone-salt hypertensive rats, *Hypertension,* 6, 27, 1984.

37. **Rosenblum, W. I., El-Sabban, F., and Loria, R. M.,** Platelet aggregation in the cerebral and mesenteric microcirculation of mice with genetically determined diabetes, *Diabetes,* 30, 89, 1981.

38. **Rosenblum, W. I. and Levasseur, J. E.,** Microvascular response of intermediate-size arterioles on the cerebral surface of diabetic mice, *Microvasc. Res.,* 28, 368, 1984.

39. **Aikawa, M., Brown, A., Smith, C. D., Tegoshi, T., Howard, R. J., Hasler, T. H., Ito, Y., Perry, B., Collins, W. E., and Webster, K.,** A primate model for human cerebral malaria: Plasmodium Coatneyi-infected rhesus monkeys, *Am. J. Trop. Med. Hyg.,* 46, 391, 1992.

40. **Dacey, R. G., Jr. and Duling, B. R.,** A study of rat intracerebral arterioles; methods, morphology and reactivity, *Am. J. Physiol.,* 243, H598, 1982.

41. **Rosenblum, W. I. and Zweifach, B. W.,** Cerebral microcirculation in the mouse brain, *Arch. Neurol.,* 9, 414, 1963.

42. **Rosenblum, W. I., Donnenfeld, H., and Aleu, F.,** Effects of increased blood pressure on cerebral vessels in mice, *Arch. Neurol.,* 14, 632, 1966.

43. **Allen, A. D. and Rosenblum, W. I.,** Effects of two methods of craniotomy on microvascular responses in the mouse brain, *Microvasc. Res.,* 27, 385, 1984.

44. **Levasseur, J. E., Wei, E. P., Raper, A. J., Kontos, H. A., and Patterson, J. L., Jr.,** Detailed description of a cranial window technique for acute and chronic experiments, *Stroke,* 6, 308, 1975.

45. **Lefer, D. J., Lynch, C. D., Lapinski, K. C., and Hutchins, P. M.,** Enhanced vasomotion of cerebral arterioles in spontaneously hypertensive rats, *Microvasc. Res.,* 39, 129, 1990.

46. **Elliott, K. A. C. and Jasper, H. H.,** Physiological salt solutions for brain surgery, *J. Neurosurg.,* 6, 140, 1949.

47. **Kuschinsky, W., Wahl, M., and Neiss, A.,** Evidence for cholinergic dilatory receptors in pial arteries of cats, *Pflug. Arch.,* 347, 199, 1974.

48. **Betz, E., Enzenross, H. G., and Vlahov, V.,** Interaction of H^+ and Ca^{++} in the regulation of local pial vascular resistance, *Pflug. Arch.,* 343, 79, 1973.

49. **Segal, S. S. and Duling, B. R.,** Conduction of vasomotor responses in arterioles: A role for cell to cell coupling?, *Am. J. Physiol.,* 256, H838, 1989.

50. **Segal, S. S. and Duling, B. R.,** Flow control among vessels coordinated by intercellular conduction, *Science,* 234, 868, 1986.

51. **Rosenblum, W. I., Weinbrecht, P., and Nelson, G. H.,** Propagated constriction in mouse pial arterioles: Possible role of endothelium in transmitting the propagated response, *Microcirc. Endoth. Lymph.,* 6, 369, 1990.

52. **Osol, G., Laher, I., and Cipolla, M.,** Protein kiknase C modulates basal myogenic tone in resistance arteries from the cerebral circulation, *Circ. Res.,* 68, 359, 1991.

53. **Baez, S.,** Recording of microvascular dimension with an image splitter television microscope, *J. Appl. Physiol.,* 21, 299, 1966.

54. **Rosenblum, W. I.,** Measurement of red cell velocity with a two-slit technique and cross correlation. Use of reflected light and either regulated DC or unregulated AC power supplies, *Microvasc. Res.*, 22, 225, 1981.

55. **Rosenblum, W. I. and El Sabban, F.,** Influence of shear rate on platelet aggregation in cerebral microvessels, *Microvasc. Res.*, 23, 311, 1982.

56. **Rosenblum, W. I.,** Erythrocyte velocity and a velocity pulse in minute blood vessels on the surface of the brain, *Circ. Res.*, 24, 887, 1969.

57. **Rosenblum, W. I.,** Effects of reduced hematocrit on erythrocyte velocity and fluorescein transit time in the cerebral microcirculation of the mouse, *Circ. Res.*, 24, 96, 1971.

58. **Shapiro, H. M., Stromberg, D. D., Lee, D. R., and Wiederhielm, C. A.,** Dynamic pressures in the pial arterial microcirculation, *Am. J. Physiol.*, 221, 279, 1971.

59. **Dirnagl, U., Villringer, A., Gebhardt, R., Haberl, R. L., Schmiedek, P., and Einhaupl, K. M.,** Three dimensional reconstruction of the rat brain cortical microcirculation *in vivo, J. Cereb. Blood Flow Metab.*, 11, 353, 1991.

60. **Rosenblum, W. I.,** Aspects of endothelial malfunction and function in cerebral microvessels, *Lab. Invest.*, 56, 252, 1986.

61. **Skarphedinsson, J. O., Harding, H., and Thoren, P.,** Repeated measurements of cerebral blood flow in rats. Comparisons between hydrogen clearance method and laser Doppler flowmetry, *Acta Physiol. Scand.*, 134, 133, 1988.

62. **Dirnagl, U., Kaplan, B., Jacewicz, M., and Pulsinelli, W.,** Continuous measurement of cerebral cortical blood flow by laser-Doppler flowmetry in a rat stroke model, *J. Cereb. Blood Flow Met.*, 9, 589, 1989.

63. **Line, P. D., Mowinckel, P., Lien, B., and Kvernebo, K.,** Repeated measurement variation and precision of laser Doppler flowmetry measurements, *Microvasc. Res.*, 43, 285, 1992.

Chapter 14

Eye Microcirculation

Peter Koch Jensen and Toke Bek

CONTENTS

INTRODUCTION

The eye is a unique organ from a microcirculatory standpoint because it contains several circulatory beds that can be viewed noninvasively. The conjunctiva is exposed to the external environment, and its microcirculation can therefore be observed by direct biomicroscopy. The retinal vascular system on the inner aspect of the eyeball can be observed through the optics of the eye, and one is only limited by the eye's imaging properties. With inclusion of angiographic techniques, aspects of the deeper-lying choroidal vascular system can also be studied. The ease with which one can study ocular vessels, as well as their frequent involvement in systemic disease, makes the eye an attractive organ to be used as a model for microcirculation research.

0-8493-4870-6/95/$0.00+$.50

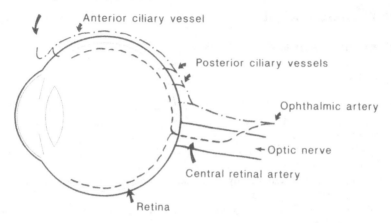

Figure 1 A schematical representation of the dual blood supply to the ocular fundus. The central retinal artery (----) supplies the inner parts of the retina, whereas the ciliary vascular system (- - -) supplies the outer parts of the retina, the choroid, and the anterior part of the eye.

I. ANATOMY AND FUNCTION

The eye receives its blood supply from the ophthalmic artery, which enters the orbita through the optic canal. Inside the orbita, anterior ciliary arteries branch off and follow the extraocular muscles to their insertion anteriorly in the sclera. Here, the main vessel penetrates the sclera to supply the anterior segment of the eye, including the ciliary body and the iris, while smaller branches leave to supply the perilimbal conjunctiva. The posterior ciliary arteries branch from the ophthalmic artery in a variable number just behind the eyeball, with two long vessels branching to the equatorial choroid, and about ten shorter vessels branching to the posterior choroid. After penetration of the sclera, the choroidal vessels branch and end in lobules with large fenestrated capillaries that are in close proximity to the retinal pigment epithelium.[1] Structural evidence suggests that choroidal lobules in the periphery are supplied by a central arteriole and are drained by venoles arranged peripherally at the lobule, whereas the reverse arrangement exists in the posterior pole.[2] The choroid has the largest blood perfusion in the body per unit tissue weight, and the resulting small oxygen extraction (5%) ensures a high ambient oxygen concentration in the outer retina supplied by this system.[3] The choroidal circulation is regulated autonomously with sympathetic innervation from the superior cervical ganglion and parasympathetic innervation from the ciliary and the pterygopalatine ganglions.[4]

The blood supply to the inner layers of the retina differs among species; but in most mammals including humans, the supply is holangiotic with a termination of the ophthalmic artery in the central retinal artery that enters the eye with the optic nerve.[5] The only anastomotic connections between the choroidal and retinal circulations exist at the optic nerve head, forming the circular plexus of Zinn. The central retinal artery branches into four larger arcade vessels, each with a diameter of about 150 μ. Two temporal arcades course around the macular area and give off branches to supply this, while two nasal arcades take a more direct course toward the periphery. The midperiphery is supplied by long radiating vessels that originate from the larger arcades. In the far periphery, adjacent radiating vessels anastomose close to the ora serrata. A central zone of about 400 μ in the foveal region is free from blood vessels. In the posterior pole, the vessels branch dichotomously, whereas the retinal midperiphery is supplied by metarterioles leaving at right angles from the long radiating vessels. The general arrangement of capillaries is

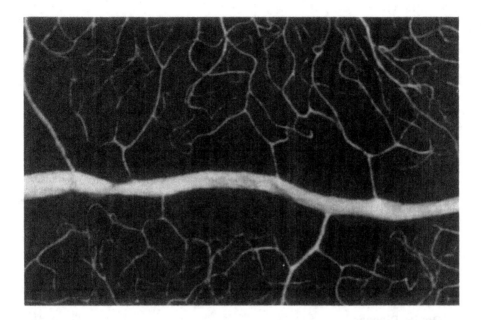

Figure 2 A vascular cast of the midperipheral retina. A larger radiating arteriole is seen to give off small branches that leave at right angle to supply the capillary network in this area. This branching pattern leads to plasma skimming, with plasma rich blood flowing into the small branches, and a flow of hemoconcentrated blood continuing in the radiating main branch to supply the retinal periphery.

two-layered, with one layer located at the level of the inner plexiform layer and a deeper layer located at the level of the outer plexiform layer, with numerous anastomoses connecting the two.[6] In the macular area, the inner capillary layer splits into a third capillary layer at the level of the ganglion cells. Furthermore, a radial peripapillary network of long thin capillaries with scarcity of anastomoses supplies the retinal nerve fiber layer close to the optic nerve head.[7] The retinal vessels receive no autonomic nerve supply, but like brain vessels, have autoregulated blood flow.

II. PATHOLOGY

A. CURRENT KNOWLEDGE
The current knowledge of the pathology of ocular microcirculation has predominantly been gained from studies of retinal vascular impairment in systemic and ocular disease in humans. This impairment has been studied *in vivo* by photographic techniques, and *in vitro* by histologic and vascular injection techniques.

1. Systemic Disease
a. Diabetic Retinopathy
In human studies, scanning laser video fluorescein angiography of the perifoveal capillary network has shown that leukocytes in normal subjects generally follow a preferential route through capillary branches; whereas, in diabetics, the leukocytes distribute more evenly among the branches,[8] presumably as a result of vasodilation. As assessed by laser Doppler velocimetry and blue-field entoptoscopy, the retinal blood flow is increased in the early stages of diabetic retinopathy, presumably because of vasodilation due to tissue ischemia, whereas retinal blood flow is decreased in the later stages of the disease,

presumably due to increased blood viscosity and occlusion of larger areas of the capillary network.[9-11]

Animal studies are hampered by the fact that no satisfactory animal model of diabetic retinopathy exists.[12] However, diabetic complications involving the retinal microcirculation that are not specific to diabetic retinopathy, such as basement membrane thickening, impaired retinal autoregulation, and barrier function, have been extensively studied.[13]

b. Arterial Hypertension

In arterial hypertension, the autoregulation of retinal blood flow leads to a vasoconstriction of larger retinal arterioles that can be seen by direct inspection of the ocular fundus. Furthermore, a videomicroscopic study of erythrocyte velocity and vascular autoregulation in the conjunctiva has demonstrated that these parameters are impaired in hypertensive patients.[14] Experimentally produced arterial hypertension in monkeys has been shown to cause focal irreversible retinal damage.[15]

c. Other Systemic Diseases

In macroglobulinemia, a microcirculatory disturbance in the retinal periphery leads to microaneurysmatic dilations, especially in this area.[16] Furthermore, using the blue-field entoptic light technique, a study has shown a significant reduction in macular blood flow in patients displaying Raynaud's phenomenon.[17]

2. Ocular Disease

a. Glaucoma

In glaucoma, the microcirculation of the optic nerve head is disturbed, but it is unknown whether this disturbance is primary or secondary to the development of the disease.[18] However, structural studies suggest that atrophy of the radial peripapillary network is involved in glaucoma damage.[19] Furthermore, fluorescein angiographic studies have shown filling defects of the optic nerve that correlate with visual loss in glaucoma,[20] and the filling rate of retinal vessels has been found decreased.[21] Additionally, using the blue-field entoptic scattering technique, results by Grunwald et al.[22] suggest a decreased autoregulation of retinal macular blood flow in glaucoma.

b. Other Ocular Diseases

Using video angiography, a study has shown reduced retinal and choroidal circulation in retinitis pigmentosa.[23] Furthermore, fluorescein iris angiography has shown filling delay of iris vessels in the post-operative period following squint surgery.[24]

B. FUTURE PERSPECTIVES

Microcirculation research on the ocular vascular beds stands out as a potentially important tool for gaining further insight into vascular pathophysiology in general and ocular disease in particular. However, a proper elucidation of the pathophysiologic problems encountered has until now been limited by some methodological constraints. To date, the most extensively studied ocular vascular system is the retinal vascular bed. The techniques employed have generally assessed larger areas of retinal microcirculation, and when localized microcirculation functions have been assessed, these have been limited to specific parts of the system, e.g., the perifoveal capillaries. Since pathologic processes in acquired retinal disease display a localized appearance, and within a broad range have a somewhat unpredictable location, it has generally not been possible to study microcirculation in retinal areas relevant for the disease state in question. Therefore, important steps toward an understanding of pathologic features of retinal microcirculation could be taken by developing appropriate new techniques that fulfill these requirements. One possible way could be the study of cells labeled with fluorochromes that would allow direct visualization of erythrocyte flow behavior in capillaries. This would require a sensitive detector system, a possible example being the real-time confocal microscope technique. Although this technique holds great promises, it needs some sort of image-stabilizing technique to compensate for eye movements before it will be clinically useful.

In the anterior segment of the eye, only a few studies have been done on microcirculation, probably due to lack of quantitative estimates of blood flow in this area, and because of detection difficulties due to ocular instability. However, a significantly unexploited potential for microcirculation research is available here in capillary beds that can be directly visualized, especially in case of the conjunctiva that is directly exposed to free air. Models for the study of specific ocular afflictions such as pterygium, corneal ingrowth of blood vessels, or ocular immunopathology could be developed, but also characteristics of general vascular responses such as inflammation and vasoactive drug action could be studied in this area.

III. MODELS AND TECHNIQUES

An array of older techniques for estimation of ocular circulation in experimental animals have been reviewed previously.[25] These include direct venous sampling, calorimetry, krypton clearance, and recording of vitreous oxygen tension by electrodes. The methods most commonly used in recent years are discussed below, emphasizing techniques that can be applied clinically.

A. SLIT LAMP BIOMICROSCOPY
It has been known for several decades that flow in the conjunctival capillaries can be observed qualitatively through the slit lamp biomicroscope by offsetting the illumination beam to the side of the viewpoint. Good contrast is obtained by scattered light from the sclera transluminating the capillaries and thereby visualizing cell flow. Due to the unevenly illuminated field and eye movements, it is very difficult to obtain clear video or film recordings.

B. MICROENDOSCOPY
The development of small bore endoscopes has enabled direct observation of the ciliary processes by an invasive procedure in experimental animals. After contrast injection, relatively high velocities of dye in the capillaries (0.8–1.0 mm/s) can be determined from video angiograms.[26]

C. CONTRAST INJECTION
The ancient principle of introducing a dye bolus into a stream has the advantage of visualizing the instantaneous mean velocity of the fluid. The use of a fluorescent compound increases the contrast significantly (at the cost of a detecting low light level) because the barrier filter eliminates the excitation light from the detection system. The interpretation in terms of flow is complicated by Taylor diffusion, smearing of the bolus, and the need for knowing the cross-sectional area of the vessel. Furthermore, in a recirculating system, the method only allows a single measurement to be made.

1. Fluorescein
This is a small molecule (MW 332 in dissociated form) that fluoresces at a wavelength of around 525 nm. It diffuses out of the microcirculation in the anterior parts of the eye, making visualization of the capillary bed here very difficult.[27] However, recently, a modification of the scanning laser ophthalmoscope (see Section D.1, next page) has facilitated observation of the circulation in the anterior eye segments.[28]

The blood-retina barrier has a low permeability for the fluorescein molecule in healthy vessels, which is the basis for the use of this method in several studies where pathology of the retinal microcirculation can be evaluated qualitatively.[29] Application of the dye-dilution technique has made it possible to calculate flow by computer analysis of the light intensity over time in defined areas located over the major vessels.[30] Processing images of the fundus may allow detection of occluded single capillaries occurring at cardiopulmonary bypass operations,[31] by analyzing capillary dropout seen on angiograms obtained post-operatively.

2. Indocyanine Green

This compound fluoresces at a wavelength of about 835 nm. This presents an advantage over fluorescein in that when used in the ocular media, there is six times less scatter of this wavelength. However, the efficiency of the fluorescence is much less, and thereby causes a severe detection problem. Indocyanine green is strongly bound to plasma proteins. It has therefore been used mainly for clinical studies of the choroidal circulation.[32]

3. Liposome Encapsulated Dyes

Release of dye from temperature-sensitive liposomes can be elicited by local laser heating, thus obtaining a sharp dye front to be used for calculation of a local flow rate.[33] The method is repeatable since recirculation is minimal. It remains to be seen whether the high laser power used is safe for human experiments.[34]

4. Labeled Cells

Although erythrocytes in retinal capillaries cannot be seen through the biological lens, they can be detected if sufficient contrast and separation is present. This condition occurs when a minute fraction of the cells are given a contrast-enhancing label. An assessment of flow can easily follow from simple counts of labeled cells passing through each capillary. Various labels have been used for erythrocytes, either calcein-loaded ghosts,[35] or fluorescein-labeled erythrocytes.[36,37] The longer wavelength of XRITC around 605 nm is advantageous in the eye because of better penetration.[38] So far, these direct methods have only been applied in experimental animals.

D. CONFOCAL TECHNIQUES

Introduction of a pinhole in the back focal plane of an objective reduces out of focus scattered light, and thereby results in a large increase in contrast. This contrast is gained at the expense of a significant reduction in light intensity and field of view. Therefore, a scanning principle is required to produce an image.

1. Scanning Laser Ophthalmoscope

With this technique, a laser beam is focused on the retina and scanned across by moving mirrors in synchrony with a video system producing live images. In larger vessels, predominantly erythrocytes are viewed in the marginal vascular zone, this explaining a lower recorded velocity than obtained by transillumination[39] or by laser Doppler velocimetry (see Section F.1, next page). In the capillary bed, however, the velocity is low enough to enable a view of particulate flow, which stands out as hyperfluorescent particles moving at a velocity of about 3 mm/s.[40] The nature of the hyperfluorescent dots is speculative, and has been presumed to be dye uptake by leukocytes,[41] thrombocytes and erythrocyte aggregates.[40]

2. Tandem Scanning Microscope

This is a principle of scanning that allows a higher temporal scanning frequency. Recording requires a sensitive, low-noise camera that can read out at real-time video rates. The elimination of out-of-focus scattered light allows penetration even through the sclera to directly visualize the choroidal circulation.[42]

E. BLUE-FIELD ENTOPTOSCOPY

There are several entoptic phenomena permitting the visualization of capillary flow.[43] The blue-light entoptic phenomenon has been utilized most widely in clinical settings.[44] The (cooperative) subject views an evenly blue illuminated screen with one eye. The flying spots presumably originate from relatively slow passage of leukocytes through the perimacular capillary network, causing a gap in the erythrocyte column. The observed field of moving dots is matched subjectively to a simulation on a computer screen presented to the other eye. It is the task of the subject in the two views to match the number of flying spots, their velocity, and (in very cooperative persons) also the pulsating velocity. The method has the drawback of being subjective and presumably measures the velocity of leukocytes that could be different from the erythrocyte velocity. The observed velocities are in the range of 0 to 2 mm/s.

F. DOPPLER SHIFT METHODS

The well-known phenomenon of an incoming wave being frequency shifted by a moving object has been used in a number of studies on circulation in the eye. Laser techniques have been reviewed recently.[45]

1. Laser Velocimetry

A laser spot is located on a major vessel (vein) and the bidirectional Doppler shift is used to calculate the velocity.[30] The method is tricky because of involuntary refixation and because the cutoff of the frequency spectrum may be hidden by noise.[46] Furthermore, the cross-section of the vessel must be known. The total flow to the region supplied by the vessel is measured. The method has been validated in pigs using the microsphere method as reference.[47]

2. Laser Flowmetry

Frequency broadening of scattered infrared laser light in a piece of tissue is affected by blood cells moving through the capillaries. In most of the circulatory beds of the eye exhibiting a layered structure, the assumption of the random orientation of capillaries[48] is violated to some degree. The tissue volume that is being sampled is uncertain. The intensity of the laser light used is presently too high for human experiments. Interestingly, perfusion of the the local optic nerve head in the cat has been found to exhibit cyclic vasomotor oscillations by this method.[49]

3. Ultrasound

The attenuation of sound in biological tissue impedes the use of frequencies above 7 to 10 MHz in the back of the eye. Thus, the spatial resolution of these instruments is limited to about 0.5 mm. A decrease of the maximum frequency shift in radioactivity-treated choroidal melanomas has been associated with tumor necrosis.[50,51] Without knowledge of vascular morphology, quantitative flow calculations are impossible, and thus the diagnostic value has to be proved.

G. MICROSPHERES

This method has the advantage of measuring the regional blood flow in all organs simultaneously in animal experiments.[52] The spheres are injected intracardially, distributed with the blood, and trapped in the peripheral capillaries. After sacrifice of the animal, the number of trapped spheres can be counted directly with a microscope or by radioactive counts. The activity is calibrated by the known aspiration rate in a large artery. The method has limitations in the number of measurements that can be made in each animal, depending on the maximum number of isotopes (3) that can be counted independently. Furthermore, the spheres streaming axially are amenable to plasma skimming, conceivably different from the erythrocytes. Thereby, the method underestimates the flow through small arteriolar side branches, i.e., in the midperipheral retina. The reproducibility is poor, however, because of the small fractional flow to the retina.[53]

H. OTHER METHODS

Indirect measures of perfusion pressures in the retinal and choroidal circulation have been obtained by oscillo-dynamography.[54] A similar technique has been used to investigate the autoregulation in glaucoma.[55] The pressure in the choroidal microcirculation has recently been measured directly by microcannulas featuring the servo-null technique,[56] and found to follow the intraocular pressure closely. The 2-deoxyglucose uptake method developed by Sokoloff measures glucose consumption by autoradiography with high spatial resolution. It has been used to study optic nerve head metabolism in monkeys.[57]

ACKNOWLEDGMENTS

The work was supported by the Benzon Research Foundation (to Dr. Jensen), and by the Danish Eye Research Foundation and the Carl and Nicoline Larsen Foundation (to Dr. Bek).

REFERENCES

1. **Torczynsky, E. and Tso, M.,** The architechture of the choriocapillaris at the posterior pole, *Am. J. Ophthalmol.,* 81, 428, 1976.
2. **Woodlief, N. F. and Eifrig, D. E.,** Initial observations on the ocular microcirculation in man. The choriocapillaris, *Ann. Ophthalmol.,* 14, 176, 1982.
3. **Bill, A.,** Blood circulation and fluid dynamics in the eye, *Physiol. Rev.,* 55, 383, 1975.
4. **Bill, A.,** Circulation in the eye, in *Handbook of Physiology,* Renkin, E. M. and Michel, C. C., Eds., Microcirculation, Part 2, Am. Physiol. Soc., 1984, 1001–1034.
5. **Michaelson, I. C.,** *Retinal Circulation in Man and Animals,* Thomas, Springfield, IL, 1954.
6. **Bek, T. and Jensen, P. K.,** Three-dimensional structure of human retinal vessels studied by vascular casting, *Acta Ophthalmol.,* 71, 506, 1993.
7. **Henkind, P.,** New observations on the radial peripapillary capillaries, *Invest. Ophthalmol. Vis. Sci.,* 6, 103, 1967.
8. **Choi, J. C., Liu, P., Sinclair, S. H., and Frambach, D. A.,** Retinal blood flow pattern at capillary bifurcation points, *Invest. Ophthalmol. Vis. Sci.,* Suppl. 33/4, 812, 1992.
9. **Grunwald, J. E., Riva, C. E., Stone, R. A., Keates, E. V., and Petrig, B. L.,** Retinal autoregulation in open angle glaucoma, *Ophthalmology,* 91, 1690, 1984.
10. **Fallon, T. J., Chowiencyzk, P., and Kohner, E. M.,** Measurement of retinal blood flow in diabetes by the blue-light entoptic phenomenon, *Br. J. Ophthalmol.,* 70, 43, 1986.
11. **Rimmer, T., Fallon, T. J., and Kohner, E. M.,** Long-term follow-up of retinal blood flow in diabetes using the blue light entoptic phenomenon, *Br. J. Ophthalmol.,* 73, 1, 1989.
12. **Frank, R. N.,** On the pathogenesis of diabetic retinopathy. A 1990 update, *Ophthalmology,* 98, 586, 1990.
13. **Bursell, S. E., Clermont, A. C., Shiba, T., and King, G. L.,** Evaluating retinal circulation using fluorescein angiography in control and diabetic rats, *Curr. Eye Res.,* 11, 287, 1992.
14. **Korber, N., Jung, F., Kiesewetter, H., Wolf, S., Prunte, C., and Reim, M.,** Microcirculation in the conjunctival capillaries of healthy and hypertensive patients, *Klin. Wochenschr.,* 64, 953, 1986.
15. **Hayreh, S. S., Servais, G. E., and Virdi, P. S.,** Cotton-wool spots (inner retinal ischemic spots) in malignant arterial hypertension, *Ophthalmologica,* 198, 197, 1989.
16. **Ashton, N.,** Ocular pathology in macroglobuliaemia, *J. Path. Bact.,* 86, 453, 1963.
17. **Salmenson, B. D., Reisman, J., Sinclair, S. H., and Burge, D.,** Macular capillary hemodynamic changes associated with Raynaud's phenomenon, *Ophthalmology,* 99, 914, 1992.
18. **Harrington, D. O.,** The pathogenesis of the glaucoma field; clinical evidence that circulatory insufficiency in the optic nerve is the primary cause of visual field loss in glaucoma, *Am. J. Ophthalmol.,* 47, 177, 1959.

19. **Kornzweig, A. L., Eliasoph, I., and Feldstein, M.,** Selective atrophy of the radial peripapillary capillaries in chronic glaucoma, *Arch. Ophthalmol.,* 80, 696, 1968.

20. **Begg, I. S., Drance, S. M., and Goldmann, H.,** Fluorescein angiography in the evaluation of focal circulatory ischaemia of the optic nervehead in relation to the arcuate scotoma in glaucoma, *Can. J. Ophthalmol.,* 7, 68, 1972.

21. **Goldmann, H. and Cabernard, E.,** Fluorescein in the human optic disc. II. The fluorescein appearance rate, *Albrecht von Graefes Arch. Clin. Exp. Ophthalmol.,* 200, 123, 1976.

22. **Grunwald, J. E., Riva, C. E., Stone, R. A., Keates, E. V., and Petrig, B. L.,** Retinal autoregulation in open angle glaucoma, *Ophthalmology,* 91, 1690, 1984.

23. **Ulrich, C., Ulrich, W. D., Vehlow, K., and Vehlow, S.,** Haemodynamische Aspekte bei der Retinitis Pigmentosa (RP), *Fortschr. Ophthalmol.,* 88/6, 642, 1991.

24. **Oliver, J. M. and Lee, J. P.,** The effects of strabismus surgery on anterior segment circulation, *Eye,* 3, 318, 1989.

25. **Alm, A. and Bill, A.,** Ocular circulation, in *Adlers Physiology of the Eye,* Moses, R. A. and Hart, W. M., Jr., Eds., C. V. Mosby, St. Louis, MO, 1987, 183.

26. **Funk, R. H. W., Wagner, W., and Wild, J.,** Microendoscopic observations of the hemodynamics in the rabbit ciliary processes, *Curr. Eye Res.,* 11, 542, 1992.

27. **Meyer, P. A. R. and Watson, P. G.,** Low dose fluorescein angiography of the conjunctiva and episclera, *Br. J. Ophthalmol.,* 71, 2, 1987.

28. **Ormerod, K. D., Fariza, E., Hughes, G. W., Doane, M. G., and Webb, R. W.,** Anterior segment fluorescein video angiography with a scanning angiographic microscope, *Ophthalmology,* 97, 745, 1990.

29. **Yanuzzi, L. A., Gitter, K. A., and Schatz, H.,** *The Macula: A Comprehensive Text and Atlas,* Williams & Wilkins, Baltimore, 1979.

30. **Riva, C. E., Grunwald, J. E., Sinclair, S. H., and Petrig, B. L.,** Blood velocity and volumetric flow rate in human retinal vessels, *Invest. Ophthalmol. Vis. Sci.,* 26, 1124, 1985.

31. **Arnold, J. V., Blauth, C. I., Smith, P. K. C., Jagoe, J. R., Wotton, R., and Taylor, K. M.,** Demonstration of cerebral microemboli occurring during coronary artery by-pass graft surgery using fluorescein angiography, *J. Audiovis. Med.,* 13, 87, 1990.

32. **Klein, G. J., Bäumgartner, R. H., and Flower, R. W.,** An image processing approach to characterizing choroidal blood flow, *Invest. Ophthalmol. Vis. Sci.,* 31, 629, 1990.

33. **Guran, T., Zeimer, R. C., Shahidi, M., and Mori, M. T.,** Quantitative analysis of retinal hemodynamics using targeted dye delivery, *Invest. Ophthalmol. Vis. Sci.,* 31, 2300, 1990.

34. **Khoobehi, B., Peyman, G. A., and Vo, K.,** Laser-triggered repetitive fluorescein angiography, *Ophthalmology,* 99, 72, 1992.

35. **Nutall, A. L.,** Techniques for the observation and measurement of red blood cell velocity in vessels of the guinea pig cochlea, *Hearing Res.,* 27, 111, 1987.

36. **Sarelius, T. H. and Duling, B. R.,** Direct measurement of microvessel hematocrit, red cell flux, and transit time, *Am. J. Physiol.,* 243, 1018, 1982.

37. **Horan, P. K. and Slezak, S. E.,** Stable cell membrane labelling, *Nature,* 340, 167, 1989.

38. **Jensen, P. K., Pokorny, K. S., Wagner, A. J., and Marsh, D. J.,** *In vivo* determination of retinal microcirculation using fluorescent erythrocytes in an animal model, *Invest. Ophthalmol. Vis. Sci.,* 31, 381, 1990.

39. **Seki, J. and Lipowsky, H. H.,** *In vivo* and *in vitro* measurement of red cell velocity under epifluorescence microscopy, *Microvasc. Res.,* 38, 110, 1989.

40. **Wolf, S., Arend, O., Toonen, H., Bertram, B., Jung, F., and Reim, M.,** Retinal capillary blood flow measurement with a scanning laser ophthalmoscope, *Ophthalmology,* 98, 996, 1991.

41. **Tanaka, T., Muraoka, K., and Shimizu, K.,** Fluorescein fundus angiography with scanning laser ophthalmoscope, *Ophthalmology,* 98, 1824, 1991.

42. **Beuerman, R. W., Chew, S. J., and Kaufman, H. E.,** Application of confocal microscopy in corneal research, *Exp. Eye Res.,* 55 (Suppl. 1), 134, 1992.

43. **Hart, W. M., Jr.,** Entoptic imagery, in *Adler's Physiology of the Eye,* Moses, R. A. and Hart, W. M., Jr., Eds., C. V. Mosby, St. Louis, MO, 378, 1987.

44. **Riva, C. E. and Loebl, M.,** Autoregulation of blood flow in the capillaries of the human macula, *Invest. Ophthalmol. Vis. Sci.,* 16, 568, 1977.

45. **Shepherd, A. P. and Öberg, P. Å.,** *Laser Doppler Blood Flowmetry,* Kluwer, Academic Press, Boston, 1990.

46. **Petrig, B. and Riva, C.,** Retinal laser Doppler velocimetry. Towards its computer-assisted clinical use, *Appl. Optics,* 27, 1126, 1988.

47. **Davies, E. G., Sullivan, P. M., Fitzpatrick, M., and Kohner, E. M.,** Validation and reproducibility of bidirectional laser Doppler velocimetry for the measurement of retinal blood flow, *Curr. Eye Res.,* 11, 633, 1992.

48. **Bonner, R. and Nissal, R.,** Model for laser Doppler measurements of blood flow in tissue, *Appl. Optics,* 20, 2097, 1981.

49. **Riva, C. E., Pournaras, C. J., Poitry-Yamate, C. L., and Petrig, B. L.,** Rhythmic changes in velocity, volume, and flow of blood in the optic nerve head tissue, *Microvasc. Res.,* 40, 36, 1990.

50. **Guthoff, R., Berger, R. W., Helmke, K., and Winckler, B.,** Doppler-monographische befunde bei intraokularen tumoren, *Fortschr. Ophthalmol.,* 86, 239, 1989.

51. **Lieb, W. E., Shields, J. A., Steven, M. C., Morton, D. A., Mitchell, D. G., Shields, C. L., and Goldberg, B. B.,** Color Doppler imaging in the management of intraocular tumors, *Ophthalmology,* 97, 1660, 1990.

52. **Alm, A. and Bill, A.,** The oxygen supply to the retina. II. Effects of high intraocular pressure and of increased arterial carbon dioxide tension on uveal and retinal blood flow in cats, *Acta Physiol. Scand.,* 84, 306, 1972.

53. **Roy, M. S., Harrison, K. S., Harvey, E., and Mitchell, T.,** Ocular blood flow in dogs using radiolabeled microspheres, *Nucl. Med. Biol.,* 16, 81, 1989.

54. **Ulrich, C. and Ulrich, W. D.,** Das saugnapfverfaren in der okulären kreislaufdiagnostik, in *Okuläre durchblutungsstörungen,* Stodtmeister, R., Christ, T., Pillunat, L. E., and Ulrich, W. D., Eds., Enke Verlag, Stuttgart, 80, 1987

55. **Pillunat, L. E. and Stodtmeister, R.,** Das normaldruckglaucom — eine mikrozirkulationsstörung, in *Mikrozirkulation in gehirn und sinnesorgan,* Stodtmeister, R. and Pillunat, R. E., Eds., Enke Verlag, Stuttgart, 1991, 124.

56. **Mäepea, O.,** Pressures in the anterior ciliary arteries, choroidal veins and choriocapillaris, *Exp. Eye Res.,* 54, 731, 1992.

57. **Sperber, G. O. and Bill, A.,** The 2-deoxyglucose method and ocular blood flow, in *Ocular Blood Flow in Glaucoma,* Lambrou, G. N. and Greve, E. L., Eds., Kugler and Ghedini, 1989.

Chapter 15

Stomach Microcirculation

Julio C. U. Coelho

CONTENTS

I. ANATOMY AND FUNCTION

A. VASCULAR ANATOMY OF THE STOMACH

The blood supply of the stomach is particularly rich (Figure 1). Six arteries provide the main blood supply: the left and right gastric arteries supply the area of the lesser curvature, the right and left gastroepiploic arteries supply the area of the greater curvature, the splenic artery via short gastric arteries (vasa brevia) supply the area of the fundus, and the gastroduodenal artery sends branches to the pylorus.[1-3]

The left and right gastric arteries form an arcade that extends along the lesser curvature.[1,2] As the left gastric artery, a major branch of the celiac axis, turns down along the lesser curvature, it divides into two branches. The anterior branch runs on the anterior wall toward the right part of the greater curvature where it divides into numerous small ramifications. The dorsal branch follows the lesser curvature and anastomoses with the right gastric artery. This artery is a branch of the hepatic artery and sends branches to the pylorus and to both adjacent walls of the stomach before it anastomoses with the dorsal branch of the left gastric artery.

The gastroepiploic arcade is formed by the left and right gastroepiploic arteries and it extends from the lower border of the first part of the duodenum to a point on the greater

0-8493-4870-6/95/$0.00+$.50
© 1995 by CRC Press, Inc.

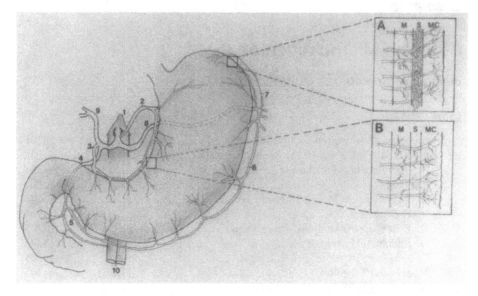

Figure 1 Schematic representation of the distribution of the main arteries supplying the stomach. The inset illustrates the arterial distribution of the gastric wall. The mucosa is supplied by arteries originating from the submucous plexus (A), except at the lesser curvature, where the mucosa is supplied by end-arteries that arise directly from the left gastric artery, without anastomoses with the submucous plexus (B). Muscle contraction at A would not occlude blood flow in the mucosal artery because of the collateral circulation. Muscular constriction at B would occlude the end-arteries and cause an area of mucosal ischemia, predisposing this area to peptic ulcer. (M = muscle layer; S = submucosa; MC = mucosa; 1 = aorta; 2 = left gastric artery; 3 = right gastric artery; 4 = gastroduodenal artery; 5 = right gastroepiploic artery; 6 = left gastric artery; 7 = short gastric arteries; 8 = splenic artery; 9 = hepatic artery; and 10 = superior mesenteric artery and vein.)

curvature just distal to the lower end of the spleen.[1,2] The left gastroepiploic artery is a branch of the splenic artery and the right gastroepiploic artery is a branch of the gastroduodenal artery. The area of the stomach on the greater curvature proximal to the gastroepiploic arcade is supplied by the short gastric arteries that are branches of the splenic artery. Usually, there are two to four short gastric arteries, but the number varies from one to nine.[1] The gastroduodenal artery is a branch of the hepatic artery and it supplies the pylorus.

Six other arteries are of secondary importance: superior pancreaticoduodenal artery, supraduodenal artery, retroduodenal artery, transverse pancreatic artery, dorsal pancreatic artery, and left inferior phrenic artery. All these arteries form a well-anastomosed network within the wall of the stomach.[1,2] Injection of contrast material into any of these arteries usually fills the whole vascular network.

The anterior and posterior walls of the stomach have a similar vascular arrangement.[3,4] Branches arise at intervals of about 1 cm from the arterial arcades on the greater and lesser curvature and pass on to the surface of the stomach. The arterial branches pierce the muscle coat, where they send off a branch. After having pierced the muscle coat, the branches subdivide into smaller branches in the outer portion of the submucosa. They, by anastomosing among themselves, form the main arterioarterial anastomotic plexus or primary arcade of arteries of 34 to 58 μ in diameter.[3,4] These branches give rise to smaller branches of 21 to 41 μ in diameter, which interconnect with each other and their parent vessels to form a secondary arcade.[3,4] The submucous plexus is continuous over the entire anterior and posterior walls and it is much less extensive near the lesser curvature. At this location, the mucosa is supplied by end-arteries that arise directly from the left gastric artery, without communication with the submucous plexus[3,5] (Figure 1). This anatomic arrangement may be important in the pathogenesis of gastric ulcer.[5,6] (See Section II.B. Pathology. Peptic Ulcer in this chapter).

The secondary arcade gives rise to smaller mucosal arteries of 14 to 19 μ in diameter, which pierce the muscularis mucosae.[3,4] Each mucosal artery divides into three or four branches, each of which in turn break up into three to six capillaries in the base of the mucosa. The capillaries form a honeycomb-like network around the gastric pits.[4] This hexagonal vascular system is generated by the terminal branching of capillaries that run along the gastric glands.[3,7]

The presence of arteriovenous communications in the gastric submucosa or mucosa is controversial. Arteriovenous anastomoses has been described by Barlow et al.[2] in human subjects and by Hase and Moss[8] and Nylander and Olerud[9] in rats, employing arterial injection techniques. However, Guth and Rosenberg[3] and Gannon et al.,[7] using vital microscopy, did not find either type of shunt, observing the gastric microcirculation of rats.

The superficial mucosal capillaries converge to form small venules that drain into collecting veins that are 21 to 24 μ in diameter.[3] These vessels drain into veins to form the venous submucosal plexus. These veins are larger than their respective arteries and are interconnected in a manner similar to the arteries. The venous pattern of the submucosa and the muscle coat follow the same course as the arterial branches.

B. MICROVASCULAR FUNCTION OF THE STOMACH

Mucosal blood flow in first-, second-, and third-order venules and capillaries is 0.075, 0.024, 0.013, and 0.005 nl/s, respectively, as determined in rats by intravital microscopy.[4] The flow velocity is pulsatile at 4 to 7 cycles/min. These pulsations do not correlate with respiration, gastric motility, or heart rate and they are supposedly due to vasomotion in the feeder arterioles or precapillary sphincters located deep down in the mucosa.[4] Vessel diameter is 14.5 μm for first-order venules, 10 μm for second-order, 7.9 μm for third-order, and 6.5 μm for capillaries.[4]

Gastric mucosal blood flow is dependent upon the systemic blood pressure. Reduction in systemic blood pressure in hemorrhagic shock is associated with a decrease in gastric mucosal blood flow.[10,11] One might anticipate that flow to a nonessential organ like the stomach would decrease proportionately more rapidly and at an earlier stage during shock to help maintain flow to essential organs such as the brain and kidney. However, a significant linear correlation between gastric mucosal blood flow and mean systemic blood pressure has been observed in the rat.[10,11]

Gastric microvessel diameters do not change with the fall of blood pressure.[10,11] Therefore, red blood cell velocity measured by *in vivo* microscopy reflects blood flow.[11]

Autonomic nerves and hormones also affect the gastric mucosal blood flow. Stimulation of parasympathetic nerve fibers increases total gastric and gastric mucosal blood flow due to dilation of gastric submucosal arterioles in cats, dogs, and rats.[12-14] Sympathetic nerve stimulation decreases mucosal blood flow through a vasoconstricting effect on the supplying submucosal arterioles in rats, as demonstrated by *in vivo* microscopy.[12] Pentagastrin increases and glucagon decreases gastric mucosal blood flow.[4,15,16] The effect of somatostatin on the gastric microcirculation is a subject of controversy. Both a reduction and no change of gastric blood flow have been reported.[17,18]

Gastric blood flow plays an important function in the normal gastric physiology. Mucosal blood flow correlates fairly closely with acid secretion, mucosal repair, and resistance to injury.[19] A direct relationship between gastric secretion and gastric blood flow has been shown in several species.[20] Decreases in gastric blood flow is accompanied by decreases in gastric secretion.

Gastric mucosal cell turnover is essential for mucosal repair and resistance. The surface epithelial cells are replaced every 3 to 6 days. This process is dependent on the mucosal blood flow.

Gastric mucosal blood flow is important to maintain a gradient of oxygen from the base toward the surface and a gradient of hydrogen ions from the surface toward the base of the mucosa.[11] Mucosal ischemia causes a reverse gradient of oxygen and hydrogen ions. Intramural pH decreases intensely due to back-diffusion of luminal hydrogen ions.[11] This further decreases mucosal blood flow and causes capillary lesions (See Pathology. Acute Gastric Mucosal Lesions in this chapter).

II. PATHOLOGY

The study of gastric microcirculation is important to understand the pathogenesis of several disease states and treatment modalities such as acute gastric mucosal lesions, gastric ulcers, upper gastrointestinal hemorrhages, radiation gastropathy, and surgical procedures.[21]

A. ACUTE GASTRIC MUCOSAL LESIONS

Acute gastric mucosal lesions may occur in patients with shock, traumatic injury, sepsis, or other types of life-threatening illness. Local ischemia may play an important role in the pathogenesis of this condition.[22] Analysis of mucosal blood volume by reflectance spectrophotometry has shown that ischemia of the gastric mucosa is the main cause of acute gastric mucosal lesions in patients with injury.[23]

Guth and Morishita studied the gastric microcirculation of rats during hemorrhagic shock employing *in vivo* microscopy.[10] They observed that, although the blood flow was slow, there was no change in superficial mucosal flow patterns during hemorrhagic shock when basic solution (Krebs solution; pH 7.4) was applied to the mucosa. However, blood flow in the superficial mucosa gradually disappeared in some microscopic fields when 0.1 N HCl was applied topically. After retransfusion, bleeding points appeared only in areas in which the blood flow had disappeared. The bleeding always occurred at a site of erosion. The converse, however, is not true. No erosions or bleeding occurred in animals in which basic solution was applied topically during hypotension and retransfusion. The mechanism by which hydrochloric acid causes acute gastric mucosal lesions in animals subjected to hypotension is unknown. Possibly, hydrochloric acid further decreases mucosal blood flow during hypotension. This may be due to an increase in back-diffusion of acid through the mucosa that could cause occlusion of supplying arterioles in the base of the mucosa by vasoconstriction or thrombus formation.[11] Thus, lowered mucosal blood flow due to hypotension could initiate the primary ischemic damage, making the mucosa susceptible to further damage due to the acid present in the stomach.

Vital microscopic observations during shock in rats confirm that the ischemia and ulcers are patchy in distribution and that bleeding only occurs after reinfusion of shed blood.[11,24] The bleeding always occurs at the border between ischemic and perfused areas of the mucosa.[24] It is possible that the vessel walls injured by ischemia and acid, rupture after restoration of blood flow due to increase hydrostatic pressure.[11,24] Formation of oxygen free radicals may also play a damaging role.[11,24]

The pathogenesis of aspirin-induced gastric mucosal erosions may be similar. Mucosal blood flow is decreased at the site of aspirin-induced ulceration despite a rise in mucosal blood flow at intervening nonulcerated sites and an increase in total gastric blood flow.[25,26] Aspirin induces back-diffusion injury, and focal hemorrhage by thrombus formation in mucosal microvessels and submucosal arteriolar constriction.[25]

B. PEPTIC ULCER

Most gastric ulcers occur along the lesser curvature at the angularis, usually on the antral side of the junction between the antral and fundic mucosae. The reason for this preferential location is not clear. Gastric mucosal microcirculation changes may be important. The mucosal and submucosal arteries are end-vessels in the lesser curvature (see vascular anatomy). It has been suggested that muscular contractions constrict these end-arteries and cause an area of mucosal ischemia[5] (Figure 1). Thus, this area would be prone to chronic ulceration.

A poor vascularity in the lesser curvature has also been demonstrated by post-mortem injection studies in man.[6] However, the mucosa in this area is visibly flatter and thinner than elsewhere, so the reduced vascularity may merely reflect a lower circulatory demand.[5]

C. UPPER GASTROINTESTINAL HEMORRHAGE

Peptic ulcers and erosive gastritis are common causes of upper gastrointestinal hemorrhage that can be difficult to control. Drugs, such as somatostatin, that decrease splanchnic blood flow, have been employed in the treatment of severe upper gastrointestinal hemorrhage. Studies of the gastric microcirculation after administration of somatostatin have been contradictory. Price et al. reported a reduction of gastric blood flow during somatostatin infusion employing radioactive microspheres in dogs.[17] However, Lunde et al., using endoscopic laser Doppler flowmetry, observed no change in the gastric microcirculation of patients during administration of somatostatin.[18]

D. RADIATION GASTROPATHY

Patients undergoing abdominal irradiation for treatment of cancer may develop acute, subacute, or chronic symptoms secondary to radiation gastropathy. Abdominal irradiation in rats causes a progressive and significant inflammatory response associated with increased microvascular permeability and vasodilation that reaches a peak at 12 h.[27] Transmural inflammation, fibrotic changes, and vasculitis predominate during subacute and chronic phases.

E. SURGICAL PROCEDURES

Gastric microcirculation may be very important in the pathogenesis of some complications after gastric operations, such as esophagogastroplasty and highly selective vagotomy.[28,29] Ischemia after esophagogastroplasty is a frequent cause of anastomotic breakdown, fistula, and stenosis at the anastomoses. Necrosis with perforation of the lesser curvature is a rare complication of highly selective vagotomy procedures. It has been suggested that this complication may be due to ischemia of the lesser curvature. Employing arteriography, Agossou-Voyene et al. observed an avascular band of 2 to 4 cm in the lesser curvature of patients subjected to highly selective vagotomy procedures.[29] Dyes employed in the gastric microcirculation could be important for elucidating the pathogenesis of these complications.

III. MODELS AND TECHNIQUES

Techniques to study the gastric microcirculation are of great interest since gastric mucosal blood flow plays a central role in the secretory process and the ability of the mucosa to protect itself against injury. Several techniques have been utilized. Most are performed in anesthetized animals or *in vitro* and give only indirect measurements. No comparative studies of the several methods are available.

A. ARTERIOGRAPHY

Arteriography was one of the first methods employed to study the gastric microcirculation. It still is commonly used today.[1,28,29] Contrast material is infused into gastric vessels before or after the animal is killed. Several contrast substances have been used, such as India ink, silicone rubber, and micropaque.[1,2,8,9,28] The stomach is then dissected and the microvessels studied using a microscope.

This method allows study of the microvessel anatomy. However, dynamic measurements such as red blood cell velocity and blood flow cannot be determined.

B. AMINOPYRINE CLEARANCE TECHNIQUE

This method was developed by Jacobson et al. in 1966.[30] It is based upon the permeability of lipid membranes to the undissociated but not the dissociated aminopyrine. After its administration, aminopyrine is present in the plasma in the undissociated state. Due to the marked pH gradient between plasma and gastric juice, aminopyrine, a weak base, is actively transported from the plasma into the lumen of the stomach. At the acid pH of gastric juice, aminopyrine ionizes and is retained in the lumen of the stomach. Aminopyrine is completely cleared from the blood on a single passage through the gastric mucosal blood flow. Thus, the clearance of aminopyrine into gastric juice is a direct measure of gastric mucosal blood flow.

Aminopyrine clearance technique measures the gastric mucosal blood flow of the entire stomach. Although its accuracy is high in the secretory stomach, measurements characteristically underestimate flow in the nonsecretory stomach.[31] Aminopyrine is toxic and may cause agranulocytosis.[32] Aminopyrine is administered intravenously at a loading dose of 20 mg/kg, followed by 5 mg/kg/h. Its concentration in gastric and plasma samples is then measured. Aminopyrine clearance is calculated using the following formula.[30]

$$C_A = \frac{G_A}{P_A} \times V_G$$

Where C_A = clearance of aminopyrine (ml/min)
         G_A = gastric aminopyrine concentration (mg/ml)
         P_A = arterial plasma aminopyrine concentration (mg/ml)
         V_G = volume of gastric fluid collected per time (ml/min)

This technique is not employed in human subjects due to the large doses of aminopyrine required. However, Guth et al. employed [^{14}C]-aminopyrine with success to measure mucosa blood flow in man.[15] Only a trace amount of [^{14}C]-aminopyrine is given intravenously: a 0.2 µCi per kilogram loading dose is followed by 0.05 µCi per kilogram per hour continuous infusion.

C. PERTECHNETATE CLEARANCE TECHNIQUE

This technique was first used by Meredith and Khan in 1967.[33] The procedure is similar to that of [^{14}C]-aminopyrine clearance; 1 mCi ^{99}Tc^m is administered intravenously and radioactivity is determined in venous and gastric juice samples. It is important to aspirate the gastric juice continuously to avoid gastric or small bowel absorption of ^{99}Tc^m. Its rapid absorption by the gastrointestinal tract may give spurious measurements, which is a disadvantage of this method. The clearance of ^{99}Tc^m is considerably less than clearance of [^{14}C]-aminopyrine in rats, dogs, and human subjects.[20]

D. RADIOACTIVE MICROSPHERE TECHNIQUE

This method measures focal blood flow with microspheres labeled with ^{85}Sr, ^{141}Ce, ^{51}Cr, and ^{46}Sc. Approximately 100,000 to 500,000 spheres, 15 ± 5 µ in diameter are injected into the left ventricle through a catheter passed into the heart via the carotid artery.[31,34] The microspheres mix in the left ventricle and then are distributed throughout the body in direct proportion to the distribution of cardiac output. Blood flow to each tissue can be calculated by comparison to a standard reference. Reference samples are collected from the carotid artery catheter using a constant-rate withdrawal pump.

Organ blood flow is calculated using the following formula:

$$\text{Organ blood flow} = \frac{\text{organ counts per minute}}{\text{reference counts per minute}} \times \text{reference blood flow}$$

Although the radioactive microsphere technique determines regional blood flow, it is inaccurate when measuring mucosal blood flow at a small foci because a single sample must contain at least 400 microspheres to avoid significant sampling error. In addition, other disadvantages include the facts that this technique allows only a limited number of measurements and uses radioactive material.

E. HYDROGEN CLEARANCE TECHNIQUE

This method was originally developed by Aukland et al. in 1964 to study cardiac and renal microcirculation.[35] In 1982, Murakami et al. modified the technique to determine focal gastric mucosal blood flow in animals and human subjects.[36] The method is noninvasive, safe, and of high precision. Measurement of mucosal blood flow at the site of the mucosa in contact with the electrode may be repeated several times with reproducible values.[36-40]

In this method, a platinum electrode serves as the probe. The electric current generated at the electrode by the oxidation of molecular H_2 to $2 H^+$ is measured. There is a linear relationship between the current generated and the concentration of H_2 dissolved in tissue.[35]

The rate of dissipation of a highly diffusible, biologically inert gas such as H_2 from a homogeneously perfused tissue is determined by the rate of blood flow that carries the gas away. Assuming that H_2 in the tissue is in an instantaneous diffusion equilibrium with H_2 in venous blood flowing through that tissue, the Fick principle can be applied to determine the blood flow.

Contact electrodes made from a 0.3-mm platinum wire are placed in contact with a target site of gastric mucosa through the channel orifice of an endoscope (human subjects) or through a small incision in the stomach (animals). A colomel reference electrode is attached to the skin of the lower extremity. The terminals of the platinum and colomel electrodes are connected to an amplifier-recorder device, and the electrode current is adjusted to zero in the absence of H_2. Stomach air is removed during measurements in order to minimize H_2 gas escape into the gastric lumen.

Pure H_2 gas is inhaled to achieve tissue saturation with hydrogen gas. Inhalation is terminated within 30 s, when a sharp increase in current is observed in the chart recorder. The electric current increases for a short period of time, attains a peak, and then decreases. The declining portion of the curve is plotted semilogarithmically at appropriate intervals. Gastric mucosal blood flow is calculated from the slope of this curve and expressed in milliliters per minute per 100 g tissue.

F. KRYPTON ELIMINATION TECHNIQUE

Ivarsson et al.[41] measured gastric blood flow by recording the elimination of intra-arterially injected Krypton-85. This method allows the measurement of total gastric blood flow and its distribution in animals and human subjects. Elimination of krypton is monitored with two external detectors: a scintillation detector recording the disappearance of γ-activity from the entire gastric wall and a G-M tube recording the disappearance of β-activity from the muscle layer only. Total and muscle layer blood flow can be calculated from the washout curves. It is possible to calculate mucosa-submucosa blood flow by knowing total and muscle blood flow and the relative weights of the mucosa, submucosa, and muscle layers. Experience with this method is very limited and its importance and accuracy have not been determined yet.

G. ENDOSCOPIC LASER DOPPLER FLOWMETRY

The use of the laser Doppler technique for blood flow measurements was first described by Riva et al. in 1972.[42] Kvernebo et al. used this technique to measure gastric blood flow.[43]

It allows one to study blood flow in different parts of the stomach in conscious human subjects. Measurements are performed endoscopically and intraoperatively.[44] The basic principle of laser Doppler flowmetry is that the frequency of light is changed when light is scattered by a moving object, such as a moving red blood cell. The magnitude of Doppler shift is dependent on the product of the number of moving red blood cells and their velocity. Fluctuations in blood flow are recorded with respiration, heart rate, gastric peristalsis, and internal vasomotion.[43] Cautions include putting too much pressure by the probe against the mucosa, and reducing the flowmeter signal or having poor contact between the probe and tissue with loss of optical coupling between the probe and tissue, which also interferes with recordings.[44]

H. REFLECTANCE SPECTROPHOTOMETRY TECHNIQUE

This noninvasive technique was used by Kamada et al. in 1982 to determine gastric mucosal blood volume in human subjects.[23] A flexible coaxial fiberoptic bundle connected to a computer-equipped spectrophotometer is passed into the stomach through an endoscope. Spectra of gastric mucosa are monitored and stored in the computer. The spectrum with the highest absorption due to hemoglobin is selected. The mucosal blood volume is determined by the difference of absorption between 569 and 650 nm in the spectra.

I. VITAL MICROSCOPY

Study of the stomach microcirculation by *in vivo* microscopy was developed by Rosenberg and Guth in 1970.[45] It allows observation of the microcirculatory architecture and measurements of vessel diameters and red blood cell velocities. The technique is employed in anesthetized animals. Two preparations may be used: (1) the exteriorized stomach to study the serosal, muscular, submucosal, and deep mucosal circulation; and (2) the everted pouch preparation to study the superficial mucosal circulation.

1. Exteriorized Stomach Preparation[3,46]

A 3-cm midline laparotomy is performed and the stomach is exteriorized. A small incision is made in the anterior wall of the stomach to insert a 3-mm fiberoptic light carrier rod into the stomach lumen. The rod is attached to a mirrored prism. With the gastric wall thus transilluminated, the microcirculation of the serosa and muscle layers can be studied. To facilitate visualization of the submucosal microcirculation, the serosa and the muscle layers of an area of 7 to 10 mm are carefully dissected and removed under stereomicroscopic observation. A concave brass disk with a 5-mm diameter hole is fixed over the exposed mucosa with a silicone adhesive through which Krebs solution (pH 7.4) at 37°C is applied to maintain constant temperature and moisture of the exposed surface. The mucosal microcirculation cannot be adequately visualized using this preparation. To do so, the everted pouch model should be employed.

2. Everted Pouch Preparation[10,11,25]

A long incision is made along the anterior wall of the stomach. A portion of the posterior wall of the corpus is everted through the gastric incision to expose the mucosal surface to direct visualization. A fiberoptic light is placed beneath the serosa of the everted stomach to transilluminate the gastric wall. A concave brass disk is fixed over the exposed mucosa for application of Krebs solution. This model allows application of various substances, such as aspirin and hydrochloric acid, on the mucosa to study the effect of these substances on the gastric mucosal microcirculation.[11,25]

The gastric preparations are studied using a microscope and are transilluminated with a xenon light source with a heat filter and a standard condenser system. A green filter is used to enhance the contrast between the red blood cell-filled microvessels and the background, thus improving optical resolution, which is otherwise reduced by the mucus. The microscope is connected to a closed-circuit television system that consists of a television camera, a videotape, and a television monitor. The studies may be videotaped and analyzed, off-line.

Red blood cell velocity is determined by playing back the videotape and determining the voltage output at two points in the vessel using an analyzer.[4,11] The signals, which vary as each red blood cell passes at a given point, are fed into a red blood cell velocity tracking correlator that continuously outputs the velocity.

Vessel diameter, actually blood column diameter, is measured from the television screen with a caliper[4] or using an image-splitting technique.[12,25] Turning the knob on the image-splitter, shears the image horizontally. When the vessel is split exactly one diameter, the value readout on the image splitter is the vessel diameter. Blood flow is calculated as the product of vessel cross-sectional area and red blood cell velocity.

The principal technical difficulties encountered when using vital microscopy to study the stomach are:[4] (1) exteriorization of the mucosal layer requires a surgical procedure and thus involves a certain amount of trauma; (2) the thickness of the stomach wall and the secreted mucus limit the transillumination, thus reducing the optical resolution; and (3) the gastric peristalsis and the anatomical relation of the stomach to the diaphragm subjects the gastric preparation to a continuous movement, making these high magnification measurements of red blood cell velocity difficult.

J. OTHER TECHNIQUES

Other techniques, such as vessel casts, 42K clearance, neutral red dye, and [^{14}C]-aniline, are mentioned but rarely employed[20,47,48] and will not be discussed in this chapter.

REFERENCES

1. **Vandamme, J. P. J. and Bonte, J.,** The blood supply of the stomach, *Acta Anat.*, 131, 89, 1988.
2. **Barlow, T. E., Bentley, F. H., and Walder, D. N.,** Arteries, veins and arteriovenous anastomoses in the human stomach, *Surg. Gynecol. Obstet.*, 93, 657, 1951.
3. **Guth, P. H. and Rosenberg, A.,** *In vivo* microscopy of the gastric microcirculation, *Am. J. Dig. Dis.*, 17, 391, 1972.
4. **Holm-Rutili, L. and Obrink, K. J.,** Rat gastric mucosal microcirculation *in vivo, Am. J. Physiol.*, 248, G741, 1985.
5. **Piasecki, C. and Wyatt, C.,** Patterns of blood supply to the gastric mucosa. A comparative study revealing an end-artery model, *J. Anat.*, 149, 21, 1986.
6. **Piasecki, C.,** The blood supply to the human gastrointestinal mucosa, with special reference to the ulcer bearing areas, *J. Anat.*, 118, 295, 1974.
7. **Gannon, B., Browning, J., and O'Brien, P.,** The microvascular architecture of the glandular mucosa of rat stomach, *J. Anat.*, 135, 667, 1982.
8. **Hase, T. and Moss, B. J.,** Microvascular changes of gastric mucosa in the development of stress ulcer in rats, *Gastroenterology*, 65, 224, 1973.
9. **Nylander, G. and Olerud, S.,** The vascular pattern of the gastric mucosa of the rat following vagotomy, *Surg. Gynecol. Obstet.*, 112, 475, 1961.
10. **Guth, P. H. and Morishita, T.,** The gastric microcirculation in shock, *Ann. N.Y. Acad. Sci.*, 597, 282, 1990.

11. **Morishita, T. and Guth, P. H.,** Effect of exogenous acid on the rat gastric mucosal microcirculation in hemorrhagic shock, *Gastroenterology*, 92, 1958, 1987.

12. **Guth, P. H. and Smith, E.,** Neural control of gastric mucosal blood flow in the rat, *Gastroenterology*, 69, 935, 1975.

13. **Swan, K. G. and Jacobson, E. D.,** Gastric blood flow and secretion in conscious dogs, *Am. J. Physiol.*, 212, 891, 1967.

14. **Martinson, J.,** The effect of graded vagal stimulation on gastric motility, secretion and blood flow in the cat, *Acta Physiol. Scand.*, 65, 300, 1965.

15. **Guth, P. H., Baumann, H., Grossman, M. I., Aures, D., and Elashoff, J.,** Measurement of gastric mucosal blood flow in man, *Gastroenterology*, 74, 831, 1978.

16. **Warrick, M. and Lin, T. M.,** Action of glucagon and atropine on mucosal blood flow of resting fundic pouches of dogs, *Life Sci.*, 17, 333, 1975.

17. **Price, B. A., Jaffe, B. M., and Zinner, M. J.,** Effect of exogenous somatostatin infusion on gastrointestinal blood flow and hormones in the conscious dog, *Gastroenterology*, 88, 80, 1985.

18. **Lunde, O. C., Kvernebo, K., Hanssen, L. E., and Larsen, S.,** Effect of somatostatin on human gastric blood flow evaluated by endoscopic laser Doppler flowmetry, *Scand. J. Gastroenterol.*, 22, 842, 1987.

19. **Whittle, B. J.,** The defensive role played by the gastric microcirculation, *Methods Find. Exp. Clin. Pharmacol.*, 11(Suppl. 1), 35, 1989.

20. **Lanciault, G. and Jacobson, E. D.,** The gastrointestinal circulation, *Gastroenterology*, 71, 851, 1976.

21. **Tsuchiya, M. and Oda, M.,** Recent advances in organ microcirculation research, *Int. Angiol.*, 6, 253, 1987.

22. **Morales, R. E., Johnson, B. R., and Szabo, S.,** Endothelin induces vascular and mucosal lesions, enhances the injury by HCl/ethanol, and the antibody exerts gastroprotection, *FASEB J.*, 6, 2354, 1992.

23. **Kamada, T., Sato, N., Kawano, S., Fusamoto, H., and Abe, H.,** Gastric mucosal hemodynamics after thermal or head injury. A clinical application of reflectance spectrophotometry, *Gastroenterology*, 83, 535, 1982.

24. **Ekman, T., Bagge, U., Bylund-Fellenius, A.-C., Soussi, B., and Risberg, B.,** Changes in gastric mucosal microcirculation and purine nucleotide metabolism during hemorrhagic shock in rats, *Scand. J. Gastroenterol.*, 26, 652, 1991.

25. **Kitahora, T. and Guth, P. H.,** Effect of aspirin plus hydrochloric acid on the gastric mucosal microcirculation, *Gastroenterology*, 93, 810, 1987.

26. **Ashley, S., Sonnenschein, L., and Cheung, L.,** Focal gastric mucosal blood flow at the side of aspirin-induced ulceration, *Am. J. Surg.*, 149, 53, 1985.

27. **Buel, M. G. and Harding, R. K.,** Proinflammatory effects of local abdominal irradiation on rat gastrointestinal tract, *Dig. Dis. Sci.*, 34, 390, 1989.

28. **Agossou-Voyeme, A. K., Hureau, J., and Germain, M. A.,** Etude des problemes vasculaires dans les oesophagoplasties gastriques apres oesophagectomie ou pharyngolaryngectomie circulaire, *J. Chir.*, 127, 141, 1990.

29. **Agossou-Voyene, A. K., Hureau, J., and Germain, M. A.,** Etude comapree de la vascularisation de l'estomac apres vagotomie hyperselective et seromyotomie anterieure, *J. Chir.*, 127, 168, 1990.

30. **Jacobson, E. D., Linford, R. H., and Grossman, M. I.,** Gastric secretion in relation to mucosal blood flow studied by a clearance technique, *J. Clin. Invest.*, 45, 1, 1966.

31. **Archibald, L. H., Moody, F. G., and Simons, M. A.,** Comparison of gastric mucosal blood flow as determined by aminopyrine clearance and γ-labeled microspheres, *Gastroenterology*, 69, 630, 1975.

32. **Taylor, T. V., Pullan, B. R., Elder, J. B., and Torrance, B.,** Observations of gastric mucosal blood flow using $^{99}Tc^m$ in rat and man, *Br. J. Surg.*, 62, 788, 1975.

33. **Meredith, J. H. and Khan, J.,** Gastric blood flow measurement by technetium clearance technic, *Am. Surg.*, 33, 969, 1967.

34. **McGreevy, J. M. and Moody, F. G.,** Focal microcirculatory changes during the production of aspirin-induced gastric mucosal erosions, *Surgery*, 89, 337, 1981.

35. **Aukland, K., Bower, B. F., and Berliner, R. W.,** Measurements of local blood flow with hydrogen gas, *Circ. Res.*, 14, 164, 1964.

36. **Murakami, M., Moriga, M., Miyake, T., and Uchino, H.,** Contact method in hydrogen gas clearance technique: A new method for determination of regional gastric mucosal blood flow in animals and humans, *Gastroenterology*, 82, 457, 1982.
37. **Mitarai, Y. and Kobayashi, M.,** Correlation between gastric microcirculation and mucosal injury after surgical therapy of esophageal varices, *Nippon Geka Gakkai Zasshi*, 91, 101, 1990.
38. **Cheung, L. Y. and Sonnenschein, L. A.,** Measurement of regional gastric mucosal blood flow by hydrogen gas clearance, *Am. J. Surg.*, 147, 32, 1984.
39. **Semb, B. K. H.,** Regional gastric flow determined by a hydrogen clearance technique in anesthetized and conscious animals, *Scand. J. Gastroenterol.*, 15, 569, 1980.
40. **Semb, B. K. H.,** Gastric flow measured with hydrogen clearance technique, *Scand. J. Gastroenterol.*, 14, 641, 1979.
41. **Ivarsson, L. E., Darle, N., Hulten, L., Lindhagen, J., and Lundgren, O.,** Gastric blood flow and distribution in anesthetized cat and man as studied by an inert gas elimination method, *Scand. J. Gastroenterolerol.*, 17, 1025, 1982.
42. **Riva, C., Ross, B., and Benedek, G. B.,** Laser Doppler measurements of blood flow in capillary tubes and retinal arteries, *Invest. Ophthalmol.*, 11, 936, 1972.
43. **Kvernebo, K., Lunde, O. C., Stranden, E., and Larsen, S.,** Human gastric blood circulation evaluated by endoscopic laser Doppler flowmetry, *Scand. J. Gastroenterol.*, 21, 685, 1986.
44. **Ahn, H., Ivarsson, L. E., Johansson, K., Lindhagen, J., and Lundgren, O.,** Assessment of gastric blood flow with laser Doppler flowmetry, *Scand. J. Gastroenterol.*, 23, 1203, 1988.
45. **Rosenberg, A. and Guth, P. H.,** A method for the *in vivo* study of the gastric microcirculation, *Microvasc. Res.*, 2, 111, 1970.
46. **Yonei, Y. and Guth, P. H.,** Effect of a leukotriene receptor antagonist on LTC_4 vasoconstriction in rat stomach, *Am. J. Physiol.*, 259, G147, 1990.
47. **Delaney, J. P. and Grim, E.,** Canine gastric blood flow and its distribution, *Am. J. Physiol.*, 207, 1195, 1964.
48. **Knight, S. E. and McIsaac, B. L.,** Neutral red as an estimator of gastric mucosal blood bow in dogs, *J. Physiol.*, 267, 45P, 1977.

Chapter 16

Heart Microcirculation

Yuan Yuan and William M. Chilian

CONTENTS

I. ANATOMY AND FUNCTION

A. VASCULAR ANATOMY OF THE HEART

The coronary arteries originate from the aorta at the base of the sinuses of Valsalva behind the cups of the aortic valve and penetrate the myocardium and proliferate in a rich network of microvessels including arterioles, capillaries, and venules. The capillaries lie between and run parallel to the myocardial fibers. Most of blood from the myocardial capillary bed is returned to the right atrium via the anterior cardiac veins or the coronary sinus, although some venous blood directly enters the ventricular cavities via thebesian channels.

Bassingthwaighte et al.[1] described the three-dimensional structure of the cardiac microvessels and made several important observations: (1) the arrangement of arterioles and venules appears to maximize concurrent flow in adjacent capillaries because arterioles and venules in the ventricular myocardium branch abruptly, and end at the capillaries in a bundle with close apposition; (2) the capillaries are long and narrow, with length-to-diameter ratios of 100:1; (3) the capillaries are arranged in bundles of parallel pathways, with many anastomotic connections; and (4) the capillary network is very dense. Capillary density in dog myocardium is 3100 to 3800/mm^3, giving intercapillary distances less than 20 μm. With the lesser density value, the capillary surface area is estimated to be 500 cm^2/g myocardium. This anatomic arrangement provides a basis mainly for concurrent flow in neighboring capillaries and diffusional exchange between inflow and outflow regions.

0-8493-4870-6/95/$0.00+$.50

B. MICROVASCULAR FUNCTION OF THE HEART
1. Regulation of Oxygen Delivery
a. Autoregulation

The coronary vascular bed exhibits an intrinsic ability to autoregulate blood flow over a wide range of arterial perfusion pressures. Metabolic dilation is the dominant mechanism in the autoregulation of myocardial perfusion; however, other mechanisms may also be involved.[15]

In vitro, coronary microvessels are able to respond directly to alterations in intraluminal pressure, with vasodilation and vasoconstriction occurring at low and high pressures, respectively. This myogenic response is primarily confined to arterioles less than 150 μm in diameter[36] where the majority of total coronary vascular resistance is located.[3] Recent *in vitro* studies on coronary microvessels obtained from the subendocardium and the subepicardium suggest that myogenic responses are less prominent in subendocardial microvessels.[26] This may account for the less-effective autoregulation in the subendocardium than in the subepicardium of the left ventricle.[18]

b. Metabolic Hyperemia

Coronary blood flow is coupled to interstitial concentrations of endogeneously produced vasoactive substances. Such metabolites dilate resistance vessels and increase local blood flow to maintain the balance between energy delivery and tissue demand. Increases in metabolism during pacing augment the diameter of all microvessels, but the magnitude of dilation is inversely related to the size of coronary microvessels.[23] The mechanisms of metabolic autoregulation are not fully understood. A large body of evidence indicates that adenosine is an important vasodilator metabolite in myocardium.[23]

It is worth noting that both metabolic and myogenic dilation are heterogeneous responses. The size of arterial microvessels responsible for the dilator response to autoregulation may not be identical. In fact, with myogenic regulation, arterial microvessels less than 100 μm in diameter dilate, whereas larger microvessels passively collapse.[36] However, Chilian and Layne found that these larger microvessels could be recruited to participate in the autoregulatory adjustment at low perfusion pressures.[8]

c. Flow-Induced Dilation

Coronary vasodilation in response to flow was initially demonstrated in large arteries of canine hearts and was found to cause modest dilation (5–10% increase in diameter).[6] Recent *in vitro* studies on isolated and cannulated coronary microvessels show that flow-dependent responses also occurred in the coronary arterioles between 40 and 80 μm in diameter.[27,28] Moreover, the dilation is very large in magnitude (increase in diameter by up to 25–30%). The dilation is not affected by indomethacin, an inhibitor of prostaglandin production, but is abolished by L-NMMA, a nitric oxide synthase inhibitor, and by denudation of endothelium from the vessels, suggesting that the flow-dependent response is mediated by endothelium-derived nitric oxide.

Even within the coronary microcirculation, gradients in the sensitivity of flow-dependent responses exist at different levels within the coronary microcirculation. Small arteries and arterioles between 80 to 150 μm are more sensitive to flow than smaller arterioles.[29] Since the smallest arterioles are the most sensitive to myogenic and metabolic stimuli,[23] vascular tone in larger microvascular segments appears to be predominantly controlled by different mechanisms.

d. Neural Control

Studies of neural control of the coronary microcirculation have been focused primarily on α-adrenergic and cholinergic mechanisms. Selective activation of α-receptors *in vivo* either by electrical stimulation of sympathetic nerves or by infusion of norepinephrine during β-blockade produces greater constriction of arterial microvessels larger than 150 μm in diameter than it does in smaller vessels.[5] α-adrenergic constriction of small coronary microvessels is modified by autoregulatory factors,[5,36] nitric oxide,[22] and adenosine.[11] In contrast, *in vivo* activation of cholinergic receptors by either vagal stimulation or acetylcholine infusion produces modest but relatively uniform dilation of all coronary microvessels.[32] *In vitro* studies indicate that in dog, acetylcholine-induced dilation of coronary microvessels is endothelial dependent.[39]

These studies suggest that α-adrenergic receptors and adrenergic regulation of coronary vascular resistance is heterogeneous across different-size arterial microvessels and modulated by intrinsic factors. Furthermore, these studies provide evidence that in the dog, acetylcholine and vagal stimulation dilate both large arteries and arterioles down to 50 μm in size.

e. Humoral Control

Effects of several humoral substances have been examined at the microcirculatory level. They include serotonin, vasopressin, norepinephrine, epinephrine, adenosine, and endothelin.[5,7,23,33,34] These humoral substances often have disparate effects on different-size arterial microvessels. For example, adenosine preferentially dilates vessels less than 150 μm in diameter; whereas, serotonin constricts microvessels greater than 100 μm in diameter, but dilates vessels less than 100 μm in diameter.[23] In contrast, vasopressin intensely constricts microvessels less than 100 μm in diameter and has either no effect or slightly dilates microvessels greater than 100 μm in diameter.[33]

The observation that different-size coronary microvessels have heterogeneous responses to important vasoactive substances, suggests that control mechanisms in microvessels above and below the 100 to 150 μm level must be strikingly different.

2. Coronary Microvascular Exchange

Using the indicator-dilution approach, investigators have measured PS product (permeability-surface area product) of various solutes including glucose, sodium, inulin, sulfate, rubidium, and sucrose.[12,43,49,50] Generally, permeability of these small molecules in the myocardium are similar to those in skeletal muscle.[42] In contrast, the rates of fluid and protein extravasation in normal myocardium are greater.[42] Laine and Granger[31] report that the transmicrovascular fluid and albumin fluxes in dog cardiac muscle are at least one order of magnitude higher per unit mass than in skeletal muscle. The high efflux of fluid and protein in this study cannot be explained fully by the larger exchange surface area in myocardium because the lymph-to-plasma concentration ratio for proteins is higher than that in skeletal muscle.

A recent methodological advance enables empirical measurements of coronary microvascular permeability.[46] Using a quantitative fluorescent microscopy technique, apparent permeability coefficient to albumin has been quantitated in isolated and perfused coronary venules ranging from 30 to 70 μm in diameter. We emphasize that venules of this size are important vessels for blood-tissue exchange of solutes and water *in vivo*. The study has revealed a permeability coefficient to albumin of 3.68×10^{-6} cm/s at an intraluminal pressure of 11 cm H_2O. Compared to other tissues,[9] both estimated true diffusive permeability and solvent drag coefficient are relatively high, indicating an active exchange activity in myocardium. Since the primary metabolic fuel for myocardium is fatty acids, which are normally bound to albumin, the high permeability coefficient for albumin in coronary venules would seem to be advantageous for the heart to meet its high metabolic demands because it would allow rapid flux of the fatty acid-albumin complex to traverse the venule into the interstitium.

The heart has the ability to simultaneously regulate its delivery and exchange functions at the microcirculatory level. In addition to flow-dependent dilation of arterioles, coronary venules facilitate the transvascular exchange of nutrients by exhibiting an increased permeability in response to increased flow. A recent *in vitro* study by Yuan et al.[47] indicates that the permeability coefficient for albumin increases by 8% with every 1 mm/s increase in flow velocity over the physiological range of flow velocities *in vivo* (Figure 1). This flow-dependent response seems to be mediated by the production of nitric

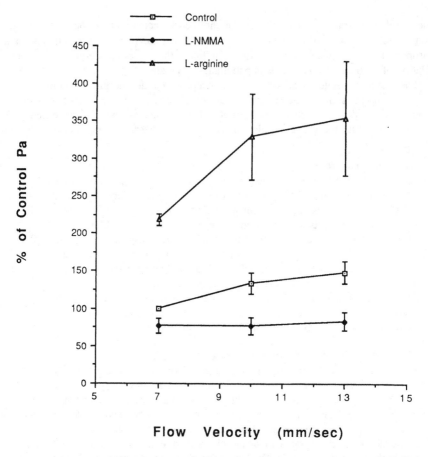

Figure 1 Albumin permeability in isolated coronary venules increased 48% as intraluminal flow increased 6 mm/s. Effect of flow on permeability was abolished by treating the same venules with NG-monomethyl-L-arginine (L-NMMA; 10^{-5} M). L-arginine (10^{-3} M) in the presence of L-NMMA restored the flow-induced permeability changes.

oxide because flow-induced increase in albumin flux is inhibited by the nitric oxide synthase inhibitor, L-NMMA, and reversed by L-arginine. These findings imply a further dynamic role for flow-dependent release of nitric oxide in facilitating the delivery of nutrients to myocardium during periods of increased demand.

II. PATHOLOGY

A. ISCHEMIA-REPERFUSION INJURY

Besides ischemic heart disease, myocardial ischemia can occur during thrombolytic therapy, angioplasty, and open heart surgery. Prolonged deprivation of blood flow in conjunction with hypoxia can lead to irreversible cellular injury, resulting from energy depletion, lactic acidosis, and inhibition of both glucose and fatty acid utilization.[24,40,41] Reperfusion following ischemia causes additional tissue damage, which is characterized by reperfusion injury.

Neutrophils have been found to accumulate in the reperfused region of the myocardium.[13,14] Adherence of neutrophils to the endothelial cells during ischemia-reperfusion is believed to be mediated by locally decreased shear stress (driving force)[19] and upregulated neutrophil-endothelial adhesion molecules such as CD11/CD18 membrane glycoprotein.[21] Once the neutrophils are activated, they release a variety of vasoactive and

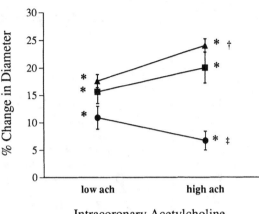

Figure 2 Average response of coronary arterioles during intracoronary infusion of low-dose and high-dose acetylcholine. Data are percent (%) change in diameter from baseline. Points represent mean ± SEM in control (■), ischemia-reperfusion (●), and preconditioned (▲) vessels. * indicates $p < 0.01$ vs. baseline; † indicates $p < 0.05$ vs. control, † indicates $p < 0.05$ vs. ischemia-reperfusion.

cytotoxic metabolites, of which reactive oxygen radicals are the major factor thought to cause myocardium injury.

Ischemia-induced changes of microvascular hemodynamics include dilation of small coronary arterioles and subsequent drop of perfusion pressure, increase of functional intercapillary distances, leukocyte capillary plugging, platelet aggregation, and microvascular hyperpermeability.[38,45] Also, endothelium-dependent vasodilatation is compromised during ischemia-reperfusion injury.[10,35]

The structural and functional conditions of the microvascular bed in the ischemic-reperfused myocardium may be an important factor in determining the final outcome and reversibility of cellular injury to the myocardium. The microvascular endothelial cell has been proposed as a major source of free radical production, and more importantly, is one of the primary targets of these radicals.[25] Recent studies in canine beating hearts by Defily and Chilian[10] demonstrate that ischemia-reperfusion significantly attenuates endothelium-dependent vasodilation of coronary arterioles, and importantly, preconditioning reduces arteriolar endothelial dysfunction after the injury (Figure 2). Therefore, preservation of microvascular function may reduce the amount of tissue necrosis and limit the reperfusion injury. (For further details, see Chapter 6 of this volume.)

B. ATHEROSCLEROSIS

Atherosclerotic microvessels display altered responses to endothelium-dependent vasodilator agonists and flow. Chilian et al.[4] showed that microvascular constriction in response to serotonin and ergonovine were enhanced in the beating heart of primates with dietary hypercholesterolemia and atherosclerosis, suggesting that endothelial function is impaired. This concept was supported by other studies[44] showing attenuated dilation to bradykinin and calcium ionophore (both are endothelium-dependent vasodilators), but not to the endothelium-independent dilators, adenosine or sodium nitroprusside, in atherosclerotic monkeys compared with controls. Moreover, the response to acetylcholine is converted from dilation to constriction. *In vitro* studies[30] in isolated coronary microvessels indicate that atherosclerotic arterioles can develop similar degrees of spontaneous tone to the control vessels, but show impaired vasodilator responses to endothelium-dependent agonists serotonin, histamine, and ADP, and fail to exhibit any vascular response to a step increase in flow rate. However, after preincubation with L-arginine, the precursor of endothelial nitric oxide, the atherosclerotic microvessels exhibit agonist- and flow-induced dilation of a similar magnitude to the normal vessels (Figure 3).

These studies suggest that atherosclerosis of large arteries is associated with major abnormalities of endothelial responsiveness in the coronary microcirculation. Atherosclerotic arterioles lose the capacity to dilate in response to flow and exhibit altered responses

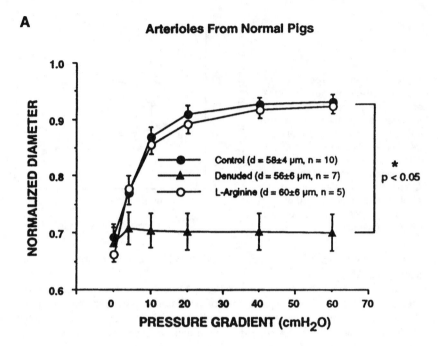

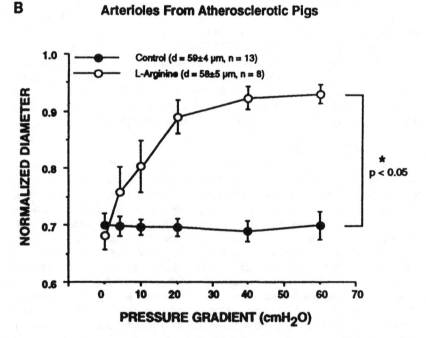

Figure 3 Comparison of flow-dependent responses in control and atherosclerotic pigs. In control pigs, flow-dependent dilation occurred under baseline conditions, was not affected by L-arginine (3 mM), but was abolished by endothelial removal. In atherosclerotic animals, flow-dependent dilation was not observed under baseline conditions, but occurred as in control pigs after L-arginine (3 mM). Lumen diameter were normalized to the diameter at the same pressure in the presence of nitroprusside (10^{-4} M).

to endogeneously occurring vasoactive agents. Restoration of normal endothelial responses by L-arginine indicates that they are due to impaired production of nitric oxide.

The pathophysiological importance of these abnormalities in the development of atherosclerosis is not clear. The loss of flow-dependent dilation may adversely influence the capacity to autoregulate during altered coronary perfusion pressure, reduce the ability to increase coronary blood flow during augmented oxygen demands, and impede the delivery of nutrients to myocardium through reduced coronary microvascular permeability. (For further information, see Chapter 2 of this volume.)

III. MODELS AND TECHNIQUES

Studies on microcirculatory control of blood flow and exchange in the heart have been hampered by the thickness of ventricular muscle and the excessive movement of microvessels during cardiac contraction. There have been three major approaches used to study the heart microcirculation: indirect study of hemodynamics *in vivo*, direct measurements of microvascular parameters *in situ* in the beating heart or isolated and perfused heart, and *in vitro* study using isolated coronary microvessel technique. We will briefly review the approaches applied to the study of the coronary microcirculation, focusing on several specific methodologies *in situ* and *in vitro*.

A. *IN VIVO* APPROACHES

Indirect approaches do not require actual visualization of the coronary microcirculation; rather, they are dependent on mathematical assumptions. Such approaches include indicator-dilution techniques, nuclide-labeled microspheres, protein-lymph solute, and microspectrophotometric analysis.

The indicator-dilution technique involves an intracoronary bolus of blood labeled with tracers (substrate, gases, vascular space indicators, etc.). Venous drainage from the heart is then analyzed for the tracer, either on-line or following rapid collection procedures with subsequent analysis of radioactive tracers. The amount of tracer appearing in the coronary sinus is normalized to the amount of tracer injected, providing information concerning the fraction of tracer that appears per unit time or the residual amount of tracer left in the tissue per unit time. The theory behind this approach has been reviewed by Bassingthwaighte and Goresky.[2]

The indicator-dilution technique can provide valuable knowledge concerning permeability-surface area product, capillary recruitment, and transport characteristics of various solutes and compounds. Because the transit time of substances can be measured, the technique can also provide estimates of vascular volume and compliance.

Another approach that has been widely used in the study of coronary microcirculation is to examine the lymphatic clearance of solutes.[31] This technique requires the measurement of cardiac lymph flow and the lymph and plasma solute concentrations in lymphatic and venous drainage from the heart. Information about microvascular exchange characteristics is gained by analyzing the relative concentrations of macromolecules of various sizes in lymph and plasma. This technique is based on an assumption that the composition of lymph is identical to that of interstitial fluid under steady-state conditions.

Although *in vivo* approaches are easier to employ and are not influenced by the thickness and motion of the heart, there are several limitations. First, measurements are based on principles that assume periods of steady-state conditions, and the time constant of such measurements is sufficiently large that it precludes documentation of transient changes. Second, the sample volume of such measurements is too large to detect localized microvascular phenomena, such as vasomotion or red cell velocities in capillaries vs. arterioles. Third, the techniques reflect "global" information and do not allow distinguishing regulatory mechanisms at different microvascular levels.

B. *IN SITU* APPROACHES

In situ direct approaches involve visualization of the coronary microcirculation in the intact heart and measurement of some parameters of microvascular dynamics, including microvascular pressure, diameter, red cell velocity, and transvascular flux of solutes. The studies utilize microscopy equipped with either epi-illumination, transillumination, or a fluorescent light source. There are two basic approaches that enable direct measurement of microvascular parameters *in situ*: beating heart preparation and isolated heart preparation. The two models can be used to study coronary microcirculation in different aspects. To investigate normal regulatory functions of the microcirculation at different vascular levels, the beating heart preparation would be preferable. In contrast, if *in situ* examination of the subepicardial and subendocardial microcirculation are necessary, studies must be completed in isolated and arrested hearts.

1. Beating Heart

The major obstacle in visualizing and measuring the diameter of epicardial coronary microvessels in the beating heart is the motion of the heart due to cardiac contraction and inflation of the lungs. Fortunately, the respiratory-imposed movements can be eliminated by ventilating experimental animals with a high-frequency jet ventilator synchronized to the cardiac cycle.[6] To control the cardiac motion due to contraction, the heart is partially restrained with several small pins inserted into the myocardium. The surface of the ventricles is epi-illuminated with a stroboscopic light source. A xenon strobe is synchronized with the cardiac cycle using the instantaneous left-ventricular pressure as a timing reference. A computer receives input from the left-ventricular pressure dP/dt, and will subsequently trigger the strobe. When the strobe flashes at the same point in time per cardiac cycle, the heart and microvasculature appear to be fixed, simply because the epicardium is in view for a short instant (15–25 µs) at the same time in the cardiac cycle. To enhance the visualization of microvessels, small bolus injections of fluorescein-isothiocyanate-labeled dextran are made into an indwelling coronary cannula, thereby increasing the contrast between the vessel and background. Measurement of microvascular caliber with fluorescence microscopy provides data on the internal diameter of the blood vessels and allows the differentiation of arterioles from venules. Furthermore, microvascular pressure can be measured using a micropuncture technique with a computer-controlled micropipette in concert with the beating heart. This approach, however, makes it impossible to obtain continuous measurements of coronary microcirculation, because the vessels are not continually visualized. The influence of the holding needles on local stress and strain is also a concern.

2. Isolated Heart

Due to the thickness of cardiac muscle, intramural and subendocardial microcirculation cannot be visualized by epi-illumination. For this reason, Chilian et al. have developed an approach to study the left-ventricular subendocardial microcirculation *in situ*.[6] A blood perfused, arrested, and isolated porcine heart is utilized for these studies. The ventricular wall is incised and the cut edges are hemostatically clamped. This enables measurements of the epicardial and endocardial microvascular diameter and pressure with the use of an intravital video microscope technique in conjunction with the servo-null pressure measuring system and micropuncture technique. Limitations of the technique include the effects of cardioplegic solution on alterations in the normal control mechanisms of microcirculatory processes in the arrested heart.

Exchange processes of the myocardium have also been assessed directly in the isolated and perfused heart.[37] Briefly, the heart is arrested and stabilized on the microscope stage for visualization of coronary capillary-venular field with a fluorescence microscope. After perfusing the heart with FITC-labeled macromolecules, a video densitometer is used to first measure fluorescence intensity over a venule, then over an adjacent capillary field. The intensity reading over the venule is called "I" and the reading outside the venule over the capillary field is called "O". The I/O ratio is calculated as a function of time. At constant capillary perfusion, an increase in this ratio is due to FITC-labeled tracer extravasation out of the coronary vascular space into the tissue space. This approach gives a simple, direct measure of macromolecular exchange in the heart, and allows a continuous assessment of microvascular function and exchange. However, the technique does not distinguish between convective and diffusive protein flux, nor can it identify which venule contributes to the leak.

C. *IN VITRO* APPROACHES

Although the aforementioned *in vivo* and *in situ* approaches are capable of providing dynamic information about the microvascular hemodynamics and exchange process in the intact heart, these measurements reflect global phenomena involving the participation of different microvascular segments subjected to different physical and chemical forces. For example, it has been an insurmountable problem to unequivocally establish *in vivo* or *in situ* that flow independently induces vasodilation and increases the permeability-surface area product, because there are often luminal pressure changes during the investigation of flow-induced responses. To directly study the function and regulation of specific microvascular segment of the heart, we have developed an *in situ* model to measure microvascular caliber, pressure, flow, and permeability in isolated and cannulated coronary arterioles and venules.[26,46,48]

Using microdissection techniques, coronary arterioles or venules of the desired size are dissected very carefully and then cannulated with two glass micropipettes (inner and outer) on the inflow end and one micropipette on the outflow end. The cannulating pipettes are connected to three reservoirs so that intraluminal pressure and flow can be adjusted independently by simultaneously changing the heights of the inflow and outflow reservoirs in equal increments. Using an inverted microscope equipped with a silicon-intensified target (SIT) camera or a charge-coupled device (CCD) camera, the image of the cannulated vessel is projected onto a high-resolution monochromatic video monitor. The diameter of the vessel can be measured on the monitor with a calibrated video caliper. The intraluminal pressure can be measured through a pressure transducer connected to the inner inflow pipette when the pipette tip is advanced into the midpoint of the vessel lumen. The intraluminal flow velocity is measured with an optical doppler velocimeter by perfusing the vessel with 1% red blood cell suspension.

Macromolecular permeability can be quantified in the isolated perfused venules with FITC-labeled tracers by measuring the ratio of the transmural flux of the tracer per unit surface area at different transmural solute concentrations.[20] With the use of an "optical window" from a video photometer positioned over the vessels on the monitor, the fluorescence intensity from the window is measured (Figure 4). In each measurement, the isolated vessel is first perfused with nonfluorescent perfusate through the outer inflow pipette to establish a baseline intensity. The vessel lumen is then rapidly filled with fluorochromes by switching the perfusion to the inner inflow pipette, which produces a step increase and, subsequently, a gradual increase in the fluorescence intensity. There is a step decrease of intensity when the fluorochromes are washed out by switching the perfusion to the outer inflow pipette. The apparent solute permeability coefficient (P) is calculated by the equation $P = (1/\Delta If)(dIf/dt)_0(r/2)$, where ΔIf is the step increase in fluorescence intensity, $(dIf/dt)_0$ is the initial rate of increase in intensity as solutes diffuse out of the vessel and into the extravascular space, and r is the vessel radius.

An important feature of this approach is that the hemodynamic and exchange properties of coronary microvessels can be studied at precisely controlled conditions. The preparation enables rapid and repeated measurements. Because intraluminal pressure and

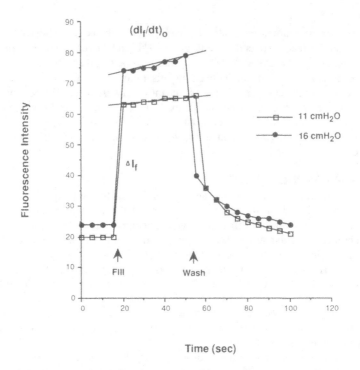

Figure 4 Measurement of apparent permeability coefficient of albumin (Pa) in an isolated coronary venule (48 μm diameter) at intraluminal pressures of 11 (□) and 16 (●) cm H_2O. Output of video photometer is plotted as a function of time. Venule was first perfused with nonfluorescent perfusate to obtain baseline fluorescence intensity. Vessel lumen was then rapidly filled (left arrow) with perfusate containing fluorescently labeled albumin by switching perfusion from outer inflow pipette to inner inflow pipette. This rapid filling produced a stepwise increase in fluorescence intensity (Δlf). Subsequent diffusion across venular wall of fluorochromes caused a gradual increase in intensity in measuring window $(dlf/dt)_o$. There was a rapid decrease in fluorescence intensity when fluorescently labeled solutes were washed (right arrow) out of vessel lumen and a subsequent gradual return of intensity to baseline level as solutes diffuse away from vessel wall. Note that increasing intraluminal pressure augments $(dlf/dt)_o$ and Pa.

flow are independently controlled, and because extrinsic factors including vasoactive agents and permeability-influencing factors are eliminated, the technique allows direct evaluation of the effects of blood components and chemical mediators on solute exchange. For example, inflammatory mediators have been implicated to increase venular solute exchange, not only by their direct effects on the vessel wall but also by the indirect effects through altering microvascular pressure and activating neutrophils, which in turn cause venular hyperpermeability.[17] With this experimental model, the direct and indirect effects of these factors can be systemically evaluated.[48]

One limitation of the isolated-microvessel technique is the size of vessels that can be successfully isolated and cannulated without causing damage to the preparation. At present, the lower limit for coronary venules is ~25 μm in diameter. For softer tissue, such as brain or hamster cheek pouch, vessels with diameter as small as 20 μm could possibly be studied. However, it is not clear whether this technique can be extended to mammalian capillaries measuring 10 μm or less in diameter. At the capillary level, the beating heart or isolated heart model may be the method of choice.

IV. SUMMARY

Studies of coronary microcirculation have established a substantial number of new concepts regarding the basic mechanisms of modulation of oxygen delivery and nutrient exchange in the myocardium. Recently developed technologies, including the *in situ* beating heart preparation and *in vitro* isolated microvessels, have enhanced our knowledge about the specialization of function within the microvasculature, i.e., the presence of vascular microdomains that act in a coordinated manner to regulate myocardial perfusion and solute exchange. Measurements of coronary pressure in different-sized arterioles have indicated a heterogeneous distribution of coronary microvascular resistance. The myocardial perfusion and exchange processes can be modulated in a nonuniform manner by a variety of physiological stimuli, including autoregulatory factors, metabolites, flow, and sympathetic stimulation. The microvascular responses to these factors are impaired in myocardial ischemia-reperfusion injury and atherosclerosis. The mechanisms responsible for these heterogeneous responses, and the consequences of their dysfunction during various pathologies require further study.

REFERENCES

1. **Bassingthwaighte, J. B., Yipintsoi, T., and Harvey, R. B.,** Microvasculature of the dog left ventricular myocardium, *Microvas. Res.*, 7, 229–249, 1974.
2. **Bassingthwaighte, J. B. and Goresky, C. A.,** Modeling in the analysis of solute and water exchange in the microvasculature, in *The Cardiovascular System*, Vol. 4: Microcirculation, Renkin, E. M. and Michel, C. C., Eds., Williams & Wilkins, Baltimore, 1984, 549–626.
3. **Chilian, W. M., Eastham, C. L., and Marcus, M. L.,** Redistribution of coronary microvascular resistance produced by dipyridamole, *Am. J. Physiol.*, 256(Heart Circ. Physiol. 25), H383–H390, 1989.
4. **Chilian, W. M., Dellsperger, K. C., Layne, S. M., Eastham, C. L., Amstrong, M. A., Marcus, M. L., and Heistad, D. D.,** Effects of atherosclerosis on the coronary microcirculation, *Am. J. Physiol.*, 258(Heart Circ. Physiol. 27), H529–H539, 1990.
5. **Chilian, W. M., Layne, S. M., Eastham, C. L., and Marcus, M. L.,** Heterogeneous microvascular coronary α-adrenergic vasoconstriction, *Circ. Res.*, 64, 376–388, 1989.
6. **Chilian, W. M. and Defily, D. V.,** Methodological approaches used for the study of the coronary microcirculation *in situ, Blood Vessels*, 28, 236–244, 1991.
7. **Chilian, W. M., Layne, S. M., Eastham, C. L., and Marcus, M. L.,** Effects of epinephrine on coronary microvascular diameters, *Circ. Res.*, 61(Suppl. II), II47–II53, 1987.
8. **Chilian, W. M. and Layne, S. M.,** Coronary microvascular responses to reductions in perfusion pressure. Evidence for persistent arteriolar vasomotor tone during coronary hypoperfusion, *Circ. Res.*, 66, 1227–1238, 1990.
9. **Curry, F. E., Joyner, W. L., and Rutledge, J. C.,** Graded modulation of frog microvessel permeability to albumin using ionophore A23187, *Am. J. Physiol.*, 258(Heart Circ. Physiol. 27), H587–H598, 1990.
10. **Defily, D. V. and Chilian, W. M.,** Preconditioning protects coronary arteriolar endothelium from ischemia-reperfusion injury, *Am. J. Physiol.*, 265(Heart Circ. Physiol. 34), H700–H706, 1993.
11. **DeFily, D. V., Patterson, J. L., and Chilian, W. M.,** Adenosine modulates α2-adrenergic constriction of coronary arterioles (Abstr.), *Circulation*, 88, I-470, 1993.
12. **Duran, W. N. and Yudilevich, D. L.,** Estimate of capillary permeability coefficients of canine heart to sodium and glucose, *Microvasc. Res.*, 15, 195–205, 1978.
13. **Engler, R. L., Schmid-Schonbein, G. W., and Pavelec, R. S.,** Leukocyte capillary plugging in myocardial ischemia and reperfusion in the dog, *Am. J. Pathol.*, 111, 98–111, 1983.
14. **Engler, R. L., Dahlgren, M. D., Morris, D. D., Peterson, M. A., and Schmid-Schonbein, G. W.,** Role of leukocytes in response to acute myocardial ischemia and reflow in dogs, *Am. J. Physiol.*, 251(Heart Circ. Physiol. 20), H314–H322, 1986.
15. **Feigl, E. O.,** Coronary physiology, *Physiol. Rev.*, 63, 1–205, 1983.

16. **Gerova, M., Gero, J., Barta, E., Dolezel, S., Smiesko, V., and Levicky, V.,** Neurogenic and myogenic control of conduit coronary arteries: A possible interference, *Bas. Res. Cardiol.*, 76, 503–507, 1981.

17. **Grega, G. J., Adamski, S. W., and Dobbins, D. E.,** Physiological and pharmacological evidence for the regulation of permeability, *Fed. Proc.*, 45, 96–100, 1986.

18. **Guyton, R. A., McClenathan, J. H., Newman, G. E., and Michaelis, L. L.,** Significance of subendocardial S-T segment elevation caused by coronary stenosis in the dog, *Am. J. Cardiol.*, 40, 373–380, 1977.

19. **Hansell, P., Borgstrom, P., and Arfors, K. E.,** Pressure-related capillary leukostasis following ischemia-reperfusion and hemorrhagic shock, *Am. J. Physiol.*, 265(Heart Circ. Physiol. 34), H381–H388, 1993.

20. **Huxley, V. H., Curry, F. E., and Adamson, R. H.,** Quantitative fluorescence microscopy on single capillaries: α-lactalbumin transport, *Am. J. Physiol.*, 252(Heart Circ. Physiol. 21), H188–H197, 1987.

21. **Jerome, S. N., Smith, C. W., and Korthuis, R. J.,** CD 18-dependent adherence reaction play an important role in the development of the no-reflow phenomenon, *Am. J. Physiol.*, 264(Heart Circ. Physiol. 33), H479–H483, 1993.

22. **Jones, C. J. H., DeFily, D. V., Patterson, J. L., and Chilian, W. M.,** Endothelium-dependent relaxation competes with a1- and α2-adrenergic constriction in the canine epicardial coronary microcirculation, *Circulation*, 87, 1264–1274, 1993.

23. **Kanatsuka, H., Lamping, K. G., Eastham, C. L., Dellsperger, K. C., and Marcus, M. L.,** Comparison of the effects of increased myocardial oxygen consumption and adenosine on the coronary microvascular resistance, *Circ. Res.*, 65, 1296–1305, 1989.

24. **Kjekshus, J. K. and Mjos, O. D.,** Effect of free fatty acids on myocardial function and metabolism in the ischemic dog heart, *J. Clin. Invest.*, 51, 1767, 1972.

25. **Kukerja, R. C. and Hess, M. L.,** Oxygen radicals, neutrophil-derived oxidants, and myocardial reperfusion injury, in *Pathophysiology of Reperfusion Injury*, Das, D. K., Ed., CRC Press, Boca Raton, FL, 1993, 221–241.

26. **Kuo, L., Davis, M. J., and Chilian, W. M.,** Myogenic activity in isolated subepicardial and subendocardial coronary arterioles, *Am. J. Physiol.*, 255(Heart Circ. Physiol. 24), H1558–1562, 1988.

27. **Kuo, L., Chilian, W. M., and Davis, M. J.,** Interaction of pressure- and flow-induced responses in porcine coronary resistance vessels, *Am. J. Physiol.*, 261(Heart Circ. Physiol. 30), H1706–H1715, 1991.

28. **Kuo, L., Davis, M. J., and Chilian, W. M.,** Endothelium-dependent, flow-induced dilation of isolated coronary arterioles, *Am. J. Physiol.*, 259(Heart Circ. Physiol. 28), H1063–H1070, 1990.

29. **Kuo, L., Davis, M. J., and Chilian, W. M.,** Response gradient for flow-induced dilation in the porcine coronary microvascular network, *FASEB J.*, 6, A2078, 1992.

30. **Kuo, L., Davis, M. J., and Chilian, W. M.,** Alteration of arteriolar responses during atherosclerosis, in *Resistance Arteries, Structure and Function*, Mulvany, M. J., et al., Eds., Elsevier, Amsterdam, 1991, 333–338.

31. **Laine, G. A. and Granger, H. J.,** Microvascular, interstitial, and lymphatic interactions in normal heart, *Am. J. Physiol.*, 249(Heart Circ. Physiol. 18), H834–H842, 1985.

32. **Lamping, K. G., Kanatsuka, H., Eastham, C. L., and Marcus, M. L.,** Cholinergic nerve stimulation and acetylcholine produce uniform dilation throughout coronary microcirculation, *FASEB J.*, 2, A495, 1988.

33. **Lamping, K. G., Kanatsuka, H., Eastham, C. L., Chilian, W. M., and Marcus, M. L.,** Nonuniform vasomotor responses of the coronary microcirculation to serotonin and vasopressin, *Circ. Res.*, 65, 343–351, 1989.

34. **Lamping, K. G. and Eastham, C. L.,** Endothelin: A potent vasoconstrictor in the coronary microcirculation, *Circulation*, 80(Suppl. II), II-212, 1989.

35. **Lefer, A. M., Tsao, P. S., Lefer, D. J., and Ma, X. L.,** Role of endothelial dysfunction in the pathogenesis of reperfusion injury after myocardial ischemia, *FASEB J.*, 5, 2029–2034, 1991.

36. **Marcus, M. L., Chilian, W. M., Kanatsuks, H., Dellsperger, K. C., Eastham, C. L., and Lamping, K. G.,** Understanding the coronary circulation through studies at the microvascular level, *Circulation*, 82, 1–7, 1990.

37. **McDonagh, P. F.,** Platelets reduce coronary microvascular permeability to macromolecules, *Am. J. Physiol.,* 251(Heart Circ. Physiol. 20), H581–H587, 1986.

38. **McDonagh, P. F and Reynolds, J. M.,** Transcoronary exchange during reperfusion after myocardial ischemia, in *Microvascular Perfusion and Transport in Health and Disease,* Karger, Basel, 1987, 169–203.

39. **Myers, P. R., Banitt, P. F., Guerra, R., and Harrison, D. G.,** Characteristics of canine coronary resistance arteries: Importance of endothelium, *Am. J. Physiol.,* 257, H603–H610, 1989.

40. **Neely, J. R., Rovetto, M. J., and Whitmer, J. T.,** Rate-limiting steps of carbohydrate and fatty acid metabolism in ischemic hearts, *Acta Med. Scand.,* 587, 9, 1975.

41. **Neely, J. R. and Grotyohann, L. W.,** Role of glycolytic products in damage to ischemic myocardium, *Circ. Res.,* 55, 816, 1984.

42. **Renkin, E. M.,** Control of microcirculation and blood-tissue exchange, in *Handbook of Physiology. The Cardiovascular System. Microcirculation,* Am. Physiol. Soc., Bethesda, MD, 1984, Sect. 2, Vol. IV, Pt. 2, Chap. 14, 627–675.

43. **Rose, C. P. and Goresky, C. A.,** Constraints on the uptake of labeled palmitate by the heart: The barriers at the capillary and sarcolemmal surface and the control of intracellular sequestration, *Circ. Res.,* 41, 534–549, 1977.

44. **Sellke, F. W., Armstrong, M. L., and Harrison, D. G.,** Endothelium-dependent vascular relaxation is abnormal in the coronary microcirculation of atherosclerotic primates, *Circulation,* 81, 1586–1593, 1990.

45. **Tillmanns, H., Leinberger, H., Neumann, F.-J., Steinhausen, M., Parekh, N., Zimmermann, R., Dussel, R., and Kubler, W.,** Microcirculation of the heart during postischemic reperfusion, *Prog. Appl. Microcirc.,* 13, 71–77, 1989.

46. **Yuan, Y., Chilian, W. M., Granger, H. J., and Zawieja, D. C.,** Permeability to albumin in isolated coronary venules, *Am. J. Physiol.,* 265(Heart Circ. Physiol.34), H543–H552, 1993.

47. **Yuan, Y., Granger, H. J., Zawieja, D. C., and Chilian, W. M.,** Flow modulates coronary venular permeability by a nitric oxide-related mechanisms, *Am. J. Physiol.,* 263(Heart Circ. Physiol. 32), H641–H646, 1992.

48. **Yuan, Y., Granger, H. J., Zawieja, D. C., DeFily, D. V., and Chilian, W. M.,** Histamine increases venular permeability via a phospholipase C-NO synthase-guanylate cyclase cascade, *Am. J. Physiol.,* 264(Heart Circ. Physiol. 33), H1734–H1739, 1993.

49. **Ziegler, W. H. and Goresky, C. A.,** Transcapillary exchange in the working dog heart, *Circ. Res.,* 29, 181–207, 1971.

50. **Ziegler, W. H. and Goresky, C. A.,** Kinetics of rubidium uptake in the working dog heart, *Circ. Res.,* 29, 208–220, 1971.

Chapter 17

Intestine Microcirculation

H. Glenn Bohlen

CONTENTS

I. ANATOMY AND FUNCTION

A. VASCULAR ANATOMY OF THE SMALL INTESTINE

The wall of the small intestine is composed of three layers, the mucosa where nutrients are absorbed, the submucosa where glandular tissue resides, and the visceral smooth muscle that mixes and moves the food. Microvascular perfusion of these layers begins as small arteries from the mesentery that pierce the muscle layer on both sides of the bowel wall and form a tree-like branching pattern on either side of the bowel wall within the superficial submucosa.[14] The venular drainage is a mirror image of the arteriolar inflow system. As shown in Figure 1, the first- and second-order arterioles are shared by all muscle layers. The 3A continues into the submucosa and sends multiple small branches to glandular structures and ultimately the 3A becomes the primary inflow vessel for a villus.

In the majority of species, including man, the single inflow vessel to a villus perfuses nearly all of the capillaries.[13,14] In dogs and cats, the capillary perfusion is predominantly from the villus apex toward the base; whereas, in rabbits and humans, the inflow vessel perfuses capillaries along its length and capillaries are oriented radially around the villus. Rodents send their inflow vessel to the villus tip where it divides into two arterioles that descend the villus and provide perfusion to a highly branched capillary network.

The lymphatic drainage of the small intestine requires two separate lymphatic systems, the mucosal-submucosal and muscularis systems, which do not communicate until they join and leave the bowel wall at the mesenteric border.[48] The submucosal portion of the mucosal-submucosal system is a vast and highly interconnected collection system, illustrated in Figure 2, which primarily receives the lymph from the lacteals of the villi.[48] In the majority of species, a single lacteal virtually fills the villus during life; in rats, multiple small lacteals are present. The muscle layer lymphatic system is far less extensive than the mucosal-submucosal system and is made up of separate rectangular geometric patterns of lymph vessels in the longitudinal and circular muscle layers. Although histological evidence interpreted as lymphatic valves has been reported for the small intestine,[27,28] practical demonstration of lymphatic valves in the intestinal system has only been successful where the muscle and mucosal-submucosal layer systems join.[48]

Mechanical propulsion of lymph through the two intestinal lymphatic systems may depend upon contractions of the bowel musculature rather than contractions of the lymphatic vessels. Visceral smooth muscle in the villi and muscularis mucosa are capable of shortening villi, which presumably pumps the lymph from the villus.[56] The outer

0-8493-4870-6/95/$0.00+$.50

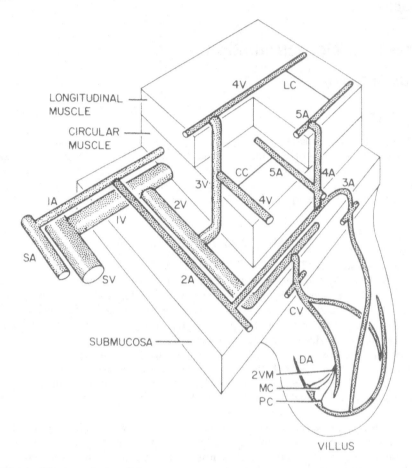

Figure 1 Microvascular branching pattern in the rat small intestine. Arterioles are consecutively numbered from largest to smallest branches; SA and SV are the small artery and vein that run parallel to the mesenteric border of the bowel and are in turn perfused by arteries in the mesentery. (Reproduced with permission of the American Heart Association; see Reference 4 for additional details.)

muscle layers are constantly moving the bowel tissue and, in doing so, compress the lymphatic structures in all bowel layers to help propel lymph.

B. FUNCTION OF INTESTINE MICROCIRCULATION

The major functions of the small intestine are digestion and absorption of food nutrients. The absorption process for most monosaccharides and amino acids depends upon maintenance of the cell sodium gradient and, therefore, active transport of sodium. Although lipid molecules enter the enterocytes by passive diffusion or a passive carrier system, packaging and molecular modification of lipids into chylomicron require a large amount of energy.[46] Therefore, no matter which nutrients the intestine may be absorbing, increased oxygen consumption is necessary, and even with an increase in blood flow, in oxygen tension mucosal tissue is typically below 5 mmHg during absorption compared to a resting tension of 15 to 20 mmHg during resting conditions.[1,2] To support the metabolic requirements of absorption, blood flow can increase 70 to 100%.[25,33,40,52]

Measurements of microvascular blood pressures in the small intestine of rats and rabbits indicate that the mucosal vasculature per se controls only 20 to 30% of the total

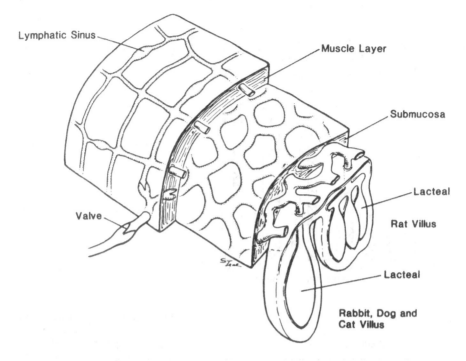

Figure 2 Lymphatic branching pattern in the small intestine. The model presented is based on studies in rats, rabbits, cats, and dogs (Reference 51), and variations in the lacteal structures are indicated. The lymphatic valves in the muscle and submucosal-mucosal layer lymphatic systems occur within the submucosa just as each system joins a common vessel that exits into the mesenteric lymphatic system. (Reproduced with the permission of the American Physiological Society from Reference 51.)

intestinal resistance.[5] Therefore, arterioles of the submucosa, which control about 50% of the resistance, must contribute to absorptive hyperemia whenever blood flow increases more than about 20%, which would exceed the ability of just the mucosal vessels to lower resistance. How this process is both regulated and communicated from the villus to submucosal layer may involve multiple mechanisms. Lipid absorption appears to induce absorptive hyperemia in part by a local neural process that may involve neural release of Substance P,[34] although contradictory evidence for a local neural control system as a contributor to any form of absorptive hyperemia has been presented.[26] Extrinsic innervation is not a major issue in the regulation of absorptive hyperemia because hyperemia readily occurs in denervated preparations.[20] A role for the dramatically increased oxygen usage in absorptive hyperemia during lipid absorption, and to a lesser extent during sodium coupled transport of carbohydrate, has been proposed.[34] However, only about one fourth of the absorptive hyperemia associated with glucose absorption can be attributed to the low tissue oxygen content,[1] and metabolite release, particularly adenosine, during absorptive hyperemia has been both supported[32] and questioned.[35]

A possible mechanism for absorptive hyperemia during sodium-coupled transport of nutrients is related to the villus hyperosmolarity during absorption,[3,18] although there are arguments against hyperosmolarity as a major cause of absorptive hyperemia.[22,30] Even at rest, the villus interstitial environment is hypertonic, such that the villus tip osmolarity may be in excess of 400 mOsm. During glucose absorption from isotonic media in the lumen, villus interstitial osmolarity can exceed 600 mOsm. In conscious animals, the osmolarity of the digested food is essentially isotonic if adequate water is available[19,21]

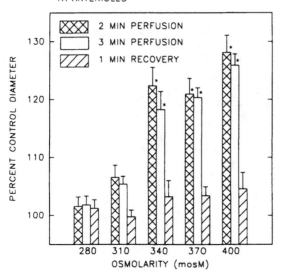

1A ARTERIOLES

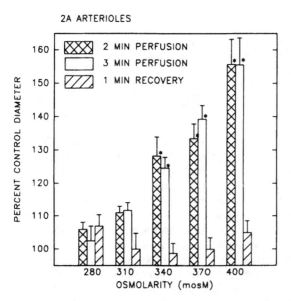

2A ARTERIOLES

Figure 3 The data illustrate the changes in diameter of large (1A, upper panel) and intermediate diameter intestinal arterioles (2A, lower panel) during perfusion of the submucosal lymphatic system with isotonic to hypertonic artificial lymph. The artificial lymph was made from Medium 199, to which calcium was added and pH adjusted with sodium bicarbonate; osmolarity was increased with sodium chloride. Isotonic media had no effect on arteriolar diameter, but hypertonic media caused a tonicity-dependent vasodilation similar at 2 and 3 min of perfusion, and virtually complete recovery occurred by 1 min after perfusion ended. (Reproduced with permission of the American Physiological Society; see Reference 43 for additional details.)

and the tissue osmolarities mentioned occurred when the lumenal environment was isotonic. The hypertonicity of the mucosa during absorption influences the osmolarity of the submucosal tissues because hypertonic blood and lymph flow from the mucosa through the permeable vessels of the submucosal layer (Figure 1).[9] Even during lipid absorption, the lymph and venous blood leaving the mucosa become mildly hypertonic.[9] Artificial elevation of the submucosal osmolarity with NaCl to the range found during glucose and oleic acid absorption causes dilation equivalent to that in natural absorptive hyperemia (Figure 3).[41] Perfusion with isotonic artificial lymph did not cause dilation. The process is particularly sensitive to sodium hyperosmolarity in that, for equal

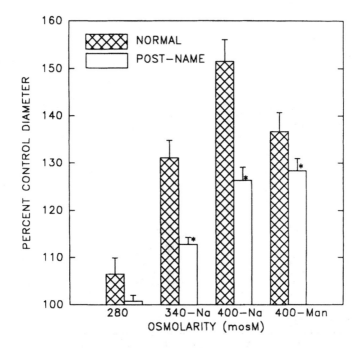

Figure 4 After the tissue was exposed to L-NAME to block the formation of nitric oxide, the vasodilation of second-order intestinal arterioles is suppressed by about half compared to normal responses during lymphatic perfusion with isotonic Media 199 (similar to Figure 3) made hypertonic with sodium chloride. In the two right bars, the dilation to 400 mOsm mannitol was compared before and after L-NAME treatment and less suppression of dilation occurred than during sodium chloride hyperosmolarity. The data indicate that sodium hyperosmolarity induces the release of nitric oxide, as well as inducing a nonspecific dilation to hyperosmolarity. For equal hypertonicities under normal conditions, mannitol was less effective in causing vasodilation than sodium chloride; but after L-NAME, mannitol and sodium chloride cause equivalent dilation. (Reproduced with permission of the American Physiological Society; see Reference 43 for additional details.)

hyperosmolarities, sodium causes about 40 to 50% greater dilation than inert mannitol (Figure 4). Furthermore, blockade of the ability of the intestinal tissues and vasculature to make nitric oxide, the putative endothelial-derived relaxing factor, decreases the response to sodium hyperosmolarity by about half and has a minor effect on dilation due to mannitol.

From a histological perspective, one might expect the intestinal vasculature to be very permeable to water and large molecules because the extensive mucosal capillary network has many mucosal capillaries with fenestrated endothelial cells. However, measurements of the capillary filtration coefficient for water and the reflection coefficient for plasma protein indicate remarkably low permeabilities.[15,16] However, during intestinal absorption, particularly of lipids, permeability increases in the intestinal vasculature.[16,17]

II. PATHOLOGY

The intestinal vasculature participates in the increased vascular resistance associated with essential hypertension, as judged by studies in the spontaneously hypertensive rat (SHR)[44,45] and evidence of microvascular structural deformities in the intestine in humans with

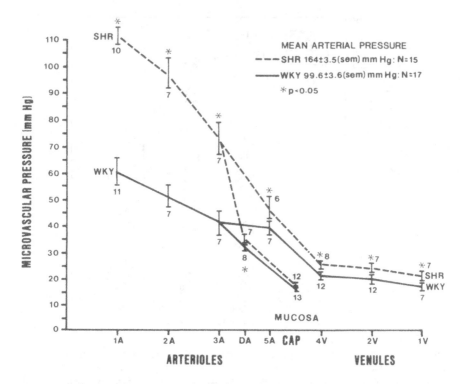

Figure 5 Microvascular pressures in the small intestine of 18- to 21-week-old SHR and WKY rats in the upper panel, and the microvascular pressures expressed as a fraction of the mean arterial pressure in the lower panel. Although arteriolar pressures are substantially increased, capillary pressures in the mucosa and muscle layer are essentially normal. On a fractional basis, the distribution of relative resistances is similar in normal and hypertensive rats, with a greater resistance in SHR in the smallest arterioles preceding the capillary beds. (Reproduced with permission of the American Heart Association; see Reference 4 for additional details.)

chronic hypertension.[38,39] However, as is the case for most organs and their vasculatures during essential hypertension, there is very little reason to believe that function of the organ is significantly compromised until late in the course of the disease. Blood flow per 100 g tissue can be near normal in the SHR because the vascular resistance increases in similar proportion to the increased arterial pressure.[44,45] Resistance is increased primarily through vasoconstriction with a very limited amount of closure, either temporary or permanent, of small arterioles.[4] Because resistance is related to the inverse of the fourth power of the inner radius, a generalized 5 to 10% constriction would be ample to explain the increased resistance in hypertension, although greater constriction is typically found in the larger arterioles.[4,8] Direct measurements in the muscle and mucosal layer capillaries in SHR indicate essentially normal capillary pressures despite severe systemic hypertension (Figure 5).[4] It is very likely that a similar situation occurs in hypertensive humans because elevated mucosal capillary pressures should cause clinical evidence of increased filtration of water into the abdominal cavity and bowel lumen.

Diabetes mellitus causes more obvious symptoms of a disease process in the gastrointestinal tract than does essential hypertension. Diarrhea, constipation, and impaired gastric emptying are common problems in humans with diabetes,[12,53] although absorption of nutrients appears to be within normal limits and could be enhanced.[10,43] In untreated insulin-dependent diabetes mellitus in animals, the bowel increases in both length, circumference, and mass,[36,49] and with essentially no formation of new arterioles; each

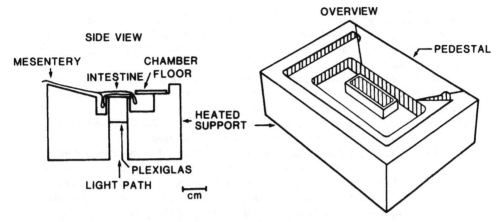

Figure 6 Tissue support device for the small intestine. Construction of this support device in brass or stainless steel (scale line shown) allows circulation of heated water through holes in the structure to warm both the bath and tissue. However, incoming suffusion fluid should be warmed as it enters the chamber, and the surface of the chamber should be covered with non-wettable insulation to help maintain uniform temperatures. (Reproduced with permission of the American Heart Association; see Reference 5 for additional details.)

existing arteriole must perfuse about 100% more tissue than normal.[49] However, there is increased formation of capillaries in the muscle layers[49] such that, despite tissue expansion, capillary diffusion distances are not doubled. There is increasing evidence that hyperglycemia per se leads to microvascular damage, including damage of the intestinal microvasculature,[6] through increased oxygen radical formation secondary to elevated prostaglandin formation.[7,23,24,42] The expression of this damage when hyperglyemia is exposed to otherwise normal tissues is increased capillary permeability[55] and impaired endothelial-derived relaxing factor dilation (EDRF).[7] In the latter case, EDRF is probably made in the endothelial cells but destroyed by reacting with oxygen or hydroxyl radicals before EDRF can cause relaxation of the vascular smooth muscle.[7]

III. MODELS AND TECHNIQUES

The mucosal vasculature can be studied in virtually any species because only the enterocytes separate the lumen from the microvessels. To study the all important vessels of the submucosa, which do most of the blood flow regulation, animals with a thin muscle layer, such as the rat and rabbit, are ideal.[5]

The muscle and submucosal layers of the small intestine can be easily studied by simply placing the bowel in a warm physiological environment that duplicates the temperature (37–38°C) and gas tensions of the abdominal cavity (pO_2 = 40–45 mmHg; PCO_2 = 40–50 mmHg; pH = 7.35–7.45). The microvessels may be seen by reflected or transmitted light, using either a stereo or conventional microscope. Isoproterenol (10^{-7}–10^{-6} g/ml) or norepinephrine (10^{-8}–10^{-7} g/ml), either separately or in combination with Dilantin (10^{-6}–10^{-5} M) (Parke-Davis Pharmaceuticals), can be used to suppress natural motility with minimal effects on the microvascular physiology.[5]

The best optical results for the muscle-submucosal microvessels and exposure of the mucosal surface requires slitting the bowel along the antimesenteric border with a small thermal cautery; electrostatic cauteries cause irreparable damage to the microvasculature and should not be used. One side of the bowel can be arranged over a rectangular or circular translucent pedestal to allow transillumination by tying small sutures to the cut edges of the bowel.[5] Figure 6 presents a general model of a tissue support device whose dimensions can be adjusted to fit virtually any size bowel. Optical magnification of 200 to 400× provides adequate details of the microvessels for visual observation, and video display of the images at a final magnification of up to 1000–1500× is useful for vessel diameter measurement.

Evaluation of the intestinal microvasculature should consider three major issues. First, there simply should be no stasis of blood flow in the capillaries, other than momentary stoppage of red cell motion, and certainly, no petechial hemorrhages of red blood cells into the spaces around capillaries or small venules. Second, within 30 to 45 min after a warm and properly maintained physiological environment has been made for the small intestine, the majority of arterioles should dilate at least 50% and blood flow should approximately triple when exposed to a topical concentration of 10^{-4} to 10^{-3} M adenosine or sodium nitroprusside.[5] Third, the microvascular preparation should be stable over a period of about 3 h in the sense of relatively constant arteriolar diameters at rest and no evidence of capillary stasis or sticking of leukocytes to the lining of small and large venules.

The study of intestinal microvascular function requires knowledge of the blood flow regulation, distribution of microvascular pressures to judge which vessels have the greatest effects on resistance, an index of tissue or blood oxygen tensions, and obviously, visual measurements of the inner diameter and numbers of microvessels. Relative changes in blood flow to the area of interest can be measured with Doppler ultrasound blood velocity probes on the intestinal arteries,[5] calculated from measurements of flow velocity and vessel diameter in microvessels using the red cell cross-correlated velocity technique,[2] and estimated from red cell flux (number of cells per unit time) using observed fluorescently labeled red blood cells in capillaries to vessels with inner diameters not greater than 25 μ.[51] In large rats and larger species, actual flow can be measured using small flow probes, such as the electromagnetic or ultrasonic flow probe methods, placed on the intestinal artery. For flow probe systems, ligation of the inflow vessels along the bowel margin and the gut wall itself at both ends of the tissue field perfused by the selected artery is essential if data on flow per mass of tissue is needed.

Measurement of microvascular pressures requires impalement of the vessel lumen with a micropipette that can be used to measure physical pressure. Two systems for such measurements, Instrumentation for Physiology and Medicine (San Diego, CA) and World Precision Instruments (Sarasota, FL), become available in 1993 and the former has been used very extensively in microcirculatory studies. The micropipettes must be sharpened to an outer tip diameter of 2 to 5 μ to facilitate penetration of the tissues and vessel wall with minimum trauma; traumatic impalement is very obvious from vessel constriction and formation of blood clots on the portion of the micropipette in the vessel. The primary use of microvascular pressure data, other than simply knowing the pressure per se, is that the ratio of microvascular to the sum of mean arterial pressure minus local venous pressure is a good index of the fraction of the total resistance up to the type of vessel penetrated.

Measurement of tissue oxygen tension with the Whalen[54] microelectrode is not a particularly difficult technique, but construction of the microelectrodes is difficult. The microelectrodes must be calibrated at oxygen tensions of 0 to 100 mmHg, with particular attention to the calibration at oxygen tensions below 40 mmHg where most tissue oxygen tensions reside.[31] Details of construction of the microelectrodes are published[54] and commercial microelectrodes are available. The principal of operation is that the gold anode, which is plated within the electrode tip, will facilitate reduction of oxygen and the higher the oxygen tension, the higher the microelectrode current; theoretical and practical aspects of electrode design and physics are available.[37] The typical current range is 10^{-11} to 10^{-9} amps at physiological oxygen tensions and, as a result of such low currents, electronic shielding equivalent to that used in membrane potential and patch clamp technology is essential.

An indirect approach to measurement of oxygen tension can be obtained with optical measurement of the percent saturation of hemoglobin in arterioles, capillaries, and venules.[11,29] The use of quantitative microscopic spectroscopy and mathematical theory for this process has been eloquently described by Pittman and co-workers[11,29] and is well beyond the scope of this chapter.

For studies that require chronic evaluation of the same microvascular region over days to months, a section of bowel can be observed in an anesthetized rat, returned to the abdominal cavity, and observation of the same tissues and vessels can be repeated at a later time.[47,49,50] This technique has been shown to have minimal, if any, effect on the microvascular and tissue growth in normal and diabetic rats. This approach has been used to follow the growth of existing microvessels in normal juvenile animals as they mature[50] and effects of diabetes mellitus on microvascular growth during juvenile life.[49]

ACKNOWLEDGMENTS

Dr. Bohlen's research has been supported by National Institutes of Health Grants HL-20605 and HL-25824.

REFERENCES

1. **Bohlen, H. G.**, Intestinal mucosal oxygenation influences absorptive hyperemia, *Am. J. Physiol.*, 239, H489–H493, 1980.
2. **Bohlen, H. G.**, Intestinal tissue PO_2 and microvascular responses during glucose exposure, *Am. J. Physiol.*, 238, H164–H171, 1980.
3. **Bohlen, H. G.**, Na^+-induced intestinal interstitial hyperosmolality and vascular responses during absorptive hyperemia, *Am. J. Physiol.*, 242, H785–H789, 1982.
4. **Bohlen, H. G.**, Intestinal microvascular adaptation during maturation of spontaneously hypertensive rats, *Hypertension*, 5, 739–745, 1983.
5. **Bohlen, H. G.**, Determinants of resting and passive intestinal vascular pressures in rat and rabbit, *Am. J. Physiol.*, 253, G587–G595, 1987.
6. **Bohlen, H. G. and Hankins, K. D.**, Early arteriolar and capillary changes in streptozotocin-induced diabetic rats and intraperitoneal hyperglycaemic rats, *Diabetologia*, 22, 344–348, 1982.
7. **Bohlen, H. G. and Lash, J. M.**, Topical hyperglycemia rapidly suppresses EDRF mediated vasodilation of normal rat arterioles, *Am. J. Physiol.*, 265, H219–H225, 1993.
8. **Bohlen, H. G. and Lash, J. M.**, Active and passive contributions to arteriolar diameter regulation in spontaneously hypertensive rats, *Hypertension*, in press, 1993.
9. **Bohlen, H. G. and Unthank, J. L.**, Rat intestinal lymph osmolarity during glucose and oleic acid absorption, *Am. J. Physiol.*, 257, G438–G446, 1989.
10. **Csaky, T. Z. and Fischer, E.**, Intestinal sugar transport in experimental diabetes, *Diabetes*, 30, 568–574, 1981.
11. **Ellsworth, M. L., Pittman, R. N., and Ellis, C. G.**, Measurement of hemoglobin oxygen saturation in capillaries, *Am. J. Physiol.*, 252, H1031–H1040, 1987.
12. **Falchuk, K. R.**, Motor and absorptive abnormalities of the gastrointestinal tract, *N.Y. State J. Med.*, May, 914–917, 1982.
13. **Gannon, B. J., Gore, R. W., and Rogers, P. A. W.**, Is there an anatomical basis for a vascular counter-current mechanism in rabbit and human intestinal villi?, *Biomed. Res.*, 2, 235–241, 1981.
14. **Gore, R. W. and Bohlen, H. G.**, Microvascular pressures in rat intestinal muscle and mucosal villi, *Am. J. Physiol.*, 233, H685–H693, 1977.
15. **Granger, D. N., Granger, J. P., Brace, R. A., Parker, R. E., and Taylor, A. E.**, Analysis of the permeability characteristics of cat intestinal capillaries, *Circ. Res.*, 44, 335–344, 1979.
16. **Granger, D. N., Korthuis, R. J., Kvietys, P. R., and Tso, P.**, Intestinal microvascular exchange during lipid absorption, *Am. J. Physiol.*, 255, G690–G695, 1988.
17. **Granger, D. N., Ulrich, M., Parks, D. A., and Harper, S. L.**, Transcapillary exchange during intestinal fluid absorption, in *Physiology of Intestinal Circulation*, Shepherd, A. P. and Granger, D. N., Eds., Raven Press, New York, 1984, 211–221.

18. **Hallback, D.-A., Jodal, M., Mannischeff, M., and Lundgren, O.,** Tissue osmolality in intestinal villi of four mammals *in vivo* and *in vitro*, *Acta Physiol. Scand.*, 143, 271–277, 1991.

19. **Houpt, T. R.,** Patterns of duodenal osmolality in young pigs fed solid food, *Am. J. Physiol.*, 261, R569–R575, 1991.

20. **Kvietys, P. R., Perry, M. A., and Granger, D. N.,** Intestinal capillary exchange capacity and oxygen delivery-to-demand ratio, *Am. J. Physiol.*, 245, G635–G640, 1983.

21. **Ladas, S. D., Isaacs, P. E. T., and Sladen, G. E.,** Post-prandial changes of osmolality and electrolyte concentration in the upper jejunum of normal man, *Digestion*, 26, 218–223, 1983.

22. **Levine, S. E., Granger, D. N., Brace, R. A., and Taylor, A. E.,** Effect of hyperosmolality on vascular resistance and lymph flow in the cat ileum, *Am. J. Physiol.*, 234, H14–H20, 1978.

23. **Mayhan, W. G.,** Impairment of endothelium-dependent dilatation of cerebral arterioles during diabetes mellitus, *Am. J. Physiol.*, 256, H621–H625, 1989.

24. **Mayhan, W. G., Simmons, L. K., and Sharpe, G. M.,** Mechanism of impaired responses of cerebral arterioles during diabetes mellitus, *Am. J. Physiol.*, 260, H319–H326, 1991.

25. **Moneta, G. L., Taylor, D. C., Helton, W. S., Mulholland, M. W., and Strandness, D. E.,** Duplex ultrasound measurement of postprandial intestinal blood flow: Effect of meal composition, *Gastroenterology*, 95, 1294–1301, 1988.

26. **Nyhof, R. A. and Chou, C. C.,** Evidence against local neural mechanism for intestinal postprandial hyperemia, *Am. J. Physiol.*, 245, H437–H446, 1983.

27. **Ohtani, O.,** Three-dimensional organization of lymphatics and its relationship to blood vessels in rat small intestine, *Cell Tissue Res.*, 248, 365–374, 1987.

28. **Ohtani, O. and Ohtsuka, A.,** Three-dimensional organization of lymphatics and their relationship to blood vessels in rabbit small intestine. A scanning electron microscopic study of corrosion casts, *Arch. Histol. Jpn.*, 48, 255–268, 1985.

29. **Pittman, R. N. and Duling, B. R.,** A new method for the measurement of percent oxyhemoglobin, *J. Appl. Physiol.*, 38, 315–320, 1975.

30. **Proctor, K. G.,** Contribution of hyperosmolality to glucose-induced intestinal hyperemia, *Am. J. Physiol.*, 248, G521–G525, 1985.

31. **Proctor, K. G. and Bohlen, H. G.,** Tonometer for calibration and evaluation of oxygen microelectrodes, *J. Appl. Physiol.*, 46, 1016–1018, 1979.

32. **Proctor, K. G. and Duling, B. R.,** Adenosine and free-flow functional hyperemia in striated muscle, *Am. J. Physiol.*, 242, H688–H697, 1982.

33. **Qamar, M. I. and Read, A. E.,** Effects of ingestion of carbohydrate, fat, protein, and water on mesenteric blood flow in man, *Scand. J. Gastroenterol.*, 23, 26–30, 1988.

34. **Rozsa, Z. and Jacobson, E. D.,** Capsaicin-sensitive nerves are involved in bileoleate-induced intestinal hyperemia, *Am. J. Physiol.*, 256, G476–G481, 1989.

35. **Sawmiller, D. R. and Chou, C. C.,** Adenosine plays a role in food-induced jejunal hyperemia, *Am. J. Physiol.*, 255, G168–G174, 1988.

36. **Schedl, H. P. and Wilson, H. D.,** Effects of diabetes on intestinal growth in the rat, *J. Exp. Zool.*, 176, 487–496, 1971.

37. **Schneiderman, G. and Goldstick, T. K.,** Oxygen electrode design criteria and performance characteristics: Recessed cathode, *J. Appl. Physiol.*, 45, 145–154, 1978.

38. **Short, D.,** Morphology of the intestinal arterioles in chronic human hypertension, *Br. Heart J.*, 28, 184–191, 1966.

39. **Short, D. S. and Thomson, A. D.,** The arteries of the small intestine in systemic hypertension, *J. Path. Bact.*, 78, 321–334, 1959.

40. **Sidery, M. B., Macdonald, I. A., Cowley, A. J., and Fullwood, L. J.,** Cardiovascular responses to high-fat and high-carbohydrate meals in young subjects, *Am. J. Physiol.*, 261, H1430–H1436, 1991.

41. **Steenbergen, J. M. and Bohlen, H. G.,** Sodium hyperosmolarity of intestinal lymph causes arteriolar vasodilation in part mediated by EDRF, *Am. J. Physiol.*, 265, H323–H328, 1993.

42. **Tesfamariam, B. and Cohen, R. A.,** Free radicals mediate endothelial cell dysfunction caused by elevated glucose, *Am. J. Physiol.*, 263, H321–H326, 1992.

43. **Thomson, A. B. R.,** Experimental diabetes and intestinal barriers to absorption, *Am. J. Physiol.*, 244, G151–G159, 1983.

44. **Tobia, A. J., Lee, J. Y., and Walsh, G. M.,** Regional blood flow and vascular resistance in the spontaneously hypertensive rat, *Cardiovasc. Res.*, 8, 758–762, 1974.

45. **Tobia, A. J., Walsh, G. M., Tadepalli, A. S., and Lee, J. Y.,** Unaltered distribution of cardiac output in the conscious young spontaneously hypertensive rat: Evidence for uniform elevation of regional vascular resistances, *Blood Vessels*, 11, 287–294, 1974.

46. **Tso, P. and Fujimoto, K.,** The absorption and transport of lipids by the small intestine, *Br. Res. Bull.*, 27, 477–482, 1991.

47. **Unthank, J. L. and Bohlen, H. G.,** Quantification of intestinal microvascular growth during maturation: Techniques and observations, *Circ. Res.*, 61, 616–624, 1987.

48. **Unthank, J. L. and Bohlen, H. G.,** Lymphatic pathways and the role of valves in lymph propulsion from the small intestine, *Am. J. Physiol.*, 254, G389–G398, 1988.

49. **Unthank, J. L. and Bohlen, H. G.,** Intestinal microvascular growth during maturation in diabetic juvenile rats, *Circ. Res.*, 63, 429–436, 1988.

50. **Unthank, J. L., Lash, J. M., and Bohlen, H. G.,** Maturation of the rat intestinal microvasculature from juvenile to early adult life, *Am. J. Physiol.*, 259, G282–G289, 1990.

51. **Unthank, J. L., Lash, J. M., Nixon, C., Sidner, R. A., and Bohlen, H. G.,** Evaluation of carbocyanine labeled erythrocytes for microvascular measurements, *Microvasc. Res.*, 45, 193–210, 1993.

52. **Vatner, S. F., Franklin, D., and Van Citters, R. L.,** Mesenteric vasoactivity associated with eating and digestion in the conscious dog, *Am. J. Physiol.*, 219, 170–174, 1970.

53. **Whalen, G. E., Soergel, K. H., and Geenen, J. E.,** Diabetic diarrhea: A clinical and pathophysiological study, *Gastroenterology*, 56, 1021–1032, 1969.

54. **Whalen, W. J., Nair, P., and Ganfield, R. A.,** Measurements of oxygen tension in tissues with a microoxygen electrode, *Microvasc. Res.*, 5, 254–262, 1973.

55. **Williamson, J. R., Ostrow, E., Eades, D., et al.,** Glucose-induced microvascular functional changes in nondiabetic rats are stereospecific and are prevented by an aldose reductase inhibitor, *J. Clin. Invest.*, 85, 1167–1172, 1990.

56. **Womack, W. A., Barrowman, J. A., Graham, W. H., Benoit, J. N., Kvietys, P. R., and Granger, D. N.,** Quantitative assessment of villous motility, *Am. J. Physiol.*, 252, G250–G256, 1987.

Chapter 18

Kidney Microcirculation

John D. Conger

CONTENTS

I. ANATOMY AND FUNCTION

A. VASCULAR ANATOMY OF THE KIDNEY

The anatomy of the conduit arterial vasculature is shown in Figure 1. Resistance vessels begin with the interlobular arteries, which give rise to lateral afferent arteriolar branches, and terminate in afferent arterioles in the superficial cortex. Near the vascular pole of the glomeruli, the smooth muscle cells of afferent arterioles are modified to renin granule-containing epithelioid cells that contain rudimentary myofibrils. Upon entering the glomerular capsule, afferent arterioles promptly divide into primary glomerular capillaries that give rise to the anastomosing capillary network (Figure 2). The outer two thirds of the capillary endothelium rests on a well-defined basement membrane. External to the basement membrane is a highly fenestrated and interdigitated epithelium. External to the visceral epithelium is the uriniferous space (Bowman's capsule), which is enclosed by the parietal layer of the epithelium. The anatomic arrangement of the glomerular capillaries restricts passage of molecules greater than 50 kDa or an effective radius of greater than 40 Å. However, molecular movement from capillary lumen to the uriniferous space is also influenced by molecular charge and shape. The hydraulic permeability coefficient for glomerular capillaries is approximately 300 times that of skeletal muscle capillaries and 50 times that of mesenteric capillaries.

Within the glomerulus, the capillaries converge to form the efferent arteriole.[1] The intraglomerular portion of the efferent arteriole is surrounded by mesangial cells. Upon exit from the glomerulus, the efferent arteriole is encircled by a relatively sparse (compared to the afferent arteriole) single layer of smooth muscle cells.

In the middle and outer cortex, efferent arterioles divide into a capillary network that surrounds the proximal and distal tubules largely from the same nephron. A similar capillary network arises from efferent arterioles in the juxtamedullary cortex. In addition, however, juxtamedullary efferent arterioles also give rise to the vasa rectae capillaries, which form hairpin loops that course into and out of the renal medulla.

0-8493-4870-6/95/$0.00+$.50

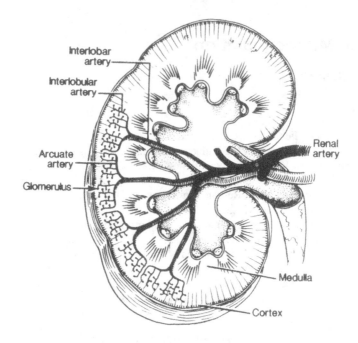

Figure 1 Arterial anatomy of the human kidney. See text for detailed description.

Venous outflow from the cortex follows the pattern of the arterial system and can be clearly identified beginning at the interlobular vessel level.

B. FUNCTION OF KIDNEY MICROCIRCULATION

While the combined weight of the kidneys is only 300 g, they receive one fifth of the cardiac output. Glomerular filtration, which is dependent on the high blood flow, is the principal process underlying the clearance function of the kidney. The process of glomerular filtration is controlled by a combination of physical forces. The vascular pressure profile through the kidney, based primarily on measurements in the rat,[2] is shown in Figure 3. The capillary hydraulic pressure of approximately 45 to 50 mmHg is maintained by variations in the preglomerular and postglomerular arteriolar resistances. At the afferent end of the glomerular capillary network, the intracapillary colloid osmotic pressure is approximately 20 mmHg. The hydraulic conductivity coefficient of glomerular capillaries measured directly in the Munich Wistar rat kidney with surface glomeruli is 2520 nl/min per mmHg per cm²,[3] The filtration process increases the plasma protein concentration and colloid osmotic pressure of the plasma remaining in the efferent end of the glomerular capillary network to approximately 35 mmHg, reducing the net driving pressure for ultrafiltration to near 0. Thus, under basal physiologic conditions, near filtration equilibrium exists in the efferent arterial end of the glomerular capillaries.

The glomerular filtration rate remains relatively constant despite variations in renal perfusion pressure. This is the result of autoregulation of renal blood flow. Over a wide range of renal perfusion pressures (estimated to be 80 to 160 mmHg in humans), renal blood flow remains nearly the same. Two mechanisms are primarily responsible for autoregulation: myogenic adjustments in preglomerular vascular resistance[4] and tubuloglomerular feedback.[5]

Several factors can increase or decrease basal renal blood flow. Table 1 gives a number of humoral factors and their influence on renal blood flow and glomerular filtration rate.

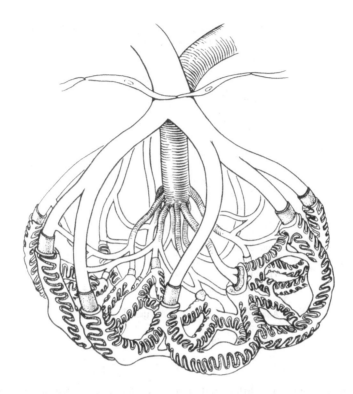

Figure 2 Illustration of the glomerular vasculature. The afferent arteriole enters through Bowman's capsule (from the left in diagram) and divides into segmental branches of the glomerular capillaries. The capillaries join within the glomerulus to form the efferent arteriole, which exists at the vascular pole adjacent to the afferent arteriole. The diagram is cut away to show the basement membrane applied to the capillary endothelium and the visceral epithelium overlying the basement membrane.

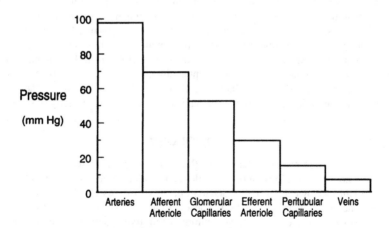

Figure 3 The hydraulic pressure profile along the renal vasculature, based on direct micropuncture measurements in rat kidneys.

Table 1 Effects of Vasoactive Agents on Renal Blood Flow and Glomerular Filtration Rate

	RBF	GFR
Catecholamines		
Norepinephrine	↓	→ or ↓
Dopamine	↑	↑
Peptides		
Antidiuretic hormone	→	→
Parathyroid hormone	↑ or →	→ or ↓
Atrial natriuretic peptide	→	→ or ↑
Angiotensin II	↓	→ or ↓
Bradykinin	↑	→
Glucagon	↑	↑
Endothelin	↓	↓
Arachidonate metabolites		
Prostaglandins E_2, I_2	↑	→
Thromboxane A_2	↓	↓
Leukotrienes C_4, D_4	↓	↓
Other		
Adenosine	↓ then ↑	↓
Histamine	↑	→
Platelet-activating factor	↓	↓
Acetylcholine	↑	→

Some of these agents have differential effects on afferent and efferent arteriolar resistances and the glomerular ultrafiltration coefficient and, therefore, can have different effects on renal blood flow and glomerular filtration rate.

In the human, glomerular filtration rate is approximately 150 l/day. Obviously, if there were no tubular reabsorption, profound volume depletion would occur. Tubular reabsorptive processes reclaim about 99% of the filtered salt and water. Tubular reabsorption involves both active and passive transport mechanisms. While volume reclamation from proximal tubular lumens is largely the consequence of active ion transport, vascular uptake of fluid from the interstitium is dependent on the high colloid osmotic pressure in the peritubular capillaries resulting from glomerular filtration, and this imparts a strong net driving force for volume reabsorption. The vasa rectae have a special exchange function. The high osmolar tonicity of the medullary interstitium is maintained by a combination of the countercurrent multiplication of sodium and urea by cycling from the ascending to the descending loops of Henle and countercurrent exchange of ions and urea from ascending to descending vasa rectae vessels. Changes in flow rates through the vasa rectae can alter the interstitial osmolality and, thereby, the maximal concentrating capacity of the kidney.

II. PATHOLOGY

If one were to include primary diseases of the glomerular capillaries, then all forms of immune and nonimmune glomerulonephritides could be included as disorders of the renal microvasculature. However, for this discussion, only diseases that have effects on the renal resistance vessels are considered. These entities can be considered in four broad categories shown in Table 2. The most common infiltrative and remodeling disorders are arteriolar nephrosclerosis (due primarily to arterial hypertension) and diabetes mellitus. Together, these two entities account for 50% of all kidney disease leading to end-stage renal failure.

Table 2 Classification of Disorders
of the Renal Microcirculation

Infiltrative and remodeling disorders
Arteriolar nephrosclerosis
Diabetes mellitus
Scleroderma
Thrombotic disorders
Hemolytic-uremic syndrome
Sickle cell nephropathy
Vasculitis
Polyarteritis nodosa
Wegener's granulomatosis
Allergic angiitis and granulomatosis
Acute renovascular dysfunction
Post-ischemia
Cyclosporine A

In arteriolar nephrosclerosis, the medium and small arteries show a process characterized by fibrous thickening of the intima with narrowing of the lumen diameter.[6] The typical glomerular lesion is one of ischemia and atrophy, reflecting the marked narrowing of the afferent arterioles.

Early diabetic nephropathy is characterized by microvasculopathy.[7] There is a progressive infiltration of advanced glycosylation products in the subintimal space of the small arterial vasculature. These vascular changes are found long before there is measurable deterioration in renal function.

Sclerodema is another disorder in which renal disease is primarily the result of a vascular infiltration and remodeling.[8] Sclerodema with progressive azotemia is frequently associated with malignant hypertension. However, the renovascular lesion of sclerodema is largely distinguishable from arteriolar nephrosclerosis and can be found in normotensive patients with this disease. The most characteristic histologic findings occur in the interlobular arteries. These changes consist of mucinous or finely collagenous deposits in the vessel intima.

Hemolytic-uremic syndrome and sickle cell nephropathy are examples of thrombotic disorders of the renal vasculature. In the hemolytic-uremic syndrome, the renal manifestations occur abruptly as anuria, hypertension, and azotemia.[9] The typical vascular lesions involve small arteries and afferent arterioles. There is intimal hyperplasia, subintimal fibrin deposition, and fibrin thrombi. In sickle cell nephropathy, the prominent renovascular lesion is RBC engorgement and thrombosis of the vasa rectae capillaries.[10]

Of the vasculitides, three diseases have frequent and significant renal involvement — polyarteritis nodosa, Wegener's granulomatosis, allergic angiitis, and granulomatosis. Polyarteritis involves small- to medium-sized arteries.[11] In a microscopic form, changes are seen primarily in arterioles, capillaries, and vessels. The essential lesion is inflammatory with leukocyte infiltration, fibrinoid necrosis, and diapedesis of red blood cells and plasma proteins. Wegener's granulomatosis, allergic angiitis, and granulomatosis, while involving arterial vessels more frequently in the lungs and other parts of the airway, are manifest in the kidneys primarily as a focal proliferative or necrotizing glomerulonephritis.[12,13]

Recently, studies carried out largely in experimental animals have focused on functional aberrations of the renal vasculature following ischemic or nephrotoxic results. These functional abnormalities have been shown to have deleterious effects on glomeruli and tubules. Loss of renal blood flow autoregulation, hypersensitivity to adrenergic nerve activity, and a blunted response to endothelium-dependent vasodilators have been found following transient renal ischemia in dog and rat models.[14-16] Continual exposure to

Table 3 Renal Microvascular Models and Techniques

Whole kidney hemodynamics and micropuncture
Perfused hydronephrotic kidney
Perfused juxtamedullary nephron
Red blood cell videomicroscopy and laser Doppler flowmetry
Isolated renal microvessels
Endothelial and smooth muscle cell cultures

cyclosporine A results in defective endothelial function. The resultant changes in vascular reactivity may lead to glomerulosclerosis, interstitial inflammation, and fibrosis.[17]

III. ROLE OF MICROCIRCULATION RESEARCH IN RENOVASCULAR DISEASE

Despite a formidable body of descriptive pathology, very little is known regarding the pathophysiology of the disorders described above. However, several avenues of investigation are providing insight into the nature of the evolutionary processes of these diseases.

In infiltrative and remodeling disorders, the roles of factors that stimulate mitogenesis are of particular interest.[18] Endothelial and non-endothelial vasoconstrictor agonists are known to be potent stimuli of smooth muscle cell growth and proliferation. Likewise, extracellular matrix deposition initiates vascular cell hyperplasia, as well as fibroblast infiltration.[19] These remodeling effects are mediated through a variety of growth factors.[20] In diabetes, the subintimal deposit of advanced glycosyation products may quench the vasodilatory and antimitogenic effects of nitric oxide leading to vasoconstriction and proliferative changes.[21] Disorders of endothelial function promote thrombus formation.[22] In addition, the role of endothelial adhesion molecules in thrombosis is currently being investigated.[23]

The role of cytokines released by activated inflammatory cells in the morphologic changes of vasculitis are of great interest. These substances, including tumor necrosis factor and interleukins, have a variety of effects on the remodeling and repair processes.[24]

Understanding the relative importance and interaction of endothelial, smooth muscle, neurogenic, and circulating factors in postischemic and nephrotoxic disorders is critical to managing aberrant vasoreactivity associated with these conditions. At present, it is uncertain to what extent these vascular abnormalities are intrinsic to the vasculature.

IV. MODELS AND TECHNIQUES

Techniques used to examine the renal microvasculature are listed in Table 3. Different methods are employed to answer different questions that focus on selected aspects of microvascular function and dysfunction.

A. WHOLE KIDNEY HEMODYNAMICS AND NEPHRON MICROPUNCTURE

para-Aminohippurate clearance estimates renal plasma flow, and inulin clearance measures glomerular filtration rate. Changes in the fractional filtration of plasma reflect changes in pre- and postglomerular arteriolar resistances. These clearance techniques are simple,[25] but can give valuable estimates of changes in pre- and postglomerular vascular resistances. More sophisticated techniques for determining renal blood flow — the electromagnetic flow probe and the radiolabeled microsphere technique — can be substituted for hippurate clearance in experimental animals.[26]

Nephron micropuncture is a technique used in anesthetized experimental animals — principally rat and dog.[27] With this method, the kidney is exposed, and the tubules and blood vessels of individual nephrons punctured with micropipettes. Tubular fluid or arteriolar blood can be collected. Hydraulic pressures can be measured in glomerular capillaries, efferent arterioles, and peritubular capillaries in mutant Wistar rats that have surface glomeruli.

B. PERFUSED HYDRONEPHROTIC KIDNEY

In this model, the ureter of a rat is ligated and the renal artery occluded for 60 min. After 3 weeks, tubules atrophy, leaving a remnant vasculature in a translucent renal cortex. The model can be studied *in vivo* or the kidney can be removed and perfused *in vitro*.[28,29] Under microscopic visualization, elements of the renal microcirculation from the interlobular arteries to peritubular capillaries can be examined. Changes in lumen diameters to neurohumoral stimuli can be determined.

Several important observations have been made with the hydronephrotic rat kidney method. The roles of the afferent and efferent arterioles in myogenic autoregulation, the importance of potential-dependent calcium entry channels in response to constrictor agonists in the pre- and postglomerular resistance vessels, and the segmental vascular responses to renal adrenergic nerve activity have been delineated with this technique.

The hydronephrotic kidney technique requires a perfusion system if studies are carried out *in vitro*. An optimal illumination source and microscope system are required to measure changes in lumen diameter. A video camera and monitor facilitate the accuracy of measurement.

C. PERFUSED JUXTAMEDULLARY NEPHRON MICROVASCULAR PREPARATION

This method takes advantage of the superficial location of a few glomeruli that lie near the inner surface of the cortex adjacent to the renal pelvis. The renal artery of an anesthetized rat is cannulated and perfused *in situ* with a plasma-like solution. After hemisection of the kidney, the papilla is reflected and renal artery branches not perfusing the study zone are ligated. The kidney is perfused either with blood from a donor rat or an artificial blood solution. Using videomicroscopy, it is possible to measure diameter changes in pre- and postglomerular arterial vessels, measure single nephron glomerular filtration rate, and obtain tubular fluid samples with micropipettes. This technique allows measurement of resistances in pre- and postglomerular vessels as in the hydronephrotic kidneys; however, it has the advantage of vascular assessment in the presence of an intact tubular system.[30]

Surgical preparation and exposure of the juxtamedullary zone of glomeruli require some microsurgery. Video imaging is similar to that with the hydronephrotic kidney. Collection of tubular fluid samples requires micromanipulators and micropipettes, the same as are required for standard nephron micropuncture.

D. RED BLOOD CELL VIDEOMICROSCOPY AND LASER-DOPPLER FLOWMETRY

Two techniques have been developed to examine the renal medullary circulation. The former method is based on the dual-slit technique for tracking RBC in peripheral vessels by videomicroscopy.[31] The papilla of rats is exposed, and the vasa rectae circulation is imaged with an epifluorescence microscope and an intensified television camera. Red blood cells are fluorescently labeled to enhance contrast. The velocity of RBCs is determined by placing two windows 10 to 25 μm apart over the vessel.

Laser Doppler flowmetry is a companion technique to the measurement of RBC velocity by videomicroscopy.[32] With this method, a signal is produced that is proportional to the flux of RBCs. The flow signal produced by laser Doppler flowmetry in the renal cortex is proportional to whole kidney blood flow measured with an electromagnetic flow probe.

The laser Doppler technique requires that the papilla be illuminated with light from a helium-neon laser. Light that interacts with moving RBCs in the tissue is shifted in frequency and creates an alternating current signal in the detection instrument.

E. ISOLATED RENAL MICROVESSELS

The isolated resistance arterial vessel technique was developed to determine the effects of vasoactive agents in the absence of confounding systemic and renal parenchymal neurohumoral influences. In addition, this model permits the determination of intrinsic vascular vs. extrinsic factors in disorders of vascular reactivity. Arterial vessels are isolated from the kidney in two ways. In the rabbit, the interlobular artery and afferent and efferent arterioles are dissected directly from slices of kidney cortex.[33] While direct dissection has been attempted to obtain rat microvessels, the yield has been unacceptably low. Therefore, a method involving sieving of glomeruli and removal of afferent and efferent arterioles from these glomeruli has been developed.[34] The microvessels are cannulated and perfused, while maintaining physiologic intraluminal pressures. Changes in vessel diameter are measured in response to vasoactive agents and the relative effects of these agents on the pre- and postglomerular vasculature determined. Recently, the isolated vessel technique has been modified further so that fluorescence measurements of smooth muscle cell calcium can be made simultaneously with changes in lumen diameter.

The basic isolated microvessel technique requires videomicroscopy capability and a microperfusion system. Measurement of changes in smooth muscle cell ions requires a fluorescence imaging system.

F. ENDOTHELIAL AND SMOOTH MUSCLE CELL CULTURES

A significant problem with the microvascular preparations described above is that the nature of the preparations does not yield sufficient tissue for biochemical measurements. Therefore, there are some questions involving cellular messengers such as phospholipases and protein kinases that are more profitably examined in vascular cell cultures. Isolated endothelial, smooth muscle and mesangial, or co-cultures of these cells can be studied for cellular mechanisms.[35]

REFERENCES

1. **Kriz, W. and Kaissling, B.,** Structural organization of the mammalian kidney, in *The Kidney: Physiology and Pathophysiology,* Seldin, D. W. and Giebisch, G., Eds., Raven Press, New York, 1991.
2. **Brenner, B. M. and Humes, H. D.,** Mechanics of glomerular ultrafiltration, *N. Engl. J. Med.,* 297, 148–154, 1977.
3. **Farquhar, M. G.,** The primary glomerular filtration barrier — basement membrane or epithelial slits?, *Kidney Int.,* 8, 197–205, 1975.
4. **Robertson, C. R., Deen, W. M., Troy, J. L., and Brenner, B. M.,** Dynamics of glomerular ultrafiltration in the rat. III. Hemodynamics and autoregulation, *Am. J. Physiol.,* 223, 1191–1200, 1972.
5. **Schnermann, J.,** Vascular tone as a determinant of tubuloglomerular feedback responsiveness, in *Symposium on the Juxtaglomerular Apparatus,* Fernstrom, E. K., Ed., A. E. G. Persson and U. Bakrg, Elsevier, Amsterdam, 1988, 393–406.
6. **Castleman, B. and Smithwick, R. J.,** The relationship of vascular disease to the hypertensive state. II. The adequacy of renal biopsy as determined from a study of 500 patients, *N. Engl. J. Med.,* 239, 729–738, 1948.
7. **Parving, H. H.,** Microvascular permeability to plasma proteins in hypertension and diabetes mellitus in man — On the pathogenesis of hypertensive and diabetic microangiopathy, *Danish Med. Bull.,* 22, 217–233, 1975.
8. **Cannon, P. J., Hassar, M., Case, D. B., Casarella, W. J., Sommers, S. C., and LeRoy, E. C.,** The relationship of hypertension and renal failure in scleroderma to structural and functional abnormalities of the renal cortical circulation, *Medicine,* 53, 1–22, 1974.

9. **Lieberman, E., Heuser, E., Donnell, G. N., Landing, B. H., and Hammond, G. C.,** Hemolytic-uremic syndrome: Clinical and pathologic considerations, *N. Engl. J. Med.*, 275, 229–240, 1966.

10. **Pitcock, J. A., Muirhead, E. E., Hatch, F. E., Johnson, J. G., and Kelly, B. J.,** Early renal changes in sickle cell anemia, *Arch. Pathol.*, 90, 403–411, 1970.

11. **Balow, J. E.,** Renal vasculitis, *Kidney Int.*, 27, 954–964, 1985.

12. **Fauci, A. S., Haynes, B. F., Katz, P., and Wolff, S. M.,** Wegener's granulomatosis. Prospective clinical and therapeutic experience with 85 patients in 21 years, *Ann. Intern. Med.*, 98, 76–85, 1983.

13. **Clutterbuck, E. J., Evans, D. J., and Pusey, C. D.,** Renal involvement in Churg-Strauss syndrome, *Nephrol. Dial. Transplant.*, 5, 161–170, 1990.

14. **Adams, P. L., Adams, P. F., Bell, P. D., and Navar, L. G.,** Impaired renal blood flow autoregulation in ischemic acute renal failure, *Kidney Int.*, 18, 68–76, 1980.

15. **Conger, J. D., Robinette, J. B., and Hammond, W. S.,** Differences in vascular reactivity in models of ischemic acute renal failure, *Kidney Int.*, 39, 1087–1097, 1991.

16. **Kelleher, S. P., Robinette, J. B., Miller, F., and Conger, J. D.,** Effects of hemmorrhagic reduction in blood pressure on recovery from acute renal failure, *Kidney Int.*, 31, 725–730, 1987.

17. **Kho, T. L., Leunissen, K. M. L., and Heidendahl, P. L.,** Cyclosporine and urinary prostaglandins, *Transplant. Proc.*, (Suppl. 3), 650–653, 1988.

18. **Folkow, B.,** The "structural factor" in hypertension with special emphasis on the hypertrophic adaptation of the systemic resistance vessels, in *Hypertension: Pathophysiology, Diagnosis and Management*, Laragh, J. H. and Brenner, B. M., Eds., Raven Press, New York, 1990, 505–581.

19. **McAnulty, R. J. and Laurent, G. J.,** Collagen synthesis and degradation *in vivo*. Evidence for rapid rates of collagen turnover with extensive degradation of newly synthesized collagen in tissues of adult rat, *Collagen Relat. Res.*, 7, 93–104, 1987.

20. **Deuel, T. F.,** Polypeptide growth factors. Roles in normal and abnormal cell growth, *Annu. Rev. Cell Biol.*, 3, 443–492, 1987.

21. **Rucala, R., Tacey, K. J., and Cerami, A.,** Advanced glycosylation products quench nitric oxide and mediate defective endothelium-dependent vasodilation in experimental diabetes, *J. Clin. Invest.*, 87, 432–438, 1991.

22. **Garg, U. C. and Hassid, A.,** Nitric oxide-generating vasodilators and 8-bromo-cyclic guanosine monophosphate inhibit mitogenesis and proliferation of cultured rat vascular smooth muscle cells, *J. Clin. Invest.*, 83, 1774–1777, 1989.

23. **Ruoslahtic, E.,** Integrins, *J. Clin. Invest.*, 87, 105–110, 1991.

24. **Smith, C. W., Marlin, S. D., Rothlein, R., Toman, C., and Anderson, D. C.,** Cooperative interaction of LFA-1 and MAC-1 with ICAM in facilitating adherence and transendothelial migration, *J. Clin. Invest.*, 83, 2008–2017, 1989.

25. **Pitts, R. F.,** *Physiology of the Kidney and Body Fluids*, Year Book Medical, Chicago, 1968.

26. **Stein, J. H.,** Regulation of the renal circulation, *Kidney Int.*, 38, 571–576, 1990.

27. **Deen, W. M., Robertson, C. R., and Brenner, B. M.,** A model of glomerular ultrafiltration in the rat, *Am. J. Physiol.*, 223, 1178–1180, 1972.

28. **Steinhausen, M., Snoei, H., Parekh, N., Baker, R., and Johnson, P. C.,** Hydronephrosis: A new method to visualize vas afferens, efferens, and glomerular network, *Kidney Int.*, 23, 794–806, 1983.

29. **Loutzenhiser, R., Hayashi, K., and Epstein, M.,** Atrial natriuretic peptide reverses afferent arteriolar vasoconstriciton and potentiates efferent arteriolar vasoconstriction in the isolated perfused rat kidney, *J. Pharmacol. Exp. Ther.*, 246, 522–528, 1988.

30. **Casellas, D. and Navar, L. G.,** *In vitro* perfusion of juxtamedullary nephrons from rats, *Am. J. Physiol.*, 246, F349–F358, 1984.

31. **Zimmerhackl, B., Tinsman, J., Jamison, R. L., and Robertson, C. R.,** Use of digital cross-correlation for on-line determination of single-vessel blood flow in the mammalian kidney, *Microvasc. Res.*, 30, 63–74, 1985.

32. **Roman, R. J. and Smits, C.,** Laser-Doppler determination of papillary blood flow in young and adult rats, *Am. J. Physiol.*, 251, F115–F124, 1986.

33. **Edwards, R. M.,** Segmental effects of norepinephrine and angiotensin II on isolated renal microvessels, *Am. J. Physiol.*, 244, F526–F534, 1983.

34. **Yuan, B. H., Robinette, J. B., and Conger, J. D.,** Effect of angiotensin II and norepinephrine on isolated rat afferent and efferent arterioles, *Am. J. Physiol.*, 258, F741–F750, 1990.

35. **Goligorsky, M.,** Role of endothelium in endotoxin blockade of voltage-sensitive calcium channels in smooth muscle cells, *Am. J. Physiol.*, 257, C875–C881, 1989.

Chapter 19

Liver Microcirculation

Ingo Marzi and Masaya Oda

CONTENTS

I. ANATOMY AND FUNCTION

A. THE HEPATIC MICROCIRCULATORY UNIT

The hepatic microcirculatory system consists of four microvascular components: the terminal portal venule (TPV) and the terminal hepatic arteriole (THA) as two afferent vessels, the sinusoids corresponding to the capillary bed, and the terminal hepatic venule (THV) as an efferent vessel. 70 to 75% of the blood flow to the liver is supplied by the portal vein, while the remaining is supplied by the hepatic artery. By intravital microscopy, the blood is seen entering the sinusoids located between the liver cell cords predominantly from the TPV, and also directly from the THA in part as a pulsatile jet stream.[1] The sinusoidal blood flow is directed in radial fashion from the periportal area (zone 1) to the middle zone (zone 2), further reaching the pericentral area (zone 3), where the blood drains into the THV.[1] This circuit pattern corresponding to the smallest hepatic microcirculatory unit has led to the concept of "liver acinus," consisting of the portal tract as an axis in the center and of the terminal hepatic venules in the periphery. From a functional point of view, the simple liver acinus more properly represents the microvascular unit of the liver than the classical hexagonal pattern of the hepatic lobule.[2]

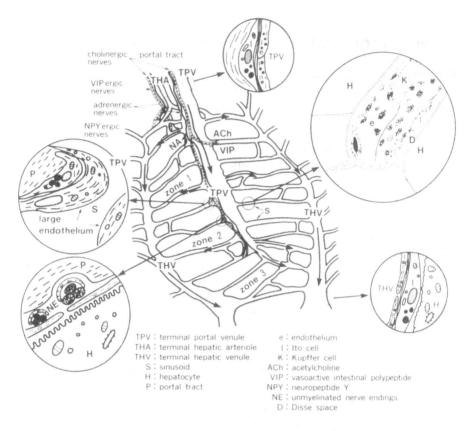

Figure 1 Summarized scheme for regulatory factors in the hepatic microcirculatory system. (From Oda, M., et al., *Prog. Appl. Microcirc.*, 19, 25, 1993.)

Ultrastructurally, the hepatic sinusoids, the major component of the hepatic microvasculature, are characterized by the presence of a large number of sieve plate-like pores in the sinusoidal endothelium, i.e., the sinusoidal endothelial fenestrae (SEF)[3] and by the absence of the basement membrane beneath the sinusoidal endothelial cells, allowing active exchange of metabolites between the sinusoidal blood and the hepatocytes via the SEF. As schematically illustrated in Figure 1, Kupffer cells are present on the luminal surface of the sinusoidal endothelial lining cells, while Ito cells (fat-storing cells, perisinusoidal cells) are located in the perisinusoidal space (the space of Dissé), partly surrounding the abluminal surfaces of the endothelial lining cells. In the process of liver cell uptake of a solute within sinusoidal blood, the solute must move out of the sinusoidal lumen and move into the space of Dissé. This movement occurs after the solute interacts with the endothelial and Kupffer cell surfaces of the sinusoid, followed by passage through the endothelial fenestrations. Therefore, the transition of a solute from the sinusoid to the space of Dissé is affected by the size and distribution of the sinusoidal endothelial fenestrae that would be mediated by intracytoplasmic Ca^{2+} caldmodulin-actomyosin system.[4]

B. REGULATION OF HEPATIC MICROCIRCULATION

The regulatory mechanism of hepatic sinusoidal blood flow has not been fully understood. There is general agreement, however, that the adrenergic and cholinergic nerves directly innervate the portal venules and arterioles in the portal tract, regulating the sinusoidal blood flow. On the other hand, there has been increasing evidence that some peptides such as vasoactive intestinal polypeptide (VIP) and neuropeptide Y (NPY) coexist with the classical neurotransmitters, (noradrenaline and acetylcholine, respectively) in the nerve terminals. The VIP-, NPY-, substance P-, and calcitonin generated peptide-immunoreactive fibers have been shown to be present in the close vicinity of the afferent vessels, portal venules, and hepatic arterioles, implying that these peptides may also be involved in neural control of the hepatic hemodynamics.

Based on the current understanding of microvascular constriction and dilatation mechanism, a potent vasoconstrictor, endothelin, and a vasodilator, EDRF (endothelium-derived relaxing factor), i.e., nitric oxide, are considered to mediate the regulation of hepatic microcirculation. It has been proposed that the inlet and the outlet sphincters may be important in the regulation of the blood flow through the hepatic sinusoids. In spite of extensive studies up to now, there has been no ultrastructural evidence for the existence of smooth muscle-like structures at the inlets and outlets of sinusoids. In recent years, intravital epifluorescence and electron microscopic studies have revealed that Ito cells are located as pericytes, not only in the perisinusoidal spaces but also along the TPVs and THVs,[5,6] possibly contributing to the control of sinusoidal blood flow. It is noteworthy that Ito cells particularly located at the junctional portions where the nonmuscular TPVs directly connect with the sinusoids would act as sphincters at the presinusoidal sites by their contractile activities recently proved *in vitro*.[7-9] This contractility of Ito cells is enhanced by endothelin 1,[8,9] that is proved to be directly bound to Ito cells *in vivo* by the recent autoradiographic study.[10] From another ultrastructural point of view, Ito cells possess long cytoplasmic processess and encircle the sinusoidal endothelial cells at the abluminal surfaces,[11] raising another possibility that Ito cells could contribute to the contraction and dilatation of hepatic sinusoids themselves, possibly in coordination with the contractile and relaxing activities of sinusoidal endothelial cells and sinusoidal endothelial fenestrae (SEF).[4] The opening and closure of the SEF would be involved in the regulatory mechanism of the sinsuoidal blood flow by controlling the sinusoidal plasma volume on the basis of filtration of plasma constituents into the perisinusoidal spaces through the SEF.[4] It has also been proposed that large endothelial cells located at the junctional portions between the TPVs and THAs and the sinusoids may function as sphincters by their contractility.[2,12] On the other hand, Kupffer cells have been demonstrated to be actively migrating on the abluminal surfaces of sinusoidal endothelial cells, not only *in vitro*[13] but also *in vivo*.[14] Kupffer cells possess an ability temporarily to block the flow of red blood cells through the sinusoid in some situations.[14] All the above-mentioned potential factors contributing to the regulation of hepatic sinusoidal blood flow are schematically illustrated in Figure 1.

II. PATHOLOGY

A. LIVER CIRRHOSIS

The most prominent structural and functional alterations of hepatic microvasculature are noted in liver cirrhosis, among a variety of human liver diseases. Cirrhosis is defined as the scarring of the liver acini in zone 3, zone 1, or in both, with the formation of the regenerating nodules and fibrous septa. The formation of scars in the liver has a most deleterious effect on the hepatic microcirculation by impending or oblitering some of its pathways. Collagenization of the space of Dissé with the appearance of a basement membrane beneath the sinusoidal endothelial cells and the formation of intrahepatic portohepatic shunts are the two major anatomical alterations. The former is called the capillarization of hepatic sinusoids.[15] Not only the deposition of glycosaminoglycans, type I, IV collagen, and laminin in the perisinusoidal space, but also the decrease of the sinusoidal endothelial fenestrae (SEF) both in number and diameter would interrupt the

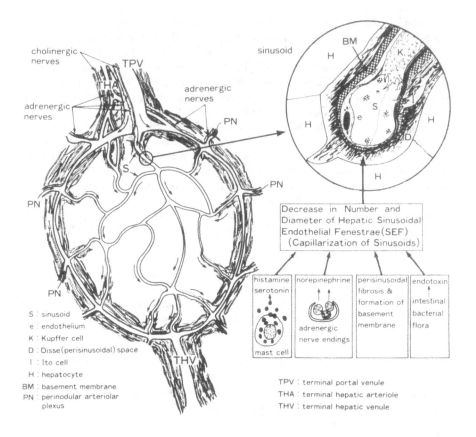

Figure 2 Schematic illustration of the hepatic microvascular alterations in liver cirrhosis. (Redrawn from Oda, M., et al., in *Microcirculation in Circulatory Disorders*, Manabe, H., Zweifach, B. W., and Messmer, K., Eds., Springer-Verlag, Tokyo, 1988, 121–133.)

transition of sinusoidal plasma into the perisinusoidal space,[16] resulting in disturbances of oxygen and nutrient supply to the hepatocytes and thereby contributing to a vicious cycle for self-perpetuating progression of liver cirrhosis, as schematically illustrated in Figure 2. These structural changes of hepatic sinusoids also contribute not only to an increase in microvascular resistance in the liver, leading to portal hypertension, but also to the formation of portohepatic shunts in the fibrous septa, clinically indicating a poor prognosis of patients with liver cirrhosis. According to a clinical study to measure hepatic local blood flow by reflectance spectrophotometry during peritoneoscopy,[17] the hepatic tissue blood hemoglobin concentration significantly decreases with progression of chronic hepatitis to cirrhosis.

It is well known that serum norepinephrine and endotoxin levels are elevated in patients with cirrhosis. The former is derived from the activated adrenergic nerve terminals in the liver, being concerned with microcirculatory derangements in liver cirrhosis. The initial responses to endotoxemia are considered to take place at the microcirculatory level in an affected organ. The low levels of gut-derived endotoxin normally present in the portal blood may modulate Kupffer cell functions and contribute to the maintenance of nonspecific resistance through the release of beneficial meditors. Higher levels of endotoxin, however, can cause the excessive release of toxic mediators and Kupffer cell dysfunction. *In vivo* microscopy reveals that the hepatic sinusoidal blood flow drops dramatically, concomitant with the changes in Kupffer cell phagocytosis, following endotoxin injection.[18] The functional failure of Kupffer cells to clean additional endotoxin from the blood would result in liver injury and systemic endotoxemia. Endotoxin may induce mast cell degranulation, probably through the activation of complements. The number of mast cells is increased with advance of liver cirrhosis. Vasoactive substances such as serotonin and histamine released from mast cells may affect sinusoidal endothelial cells and Kupffer cells, as well as microvascular functions. Thus, a general inflammatory response, adhesion of leukocytes, disturbances of blood flow, and Kupffer cell dysfunction, has been observed under such conditions.[19,20] The above-mentioned hepatic microvascular alterations and their related factors are schematically summarized in Figure 2. In acute ethanol challenge to the liver, changes of blood flow were reported to be heterogenous.[20] However, there is recent evidence that endothelin and nitric oxide are involved in ethanol-induced vasoconstriction.[21]

B. FULMINANT HEPATITIS

Pathological fulminant hepatitis is characterized by massive bridging necrosis extending from zone 3 to zone 1. It has been pointed out that disseminated intravascular coagulation (DIC) is related to the massive collapse of hepatocytes in this pathological state. It seems likely that platelet aggregations take place in the sinusoids, extensively blocking the sinusoidal blood flow and thereby causing massive cell necrosis. The mechanism of microthrombus formation within the sinusoids remains to be further elucidated. In recent years, continuous infusion of prostaglandin (PG)E_1 has been reported to be beneficial to the rescue of patients with fulminant hepatitis.[22] The efficacy of this treatment is considered to be due to the improvement of hepatic microcirculatory disturbances by PGE_1-induced vasodilating action.

C. SHOCK LIVER

Autoregulation works to some extent in the hepatic microcirculatory system to maintain a constant blood flow through the liver in response to hemorrhagic shock. In severe hemorrhagic shock exceeding this autoregulatory capacity of the liver, sinusoidal blood is decreased, leading to hepatocellular injury in zone 3 (centrilobular necrosis) according to the decreasing oxygen gradient. However, there is evidence that oxygen radical-mediated injury is highest in zone 2.[23,24] Dual digital microfluographic analysis using rhodamine-123 and propidium iodide indicates that during low-flow hypoxia, mitochondrial dysfunction in zone 3 may be essential for inducing xanthine oxidase-mediated oxidative liver cell damage in zone 2.[23,25]

Following hemorrhagic shock, depressed sinusoidal blood flow was reported earlier using a transillumination technique.[26] Applying indocyanine green clearance method, Wang et al.[27] have demonstrated a significant decrease of effective hepatic blood flow after hemorrhagic shock in the rat. Sequential alterations of sinusoidal perfusion and leukocyte margination after hemorrhagic shock have been shown by epi-fluorescence microscopy, further evidence that inflammatory mediators (e.g., leukotrienes and TNF) contribute to liver microcirculatory dysfunction.[28,29] Using such models, therapeutic approaches to improve liver microvascular failure are evaluated.[29-31]

D. ISCHEMIA/REPERFUSION INJURY AND TRANSPLANTATION

Based on the current concept of ischemia/reperfusion injury, reoxygenation of tissue after prolonged ischemia enhances ischemia-induced cell damage concomitant with microvascular injury.[32] Recently, epi-fluorescence microscopy was applied for assessment of the microcirculatory events following ischemia and reperfusion of the liver under various conditions. In the first studies following liver transplantation, severe microcirculatory disturbances and pathological adhesion of leukocytes were demonstrated in the rat model.[33-35] In subsequent studies, different patterns of leukocyte-endothelial interactions in liver sinusoids were observed, depending on the duration of ischemia and reperfusion.[36-38] There is strong evidence that oxygen radicals contribute to pathological adhesion of leukocytes to the sinusoidal endothelium, either by direct injury or induction of adhesion receptors.[36] Moreover, Kupffer cells activated during the post-ischemic reperfusion period in liver grafts have direct impact on sinusoidal leukocyte adhesion, involving calcium and most likely various inflammatory mediators.[39,40] Interestingly, it was demonstrated that pathological leukocyte adhesion in liver sinusoids is most pronounced in zone 1 and 2 of the liver acinus, where most of the Kupffer cells are located,[41] suggesting a paracrine regulation of leukocyte adhesion in the liver. Following warm ischemia of the liver, microcirculatory disturbances and increased leukocyte adhesion, including a no reflow-phenomenon, were observed.[42] Such a model was investigated earlier by Clemens and co-workers,[43,44] demonstrating beneficial effects of ATP –MgCl$_2$ and conjugated desferoxamine on hepatic microvascular injury after warm liver ischemia.

III. MODELS AND TECHNIQUES

There are *in vitro* and *in vivo* approaches to study liver microcirculation. Using *in vitro* methods such as isolated liver perfusion models, the metabolism up to sublobular compartments of the liver can be determined in addition to microcirculatory aspects. However, a major disadvantage of *in vitro* approaches appears to be that any influence of systemic circulation is excluded. *In vivo* methods such as laser Doppler flowmetry (LDF) or washout approaches allow for unspecific assessment of the hepatic microcirculation. For detailed studies requiring high resolution and magnification, intravital microscopy of the liver is a powerful and fascinating approach. It allows morphological and functional studies by use of either trans-illuminescence or epi-illuminescence techniques.

A. *IN VITRO* METHODS
1. Liver Perfusion
Most studies with isolated perfusion of the liver are performed in a nonrecirculating bloodless manner,[45] but also studies in a circulating system with blood or blood components are possible. While the majority of these studies were undertaken for assessment of biochemical functions, microcirculation and Kupffer cell functions were also investigated in sublobular regions of the liver.[46-48] The isolated rat liver perfusion (IRLP) in a bloodless nonrecirculating system is the most commonly used model.[45] Using this model, numerous functional parameters (e.g., oxygen uptake, bile flow), biochemical parameters (e.g., carbohydrate metabolism), and markers of injury (e.g., lactate dehydrogenase release) allow overall monitoring of the liver during the experiments. While most of these markers indicate parenchymal functions, evaluation of Kupffer cell activity is possible by addition of colloidal carbon to the perfusion solution and continuous spectrophotometric assessment of the outflowing perfusate at 623 nm.[49] As a rough method for assessment of perfused liver tissue, addition of trypan blue (200 μM) to the perfusate prior to fixation of the liver allows histological quantification of viable and nonviable (stained) liver cells in perfused sublobular regions.[50] To include blood or blood components into the liver perfusion system, the IRLP has to be modified into a recirculating system.[51]

2. Assessment of Microcirculation in Perfused Liver
Micro-Light Guides
Lobular and sublobular microcirculation can be estimated on the liver surface by addition of fluorescein isothiocyanate dextran (64 kDa, 12 μM) to the Krebs-Henseleit perfusion solution. Placing micro-light guides with tip diameters of 2 mm, 400 μm, or 170 μm onto the surface of the liver, fluorescence from fluorescein-dextran can be measured with a

photomultiplier. Excitation wavelengths of 400 to 460 nm are produced with a xenon lamp and light at wavelengths less than 515 nm is removed by appropriate filters. With the larger tips, lobular liver perfusion, and with the smaller one, sublobular perfusion can be successfully applied.[52] The rationale for these measurements is that the extracellular space in the liver consists of the vascular space and the space of Dissé (less than 20%). Thus, dilution of fluorescein dextran, confined largely to the extracellular space, reflects mainly the vascular space in the perfused liver, determined as 34% of the total liver volume. Interestingly, it has been demonstrated that the vascular space is about 60% larger in the pericentral region than in the periportal region.[46,52]

3. Reflectance Spectrophotometry

Reflectance spectrophotometry allows determination of hepatic tissue blood flow *in situ* (IHb) and oxygen saturation of hemoglobin in regional hepatic tissue capillaries (ISO_2).[53] Briefly, IHb is determined by the difference in absoption between 569 and 650 nm in the reflectance spectra, since a good correlation between the local tissue hemoglobin concentration and IHb has been established. A light-conducting fiber-optic bundle consisting of fibers for incident and reflected light is gently placed on the surface of the liver and measurements at several randomly selected points or in sublobular regions are taken.[53,54] This method is applicable for *in vitro* liver perfusion in a recirculating system with blood or *in vivo*.[55]

B. *IN VIVO* GLOBAL METHODS

There are several methods allowing evaluation of global and relative changes of the hepatic microcirculation, in part with additional topographical and functional information. Blood pressure can be measured directly in both portal veins and collecting hepatic venules by micropuncture in the trans-illuminated rat liver.[56]

1. Optical Methods
Laser Doppler Flowmetry

The principle of laser Doppler flowmetry is that an infrared laser with a wavelength of 780 ± 20 nm (1.6 mW) emits and penetrates up to 1 mm. Optical fibers of the flow probe conduct the laser beam to the tissue and the reflected light back to the photodetectors. Since the photons interact with moving red blood cells and stationary tissue cells, the portion of photons reflected and Doppler shifted indicates proportionally the moving microvascular blood volume and, by the frequency, the red blood cell velocity without indication of flow direction. A laser Doppler blood perfusion monitor and a flow probe available in different angles may be used for investigation of the liver surface following laparotomy.[57] However, absolute measurements of blood flow are questionable so that relative measurements are recommended.[58] Thus, LDF allows for monitoring tissue perfusion when a sufficient number of representative areas are scanned.[59] For reflectance spectrophotometry *in vivo*, see previous section.

2. Clearance Measurement Methods

Indocyanine green (ICG) is the most important clearance measurement method to estimate liver blood flow. The method is based on the Fick's principle and described, for example, by Keiding.[60] Usually, ICG (0.333 mg/kg body weight in 0.05 ml; Cardio-Green, Becton Dickinson Microbiology Systems, Cockeysville, MD) is injected intravenously and the clearance curve of ICG is measured by spectrometry or HPLC from blood samples withdrawn.[61] Also continuous recording using a hemoreflectometer and computer-assisted data acquisition system was described;[62] however, under pathological conditions such as cirrhosis, a decreased extraction of ICG may occur.[60]

In the hydrogen gas clearance method, platinum electrodes are inserted into right and middle liver lobe, respectively, and a reference electrode is placed in the abdominal cavity. Hydrogen gas is inhaled from the nasopharynx of the animal and hepatic regional blood flow (ml/min/100 g liver tissue) is determined by continuous recording of hydrogen gas clearance rate using a tissue blood flowmeter (Unique Medical MHG-D1). Such techniques have been reported in liver transplantation models.[63] Other methods applied are [85]Krypton clearance,[59] [133]Xenon washout curve, or galactosamine washout.[60,64]

3. Electromagnetic Flowmetry and Magnetic Resonance Imaging (MRI)

Electromagnetic flowmetry allows assessment of arterial and venous contributions to the hepatic blood flow and shows a higher accuracy than the ICG method.[61] It is, however, restricted to direct access to the liver with complete dissection of the vessels from surrounding tissue. Different flow probes connected to a electromagnetic blood flowmeter (e.g., Carolina Medicals Electronics, King, NC) are required to fit most precisely around the vessel.[65] Magnetic resonance imaging (MRI) offers a new noninvasive approach for determination of liver perfusion.[66]

C. IN VIVO METHODS: INTRAVITAL MICROSCOPY

The most powerful approach to investigate hepatic microcirculation under physiological and pathological conditions is intravital microscopy of the liver because it allows direct visualization of blood flow as well as of the vascular sinusoidal bed. Transillumination techniques allow for direct investigation of blood flow, white blood cell movements, and regulation of the sinusoids. A major disadvantage is that investigations must be performed on the thin edge of the liver, which is often irrepresentatively perfused under pathological conditions. Alternatively, epi-illuminescence microscopy may be applied, which generally requires injection of fluorescence dyes of plasma of specific blood cells for contrast enhancement.

1. Transilluminescence Technique

Following anesthesia, the edge of a small laboratory animal (e.g., mouse or rat) is gently exteriorized through a 2-cm right subcostal incision and positioned over a window in a specially designed plexiglass stage. The window overlies a long-working distance condenser of a modified microscope (e.g., Leitz Panphot or Nikon TMD inverted microscope). The liver is further covered by a piece of Saran Wrap® fixed to a movable U-shaped frame. This construction limits movements induced by respiration and heart beat; however, it is flexible enough not to cause impairment of hepatic microcirculation. Homeostasis is achieved by continuous irrigation with Ringers's solution and additional temperature control (37°C). Transillumination of the liver can be performed with monochromatic light (550–750 nm) from a prism monochrometer equipped with a Xenon lamp (Leitz, XBO-150). The microscope tube is positioned over the transilluminated area and microscopic images of the microvasculature allowed magnifications of 200 to 1350× using appropriate objectives of 8 to 100×. Optical images are recorded using a low-light video camera and video recording system (for further details see References 19, 67, and 68). A high-resolution Chalnicon camera (Hamamatsu) connected to an image processor incorporating analog enhancement (Hamamatsu Argus 100/VEC) leads to further improvement of the system.[4]

2. Epi-Illuminescence Technique

The rat is turned with the abdomen opened and adhesions dissected to the left side on a specially designed plexiglass stage, allowing gentle exteriorization of the left liver lobe with the plane lower surface uppermost.[35] The liver surface is continuously irrigated with

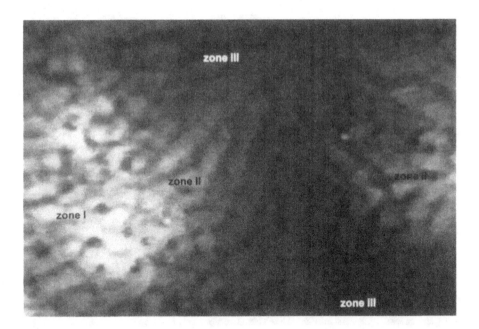

Figure 3 Intravital micrograph of a rat liver lobule in using epi-illuminescence microscopy. Bright areas indicate zone I, where the fluorescence dye is taken up first. Note network-like arrangement in zone I and a radial arrangement of sinusoids in zone 3 draining into the THV. Optical magnification was 330×.

Ringer's lactate at 37°C and covered with plastic foil (Saran Wrap) to prevent drying or surface injury. The hepatic microcirculation is then investigated using a fluorescence microscope (e.g., Nikon MM-11) with the following configuration: 100-W mercury lamp, 545-nm filter, 12× ocular, 10× and 20× (40×) water immersion objectives, 0.7–2.25 zoom objective. The experiments are recorded with a low-light CCD camera (FK6990, Pieper, Schwerte, Germany) that is connected to the microscopic system by a C-mount adapter, a serial time date generator (VTG 33, FOR-A company, Tokyo, Japan), and a SVHS video recording system (Panasonic, FS1, Tokyo, Japan).[28,36,39]

Acridine orange (1 μmol/kg, Sigma, St. Louis) is given as fluorescence marker of leukocytes, allowing assessment of sinusoidal perfusion and leukocyte endothelial interactions.[69] For determination of red blood cell velocity, *ex vivo* FITC-labeled erythrocytes are used, as originally described by Zimmerhackl et al. in a modified technique.[70] The labeled cells are stored at +4°C after addition of citrate-phosphate-dextrose (1.4:10) up to 5 days. Two min prior to liver microscopy, 0.05 ml red cells, 1:1 diluted with normal saline, are injected into the isogenic recipient animals. For investigation of macrophage function, fluorescence-labeled latex particles of approximately 1-μm diameter (Polysciences) are injected intravenously, as described earlier.[39,67]

Different lobules of the livers are recorded during a 30-s period for dynamic evaluation of microvascular events (Figure 3). Thereafter, central venules are brought into the center of the image and the pericentral region is recorded for comparable determination of sinusoidal diameters (Figure 4). Evaluation of intravital microscopy is performed using a computer-based image analysis system (e.g., Lobulus, medvis, Saarlouis, Germany), allowing standard morphometric measurements and projection of overlays onto the digitized images; for example, at a specimen to mointor ratio of 1050:1 using the 10×

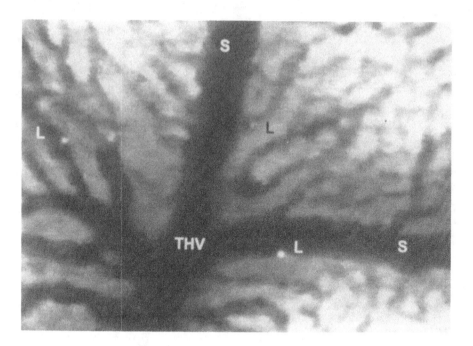

Figure 4 Intravital micrograph of zone 2 and 3 of a rat liver lobule using epi-fluorescence microscopy. White spots indicate leukocytes (L) adhering to the endothelial wall in liver sinusoids (S) or rolling in the THV. Optical magnification was 330×.

objective. Overlays are individually generated to identify the periportal, midzonal, and pericentral region by using one third of the distance between the center of the portal and central vein of each lobule. The following parameters may be evaluated as earlier defined:[28,36,39] (1) diameters of sinusoids, (2) acinar perfusion index,[71] (3) velocity of moving, nonadhering leukocytes and erythrocytes, (4) calculation of volumetric blood flow, (5) temporary adherent leukocytes, defined as leukocytes observed stationary at the sinusoidal wall between 0.2 and 20 s, (6) permanently adherent leukocytes, defined as leukocytes being stationary at the sinusoidal wall for a miminum of 20 s during the observation period, (7) slow rolling of leukocytes in THVs, and (8) phagocytic activity of Kupffer cells in portal and central regions.

The combination of the transillumination technique using an oblique illumination, together with epifluorescence, was recently applied to the liver with very high resolution, thus allowing magnifications up to the capacity of low-power electron microscopy.[14] This approach seems powerful to investigate sinusoidal pathophysiology at the cellular level.

IV. CONCLUSION

Various approaches for the investigation of hepatic microcirculation *in vitro* and *in vivo* are available. Depending on the investigative interest, global, regional, or sinusoidal microcirculation of the liver can be addressed specifically. For most of the clinically relevant situations, it should be possible to combine a clinically relevant model with one of the outlined investigative methods to understand the relevance of the hepatic microcirculation.

REFERENCES

1. **Rappaport, A. M.,** The microcirculatory hepatic unit, *Microvasc. Res.,* 6, 212, 1973.
2. **Oda, M., Nakamura, M., Watanabe, N., Ohya, Y., Sekizuka, E., Tsukada, N., Yonei, Y., Komatsu, H., Nagata, H., and Tsuchiya, M.,** Some dynamic aspects of the hepatic microcirculation — Demonstration of sinusoidal endothelial fenestrae as a possible regulatory factor, in *Intravital Observation of Organ Microcirculation,* Tsuchiya, M., Wayland, H., Oda, M., and Okazaki, I., Eds., Excerpta Medica, Amsterdam, 1984, 105–138.
3. **Wisse, E.,** An electron microscopic study of fenestrated endothelium lining of rat liver sinusoids, *J. Ultrastruct. Res.,* 31, 125, 1970.
4. **Oda, M., Azuma, T., Watanabe, N., Nishizaki, Y., Nishida, J., Ishii, K., Suzuki, H., Komatsu, H., Tsukada, N., and Tsuchiya, M.,** Regulatory mechanisms of the hepatic mirocirculation — Involvement of the contraction and dilatation of sinusoids and sinusoidal endothelial fenestrae, *Prog. Appl. Microcirc.,* 17, 103, 1990.
5. **Suematsu, M., Oda, M., Suzuki, H., Kaneko, H., Watanabe, N., Furusho, T., Masushige, T., and Tsuchiya, M.,** Intravital and electron microscopic observation of Ito cells in the rat hepatic microcirculation, *Microvasc. Res.,* 46, 28, 1993.
6. **Oda, M., Kaneko, H., Suematsu, M., Suzuki, H., Kazemoto, S., Honda, K., Yonei, Y., and Tsuchiya, M.,** A new aspect of the hepatic microcirculation: Electron microscopic evidence for the presence of Ito cells around the portal and hepatic venules as pericytes, *Prog. Appl. Microcirc.,* 19, 25, 1993.
7. **Pinzani, M., Failli, P., Ruocco, C., Casini, A., and Mitani, S.,** Fat-storing cells as liver-specific pericytes. Spatial dynamics of agonist-stimulated intracellular calcium transients, *J. Clin. Invest.,* 90, 642, 1992.
8. **Sakamoto, M., Ueno, T., Kin, M., Ohira, H., Torimura, T., Inuzuka, S., Sata, M., and Tanikawa, K.,** Ito cell contraction in response to endothelin-1 and substance P, *Hepatology,* 18, 978, 1993.
9. **Takaishi, H., Oda, M., Yokomori, H., Kaneko, H., Kazemoto, S., Suzuki, H., Suematsu, M., Komatsu, H., and Tsuchiya, M.,** A role of Ito cells in the hepatic microcirculation. Evidence for their contractility and actin filaments in primary culture, *Microcirc. Annu.,* 9, 99, 1993.
10. **Gondo, K., Uono, T., Sakamoto, M., Sakizaka, M., Sakizaka, S., Sata, M., and Tanikawa, K.,** The endothelin-1 binding site in rat liver tissue: Light- and electron-microscopic autoradiographic studies, *Gastroenterology,* 104, 1745, 1993.
11. **Ito, T.,** Participation of Ito cells in sinusoidal blood flow, in *Microcirculation — An Update,* Tsuchiya, M., Asane, M., Mishima, Y., and Oda, M., Eds., Excerpta Medica, Amsterdam, 1987, 321–324.
12. **Burkel, W. E.,** The fine structure of the hepatic arterial system of the rat, *Anat. Rec.,* 167, 329, 1970.
13. **Oda, M., Nishida, J., Honda, K., Nishizaki, Y., Yokomori, H., Ishii, K., Kaneko, H., Inoue, J., Watanabe, N., Nakamura, M., and Tsuchiya, M.,** Relation between sinusoidal endothelial cells and Kupffer cells in hepatic defence mechanisms, in *Frontiers of Mucosal Immunology,* Tsuchiya, M., Nagura, H., Hibi, T., and Moro, I., Eds., Excerpta Medica, Amsterdam, 1991, 193–196.
14. **Mac Phee, P., Schmidt, E. E., and Groom, A. C.,** Organization and flow in the liver microcirculation, *Prog. Appl. Microcirc.,* 19, 52, 1983.
15. **Schaffner, F. and Popper, H.,** Capillarization of hepatic sinusoid in man, *Gastroenterlogy,* 44, 234, 1963.
16. **Oda, M., Tsukada, N., Komatsu, H., Honda, K., Kaneko, K., Azuma, T., Ueno, M., Watanabe, N., Nakamura, M., Okazaki, I., and Tsuchiya, M.,** Abnormalities in the hepatic sinusoids: Pathological basis of self-perpetuation of liver cirrhosis, in *Microcirculation in Circulatory Disorders,* Manabe, H., Zweifach, B. W., and Messmer, K., Eds., Springer Verlag, Tokyo, 1988, 121–133.
17. **Sato, N., Hayashi, N., Kawano, S., Kamada, T., and Abe, H.,** Hepatic hemodynamics in patients with chronic hepatitis or cirrhosis as assessed by organ-reflectance spectrophotometry, *Gastroenterology,* 84, 611, 1983.

260

18. **McCuskey, R. S.,** Hepatic microvascular dysfunction during sepsis and endotemia, in *Cytoprotection and Cytobiology,* Tsuchiya, M., Ed., Excerpta Medica, Amsterdam, 1986, 3–17.

19. **McCuskey, R. S. and Reilly, F. D.,** Hepatic microvasculature: Dynamic structure and its regulation, *Semin. Liver. Dis.,* 13, 1, 1993.

20. **McCuskey, R. S.,** Hepatic microcirculation in disease, in *Sinusoids in Human Liver: Health and Disease,* Bioulac-Sage, P. and Balabaud, C., Eds., Kupffer Cell Foundation, Leiden, The Netherlands, 1988, 315–321.

21. **Oshita, M., Takei, Y., Kawano, S., Yoshihara, H., Hijioka, T., Fukui, H., Goto, M., Masuda, E., Nishimura, Y., Fusamoto, H., and Kamada, T.,** Roles of endothelin-1 and nitric oxide in the mechanism for ethanol-induced vasoconstriction in rat liver, *J. Clin. Invest.,* 91, 1337, 1993.

22. **Sinclair, S. R., Greig, P. D., Blendis, L. M., Abecassis, M., Roberts, E. A., Phillips, M. J., Cameron, R., and Levy, G. A.,** Biochemical and clinical response of fulminant hepatitis to administration of prostaglandin E, *J. Clin. Invest.,* 84, 1063, 1989.

23. **Marotto, M. E., Thurman, R. G., and Lemasters, J. J.,** Early midzonal cell death during low-flow hypoxia in the isolated, perfused rat liver: Protection by allopurinol, *Hepatology,* 8, 585, 1988.

24. **Komatsu, H., Koo, A., and Guth, P. H.,** Leukocyte flow dynamics in the rat liver microcirculation, *Microvasc. Res.,* 40, 1, 1990.

25. **Suematsu, M., Suzuki, H., Ishii, H., Kato, S., Hamamatsu, H., Miura, S., and Tsuchiya, M.,** Topographic dissociation between mitochondrial dysfunction and cell death during low-flow hypoxia in perfused rat liver, *Lab. Invest.,* 67, 434, 1992.

26. **Koo, A. and Liang, I. Y. S.,** Blood flow in hepatic sinusoids in experimental hemorrhagic shock in the rat, *Microvasc. Res.,* 13, 315, 1977.

27. **Wang, P., Ba, Z. F., Dean, R. E., and Chaudry, I. H.,** Diltiazem administration after crystalloid resuscitation restores active hepatocellular function and hepatic blood flow after severe hemorrhagic shock, *Surgery,* 110, 390, 1991.

28. **Marzi, I., Bauer, C., Hower, R., and Bühren, V.,** Leukocyte-endothelial cell interactions in the liver after hemorrhagic shock in the rat, *Circ. Shock,* 40, 105, 1993.

29. **Marzi, I., Bauer, M., Secchi, A., Redl, H., and Bühren, V.,** Tumor necrosis factor and leukocyte adhesion to the sinusoidal endothelium after hemorrhagic shock in the rat, in *Cells of the Hepatic Sinusoid, Vol. 4,* Wisse, E. and Knook, D. L., Eds., Kupffer Cell Foundation, Leiden, The Netherlands, 1993, 321–325.

30. **Flynn, W. J., Cryer, H. G., and Garrison, R. N.,** Pentoxifylline but not saralasin restores hepatic blood flow after resuscitation from hemorrhagic shock, *J. Surg. Res.,* 50, 616, 1991.

31. **Bauer, M., Marzi, I., Ziegenfuß, T., Seeck, G., Bühren, V., and Larsen, R.,** Comparative effects of crystalloid and small volume resuscitation on hepatic microcirculation after hemorrhagic shock, *Circ. Shock,* 40, 187, 1993.

32. **Granger, D. N.,** Role of xanthine oxidase and granulocytes in ischemia-reperfusion injury, *Am. J. Physiol.,* 255, H1269, 1988.

33. **Takei, Y., Marzi, I., Gores, G. J., Currin, R. T., Lemasters, J. J., and Thurman, R. G.,** Video microscopy of transplanted rat livers, in *Optical Microscopy for Biology,* Herman, B. and Jacobson, K., Eds., Wiley-Liss, New York, 1990, 487–496.

34. **Takei, Y., Marzi, I., Gores, G. J., Lemasters, J. J., and Thurman, R. G.,** Leukocyte adhesion and cell death following orthotopic liver transplantation in the rat, *Transplantation,* 51, 959, 1991.

35. **Marzi, I., Takei, Y., Knee, J., Menger, M. D., Gores, G. J., Bühren, V., Trentz, O., Lemasters, J. J., and Thurman, R. G.,** Assessment of reperfusion injury by intravital fluorescence microscopy following liver transplantation in the rat, *Transplant. Proc.,* 22, 2004, 1990.

36. **Marzi, I., Knee, J., Bühren, V., Menger, M. D., and Trentz, O.,** Reduction by superoxide dismutase of leukocyte-endothelial adherence after liver transplantation, *Surgery,* 111, 90, 1992.

37. **Marzi, I., Walcher, F., Bühren, V., Menger, M. D., Knee, J., and Trentz, O.,** Microcirculatory disturbances and leucocyte adherence in transplanted livers after cold storage in Euro-Collins, UW and HTK solutions, *Transpl. Int.,* 4, 45, 1991.

38. **Marzi, I., Knee, J., Bühren, V., Menger, M. D., Harbauer, G., and Trentz, O.,** Hepatic microcirculatory disturbances due to portal vein clamping in the orthotopic rat liver transplantation model, *Transplantation,* 52, 432, 1991.

39. **Marzi, I., Walcher, F., and Bühren, V.,** Macrophage activation and leukocyte adhesion after liver transplantation, *Am. J. Physiol.,* 265, G172, 1993.

40. Goto, M., Takei, Y., Kawano, S., Kashiwagi, T., Yoshihara, H., Tsuji, S., Fukui, H., Fushimi, H., Nishimura, Y., Fusamoto, H., and Kamada, T., Tumor necrosis factor and endotoxin are involved in the pathogenesis of liver and pulmonary injuries following orthotopic liver transplantation in the rat, *Hepatology*, 16, 487, 1992.

41. Bouwens, L., Baekeland, M., de Zanger, R., and Wisse, E., Quantitation, tissue distribution and proliferation kinetics of Kupffer cells in normal rat liver, *Hepatology*, 6, 718, 1986.

42. Koo, A., Komatsu, H., Tao, G., Inoue, M., Guth, P. H., and Kaplowitz, N., Contribution of no-reflow phenomenon to hepatic injury after ischemia-reperfusion: Evidence for a role for superoxide anion, *Hepatology*, 15, 507, 1991.

43. Clemens, M. G., McDonagh, P. F., Chaudry, I. H., and Baue, A. E., Hepatic microcirculatory failure after ischemia and reperfusion: Improvement with ATP-MgCl$_2$ treatment, *Am. J. Physiol.*, 248, H804, 1985.

44. Drugas, G. T., Paidas, C. N., Yahanda, A. M., Ferguson, D., and Clemens, M. G., Conjugated desferoxamine attenuates hepatic microvascular injury following ischemia/reperfusion, *Circ. Shock*, 34, 278, 1991.

45. Scholz, R., Hansen, W., and Thurman, R. G., Interaction of mixed-function oxidation with biosynthetic processes, *Eur. J. Biochem.*, 38, 64, 1973.

46. Conway, J. G., Popp, J. A., and Thurman, R. G., Microcirculation in periportal and pericentral regions of lobule in perfused rat liver, *Am. J. Physiol.*, 249, G449, 1985.

47. te Koppele, J. M. and Thurman, R. G., Phagocytosis by Kupffer cells predominates in pericentral regions of the liver lobule, *Am. J. Physiol.*, 259, G814, 1990.

48. Matsumura, T., Kauffman, F. C., Meren, H., and Thurman, R. G., O$_2$ uptake in periportal and pericentral regions of liver lobule in perfused liver, *Am. J. Physiol.*, 250, 800, 1986.

49. Cowper, K. C., Currin, R. T., Dawson, T. L., Lindert, K., Lemasters, J. J., and Thurman, R. G., A new method to monitor Kupffer-cell function continuously in the perfused rat liver, *Biochem. J.*, 266, 141, 1990.

50. Bradford, B. U., Marotto, M., Lemasters, J. J., and Thurman, R. G., New, simple models to evaluate zone-specific damage due to hypoxia in perfused rat liver: Time course and effect of nutritional state, *J. Pharmacol. Exp. Ther.*, 236, 263, 1986.

51. Clavien, P. A., Harvey, P. R., Sanabria, J. R., Cywes, R., Levy, G. A., and Strasberg, S. M., Lymphocyte adherence in the reperfused rat liver: Mechanisms and effects, *Hepatology*, 17, 131, 1993.

52. Ji, S., Lemasters, J. J., and Thurman, R. G., A non-invasive method to study metabolic events within sublobular regions of hemoglobin-free perfused liver, *FEBS Lett.*, 113(1), 37, 1980.

53. Sato, N., Matsumura, T., Shichiri, M., Kamada, T., Abe, H., and Hagihara, B., Hemoperfusion, rate of oxygen consumption and redox levels of mitochondrial cytochrome c (+c1) in liver *in situ* of anesthetized rat measured by reflectance spectrophotometry, *Biochim. Biophys. Acta*, 634, 1, 1981.

54. Chen, S. S., Yoshihara, H., Harada, N., Seiyama, A., Watanabe, M., Kosaka, H., Kawano, S., Fusamoto, H., Kamada, T., and Shiga, T., Measurement of redox states of mitochondrial cytochrome aa3 in regions of liver lobule by reflectance microspectroscopy, *Am. J. Physiol.*, 264, G375, 1993.

55. Goto, M., Kawano, S., Yoshihara, H., Takei, Y., Hijioka, T., Fukui, H., Matsunaga, T., Oshita, M., Kashiwagi, T., Fusamoto, H., Kamada, T., and Sato, N., Hepatic tissue oxygenation as a predictive indicator of ischemia-reperfusion liver injury, *Hepatology*, 15, 432, 1992.

56. Nakata, K., Leong, G. F., and Brauer, R. W., Direct measurement of blood pressures in minute vessels of the liver, *Am. J. Physiol.*, 105, 1984, 1960.

57. Shepherd, A. P., Riedel, G. L., Kiel, J. W., Haumschild, D. J., and Maxwell, L. C., Evaluation of an infrared laser-Doppler blood flowmeter, *Am. J. Physiol.*, 15, G832, 1987.

58. Smits, G. J., Roman, R. J., and Lombard, J. H., Evaluation of laser-Doppler flowmetry as a measure of tissue blood flow, *J. Appl. Physiol.*, 61, 666, 1986.

59. Almond, N. E. and Wheatley, A. M., Measurement of hepatic perfusion in rats by laser Doppler flowmetry, *Am. J. Physiol.*, 25, G203, 1992.

60. Keiding, S., Hepatic clearance and liver blood flow, *J. Hepatol.*, 4, 393, 1987.

61. Nxumalo, J. L., Teranaka, M., and Schenk, W. G., Hepatic blood flow measurement, *Arch. Surg.*, 113, 169, 1978.

62. Hauptman, J. G., DeJong, G. K., Blasko, K. A., and Chaudry, I. H., Measurement of hepatocellular function, cardiac output, effective blood volume, and oxygen saturation in rats, *Am. J. Physiol.*, 257, R439, 1989.

63. **Manner, M., Shult, W., Senninger, N., Machens, G., and Otto, G.,** Evaluation of preservation damage after porcine liver transplantation by assessment of hepatic microcirculation, *Transplantation,* 50, 940, 1990.
64. **Lalonde, C., Knox, J., Youn, Y.-K., and Demling, R.,** Relationship between hepatic blood flow and tissue lipid peroxidation in the early postburn period, *Crit. Care Med.,* 20, 789, 1992.
65. **Paulsen, A. W. and Klintmalm, G. B. G.,** Direct measurement of hepatic blood flow in native and transplanted organs, with accompanying systemic hemodynamics, *Hepatology,* 16, 100, 1992.
66. **Moore, J. R., Finn, J. P., and Edelman, R. R.,** Measurement of visceral blood flow with magnetic resonance imaging, *Invest. Radiol.,* 27, S103, 1992.
67. **McCuskey, R. S., Urbaschek, R., McCuskey, P. A., and Urbaschek, B.,** *In vivo* microscopic studies of the responses of the liver to endotoxin, *Klin. Wochenschr.,* 60, 749, 1982.
68. **McCuskey, R. S., Reilly, F. D., McCuskey, P. A., and Dimlich, R. V. W.,** *In vivo* microscopy of the hepatic microvascular system, *Biblthca. Anat.,* 18, 73, 1978.
69. **Jahanmehr, S. A. H., Hyde, K., Geary, C. G., Cinkotai, K. I., and Maciver, J. E.,** Simple technique for fluorescence staining of blood cells with acridine orange, *J. Clin. Pathol.,* 40, 926, 1987.
70. **Zimmerhackl, B., Parekh, N., Brinkhus, H., et al.,** The use of fluorescent labeled erythrocytes for intravital investigation of flow and local hematocrit in glomerular capillaries in the rat, *Int. J. Microcirc. Clin. Exp.,* 2, 119, 1983.
71. **Post, S., Menger, M. D., Rentsch, M., Gonzalez, A. P., Herfarth, C., and Messmer, K.,** The impact of arterialization on hepatic microcirculation and leukocyte accumulation after liver transplantation in the rat, *Transplantation,* 54, 789, 1992.

Chapter 20

Lung Microcirculation

Andrew M. Roberts and Dick W. Slaaf

CONTENTS

INTRODUCTION

Intravital microscopy has been widely used to directly observe microvascular blood flow and to measure microvascular hemodynamic variables in a number of vascular beds during physiological and pathophysiological circumstances. This basic technique has been adapted for use in the intact *in situ* lung. There are a number of challenges due to the dynamic characteristics of the lung and the unique anatomy of this vascular bed. Methods generally require opening the chest, controlling ventilation, and stabilizing movement. A number of approaches have been developed that enable observation of microvessels at the pleural surface in the intact lung during both static and dynamic conditions with the chest open or closed. Information about microvascular networks, blood flow, capillary transit time, permeability, and vascular responses during various conditions has been provided by the different preparations that have been used.

I. ANATOMY AND FUNCTION

A. VASCULAR ANATOMY

The pulmonary circulation consists of the output of the right ventricle which, via the pulmonary artery and its branches, sends mixed venous blood to the pulmonary capillaries where it undergoes gas exchange, and returns it via the pulmonary veins to the left atrium. Gas exchange is the primary function of the lungs and is achieved by the close approximation of pulmonary capillaries and alveoli. The other blood supply to the lungs is the bronchial circulation, which is a small fraction of the output of the left ventricle. It branches from the thoracic aorta or intercostal arteries and supplies arterial blood to the conducting airways and other structures such as the visceral pleura, esophagus, large blood vessels and nerves, and lymph nodes. Bronchial veins drain into pulmonary veins and also into systemic veins (the azygos and hemiazygos veins, which drain into the superior vena cava). Anastomoses between the bronchial and pulmonary circulations have been found in larger vessels between bronchial and pulmonary arterial branches, and

0-8493-4870-6/95/$0.00+$.50
© 1995 by CRC Press, Inc.

at the microcirculatory level between bronchial and pulmonary capillaries. Further discussion of the pulmonary and bronchial circulation is beyond the scope of this chapter, and the reader is referred to other articles.[9,14]

Each pulmonary artery branches to supply the various lobes of each lung as the arteries enter at the hila. Unlike in other tissues where one usually observes paired arteries and veins, pulmonary arteries branch and follow the bronchi centrally within the lobules, eventually distributing blood to the alveoli; pulmonary venules collect blood from the capillaries and drain into interlobular veins, which in many species run between lobules and come together to form larger veins, which exit the lungs at the hila.[20] Branching is not symmetrical and although successive branches are generally smaller, this is not always the case. At a particular level or generation, there is considerable variation in vessel size. Thus, especially where smaller arterioles form many branches, classification according to vessel size may put vessels of similar diameter at different generations of branching. The same holds for the centrifugal ordering method in which the generation number is increased at every branching point. Therefore, a functional branching ordering is often used, which increases the number of the branching order only if the vessel bifurcates into two (or more) branches of distinctly smaller diameter. In that case, a main feeder vessel will have the same order over a considerable length, although many (smaller) vessels of a different order might be fed. In a preparation such as the lung, where the feeding vessels cannot always be located, an alternate, centripetal ordering method may be used.[36] Ordering starts at the most distal branches and counts upwards from the alveolar capillaries. According to this scheme, when branches of different orders meet, the order of the larger branch does not change. Since the order does not change at every junction, side branches of similar size may join larger branches at different regions and be counted in the same order. Thus, vessels with similar characteristics such as diameter can be grouped together.

Morphological studies have shown that pulmonary arteries have thinner walls and less smooth muscle than systemic arteries of similar diameter.[6,20] The media of the largest pulmonary arteries has considerable elastic tissue in addition to smooth muscle, while the media of muscular pulmonary arteries has predominantly smooth muscle. Smaller arteries, unlike similar-sized systemic arteries, have a thinner media and relatively less smooth muscle. Pulmonary arteries generally have less smooth muscle as they become smaller and vessels may be classified as muscular, partially muscular (in that there is muscle in only part of the wall), or nonmuscular.[20,30] The proportion of elastic, muscular, partially muscular, or non-muscular arteries varies with diameter, and vessels less than 150 μm form a mixed population.[30] Although there is considerable species variation, pulmonary arterioles smaller than about 20 μm generally lack smooth muscle.[20] Cells with filaments that are capable of contraction have been found in nonmuscular regions of arteries, suggesting that these vessels may be capable of some contractile activity.[30]

A number of capillaries branch from each precapillary arteriole and may supply several alveoli. Capillary networks are an integral part of the alveolar wall and their configuration is largely influenced by the balance of transmural forces. Pulmonary capillaries are relatively short and are often flattened. In addition, they are so numerous that a popular concept is to describe alveolar blood flow as a sheet of fluid with posts (connective tissue) between alveolar walls.[13] Capillary blood is collected by very thin-walled venules. Larger pulmonary veins have elastic fibers, collagen, and smooth muscle in various amounts depending on size and species.[20]

B. VASCULAR FUNCTIONS

Compared to the systemic circulation, the pulmonary circulation is a low-pressure, low-resistance circuit with a relatively uniform function of supplying blood to the alveoli for gas exchange. Pulmonary blood vessels are effective in attenuating pressure and flow oscillations, and the mechanics of the pulmonary circulation are largely influenced by the interaction of a number of mechanical forces within the lungs and thorax.[6,7] Passive mechanisms, such as distension and recruitment of vessels, help to regulate pulmonary vascular resistance and are important for overall alveolar perfusion. Although the pulmonary vascular bed is capable of some neural regulation[10,12,18,34] and responds to a number of humoral substances,[2,29] under normal circumstances active vascular responses play a much smaller role in regulating tone than in the systemic circulation. Large active changes in dimensions are usually not seen as they are in systemic vessels and vascular regulation is largely affected by physical forces.[6] Although pulmonary arterioles are capable of active responses, they normally have a low tone and offer relatively little resistance to blood flow compared to the component due to larger arteries or the microvascular segment between the smallest arterioles and venules.[4,24,31] During pathophysiological conditions, however, active mechanisms may have a more significant influence on the tone of vascular smooth muscle and affect the overall pressure distribution and resistance.

II. PATHOLOGY

For a detailed description of lung pathology, refer to Chapter 7.

III. MODELS AND TECHNIQUES

Examination of the microcirculation of the lung presents unique technical challenges related to its relative inaccessibility within the thoracic cavity and to its inherent respiratory, as well as cardiogenic motion. Although its overall function is homogeneous, it is affected by the interrelationship of a number of dynamic mechanical factors, such as intravascular, intrapleural, and alveolar pressures, lung volume, and gravity, that cause regional variation. In addition to its complex anatomical arrangement, the vital function of the lung makes experimental manipulation difficult. Investigators have developed selective approaches for examination of certain factors and questions under controlled conditions, while excluding others. The applicability and limitations of some of the various measurement techniques used to study lung microcirculation are briefly discussed, and some methods for observing microvessels at the pleural surface in the intact lung using intravital microscopy are described.

The isolated perfused lung preparation has been reviewed in detail[3] and adapted for use in a number of species. It has been especially useful for investigating the pathophysiology of lung-liquid exchange and various types of lung injury because measurements of blood flow, vascular and interstitial pressures, and fluid accumulation can be determined under a variety of circumstances. The lungs (or an isolated lobe) can be perfused *in situ* or removed and variables can be controlled or altered. In general, catheters are placed in the pulmonary artery and left atrium (or a pulmonary vein) for connection to the perfusion circuit, and the lungs (or a lobe) are ventilated through a catheter inserted into the trachea (or a bronchus). For microvascular observations or measurements such as micropuncture,[5] the lung can be held statically inflated at a constant pressure. Pulmonary artery pressure, blood flow, venous pressure, and alveolar pressure or volume can be adjusted and the lungs can be perfused with constant flow or pressure. Thus, experimental interventions and measurements that would be extremely difficult to carry out in the intact lung may be possible in the isolated perfused preparation. Microvascular pressure profiles[3] and interstitial pressure gradients have been determined using micropipettes to puncture subpleural microvessels or the perimicrovascular interstitium. In isolated perfused rabbit lungs, the micropuncture method has also been used to measure pressure in larger microvessels (300–700 μm in diameter) approximately 2 to 3 mm below the pleura after exposing them by microsurgery.[32] This technique, while allowing direct measurement of pressure in intermediate-sized microvessels, causes trauma to the tissue surrounding a particular vessel, but has provided information about microvascular resistance and site of liquid filtration.

An advantage of the isolated preparation is that substances can be given intravascularly and responses are separated from confounding secondary systemic effects that may indirectly affect the lung. Because of the mechanical influence of changes in blood pressure on the pulmonary circulation, this technique may be particularly useful when examining vascular responses of chemicals. Like other isolated preparations, disadvantages include altered responsiveness and manipulation of physiological variables. Special considerations include effects of altering normal transpulmonary pressure relationships caused by opening the chest and establishing positive pressure ventilation.

Subpleural microvessels can also be directly examined in the *in situ* lung or in isolated perfused lungs using a laser Doppler technique. This method is based on the principle that light scattered by red blood cells undergoes a Doppler shift related to the flow velocity. By placing a "floating" laser probe on the surface of the lung, regional subpleural blood flows have been measured and effects of vasoactive agents have been studied.[15] Flow measurements reflect average tissue perfusion in an area below the probe and are usually given as arbitrary units. They are a function of probe position as well as the refractive index of the tissue. Whereas regional flows can be determined, a variety of vessels are included in the sample. However, measurement of blood flow velocity in individual pulmonary microvessels of the exposed lung has been accomplished in frogs with a laser Doppler microscope.[17] This technique incorporates optical methods to deliver and collect laser light, and allows quantitative measurements of blood flow velocity and pulsatile flow patterns in arterioles, venules, and capillaries that are visualized at the lung surface.

Whereas most techniques for examining the microcirculation of the lung are limited to vessels that can be visualized at the pleural surface, an X-ray angiographic method has been used to examine relatively small (100–150 μm) intraparenchymal arteries and veins in thick layers of tissue.[1,35] From videotaped sequential images recorded by an X-ray sensitive camera, it is possible to measure internal vascular diameter, cross-sectional area, flow velocity, volume flow, transit time, and to quantitate patterns of responses to vasoactive agents. The lung is positioned between an X-ray generator and an X-ray sensitive video camera of the imaging system. During measurements, ventilation is usually held constant for a brief period, while contrast medium is injected and images are obtained. As with other techniques, cardiovascular and respiratory variables can be monitored simultaneously. Although it is possible to obtain an overview of a range of vessels in a region, there are limitations due to rates of dynamic changes of radiopaque contrast medium in vessels, hemodynamic effects of contrast medium, precise localization, and absolute measurements of vessel dimensions. A great advantage, however, is that it is possible to visualize vessels at the surface or within the lung.

Others[8,41,42,44,45] have used fluorescence video microscopy to measure arterial or pulmonary capillary transit times through the subpleural microcirculation and to examine effects of variables such as gravity, airway pressure, lung inflation, and blood flow. Basically, this technique consists of injecting a bolus of fluorescent dye such as a fluorescein sodium solution and measuring the time for the dye to pass from arterioles to venules. An appropriate light source, filters, light-sensitive camera, and recording apparatus is required. Fluorescence microscopy has also been used to directly measure the transit of individual fluorescently labeled neutrophils through the pulmonary microcirculation and effects of hemodynamic changes on their sequestration.[26,27] Neutrophil transit times were compared to the rate of blood flow (plasma transit time) through the microvessels by determining the transit time of fluorescently labeled dextran. When used in conjunction with bright field illumination, microvascular networks can be examined and recorded with conventional video microscopy, thus combining analysis of flow patterns with morphology. Fluorescently labeled red blood cells have also been used to visualize blood flow and to measure red blood cell velocities and other microhemodynamic variables in pulmonary microvascular networks.[23-25] By injecting fluorescently labeled (fluorescein isothiocyanate) albumin and rhodamine dye (a fluorescent marker with a different molecular weight and excitation wavelength), it is also possible to use digital image analysis to examine the progression of macromolecular leakage of different-sized molecules from the pulmonary microcirculation into the alveoli.[11] As with other fluorescence methods, it is also possible to assess internal vascular diameters.

By modifying basic techniques that have been used to examine microvessels in peripheral vascular beds, it is possible to observe vessels and alveoli at or near the surface of the intact lung. After gaining access to the lungs and positioning a suitable microscope, light source, and filters, accommodations must be made for respiratory and cardiac motion of the tissue, while maintaining ventilation and a viable preparation. Early widely used methods, where the thorax was opened and the margin of a lobe was directly illuminated or transilluminated and examined with a compound microscope, have been summarized along with key developments that evolved.[43] Variations of this basic preparation have included viewing a relatively quiet lobe of the exposed lung in the open thorax during modified diffusion respiration to avoid respiratory movements or using an isolated perfused lung,[16,19,28] locally immobilizing the external surface of an artificially ventilated lung with a cover glass held *in situ* during a method of mechanical ventilation and continuous respiration,[39] viewing the lung through the intact parietal pleura without creating a pneumothorax,[46] or installing a thoracic window[22,38,43] and then closing the chest. In the thoracic window technique, when air is removed from the chest cavity, the lung re-expands and can be brought up to the window for examination with a dissecting or compound microscope. With this method, a relatively motionless area of lung tissue can be observed during spontaneous respiration using incident illumination.[40,43] A suction ring within the window has been incorporated to apply radial traction across the observation field and further reduce cardiorespiratory movement enabling high-resolution microscopy at greater magnification.[40] Although the window procedure has mainly been used for acute observations, it has been modified and designed so that it is possible to make repeated microscopic observations in the closed chest over longer times.[11,22,40]

Fluorescence video microscopy has been used in conjunction with a modified window technique to trace microvascular networks in the lung and to make morphometric and microhemodynamic measurements as well as to observe movement of fluorescently labeled cells.[23-27] In anesthetized rabbits and dogs, a transparent window was implanted in the chest wall, and various measures were taken to protect the lung surface. Negative pressure was applied inside the window so that part of the lung was moved flush to the window. In anesthetized rabbits whose lungs were ventilated with an oxygen mixture, intravenous injection of fluorescently labeled red blood cells enabled visualization of blood flow and allowed measurement of arteriolar and venular diameters, segment lengths, branching patterns, red blood cell velocity and flux, and capillary transit time.[23-25] These measurements were related to arterial blood pressure, pulmonary arterial pressure, left atrial pressure, and cardiac output, which were monitored simultaneously. A xenon lamp attached to a Ploemopak illuminator with a filter block (Leitz) for fluorescence was used for epi-illumination. Images were recorded onto videotape by a silicon-intensified target video camera that was mounted on a modified Leitz-Orthoplan microscope. Using a long focal length objective (10×) or a salt water immersion objective (25×), the total magnification on the video monitor was 360× or 930×. To avoid motion, observations were made during inspiration using an inversed (inspiratory to expiratory) ventilation ratio of 2 to 1 at a frequency of approximately 22 breaths per minute.

While the open chest preparation has advantages of accessibility, enabling larger areas and a number of different fields to be examined; the closed chest preparation affords the possibility of observing the lungs during conditions that are more physiologic, although there may be a certain amount of trauma associated with the procedures. In both preparations, it is possible to observe the lung microcirculation, either briefly during regular ventilation or for longer periods during intervals when the lungs are statically inflated. Breathing movements can be inhibited for a relatively longer time by a method involving tracheal insufflation or by keeping the lungs inflated to a regulated constant pressure with oxygen or an oxygen-rich mixture. Each of these preparations has been developed with specific goals in mind and has led to significant advances in knowledge about the lungs. The availability of sensitive video cameras has made it possible to work at relatively low light levels. The method of choice is the one that allows for the required time of observation, convenient illumination, and enough contrast and resolution to resolve structures of interest.

With a compound microscope and relatively low magnification objective lenses (4 to 25×), blood flow in arterioles, capillaries, and veins can be seen and the alveoli and related blood vessels can be examined. In general, at the pleural surface it is possible to directly observe responses of smaller blood vessels (usually less than 100 µm) and their flow under different conditions, or in response to chemicals applied locally or injected into the circulation. Arterioles and their branches can usually be found at the margins of the lobes where they can be seen coming up to the surface of the lung and identified by the direction of blood flow and branching structure relative to vessel size. Venules are identified as they collect blood from alveolar capillaries and join larger venules that go below the surface. Fine structural details can be examined using higher magnification if motion of the tissues can be minimized.

A. A METHOD TO EXAMINE PULMONARY MICROVESSELS IN THE INTACT LUNG USING A DIPPING CONE

The following is a description of a basic intravital microscopic technique for use in the *in situ* lung with the chest open. A modified dipping cone attached to the objective lens provides mobility with advantages of a coverglass or window and adds stability without using a suction ring. We have used this method for measuring changes in diameter of individual pulmonary arterioles and venules in response to vasoactive substances. The surface of small areas of the lung can be held steady and there is good resolution of vessels and vessel walls with epi-illumination and a polarized light. In addition, fluorescence microscopic techniques are applicable.

B. GENERAL METHODS AND SURGICAL PREPARATION

Experiments are carried out acutely in rats (about 250 g body wt.) anesthetized with sodium pentobarbital (40–50 mg/kg, i.p.). Anesthetic supplements (10–15 mg/kg, i.p.) are given as needed to maintain an adequate level of anesthesia. Subsequent to the anesthesia, the trachea is cannulated below the larynx (with PE 240, which is tied in place) and the rats breathe room air spontaneously. Arterial blood pressure and pulse rate are recorded through a catheter placed in the left carotid artery. When the lung is held inflated (apnea) at a constant pressure (see below) for brief periods, during intravital microscopy, tracheal pressure is recorded from a side arm at the tracheal cannula. Signals representing arterial blood pressure, pulse rate, tracheal pressure, or other variables, are recorded by a polygraph (Grass model 7D).

After placing the animal on its left side on a heating pad attached to a separate stage that allows movement in three directions (X, Y, and Z adjustments), the lungs are ventilated with air by a cycle-triggered ventilator (CWE model CTP-903). Tidal volume and frequency are set according to a nomogram[21] and adjusted with regard to blood

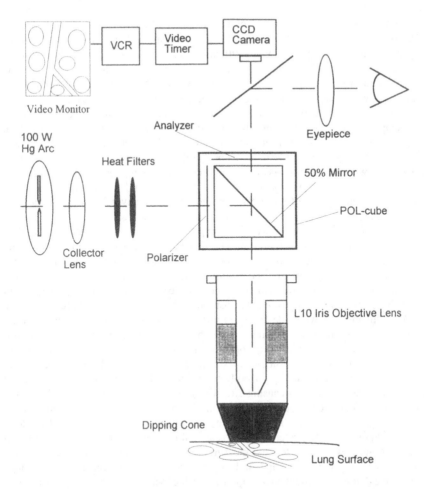

Figure 1 Schematic of microscope and video recording system with dipping cone and epi-illumination system.

pressure, arterial blood gas measurements, and visual inspection of the lungs. The right side of the chest is usually opened between the sixth and eighth ribs, taking care not to touch the lung, and spread so that the microscope objective can be positioned above the right lung. Microvessels and alveoli at the pleural surface are observed using closed-circuit video microscopy when the lung is held inflated by switching from the ventilator to a system that delivers oxygen or an oxygen mixture at a constant pressure of about 10 cm H_2O. The system consists of an outflow tube from a pressurized gas cylinder that is divided so that one branch is connected to a tube that can be adjusted to various depths in a plexiglass cylinder containing a column of water that is open to the atmosphere. The other branch has a sidearm attached to a water manometer and is used to inflate the lungs. Inflation pressure is regulated by raising or lowering the tube in the column of water. Adjustments are easily made by reading the level of the manometer and the recorded tracheal pressure.

C. VIDEOMICROSCOPY SYSTEM

Microscopic images are obtained using a trinocular microscope (Leitz) designed for incident illumination (Figure 1). A color CCD video camera (Sony DXC-101; 2/3 inch) is positioned in the image plane of the objective lens (Leitz: L10 iris, numerical aperture 0.22). Total optical magnification is 10×. Images are displayed on a color video monitor (Sony Trinitron; 12-inch model PVM 1390) and stored on videotape for off-line analysis using a video cassette recorder (JVC HR-D66OU). Total magnification of the image on the video monitor is 680× with a field of view of 380 × 285 μm. Incident illumination is achieved using a Leitz Ploemopak system (tube-factor 1×) equipped with a POL-cube (see Figure 1). The light source is a 100-W mercury arc lamp connected to a stabilized power supply (Leitz HBO 100 #990014). The light passes a heat absorption and a heat reflection filter that minimizes heating the preparation. The light passes a polarizer and is brought to the optical axis of the microscope by reflection from a 50% mirror positioned at a 45° angle with the optical axis of the microscope. Light coming from the preparation passes the 50% reflective mirror and a crossed analyzer and forms an image on the camera. The combination of the polarizer and crossed analyzer cancels all directly reflecting light.[37]

The objective lens is equipped with a dipping cone that consists of a length of optical glass mounted on the lens (Figure 1). The distance between the dipping cone and objective lens can be adjusted so that the focal plane of the lens is just below the surface of the dipping cone. By lowering the dipping cone gently to the lung surface, (1) the movements of the lung are restricted and (2) focus is easily maintained. Fine adjustment of focus has to be done by adjusting the position of the dipping cone with respect to the lens. With this method, when the lungs are inflated with oxygen or an oxygen mixture, vessels can be visualized for several minutes before switching back to the ventilator. Between observations, the microscope objective is raised and the light source is blocked to avoid photo damage. The surface of the lung is kept moist by spraying it with physiological saline solution kept at body temperature. Repeated observations can be made at the same site without causing alterations in vessel diameter or size of alveoli.

Vessels are identified by observing the direction of flow and bifurcation pattern: arterioles (Figure 2) distribute blood to successive branches, while venules collect blood (Figure 3). Parent branches refer to the largest visible portion of a vessel at the pleural surface. Internal vessel diameters are measured off-line directly from the screen of the video monitor using a vernier caliper and a calibration factor determined from the image of a graticule that was recorded on the tape with each experiment. Images of microvessels are recorded continuously. During control, diameter should be fairly constant. Measurements are made during a control period and throughout the stimulation period, using the "stop-action" feature of the video recorder.

D. APPLICATION OF CHEMICALS

Chemicals can be injected into the pulmonary circulation through a catheter placed in the right atrium via the right jugular vein or applied to the lung topically. Topical application can avoid systemic effects but may be limited by diffusion of the substance through the pleural membrane. The choice of administration route depends on the particular protocol. Constriction of an arteriole in response to topically applied $PGF_2\alpha$ is shown in Figure 4. After inflating the lungs with oxygen at constant pressure (10 cm H_2O) and gently lowering the dipping cone to the lung surface, a pulmonary arteriole was identified and observed during a control period over which diameter was stable. $PGF_2\alpha$ (1 μg in 0.1 ml saline) was applied to the lung surface over the vessel using a 1.0-ml syringe with a 26-gauge needle without touching the lung, while the dipping cone was slightly lifted. The dipping cone was then lowered and the arteriole and its branches were observed for several minutes before lifting the dipping cone and returning to mechanical ventilation. Vehicle controls (saline) applied according to the same protocol had no observable effect over the same time course.

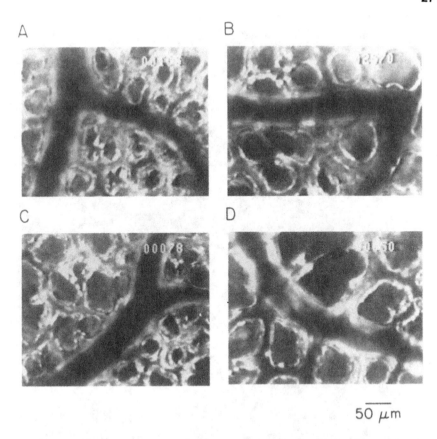

50 μm

Figure 2 Photographs (taken from videotape) of typical configurations of pulmonary arterioles observed at the surface of four different rat lungs. *A* and *B*, parent branch comes up and runs parallel to the pleural surface as it branches; *C* parent branch runs along the surface and divides further downstream; *D* parent arteriole runs across surface with no major branches visible.

IV. SUMMARY

Although there are limitations due to accessibility and movement of the tissue, intravital microscopy has been adapted for observation of microvessels and alveoli at the surface of the lungs in a variety of preparations. The method of ventilation is an important consideration as it relates to the control of blood gases, pulmonary and systemic pressures, as well as enabling microscopy at sufficient magnification. With current video imaging techniques, it is possible to measure vessel dimensions in conjunction with relevant hemodynamic variables. Models have been developed to determine the distribution of pressure and flow, and it is possible to examine transit time and permeability across microvascular networks. This has improved the ability to characterize the lung microcirculation and its responses during different physiological and pathophysiological conditions and enables a direct quantitative approach. A significant advantage of this technique is that blood flow can be observed in the region of gas exchange. On the other hand, since it is only possible to examine vessels that are close to the pleural surface, some branches, larger vessels, and microcirculation of deeper regions are excluded from observation. However, although vessels close to the pleural surface may not be representative of the entire lung, they appear to reflect general microvascular and physiological relationships.[15,33] Thus, intravital microscopy offers a method to directly observe how

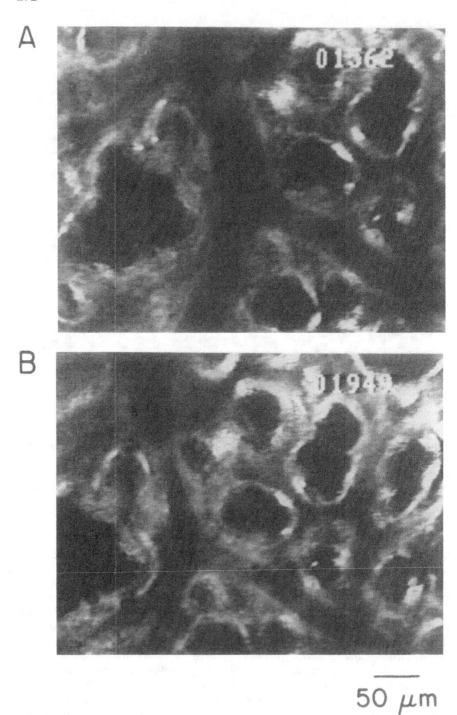

Figure 3 Photographs (taken from videotape) of venules observed in two different rats at the margin of the right lung. *A*, 2 venular branches coming together to form a larger venule. *B*, post-capillary venules draining into a larger venule.

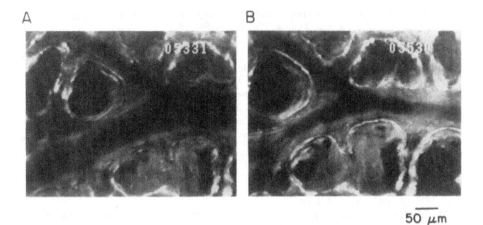

50 μm

Figure 4 Constriction of a pulmonary arteriole and its branch. A, control; B, 68 s after topical application of PGF₂α (1 μg in 0.1 ml) after constriction had reached a peak.

various stimuli and substances affect specific elements of the lung microcirculation and to study mechanisms of various diseases, abnormal function, and possible therapeutic interventions.

REFERENCES

1. **Al-Tinawi, A., Krenz, G. S., Rickaby, D. A., Linehan, J. H., and Dawson, C. A.,** Influence of hypoxia and serotonin on small pulmonary vessels, *J. Appl. Physiol.*, 76(1), 56–64, 1994.

2. **Bergofsky, E. H.,** Humoral control of the pulmonary circulation, *Ann. Rev. Physiol.*, 42, 221–233, 1980.

3. **Bhattacharya, J.,** The isolated perfused lung preparation, in *CRC Handbook of Animal Models of Pulmonary Disease*, Vol. II, 231–239, 1989.

4. **Bhattacharya, S., Glucksberg, M. R., and Bhattacharya, J.,** Measurement of lung microvascular pressure in the intact anesthetized rabbit by the micropuncture technique, *Circ. Res.*, 64, 167–172, 1989.

5. **Bhattacharya, J. and Staub, N. C.,** Direct measurement of microvascular pressures in the isolated perfused dog lung, *Sci. Wash. D.C.*, 210, 327–328, 1980.

6. **Caro, C. G., Pedley, T. J., Schroter, R. C., and Seed, W. A.,** The pulmonary circulation, in *The Mechanics of the Circulation*, Oxford University Press, Oxford, 1978, Chapter 15, 476–514.

7. **Culver, B. H. and Butler, J.,** Mechanical influences on the pulmonary microcirculation, *Annu. Rev. Physiol.*, 42, 187–198, 1980.

8. **Dawson, C. A., Capen, R. L., Latham, L. P., Hanson, W. L., Hofmeister, S. E., Bronikowski, T. A., Rickaby, D. A., and Wagner, W. W., Jr.,** Pulmonary arterial transit times, *J. Appl. Physiol.*, 63(2), 770–777, 1987.

9. **Deffebach, M. E., Charan, N. B., Lakshminarayan, S., and Butler, J.,** The bronchial circulation: Small but a vital attribute of the lung, *Am. Rev. Resp. Dis.*, 135, 463–481, 1987.

10. **Downing, S. E. and Lee, J. C.,** Nervous control of the pulmonary circulation, *Annu. Rev. Physiol.*, 42, 199–210, 1980.

11. **Fingar, V. H., Taber, S. W., and Wieman, T. J.,** A new model for the study of pulmonary microcirculation: Determination of pulmonary edema in rats, *J. Surg. Res.*, 57(3), 385–393, 1994.

12. **Fishman, A. P.,** Vasomotor regulation of the pulmonary circulation, *Annu. Rev. Physiol.*, 42, 211–220, 1980.

13. **Gil, J.,** Organization of microcirculation in the lung, *Annu. Rev. Physiol.*, 42, 177–186, 1980.

14. **Grover, R. F., Wagner, W. W., Jr., McMurtry, I. F., and Reeves, J. T.,** Pulmonary circulation, in *Handbook of Physiology. The cardiovascular system, peripheral circulation and organ blood flow*, Am. Physiol. Soc., Bethesda, MD, 1983, Sect. 2, Vol. 3, Part 1, Chapter 4, 103–136.

15. **Hakim, T. S.,** Is flow in subpleural region typical of the rest of the lung? A study using laser-Doppler flowmetry, *J. Appl. Physiol.,* 72(5), 1860–1867, 1992.

16. **Hall, H. L.,** A study of the pulmonary circulation by the trans-illumination method, *Am. J. Physiol.,* 72, 446–457, 1925.

17. **Horimoto, M., Koyama, T., Mishina, H., Asakura, T., and Murao, M.,** Blood flow velocity in pulmonary microvessels of bullfrog, *Respir. Physiol.,* 37, 45–59, 1979.

18. **Hyman, A. L., Lippton, H. L., and Kadowitz, P. J.,** Autonomic regulation of the pulmonary circulation, *J. Cardiovasc. Pharm.,* 7(Suppl. 3), S80–S95, 1985.

19. **Irwin, J. W., Burrage, W. S., Aimar, C. E., and Chesnut, R. W., Jr.,** Microscopical observations of the pulmonary arterioles, capillaries and venules of living guinea pigs and rabbits, *Anat. Rec.,* 119, 391–407, 1954.

20. **Kay, J. M.,** Pulmonary vasculature and nerves: comparative morphological features of the pulmonary vasculature of mammals, *Am. Rev. Respir. Dis.,* 128, S53–S57, 1983.

21. **Kleinman, L. I. and Radford, E. P., Jr.,** Ventilation standards for small mammals, *J. Appl. Physiol.,* 19(2), 360–362, 1964.

22. **Krahl, V. E.,** A method of studying the living lung in the closed thorax, and some preliminary observations, *Angiology,* 14, 149–159, 1963.

23. **Kuhnle, G. E. H., Groh, J., Leipfinger, F. H., Kuebler, W. M., and Goetz, A. E.,** Quantitative analysis of network architecture, and microhemodynamics in arteriolar vessel trees of the ventilated rabbit lung, *Int. J. Microcirc.: Clin. Exp.,* 12, 313–324, 1993.

24. **Kuhnle, G. E. H., Pries, A. R., and Goetz, A. E.,** Distribution of microvascular pressure in arteriolar vessel trees of ventilated rabbit lungs, *Am. J. Physiol.* (Heart Circ. Physiol. 34), H1510–H1515, 1993.

25. **Kuhnle, G. E. H., Leipfinger, F. H., and Goetz, A. E.,** Measurement of microhemodynamics in the ventilated rabbit lung by intravital fluorescence microscopy, *J. Appl. Physiol.,* 74(3), 1462–1471, 1993.

26. **Lien, D. C., Wagner, W. W., Jr., Capen, R. L., Haslett, C., Hanson, W. L., Hofmeister, S. E., Henson, P. M., and Worthen, G. S.,** Physiological neutrophil sequestration in the lung: visual evidence for localization in capillaries, *J. Appl. Physiol.,* 62(3), 1236–1243, 1987.

27. **Lien, D. C., Worthen, G. S., Capen, R. L., Hanson, W. L., Checkley, L. L., Janke, S. J., Henson, P. M., and Wagner, W. W., Jr.,** Neutrophil kinetics in the pulmonary microcirculation: effects of pressure and flow in the dependent lung, *Am. Rev. Respir. Dis.,* 141, 953–959, 1990.

28. **MacGregor, R. G.,** Examination of the pulmonary circulation with the microscope, *J. Physiol.,* 80, 65–77, 1933–1934.

29. **Mathew, R. and Altura, B. M.,** Physiology and pathophysiology of pulmonary circulation, *Microcirc. Endoth. Lymphatics,* 6, 211–252, 1990.

30. **Meyrick, B. and Reid, L.,** Ultrastructural features of the distended pulmonary arteries of the normal rat, *Anat. Rec.,* 193, 71–98, 1979.

31. **Negrini, D. A., Gonano, C., and Miserocchi, G.,** Microvascular pressure profile in intact *in situ* lung, *J. Appl. Physiol.,* 72(1), 332–339, 1992.

32. **Onizuka, M., Wagner, L., Nicolaysen, G., and Staub, N. C.,** Micropuncture pressure in small arteries or veins of perfused rabbit lungs, *J. Appl. Physiol.,* 68(5), 1838–1843, 1990.

33. **Overholser, K. A., Bhattacharya, J., and Staub, N. C.,** Microvascular pressures in the isolated perfused dog lung: comparison between theory and measurement, *Microvasc. Res.,* 23, 67–76, 1982.

34. **Richardson, J. B.,** Nerve supply to the lungs, *Am. Rev. Resp. Dis.,* 119(1), 785–802, 1979.

35. **Sada, K., Shirai, M., and Ninomiya, I.,** X-ray TV system for measuring microcirculation in small pulmonary vessels, *J. Appl. Physiol.,* 59(3), 1013–1018, 1985.

36. **Singhal, S., Henderson, R., Horsfield, K., Harding, K., and Cumming, G.,** Morphometry of the human pulmonary arterial tree, *Circ. Res.,* 33, 190–197, 1973.

37. **Slaaf, D. W., Tangelder, G. J., Reneman, R. S., Jäger, K., and Bollinger, A.,** A versatile incident illuminator for intravital microscopy, *Int. J. Microcirc. Clin. Exp.,* 6, 391–397, 1987.

38. **Terry, R. J.,** A thoracic window for observation of the lung in a living animal, *Science,* 90, 43–44, 1939.

39. **Valdivia, E., Olson, W., and Simon, S.,** Direct illumination method to visualize pulmonary vessels, *Angiology,* 12, 462–468, 1961.

40. **Wagner, W. W., Jr.,** Pulmonary microcirculatory observations *in vivo* under physiological conditions, *J. Appl. Physiol.*, 26(3), 375–377, 1969.

41. **Wagner, W. W., Jr., Latham, L. P., Gillespie, M. N., Guenther, J. P., and Capen, R. L.,** Direct measurement of pulmonary capillary transit times, *Science Wash., D.C.*, 218, 379–381, 1982.

42. **Wagner, W. W., Jr., Latham, L. P., Hanson, W. L., Hofmeister, S. E., and Capen, R. L.,** Vertical gradient of pulmonary capillary transit times, *J. Appl. Physiol.*, 61(4), 1270–1274, 1986.

43. **Wagner, W. W., Jr. and Filley, G. F.,** Microscopic observation of the lung *in vivo, Vascular Dis.*, 2(5), 229–241, 1965.

44. **Wang, P. M., Fike, C. D., Kaplowitz, M. R., Brown, L. V., Ayappa, I., Jahed, M., and Lai-Fook, S. J.,** Effects of lung inflation and blood flow on capillary transit time in isolated rabbit lungs, *J. Appl. Physiol.*, 72(6), 2420–2427, 1992.

45. **Wang, P. M., Yang, Q.-H., and Lai-Fook, S. J.,** Effect of positive airway pressure on capillary transit time in rabbit lung, *J. Appl. Physiol.*, 69(5), 2262–2268, 1990.

46. **Wearn, J. T., Ernstene, A. C., Bromer, A. W., Barr, J. S., German, W. J., and Zschiesche, L. J.,** The normal behavior of the pulmonary blood vessels with observations on the intermittence of the flow of blood in the arterioles and capillaries, *Am. J. Physiol.*, 109, 236–256, 1934.

Chapter 21

Peripheral Nerve Microcirculation

John Firrell

CONTENTS

I. ANATOMY AND FUNCTION

A. VASCULAR ANATOMY

The majority of the cellular activity of a peripheral nerve occurs in the endoneurium inside the fascicles where densely packed axons, Schwann cells, and other connective tissue cells are situated. The capillaries servicing the endoneurium are generally orientated longitudinally and have many connections with small arterioles and venules.[1] Each fascicle is surrounded completely by a thin but relatively impermeable connective tissue layer — the perineurium. There is a rich vascular plexus in the epineurium, the connective tissue that binds the fascicles together, and these vessels connect with those in the endoneurium via arterioles and venules traversing the perineurium. Interconnections along the length of the nerve within the endoneurium are important since stripping the epineurium away for short distances does not markedly affect flow in the endoneurium. The epineurium is supplied at intervals along the nerve by larger vessels derived from adjacent arteries and veins and from the vessels in the tissues that are innervated by that nerve. The manner in which the microvessels penetrate the perineurium from the epineurial plexus may make them susceptible to kinking, causing restriction to flow when the nerve is stretched or when the endoneurium swells.[2] Lymphatics have not been identified within the endoneurium, but are present in the epineurium.

B. MICROVASCULAR FUNCTION

Since the primary function of the nerve is the transmission of electrical signals, microvascular function and control are undoubtably linked to the level of metabolism required to sustain transmission. However, it is not clear how much of the metabolism is related to the continual activity necessary to support axonal transport of cellular materials and molecules in both directions along the nerve. Furthermore, it is not known how much the metabolism of the myelin-producing Schwann cells contribute to that of the total nerve.

0-8493-4870-6/95/$0.00+$.50

Blood flow to the nerve increases when it is electrically stimulated.[3] Additional capillaries are recruited in this situation and can be seen directly under intravital microscopy in the rabbit sciatic tibial nerve.[3] Stimulation of the nerve also causes significant blood flow changes in the spinal cord and in the nerve roots of that nerve,[4] where the major biochemical processing sites for the whole nerve are situated.

The control of blood flow to the nerve has not been worked out in detail. One feature that has been noticed is the network of anastomosing arteries and veins that allow the flow to be readily redistributed.[3] The extrinsic vessels that join the nerve along its length help maintain intravascular pressure. The nerve gets stretched in the normal course of motion but the influence on blood flow has not been assessed. Static studies have shown that stretching the nerve slowly by 15% causes flow to stop, probably by kinking certain vessels. Whether this is in the endo- or epineurium is not known. There has been no systematic study of the pressures and diameters of the microvessels in the peripheral nerve. The relative contributions of the various levels of the microcirculation to the resistance of the circulation therefore has not been established.

The microcirculation of the nerve is under both central nerve-mediated and local metabolic control. Histologic evidence suggests that blood vessels in the epineurium are innervated by adrenergic, serotoninergic, and peptidergic fibers of the sympathetic system.[5] Adrenergic nerves are closely associated with vessels around the perineurium.[6] Sympathetic tone is lowered by chemical sympathectomy with guanethidine.[7] Stimulation of the sympathetics has a vasoconstrictor action on the vessels in the epineurium[8] and direct addition of norepinephrine causes constriction.[9] Intraarterial injections of norepinephrine also reduces blood flow.[10] The vessels in the epineurium influence the flow in the endoneurial tissue.[11] Topical agents therefore affect endoneurial flow through the actions of the epineurial vessels.[12] Autoregulation does not significantly occur when systemic pressure changes.[13] The microcirculation does respond to changing carbon dioxide levels in the blood in decerebrate rather than anesthetized preparations.[14]

The exchange of small solutes and oxygen occurs freely by diffusion. Capillaries appear to be fewer than in other tissues with similar basal flow. In human median nerve, the capillaries are 6 to 10 μm in diameter, which is large compared to those in skeletal muscle. Low and co-workers[13] have extensively studied small solute exchange. In addition to receiving oxygen through the capillary wall, there can also be significant diffusion of oxygen from the surrounding tissue fluid.[15] At least in frogs, ionic transport in the peripheral nerve capillaries does not appear to be facilitated, as it is for the capillaries in the brain.[16]

Permeability to large molecules has been evaluated using tracers such as albumin labeled with Evans blue dye. The endothelium appears to be quite impermeable, but there are species differences in this permeability.[17] It should be noted that the permeability can change quickly even from something as simple as just exposing the nerve.

The vascular leakage of protein is important in terms of fluid exchange. Since there are no lymphatics in the endoneurium, accumulation of proteins can easily cause fluid to accumulate. This makes the nerve susceptible to local compression problems since tissue pressure would increase and eventually close capillaries within the nerve. Even normal intraneural pressures were found to be 2 mmHg higher than in most tissues when measured with a micropipette.[18]

II. PATHOLOGY

A number of pathologic conditions in the nerve are considered to have a microcirculation component. One of the most common disease entities is nerve compression syndrome. A localized compression of the nerve causes a disruption of blood flow producing at first paresthesias but also numbness, and pain if prolonged. If the compression occurs over extensive periods, the axons become permanently damaged, disrupting transport of materials across the site. Eventually, demyelination and cell death occur distal to the compression site. This disruption may affect proximal sites. Microcirculation changes include increased vascular permeability that may precede changes in flow.[19] Higher endoneurial pressure led to lower flow conditions. Much of the evidence for these findings is circumstantial and has not been proved in the clinical situation.

The ischemic condition can occur without compression. Focal ischemic neuropathy may occur in limbs with compromised vascular patency. Experiments with animals have been able to produce degenerative changes in the central region of nerves that have insufficient blood supply.[20,21] Plugging the microcirculation with excessive microspheres can also result in ischemic neuropathies.[22] Interestingly, the changes seen in other models of compression suggest that it is the periphery of the nerve that is affected most.[19,23]

Diabetic neuropathy has long been considered a microcirculatory pathology. Although metabolic disturbances are undoubtably present, the involvement of the microcirculation is becoming clear. Biopsies have suggested that endoneurial perfusion[24] and capillary density[25] are not as high as normal, and the multifocal fiber degeneration seen is consistent with ischemia.[26] Capillary abnormalities, including thickened basement membrane, endothelial cell, and interstitial diffusion barriers, all create a decreased oxygen diffusion capacity.[25]

Other neuropathies may also be of ischemic origin. For instance, hexachlorophene in large doses produces both elevated endoneurial pressure and decreased blood flow in rats.[27]

Ischemia caused by tourniquet can result in temporary or sometimes even permanent disturbances in the peripheral nerve. How much of that is due to distortion of the nerve and how much from ischemic trauma at the level of the microcirculation is still unclear.

The regeneration process can have profound effects on the microcirculation. The nerve that is injured and subsequently regenerating undergoes an enormous increase in blood flow and the same is observed in nerve grafts in the early stages after surgery.[28,29] This is primarily due to ingrowth of new vessels since it also is seen in nonvascularized grafts after an initial delay of several days.[28]

Other clinical conditions that could affect the nerve microcirculation are when regional or local anesthesia is given. An injection of local anesthetic such as Lidocaine usually has a vasodilatory effect on most smooth muscles, but it seems to have a mild vasoconstrictor effect on the nerve microcirculation.[12] This is greatly accentuated when norepinephrine is included. This combination is often used clinically for performing local anesthesia. Some of the effect of the anesthetic could be ischemia related.

Microcirculation investigative techniques have potential utility in the management of disease states or clinical situations. Although peripheral nerves are difficult to evaluate without exposure, intraoperative studies may be useful. Clinical evaluations of nerves using histological techniques cause loss of function to the area innervated by that nerve, but this technique has been used on minor nerves such as the sural nerve, which leaves only a small deficit in sensibility.

The tools to perform much intraoperative investigation of the microcirculation of peripheral nerves are lacking in sophistication. However, advances in fiber-optic technology may enable great strides in this approach. Too much manipulation of the nerve occasionally leads to the risk of scar formation around the nerve and the potential complication for local compression neuropathy. Currently, blood flow has been successfully evaluated with the laser Doppler.[30] An increase in flow in the median nerve was found following carpal tunnel release. This approach could aid in the determination of completeness of release of compression or in the degree of ischemic involvement in that particular case. The etiology of nerve compression is still unclear and needs to be followed with studies such as these.

Another potential clinical study would be to evaluate how damaged nerve tissue is doing following injury. Current clinical assessment of nerve viability in an injured tissue is usually done by gross visual inspection or by cutting back to see if it bleeds. A more objective approach could be to evaluate the microcirculation directly or to look at vascular permeability from intravascular tracers.

The basis of much peripheral nerve surgery is to provide a better environment for the nerve by avoiding tension or tethering and to place the nerve in a well-vascularized bed. It would be very advantageous to the surgeon if the nerve could be positioned and monitored for functioning blood flow at the same time. Similarly, in cases where the surgeon performs a vascular nerve graft (either as a free or pedicle nerve graft), it would be useful to determine the integrity of the circulation by monitoring the microcirculation. The advances in endoscopic surgery may lead to techniques to aid the surgeon in assessing the state of the nerves prior to extensive surgery. Coupled with objective measures of flow such as laser Doppler and other potential photometric techniques to assess the oxygenation of the issue, useful information in the diagnosis and treatment should be possible.

III. MODELS AND TECHNIQUES[4]

A. HUMAN MODELS

The methods of studying the dynamic events of the microcirculation in the peripheral nerve are currently limited to intraoperative situations. The only measurement of nerve blood flow in humans thus far has been with the laser Doppler technique.[30] This technique consists of placing a 2.2-mm diameter probe of a helium-neon laser on the median nerve underneath the transverse carpal ligament. The laser Doppler provides a pulsatile signal related to blood flow within a 1- to 1.5-mm hemisphere of the nerve. Since this technique can detect changes rapidly, it can therefore guide the surgeon in manipulations of the nerve.

Other techniques in humans relate to indirect manipulation of the microcirculation rather than direct measurement. Stopping the circulation by a tourniquet applied to an extremity causes a more rapid onset of parasthesias in an already compromised nerve. Paradoxically, this test does not apply to the diabetic patient who is able to tolerate the ischemia better because of higher plasma glucose levels.

Histology of the microcirculation of nerves in the human can only be satisfactorily done on fresh cadavers or amputated specimens. Care must be taken to perfuse the limb at physiological pressures. After perfusing with saline, the lumens can be filled by using microfil latex solution or Batson's 17 plastic solution diluted with solvent to reduce the viscosity to get good capillary filling.[31] A good and cheap alternative is an India ink solution in warmed 20% gelatin solution that solidifies when cooled. The nerve specimens are harvested carefully when the intravascular injection is hardened.

Using cross-sections of nerves to determine vascular morphometry is a painstaking method, but computer software making this task easier is becoming more readily available and can provide three-dimensional reconstructions of serial sections. Consideration of fixation artifacts are important in precise morphometry.

B. ANIMAL MODELS OF MICROCIRCULATION IN THE NERVE

1. Direct *In Vivo* or *In Situ* Observation Models

Lundborg[3] popularized the rabbit sciatic-tibial nerve preparation as an excellent way to directly observe and evaluate the *in vivo* microcirculation. The preparation requires an incision to be made on both the medial and lateral aspects of the leg, followed by freeing the nerve from adherent loose tissue for a distance of 4 to 5 cm. By placing the nerve directly on a piece of plexiglass, the light through the microscope condenser lens can be transmitted

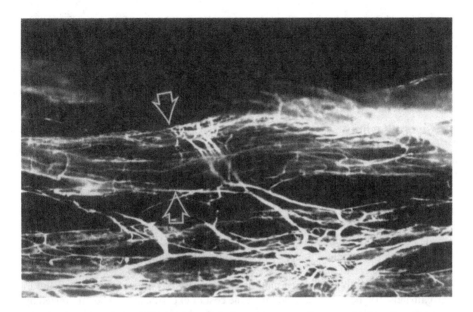

Figure 1 Microangiographic photograph of contrast-filled microcirculation of nerve. (From Lundborg, G., Intraneural microcirculation, *Orthoped. Clin. N. Am.*, 19(1), 1–11, 1988.)

through the nerve, creating an image that can be captured by an objective of a standard intravital microscope[3] (Figure 1). The tissue must be kept moist with appropriate physiological solutions. The model also has been used to observe the microcirculation under a number of experimental circumstances. In one model, compression to the nerve was applied by thin inflatable cuffs. Other situations have involved evaluating the circulation at the cut end of a nerve to understand the changes occurring after injury, after stimulation of the sympathetic supply, and after topical application or intraarterial injections of vasoactive agents were done to study the controlling mechanisms of nerve blood flow.[3]

Another model to study the microcirculation, which employs direct observation techniques, is the cauda equina of the pig.[32] The cauda equina, the extension of the spinal cord but consisting of the nerve roots of the peripheral nerves, is exposed through a laminectomy of the first and second coccygeal vertebrae after removing the relevant ligaments, fat, and cartilage. The circulation can be observed with an intravital microscope using epillumination through plexiglass plates pinned to the vertebrae to stabilize the preparation. Images of the microcirculation can be videotaped to be analyzed off-line. The model has been useful to study the effects of nerve compression and ischemia using special balloons that can be inflated to controlled pressures while continually monitoring the flow and diameters of the microvessels. For a full review of cauda equina circulation and nerve compression, see Reference 33.

2. Indirect Blood Flow Measurements

Various techniques that indirectly evaluate blood flow in the nerve have been used. They each have their own advantages and disadvantages.

a. Hydrogen Washout

This technique has been used for many years and involves the exposure of the nerve and the introduction of a micropipette into the nerve fascicles. Two variations of the technique exist. One is to generate hydrogen at the site through electrolysis, and the other is to let the animal breathe hydrogen gas. By measuring the rate of washout of hydrogen from the tissue, the local blood flow can be determined since it is related to the rate of washout. Equipment needed for this technique includes reference and hydrogen-sensitive electrodes, necessary electronics, and a source of hydrogen gas. If the hydrogen is generated locally, a current has to be supplied through the same hydrogen electrode. However, the procedures have to be done very carefully to avoid artifacts and disturbances in the nerve when introducing the electrodes. The nerve is usually bathed in warmed mineral oil. The epineurium needs to be incised before putting the electrode in.

b. Xenon Washout

This technique depends on the same principles as H_2 washout. However, ^{133}Xe is injected into the nerve and its clearance is monitored by a gamma-detector positioned above the nerve. This may avoid the continual irritation of an electrode needed for the H_2 technique. Changes in rates over time are possible with Xenon washout.

c. Microspheres

The microsphere technique has the advantage that it is noninvasive to the tissue under investigation. Its limitations include that it can only provide a momentary snapshot of blood flow unless multiple isotopes are used. At first, the canine sciatic nerve was studied since large numbers of microspheres were considered necessary.[34,35] The number of microspheres originally considered minimally necessary has been revised downward to approximately 100 per sample. In addition, the cost of experiments can be minimized by using less microspheres and less-expensive animals like rabbits, provided the injections can be given into the dorsal aorta and good mixing is achieved.[36]

d. Uptake Method

This technique depends on the complete uptake of either ^{14}C iodoantipyrine or ^{14}C butanol into the tissue as blood circulates through, without allowing any recirculation. The method requires knowing the concentration in the blood, the blood/tissue partition coefficient, and the final amount in the tissue. It has proven to be effective but provides only one time point of blood flow. These tracers are injected into a vein over a 40-s period. The arterial blood is sampled to determine the concentration, the animal is immediately sacrificed, and the nerve is harvested.[37]

e. Laser Doppler

The laser Doppler has been used in a number of different preparations, including the rat sciatic nerve. Although it requires exposure of the nerve, it is relatively noninvasive although surface contact of the nerve is required. It provides a continuous measure of flow but it cannot provide a truly quantitative value. Combined with other quantitative techniques, it has been very effective in showing changes in flow.[9,37]

One of the pitfalls of investigating the nerve microcirculation is the fact that just exposing the tissue is enough to change the blood flow. In addition, the influence of anesthesia can profoundly affect the control mechanisms. When studying control systems, it is therefore advisable to use decerebrate animals rather than anesthetized animals.

3. Exchange Studies

Evaluation of the oxygen exchange in the microcirculation of nerve has been extensively studied by Low and co-workers.[13] A technique for measuring oxygen concentration in the nerve has been clearly described.[38] Using platinum microelectrodes at the appropriate polarization potentials, both O_2 and H_2 can be measured for blood flow determination.

Permeability of small molecules has been determined from standard clearance methods.[13,39,40] The use of extracellular markers (^{14}C sucrose or ^{14}C mannitol) allow for calculation of permeability surface area products.[41,42]

Macromolecular permeability has been evaluated by standard molecular tracers. Evans Blue dye binds very tightly to serum albumin and emits fluorescence in the red wavelength. Typically, macromolecular tracers are given intravenously and the tissue is sampled at specific times afterward. Tissues are prepared as frozen sections fixed in formalin. Care needs to be taken to keep the dye totally bound to serum albumin. Unbound dye can be removed by gel filtration through standard, commercially available products. This technique has been used and described extensively by Olsson.[17,43] It is also important to note that the degree of leakage can vary among species.

REFERENCES

1. **Lundborg, G.,** Intraneural microcirculation, *Orthoped. Clin. N. Am.*, 19(1), 1–11, 1988.
2. **Myers, R. R., Murakami, H., and Powell, H. C.,** Reduced nerve blood flow in edematous neuropathies: A biomechanical mechanism, *Microvasc. Res.*, 32(2), 145–151, 1986.
3. **Lundborg, G.,** Ischemic nerve injury. Experimental studies on intraneural microvascular pathophysiology and nerve function in a limb subjected to temporary circulatory arrest, *Scand. J. Plast. Reconstr. Surg. Suppl.*, 6, 3–113, 1970.
4. **Takahashi, K., Nomura, S., Tomita, K., and Matsumoto, T.,** Effects of peripheral nerve stimulation on the blood flow of the spinal cord and the nerve root, *Spine*, 13(11), 1278–1283, 1988.
5. **Appenzeller, O., Dhital, K. K., Cowen, T., and Burnstock G.,** The nerves to blood vessels supplying blood to nerves: The innervation of vasa nervorum, *Brain Res.*, 304, 383–386, 1984.
6. **Rechthand, E., Hervonen, A., Sato, S., and Rapoport, S. I.,** Distribution of adrenergic innervation of blood vessels in peripheral nerve, *Brain Res.*, 374, 185–189, 1986.
7. **Zochodne, D. W., Huang, Z., Ward, K. K., and Low, P. A.,** Guanethidine-induced adrenergic sympathectomy augments endoneurial perfusion and lowers endoneurial microvascular resistance, *Brain Res.*, 519, 112–117, 1990.
8. **Lundborg, G. and Brånemark, P. I.,** Microvascular structure and function of peripheral nerves — Vital microscopic studies of the tibial nerve in the rabbit, *Adv. Microcirc.*, 1, 66–88 1968.
9. **Zochodne, D. W. and Low, P. A.,** Adrenergic control of peripheral nerve, *Exp. Neurol.*, 109, 300–307, 1990.
10. **Selander, D., Mansson, L. G., Karlsson, L., and Svanvik, J.,** Adrenergic vasoconstriction in peripheral nerves of the rabbit, *Anesthesiology*, 62, 6–10, 1985.
11. **Kihara, M. and Low, P. A.,** Regulation of rat nerve blood flow: Role of epineurial α-receptors, *J. Physiol.*, 422, 145–152, 1990.
12. **Myers, R. R. and Heckman, H. M.,** Effects of local anesthesia on nerve blood flow: Studies using lidocaine with and without epinephrine, *Anesthesiology*, 71, 757–762, 1989.
13. **Low, P. A., Lagerlund, T. D., and McManis, P. G.,** Nerve blood flow and oxygen delivery in normal, diabetic, and ischemic neuropathy, *Intl. Rev. Neurobiol.*, 31, 355–439, 1989.
14. **Rechthand, E., Sato, S., Oberg, P. A., and Rapoport, S. I.,** Sciatic nerve blood flow response to carbon dioxide, *Brain Res.*, 446, 61–66, 1988.
15. **Lagerlund, T. D. and Low, P. A.,** A mathematical simulation of oxygen delivery in rat peripheral nerve, *Microvasc. Res.*, 34, 211–222, 1987.
16. **Weerasuriya, A.,** Permeability of endoneurial capillaries to K, Na and Cl and its relation to peripheral nerve excitability, *Brain Res.*, 419, 188–189, 1987.
17. **Olsson, Y.,** Studies on vascular permeability in peripheral nerves. IV. Distribution of intravenously injected protein tracers in the peripheral nervous system of various species, *Acta Neuropathol.*, 17, 114–126, 1971.
18. **Lundborg, G., Myers, R., and Powell, H.,** Nerve compression injury and increased endoneurial fluid pressure: A "miniature compartment syndrome", *J. Neurol. Neurosurg. Psych.*, 46, 1119–1124, 1983.
19. **Mackinnon, S. E., Dellon, A. L., Hudson, A. R., and Hunter, D. A.,** Chronic nerve compression — An experimental model in the rat, *Ann. Plast. Surg.*, 13(2), 112–120, 1984.
20. **Hess, K., Eames, R. A., Darveniza, P., and Gilliatt, R. W.,** Acute ischemic neuropathy in the rabbit, *J. Neurol. Sci.*, 44, 19–43, 1979.
21. **Adams, W. E.,** The blood supply of nerves. II. The effects of exclusion of its regional sources of supply on the sciatic nerve of the rabbit, *J. Anat.*, 77(3), 243–250, 1943.
22. **Nukada, H. and Dyck, P. J.,** Microsphere embolization of nerve capillaries and fiber degeneration, *Am. J. Pathol.*, 115(2), 275–287, 1984.

23. **Mackinnon, S. E. and Dellon, A. L.,** Experimental study of chronic nerve compression: Clinical implications, *Hand Clinics*, 2(4), 639–650, 1986.

24. **Nukada, H., Dyck, P. J., and Karnes, J. L.,** Spatial distribution of capillaries in rat nerves: Correlation to ischemic damage, *Exp. Neurol.*, 87, 369–376, 1985.

25. **Malik, R. A., Newrick, P. G., Sharma, A. K., Jennings, A., Ah-See, A. K., Mayhew, T. M., Jakubowski, J., Boulton, A. J. M., and Ward, J. D.,** Microangiography in human diabetic neuropathy: Relationship between capillary abnormalities and the severity of neuropathy, *Diabetologia*, 32, 92–102, 1989.

26. **Dyck, P. J., Karnes, J. L., O'Brien, P., Okazaki, H., et al.,** The spatial distribution of fiber loss in diabetic polyneuropathy suggests ischemia, *Ann. Neurol.*, 19, 440–449, 1986.

27. **Myers, R. R., Mizisin, A. P., Powell, H. C., and Lampert, P. W.,** Reduced nerve blood flow in hexachlorophene neuropathy. Relationship to elevated endoneurial fluid pressure, *J. Neuropath. Exp. Neur.*, 41, 391–399, 1982.

28. **Lux, P., Breidenbach, W., and Firrell, J.,** Determination of temporal changes in blood flow in vascularized and nonvascularized nerve grafts in the dog, *Plast. Reconstr. Surg.*, 82(1), 133–142, 1988.

29. **Wood, M. B.,** Neurovascularization of nerve grafts — A quantitative study in the canine, presented at the *Orthopedic Research Society* (Abstract), 1984.

30. **Seiler, J. G., III, Milek, M. A., Carpenter, G. K., and Swiontkowski, M. F.,** Intraoperative assessment of median nerve blood flow during carpal tunnel release with laser Doppler flowmetry, *J. Hand Surg.*, 14A, 986–991, 1989.

31. **Nopanitaya, W., Aghajanian, J. G., and Gray, L. D.,** An improved plastic mixture for corrosion casting of the gastrointestinal microvascular system, *Scanning Electron Microscopy*, 3, 751–755, 1979.

32. **Olmarker, K., Rydevik, B., Holm, S., and Bagge, U.,** Effects of experimental graded compression on blood flow in spinal nerve roots. A vital microscopic study on the porcine cauda equina, *J. Orthop. Res.*, 7, 817–823, 1989.

33. **Olmarker, K.,** Spinal nerve root compression: Nutrition and function of the porcine cauda equina compressed *in vivo, Acta Orthop. Scand. Suppl. 242*, 62, 1–27, 1991.

34. **Tschetter, T. H., Klassen, A. C., Resch, J. A., and Meyer, M. W.,** Blood flow in the central and peripheral nervous system of dogs using a particle distribution method, *Stroke*, 1, 370–374, 1970.

35. **Riggi, K., Wood, M. B., and Ilstrup, D. M.,** Dose-dependent variations in blood flow evaluation of canine nerve, nerve graft, tendon, and ligament tissue by the radiolabelled microsphere technique, *J. Orthop. Res.*, 8, 909–916, 1990.

36. **Maki, Y., Breidenbach, W. C., and Firrell, J. C.,** Evaluation of a local microsphere injection method for measurement of blood flow in the rabbit lower extremity, *J. Orthop. Res.*, 11(1), 20–27, 1993.

37. **Rundquist, I., Smith, Q. R., Michel, M. E., Ask, P., Oberg, P. A., and Rapoport, S. I.,** Sciatic nerve blood flow measured by laser Doppler flowmetry and ^{14}C iodoantipyrine, *Am. J. Physiol.*, 248, H311–H317, 1985.

38. **Tuck, R. R., Schmelzer, J. D., and Low, P. A.,** Endoneurial blood flow and oxygen tension in the sciatic nerves of rats with experimental diabetic neuropathy, *Brain*, 107, 935–950, 1984.

39. **Ohno, K., Chiueh, C. C., Burns, E. M., Pettigrew, K. D., and Rapoport, S. I.,** Cerebrovascular integrity in protein-deprived rats, *Brain Res. Bull.*, 5(3), 251–255, 1980.

40. **Phillips, S. C. and Cragg, B. G.,** Weakening of the blood-brain barrier by alcohol-related stresses in the rat, *J. Neurol. Sci.*, 54(2), 271–278, 1982.

41. **Day, T. J., Schmelzer, J. D., and Low, P. A.,** Aortic occlusion and reperfusion and conduction, blood flow, and the blood-nerve barrier of rat sciatic nerve, *Exp. Neurol.*, 103, 173–178, 1989.

42. **Rechthand, E., Smith, Q. R., Latker, C. H., and Rapoport, S. I.,** Altered blood-nerve barrier permeability to small molecules in experimental diabetes mellitus, *J. Neuropathol. Exp. Neurol.*, 46, 302–314, 1987.

43. **Olsson, Y.,** Studies on vascular permeability in peripheral nerves. I. Distribution of circulating fluorescent serum albumin in normal, crushed and sectioned rat sciatic nerve, *Acta Neuropathol.*, 7, 1–15, 1966.

Chapter 22

Pancreas Microcirculation

Michael D. Menger and Brigitte Vollmar

CONTENTS

I. ANATOMY AND FUNCTION

A. MICROVASCULAR ANATOMY

The pancreas contains a highly specialized microvascular system that includes two distinguished capillary beds, interacting with each other, and guarantees adequate exocrine and endocrine organ function. The gland contains exocrine, endocrine, and ductular tissue, supporting the digestion and absorption processes by release of various enzymes, and maintaining glucose homeostasis by a complex interplay of different hormones, i.e., insulin, glucagon, and somatostatin. Despite a general interest in understanding the anatomy and physiology of the pancreas as a whole organ system, little is known about its microvasculature or microcirculatory function.

The vascular supply of the pancreas includes pancreaticoduodenal and splenic, as well as gastric, omental, and epiploic vessels. The unit of a pancreatic lobule (acinar tissue)

0-8493-4870-6/95/$0.00+$.50

is fed by two intralobular arteries, branching from interlobular vessels, which then form terminal arterioles, breaking into a honeycomb-like capillary network with the junctions about 25 to 50 µm apart. In addition to these nutritive supply vessels, terminal arterioles also continue with an arcade-like vessel, which allows the blood to bypass the capillaries as a preferential pathway. From capillaries (4–8 µm in diameter), as well as from preferential pathways (9 µm in diameter), blood is drained into postcapillary venules and, finally, into intralobular and interlobular veins.[1]

While in primitive vertebrates, the endocrine cells are found exclusively within the mucosa of the gastrointestinal tract, in humans about 1,000,000 islets of Langerhans, containing about 5000 endocrine cells each, are scattered throughout the exocrine pancreas, amounting to 1 or 2% of the volume of the gland. The islets have a round or ovoid structure and contain four major types of cells, which synthesize and secrete insulin (B-cell), glucagon (A-cell), somatostatin (D-cell), and the pancreatic polypeptide (PP-cell). While B-cells occupy primarily the central mass of each islet, the other three cell types are located in the periphery (mantle). The microvasculature of the islets can be distinguished easily from that of the exocrine tissue; the islets are supplied by one or two individual arterioles, which enter into the islet at discontinuities of the non-B-cell mantle, and branch into capillaries (about 5 µm in diameter) within the B-cell core.[2] The capillaries, tortuous in structure, form a glomerulum-like network, presenting with higher density as compared to the honeycomb-like meshwork of the acinar tissue. Thereby, each islet cell is in close proximity to at least one capillary.

Intra-islet cellular communication is predicted by the sequence of islet-cellular perfusion (intra-islet portal system): the order of islet capillary perfusion (core-to-mantle perfusion) provides blood supply initially to the B-cells located within the core of the islets, followed by capillary perfusion of A- and D-cells within the mantle of the islets.[3]

Capillary blood flow is drained by individual venules as well as by intercapillary insulo-acinar (insulo-acinar portal system) and insulo-ductular (insulo-ductular portal system) anastomoses. The islets are not surrounded by capsules or basal membranes; therefore, close contact exists between insular and acinar tissue. The microvasculature of acinar cells adjacent to the islets (peri-insular acini) can be distinguished easily from teleinsular acini due to the peri-insular "halo", characterized by only a few microvessels surrounding the relatively dense capillary network of the islets (see Reference 4).

Pancreatic capillary endothelium contains fenestrae (approximately 15 fenestrae/mm^2 — 6% of the endothelial surface), however, varying in size and number in exocrine and endocrine tissue. It is proposed that the number of fenestrae of exocrine capillaries exceeds that of endocrine capillaries by a factor of seven and includes variations in diameter of single fenestrae between 200 and 500 Å.

Microhemodynamic Parameters

Blood flow rate in the pancreas is relatively high, as is similar for other secretory organs; values of experimental measurements range from 50 to 100 ml/min/100 g tissue without significant differences between the head, corpus, and tail of the gland. However, blood flow through the islets is considerably higher when compared to acinar flow presenting with values between 800 and 1700 ml/min/100 g tissue, and single islet blood flow of 5 to 20 nl/min, respectively. Therefore, islets of Langerhans, although representing only 1 to 2% of the volume of the pancreas, conceive 10 to 23% of total pancreatic blood flow.[5]

In addition, blood flow through insular and acinar capillaries is characterized by its variability and intermittency. Capillary blood cell velocity varies from rapid (>1.5 mm/s) to zero, and is rarely the same in two adjacent microvessels. Flowmotion (intermittency of capillary blood flow) is a common phenomenon in both insular and acinar capillaries, and was considered an important criterion for the integrity of the microcirculation.[1] In contrast to previous observations, recent experimental studies from our own laboratory revealed that capillary flow intermittency, characterized by a distinct rhythm and induced by vasomotion of upstream arterioles, appears under conditions of restricted blood perfusion, probably with the aim to counteract the alteration of nutritive blood flow.[5a]

Pressure in pancreatic capillaries range between 9 and 11 mmHg; however, pressure increases to values above 20 mmHg during maximal vasodilation, probably due to the relaxation of precapillary resistance vessels. Capillary permeability (fenestrated endothelium) ranges between 0.1 and 0.3 ml/min/100 g/mmHg, and is found increased during maximal dilation by a factor of five. This high capillary filtration coefficient may be due to a combination of the fenestration of the endothelial lining and the high capillary density (see Reference 6).

B. MICROVASCULAR FUNCTIONS OF THE PANCREAS

The pancreatic islets and the associated acini are highly complex tissues, the regulation of which is dependent upon nervous vasomotor control and local action of hormones.

1. Vasomotor Control of Exocrine Pancreas

The pancreatic vasculature, in particular the arteriolar system, contains a redundant sympathetic, adrenergic innervation; however, there is apparently no adrenergic innervation of acini. As studied on the basis of adrenergic effects on the pancreatic microcirculation, the decrease of blood perfusion is accompanied by reduced pancreatic juice production. The inhibition of pancreatic secretion after adrenergic stimulation is probably caused by α-receptor-mediated vasoconstriction of precapillary arterioles. By contrast, parasympathetic stimulation results in pancreatic arteriolar vasodilation that, however, may not be mediated on the vascular level, inasmuch as pancreatic blood vessels seem to lack cholinergic innervation. Other factors, such as the action of peptidergic neurons, tissue osmolarity, kinin-forming enzymes, bradykinin, kallikrein, and accumulation of secretory enzymes and respective metabolites, are discussed to be causative for parasympathetic vasodilation. In general, an increased secretion of pancreatic juice is usually accompanied by vasodilation, and vagally induced secretion of pancreatic juice consequently results in vasodilation. However, acetylcholine (a potent vasodilator) probably enhances pancreatic juice production by direct acinar action because papaverine- and histamine-induced vasodilation are not accompanied by an increase of exocrine secretion (see Reference 6).

2. Vasomotor Control of Endocrine Pancreas

The microcirculation of islets of Langerhans is markedly inhibited by sympathomimetic agents, such as epinephrine, where the blood flow is almost totally stopped; norepinephrine has been shown to be a less potent inhibitor of islet blood flow. Epinephrine- and ephedrine-induced vasoconstriction of afferent and efferent vessels of the islets results in interruption of the circulation in the intrainsular capillary plexus, and, consequently, increased blood glucose levels. In contrast, parasympathetic stimulation (metacholine chloride) causes vasodilation of the afferent and efferent vessels of the islets along with slower but continuous blood flow in the intrainsular capillary plexus, and decreased blood glucose levels (see Reference 4).

These changes in the microcirculation of the islets prove that one of the mechanisms of glucose homeostasis is mediated through the autonomic nervous system by alteration of the blood supply to the islets, which had been classified as a neurovascular homeostatic regulator.[7]

Inasmuch as the inhibition of islet blood flow due to norepinephrine can be blocked by phentolamine, norepinephrine-induced inhibition seems to be mediated by α-adrenoceptors. Since the α_2-adrenoceptor agonist clonidine has no effect on islet blood flow, it is suggested that norepinephrine-induced decrease of islet blood flow is caused by α_1-adrenoceptor stimulation (see Reference 4).

3. Action of Hormones on Exocrine Pancreas

Hormonal control of the pancreatic microcirculation has gained particular interest because the pancreas is both a producer and target of these substances. Both secretin and cholecystokinin (CCK) induce vasodilation and secretin is known to increase pancreatic juice secretion and oxygen consumption. However, the mechanism of action of these two hormones is as yet unknown.

Based on the theory of the insulo-acinar portal system, it is conceivable that islet hormones are secretagogues on the pancreas itself, and they are carried to the exocrine tissue by the efferent capillaries of the islets to exert their action upon the pancreas at a very high concentration. Insulin induces long-term effects on the regulation of the biosynthesis of pancreatic digestive enzymes and short-term effects on the potentiation of pancreatic secretory response. In addition, further actions of insulin on the exocrine pancreas are described, including an increase in glucose transport and protein synthesis, a potentiation of CCK-induced secretion, as well as regulating CCK receptors and acinar cell insulin receptors (see Reference 4).

Other islet hormones and peptides (i.e., glucagon, somatostatin, and the pancreatic polypeptide) act as inhibitory regulators of the pancreas via the insulo-acinar portal system. Although little is known concerning the site of action of these peptides, *in vivo* experiments revealed an inhibitory effect of glucagon on the pancreatic secretory response induced by CCK and secretin. Similarly, somatostatin and pancreatic polypeptide inhibit exocrine pancreatic secretion *in vivo*, but not in either isolated pancreatic acini or pancreatic lobules, indicating the importance of an intact vascular system.

In addition, the pancreatic microcirculation provides an insulo/acinar-ductal portal system, receiving islet hormones, which may regulate the volume of the pancreatic juice.

4. Action of Hormones on Endocrine Pancreas

In addition to the insulo-acinar portal system and the insulo/acinar-ductal portal system, the islets of Langerhans provide a third *in situ* microvascular portal system confined within the islets itself. This intra-islet portal system regulates islet hormone secretion by directing blood flow in a B-A-D cellular sequence.[3] Microvascularly, the B-cell is the primary glucose sensor and hyperglycemia-induced insulin secretion plays a vital role in inhibiting A-cell secretion. Via the microvascular route, A-cells stimulate D-cells; however, D-cells are vascularly neutral within the islet. Inasmuch as islet somatostatin does not possess paracrine function, its role is not within the islet, but may be directed locally upon exocrine tissue via the insulo-acinar portal system.[8]

II. PATHOLOGY

A. DISEASES OF THE ENDOCRINE/EXOCRINE PANCREAS
1. Pancreatic Microcirculation in Diabetes Mellitus/Hyperglycemia

The influence of diabetes mellitus on the microcirculation of pancreatic islets was discussed already in the 1950s. While Bunnag et al.[9] reported no change in capillary diameter either after glucose administration or after injection of diabetic substances (alloxan, dithizone), several investigators demonstrated an increase in both the diameter and the number per unit area of the capillaries in the islets in congenital diabetic mice when compared with normal animals.[10,11] Using the microsphere technique in rats, Jansson and Hellerström[12] confirmed that hyperglycemia increases microvascular blood perfusion in islets of Langerhans *in situ*. After glucose injection, the increase in pancreatic *blood flow* resulted mainly from an increased flow to the tail of the pancreas, and within the tail preferentially to the islets. In contrast, injection of a nonmetabolizable glucose derivate, 3-0-methyl-D-glucose affected neither the pancreatic nor the islet blood flow.[12]

The increase in pancreatic islet blood flow during hyperglycemia in diabetes can be best interpreted as an adaptation to the increased functional demand of the islet cell under diabetic conditions.

Hyperglycemia-induced increase of microvascular blood flow of pancreatic islets is thought to be mediated either by local and/or nervous and humoral mechanisms. Since glucose stimulates B-cell metabolic rate, local thermogenesis and local decrease in blood oxygen saturation may enhance microvascular blood perfusion of pancreatic islets. Several lines of evidence suggest that the glucose-sensitive control mechanism is located at an extrapancreatic site. Jansson and Hellerström[13] emphasized the particular role of the central nervous system in the induction of glucose-selective increase of islet blood flow. Inasmuch as an increase of islet blood flow due to hyperglycemia was abolished by vagotomy or administration of atropine, the authors hypothesized either cholinergic vasodilation of the arterioles supplying the islets, or cholinergic release of vasoactive substances.[13]

2. Microcirculation in Acute Pancreatitis

During the last few years, particular interest has focused on the vascular factors involved in the development of acute pancreatitis.[14] The question posed is whether the necrotizing injury is caused by enzymes or by ischemia. Experimentally, induction of acute pancreatitis results in arteriolar vasoconstriction, capillary perfusion failure as a consequence of hemoconcentration with the result of stasis, local fibrin clotting, leukocyte adherence to the endothelial lining, and vessel rupture.[6,14]

Reactive oxygen metabolites contribute to pancreatitis-induced tissue injury.[15] Besides desintegration of cell membranes by lipid peroxidation, these metabolites trigger the extravasation of polymorphonuclear leukocytes into the surrounding parenchyma. The initial margination of leukocytes within the microvasculature, in particular in postcapillary venules, may represent a key factor in manifestation of endothelial damage and capillary perfusion failure.

The increase in interstitial pressure during pancreatitis, probably caused by the obstruction of lymph drainage, further compromises pancreatic microperfusion. A variety of experimental studies have demonstrated universally a decrease in total pancreatic blood flow due to progressive reduction of capillary perfusion. This begins during the first minutes after induction of pancreatitis, with only single nutritive capillaries remaining perfused after 3 h. Perfusion of arterio-venous shunts has been suggested to explain the fall in oxygen uptake and, indeed, *in vivo* microscopic analyses of the pancreatic microcirculation during the development of pancreatitis demonstrated constant flow via preferential pathways, but progressive failure of nutritive capillary perfusion.[1] Today, focal ischemia due to microcirculatory perfusion failure is accepted as one of the major pathomechanisms involved in the development of acute necrotizing pancreatitis.[14]

3. Microcirculation in Pancreas and Islet Transplantation

Adequate nutritional microvascular perfusion is a prerequisite for successful pancreas/pancreatic islet transplantation for insulin-dependent diabetes mellitus. Using a rat model and the nonradioactive microspheres technique, recent studies demonstrate that not only whole pancreatic blood flow, but also the islet blood flow within the pancreatic graft are significantly higher in transplanted organs when compared to native organs.[16] In parallel, analysis of microvascular perfusion of freely transplanted islet grafts demonstrated comparable single islet blood flow (35 nl/islet/min) of the grafts when compared to pancreatic islets *in situ* (5 to 20 nl/islet/min).[17] However, it should be taken into account that, in contrast to the whole organ pancreatic graft, which is revascularized immediately upon reperfusion, freely transplanted islets require the process of angiogenesis and revascularization to achieve adequate nutritional blood supply.[18] Using *in vivo* fluorescence microscopy, we have demonstrated that the process of vascularization of the islet grafts is completed within a 10-day period after transplantation,[18] demonstrating a glomerulum-like network of capillaries similar to what is known for pancreatic islets *in situ*.[2] After syngeneic transplantation, first signs of angiogenesis are observed at day 2 (Figure 1a), characterized by capillary sprouts originating from the venular segments of host capillaries and postcapillary venules. Blood flow within the newly formed microvessels can be demonstrated after 3 to 6 days (Figures 1b,c). The islets form a glomerulum-like network of capillaries (day 6), and complete revascularization of the graft (including individual arteriolar supply), nutritive capillaries, and blood drainage by individual venules and intercapillary anastomoses, is achieved within 10 to 14 days (Figure 1d). Hyperglycemia of the recipient does not alter revascularization of the grafts,[19] but increases capillary perfusion, comparable to what has been reported for pancreatic islets *in situ*.[12]

Cyclosporin A (CyA), in combination with azathioprine and prednisolone, is the most commonly used immunosuppressant in organ transplantation. However, this compound may exert toxic effects, in particular on endocrine pancreatic tissue, with marked degranulation and functional impairment of the islets. Recent studies indicate that CyA also affects the pancreatic microcirculation: pancreatic blood flow was found to be decreased in transplanted pancreas, including depression of islet blood perfusion.[16] In addition, in free islet transplantation, CyA inhibits vascular ingrowth, which results in decreased microvascular blood perfuson of the transplanted islets.[20,21]

4. Microcirculation in Malignant and Nonmalignant Pancreatic Tumors

Little is known about the microcirculation of malignant and nonmalignant pancreatic tumors. However, there might be an experimental approach for the study of pancreatic tumor microcirculation. Dawiskiba et al.[22] have reported induction of both exocrine pancreatic adenocarcinomas and benign tumors by N-nitrosobis(2-oxopropyl)amine (BOP) in hamsters, which may allow for the study of the microcirculation by means of intravital microscopy, laser Doppler flowmetry, microspheres, dyes, and clearance techniques. In addition, using the skinfold chamber technique with severe combined immunodeficient mice, angiogenesis, and vascularization of human pancreatic tumor cell lines may be studied, as has been reported for human colon adenocarcinoma.[23]

B. STUDY OF THE PANCREATIC MICROCIRCULATION IN CLINICAL DISEASE

The anatomic location of the pancreas, the close contact with the diaphragm, and the thickness of the organ make *in vivo* analysis of the microcirculation in clinical disease with currently available techniques very difficult if not impossible. The only approach may be the use of laser Doppler flowmetry during operative procedures. The difficulty in studying the pancreatic microcirculation in patients underlines the necessity for adequate experimental models to gain further insights in microcirculatory pathomechanisms in pancreatic diseases.

III. MODELS AND TECHNIQUES

A. MODELS FOR EXPERIMENTAL STUDIES OF PANCREATIC DISEASES

1. Diabetes Mellitus/Hyperglycemia

For the induction of acute experimental hyperglycemia, glucose may be administered intravenously. For induction of long-term hyperglycemia, pharmacological compounds, such as streptozotocin or alloxan, respectively, may be applied. However, these models only simulate hyperglycemic conditions, but do not manifest true diabetic disease. To

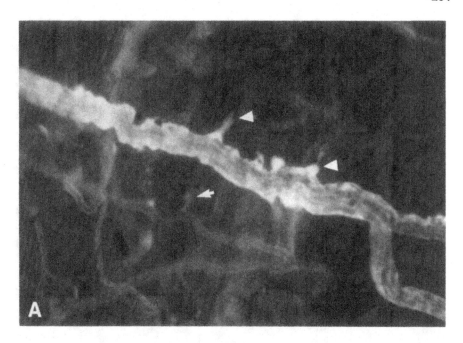

Figure 1a Striated muscle capillaries and postcapillary venule of the hamster dorsal skinfold chamber within an area where a syngeneic islet was transplanted 2 days before. Note the very beginning of angiogenesis and revascularization, i.e. capillary sprouts, demonstrated by the irregularities of the microvessel wall of the capillaries (→) and postcapillary venule (▶) of the host tissue.

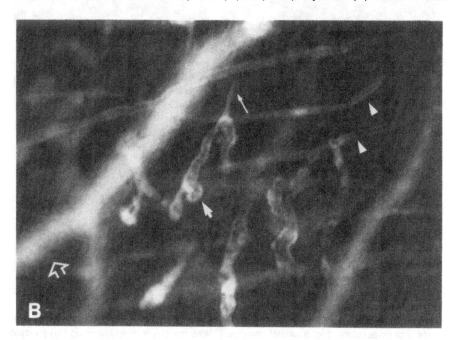

Figure 1b Microvasculature of a syngeneic pancreatic islet 3 days after transplantation. The process of revascularization is characterized by sinusoidal microvascular formations (♦) and capillary sprouts (→), originating from the venular segments of the striated muscle capillaries (▶) and the postcapillary venules (⇒) of the host's microvasculature.

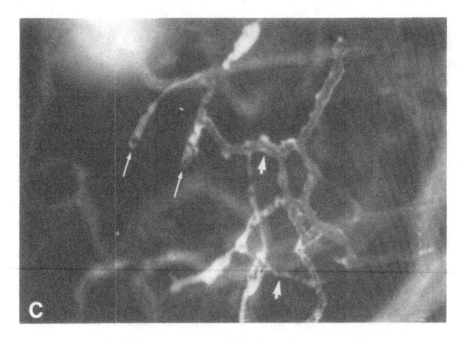

Figure 1c Microvasculature of a syngeneic pancreatic islet 4 days after transplantation. Note the formation of intercapillary anastomoses (♦), which allow for the restoration of blood flow. Further sprouting of new capillaries (→) demonstrates the persistent growth of the microvascular network.

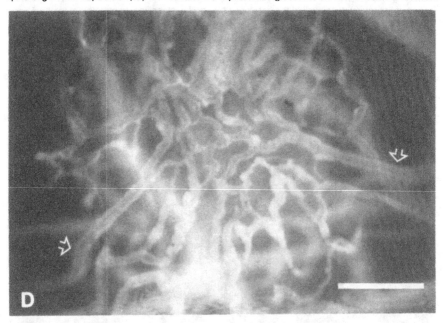

Figure 1d Microvasculature of a syngeneic pancreatic islet 10 days after transplantation. The process of revascularization is almost completed. Note the two feeding arterioles (⇒) piercing into the center of the graft, and the dense glomerulum-like network of capillaries presenting with an angio-architecture, similar as known for the microvascular network of pancreatic islets *in situ*. Intravital fluorescence microscopy, contrast enhancement by FITC-dextran 150,000 i.v.; bar represents 100 μm. (With permission from Reference 37).

approximate more appropriately the clinical disease of diabetes mellitus, the use of particular animal strains, such as ob/ob mice or non-obese diabetic (NOD) mice, provides a more distinct approach for the study of diabetes-induced pathomechanisms.

2. Acute and Chronic Pancreatitis

A variety of established and generally recognized models are known to induce variable degrees of pancreatitis, and are based on different pathophysiological mechanisms, which are discussed as possible factors initiating acute pancreatitis in man. These include (1) the closed duodenal loop technique, (2) bile duct ligation/obstruction, (3) bile, bile salt, and/ or enzyme-induced pancreatitis, (4) hormone-induced pancreatitis, (5) diet-induced pancreatitis, and (6) ischemia-induced pancreatitis.

a. Closed Duodenal Loop Technique

This technique is considered the classic experimental model for the induction of acute pancreatitis secondary to duodenal reflux. After ligation of the common bile duct, bile is diverted by cannula to the jejunum, and the duodenum is then surgically closed at the proximal and distal site of the orifice of the pancreatic duct. Following marked distension of the closed duodenal loop, the head and body of the pancreas become edematous (4 h after ligation), hemorrhagic pancreatitis develops after a 9- to 11-h period, and most of the experimental animals die within 26 h (see Reference 24). However, the role of duodenal reflux in the pathogenesis of acute pancreatitis is a matter of controversy and the clinical relevance of the model seems to be only minor.

b. Bile Duct Ligation/Obstruction

Under experimental conditions, ligation of the pancreatic duct and post-operative stimulation with secretin results in increased pancreatic duct pressure, interstitial edema, and release of pancreatic enzymes in lymph and blood vessels draining the pancreas. The inflammatory response involves large numbers of macrophages, fibroblasts, as well as leukocytes, and the final appearance of the organ after weeks and months is characterized by loss of acinar tissue and fibrosis (chronic pancreatitis). Clinical experience demonstrates that obstruction of the pancreatic duct rarely induces acute, but more commonly induces chronic pancreatitis/fibrosis; therefore, this model may have preferential relevance for the study of chronic pancreatitis/fibrosis.[25]

c. Bile/Enzyme-Induced Pancreatitis

The long-standing clinical evidence for the association of biliary diseases and pancreatitis, together with the hypothesis that bile reflux into the pancreatic duct due to obstruction of the papilla of Vater ("common channel theory"), combine to form the theoretical concept for bile/enzyme-induced pancreatitis models. Bile salts with or without activated pancreatic enzymes are injected/infused retrogradely into the pancreatic duct. The severity of the induced lesion can be altered by varying either the pressure or the concentration of the bile salts used. Pancreatitis evolves rapidly over 2 to 24 h, characterized by edema formation, hemorrhage, and necrosis.[26,27] Both local and remote manifestations of pancreatitis may be studied by the use of this model, which has become the "gold standard" of experimental biliary pancreatitis.

d. Hormone-Induced Pancreatitis

Excessive neural stimulation of the pancreas has been advanced as a possible pathomechanism of acute pancreatitis. Infusion of synthetic peptides (e.g., ceruletide, cholecystokinin, carbamylcholine) results dose-dependently in structural and functional changes of the exocrine pancreas with a significant increase of the pancreatic enzymes in the blood circulation, and vacuolization and destruction of acinar cells. Discharge of secretory proteins into the interstitial space is accompanied by edema formation and inflammatory response (accumulation of neutrophils, lymphocytes, and macrophages), resulting in destructive changes of acinar cells and cell necrosis.[28] The structural changes of acinar cells in human acute pancreatitis share many common features with secretagogue-induced pancreatitis in animals; however, the relevance of the model may be questioned, since it is in doubt whether acute pancreatitis in man occurs as a result of intense hormonal or neural stimulation.

e. Diet-Induced Pancreatitis

Despite the differences between pathogenesis of pancreatitis induced by feeding a choline-deficient, ethionine-supplemented diet in mice compared to human disease, the experimental mouse pancreatitis and the human clinical pancreatitis share several pathophysiological features.[29] The gross and histological appearance of the pancreatic and peripancreatic inflammation, as well as the clinical and biochemical course of diet-induced pancreatitis, resemble human disease. Mortality in this model can be controlled at any desired level between 0 and 100%. Ascites, acidosis, hypoxia, and hypovolemia occur in this model, as well as in human pancreatitis. The drawback of this very simple model is the restriction to solely female Swiss Webster, CD-1 or NMRI mice.

f. Ischemia-Induced Pancreatitis

Vascular mechanisms, defined as any impairment of pancreatic inflow and outflow, or as disturbances of the pancreatic microcirculation, have been advocated as a key element in the initiation and progression of acute pancreatitis. Especially, focal ischemia/reperfusion may result in formation of toxic reactive metabolites and release of a variety of potent mediators from leukocytes, resulting in direct injury of vessel wall, intravascular coagulation, and increased endothelial permeability with interstitial edema formation, hemoconcentration and impaired venous drainage. Experimental models of ischemia-induced pancreatitis include arterial inflow and venous outflow occlusion, embolization of nutritive microvessels by wax/oil droplets or microspheres,[30] or direct tissue clamping.[31] Due to the increasing evidence that focal ischemia is the critical factor in the early phase of acute pancreatitis,[14] today, this model is proposed to be of high clinical relevance for the study of initial pathomechanisms of the disease.

3. Pancreas and Free Islet Transplantation

For pancreaticoduodenal transplantation in small animal models, such as rodents, the whole pancreas, duodenum, and small intestine is dissected and excised after aortic flush with cold preservation solution (e.g., University of Wisconsin solution). The pancreaticoduodenal graft is anastomosed to the aorta/vena cava (suture) or to the renal vessels (cuff technique). Both techniques provide an ideal topographical access to the transplanted organ for the study of the microcirculation.

For microcirculatory analysis of freely transplanted pancreatic islet grafts, islets are isolated by collagenase digestion,[32] and transplanted (1) into the liver via the portal route,[33,34] (2) beneath the kidney capsule,[17,20] or (3) on striated muscle.[35] The microcirculation may be studied by intravital microscopy (transplantation to muscle,[35] kidney capsule[20]), nonradioactive microspheres (transplantation to liver,[34] kidney capsule[17]), or histology (transplantation to liver,[33] muscle[19,35]). The use of the skinfold chamber model with in vivo microscopy is the only approach that allows for repeated/continuous analyses of angiogenesis and vascularization of freely transplanted islet grafts.

4. Malignant and Nonmalignant Pancreatic Tumors

The microcirculation of pancreatic tumors may be studied after induction of tumor growth by N-nitrosobis(2-oxopropyl)amine (BOP) within the pancreatic gland, or by the use of the skinfold chamber technique and transplantation of pancreatic tumor cell lines (see Section III.A.4).

B. TECHNIQUES FOR THE STUDY OF PANCREATIC AND ISLET MICROCIRCULATION

The accuracy of the technique used for the study of the microcirculation, the variations in the surgical preparations, and, undoubtedly, the complexity/variations in vascular supply influence the measurements of nutritional perfusion of the pancreas. Tissue perfusion in the gland can be assessed qualitatively by thermocouples, and quantitatively by isotope fractionation, distribution of microspheres, hydrogen desaturation, and clearance of either xenon or krypton (reviewed in Reference 36). In addition, laser Doppler flowmetry represents a valuable, noninvasive tool for the assessment of microvascular perfusion, allowing for repeated/continuous measurements over a prolonged period of time. However, intravital microscopy is the only technique that provides direct access to the microcirculation. Visualization of the individual segments of the microcirculation, i.e., arterioles, capillaries and postcapillary and collecting venules of both acinar and insular tissue, allows for repeated/continuous analyses of dynamic processes, such as red blood cell velocity and flux, vessel diameter, and capillary density.[1,19,35] In addition, the technique allows for the assessement of cell-cell interaction, including leukocytes, thrombocytes, and endothelial cells. *In vivo* microscopy may be applied not only for the study of the microcirculation of native exocrine and endocrine tissue, but also in malignant and nonmalignant pancreatic tumors as well as pancreatic and islet transplants.

REFERENCES

1. **Klar, E., Endrich, B., and Messmer, K.,** Microcirculation of the pancreas. A quantitative study of physiology and changes in pancreatitis, *Int. J. Microcirc.: Clin. Exp.*, 9, 85–101, 1990.
2. **Bonner-Weir, S. and Orci, L.,** New perspectives on the microvasculature of the islets of Langerhans in the rat, *Diabetes*, 31, 883–889, 1982.
3. **Stagner, J. I. and Samols, E.,** The vascular order of islet cellular perfusion in the human pancreas, *Diabetes*, 41, 93–97, 1992.
4. **Menger, M. D., Hammersen, F., and Messmer, K.,** The microcirculation of the islets of Langerhans: State of the art, *Prog. Appl. Microcirc.*, 17, 192–215, 1990.
5. **Lifson, N., Kramlinger, K. G., Mayrand, R. R., and Lender, E. J.,** Blood flow to the rabbit pancreas with special reference to the islets of Langerhans, *Gastroenterology*, 79, 466–473, 1980.
5a. **Vollmar, B., Preissler, G., and Menger, M. D.,** Hemorrhagic hypotension induces arteriolar vasomotion and intermittent capillary perfusion in rat pancreas, *Am. J. Physiol.*, 267, H1936–H1940, 1994.
6. **Endrich, B., Klar, E., and Hammersen, F.,** The microcirculation of the pancreas: State of the art, *Prog. Appl. Microcirc.*, 17, 144–174, 1990.
7. **Bunnag, S. C., Warner, N. E., and Bunnag, S.,** Vasomotor reactions in the islets affecting the blood glucose levels, *Bibl. Anat.*, 16, 445–449, 1977.
8. **Samols, E., Stagner, J. I., and Nakagawa, A.,** Intra-islet and islet-acinar portal systems — Relevance to transplantation, *Diab. Nutr. Metab.*, 5(Suppl. 1), 3–7, 1992.
9. **Bunnag, S. C., Bunnag, S., and Warner, N. E.,** Microcirculation in the islets of Langerhans of the mouse, *Anat. Rec.*, 146, 117–123, 1963.
10. **Kracht, J., Lo, Y. C., and Rall, J.,** Über Beziehungen zwischen Inselkapillaren und B-Zellfunktion, *Endokrinologie*, 39, 35–43, 1960.
11. **Hellerström, C. and Hellman, B.,** The blood circulation of the islets of Langerhans visualized by the fluorescent dye vasoflavine, *Acta Soc. Med. Ups.*, 66, 88–94, 1961.
12. **Jansson, L. and Hellerström, C.,** Stimulation by glucose of the blood flow to the pancreatic islets of the rat, *Diabetologia*, 25, 45–50, 1983.
13. **Jansson, L. and Hellerström, C.,** Glucose-induced changes in pancreatic islet blood flow mediated by central nervous system, *Am. J. Physiol.*, 251, E644–E647, 1986.
14. **Klar, E., Messmer, K., Warshaw, A. L., and Herfarth, C.,** Pancreatic ischaemia in experimental pancreatitis: Mechanism, significance, and therapy, *Br. J. Surg.*, 77, 1205–1210, 1990.

15. **Schoenberg, M. H., Büchler, M., Schädlich, H., Younes, M., Bültmann, B., and Beger, H. G.,** Involvement of oxygen radicals and phospholipase A_2 in acute pancreatitis of the rat, *Klin. Wochenschr.*, 67, 166–170, 1989.

16. **Jansson, L., Korsgren, O., Wahlberg, J., and Andersson, A.,** Effects of cyclosporin A on the blood flow of the native and transplanted rat pancreas and duodenum, *Transplant. Int.*, 6, 143–147, 1993.

17. **Sandler, S. and Jansson, L.,** Blood flow measurements in autotransplanted pancreatic islets of the rat. Impairment of the blood perfusion of the graft during hyperglycemia, *J. Clin. Invest.*, 80, 17–21, 1987.

18. **Menger, M. D., Jaeger, S., Walter, P., Feifel, G., Hammersen, F., and Messmer, K.,** Angiogenesis and hemodynamics of microvasculature of transplanted islets of Langerhans, *Diabetes*, 38(Suppl 1), 199–201, 1989.

19. **Menger, M. D., Vajkoczy, P., Leiderer, R., Jäger, S., and Messmer, K.,** Influence of experimental hyperglycemia on microvascular blood perfusion of pancreatic islet isografts, *J. Clin. Invest.*, 90, 1361–1369, 1992.

20. **Rooth, P., Dawidson, I., Lafferty, K., Diller, K., Armstrong, J., Pratt, P., Simonsen, R., and Täljedal, I. B.,** Prevention of detrimental effect of cyclosporin A on vascular ingrowth of transplanted pancreatic islets with verapamil, *Diabetes*, 38(Suppl 1), 202–205, 1989.

21. **Menger, M. D., Wolf, B., Höbel, R., Schorlemmer, H. U., and Messmer, K.,** Microvascular phenomena during pancreatic islet graft rejection, *Langenbecks Arch. Chir.*, 376, 214–221, 1991.

22. **Dawiskiba, S., Pour, P. M., Stenram, U., Sundler, F., and Andren-Sandberg, A.,** Immunohistochemical characterization of endocrine cells in experimental exocrine pancreatic cancer in the Syrian golden hamster, *Int. J. Pancreatol.*, 11, 87–96, 1992.

23. **Leunig, M., Yuan, F., Menger, M. D., Boucher, Y., Goetz, A. E., Messmer, K., and Jain, R. K.,** Angiogenesis, microvascular architecture, microhemodynamics, and interstitial fluid pressure during early growth of human adenocarcinoma LS174T in SCID mice, *Cancer Res.*, 52, 6553–6560, 1992.

24. **Adler, G., Kern, H. F., and Scheele, G. A.,** Experimental models and concepts in acute pancreatitis, in *The Exocrine Pancreas Biology, Pathobiology, and Diseases*, Go, V. L. W., Gardner, J. D., Brooks, F. P., Lebenthal, E., DiMagno, E. P., and Scheele, G. A., Eds., Raven Press, New York, 1986, 407–421.

25. **Reber, H. A., Karanjia, N. D., Alvarez, C., Widdison, A. L., Leung, F. W., Ashley, S. W., and Lutrin, F. J.,** Pancreatic blood flow in cats with chronic pancreatitis, *Gastroenterology*, 103, 652–659, 1992.

26. **Senninger, N.,** Bile-induced pancreatitis, *Eur. Surg. Res.*, 24, 68–73, 1992.

27. **Vollmar, B., Waldner, H., Schmand, J., Conzen, P. F., Goetz, A. E., Habazettl, H., Schweiberer, L., and Brendel, W.,** Release of arachidonic acid metabolites during acute pancreatitis in pigs, *Scand. J. Gastroenterol.*, 24, 1253–1264, 1989.

28. **Niederau, C., Ferrell, L. D., and Grendell, J. H.,** Caerulein-induced acute necrotizing pancreatitis in mice: Protective effects of proglumide, benzotript, and secretin, *Gastroenterology*, 88, 1192–1204, 1985.

29. **Niederau, C., Lüthen, R., Niederau, M. C., Grendell, J. H., and Ferrell, L. D.,** Acute experimental hemorrhagic-necrotizing pancreatitis induced by feeding a choline-deficient ethionine-supplemented diet, *Eur. Surg. Res.*, 24, 40–54, 1992.

30. **Vollmar, B., Waldner, H., Schmand, J., Conzen, P. F., Goetz, A. E., Habazettl, H., Schweiberer, L., and Brendel, W.,** Oleic acid-induced pancreatitis in pigs, *J. Surg. Res.*, 50, 1–9, 1990.

31. **Waldner, H.,** Vascular mechanisms to induce acute pancreatitis, *Eur. Surg. Res.*, 24(Suppl. 1), 62–67, 1992.

32. **Menger, M. D. and Messmer, K.,** Pancreatic islet transplantation: Isolation, separation, and microvascularization, *Wien. Klin. Wochenschr.*, 104, 429–433, 1992.

33. **Griffith, R. C., Scharp, D. W., Hartman, B. K., Ballinger, W. F., and Lacy, P. E.,** A morphologic study of intrahepatic portal-vein islet isografts, *Diabetes*, 26, 201–214, 1977.

34. **Andersson, A., Korsgren, O., and Jansson, L.,** Intraportally transplanted pancreatic islets revascularized from hepatic arterial system, *Diabetes*, 38(Suppl. 1), 192–195, 1989.

35. **Menger, M. D., Jäger, S., Walter, P., Hammersen, F., and Messmer, K.,** A novel technique for studies on the microvasculature of transplanted islets of Langerhans *in vivo*, *Int. J. Microcirc.: Clin. Exp.*, 9, 103–117, 1990.

36. **Studley, J. G. N., Mathie, R. T., and Blumgart, L. H.,** Blood flow measurement in the canine pancreas, *J. Surg. Res.*, 42, 101–115, 1987.

37. **Menger, M. D. and Messmer, K.,** The microvasculature of free pancreatic islet grafts, in *Pathways to Applied Immunology*, Messmer, K. and Stein, M., Eds., Springer, Berlin, 1991, 109–126.

Chapter 23

Skeletal Muscle Microcirculation

Michael A. Hill and Gerald A. Meininger

CONTENTS

I. ANATOMY AND FUNCTION

Under normal conditions, skeletal muscle is the major component of body mass (30–40% of total). As a consequence, skeletal muscle represents the largest single vascular bed and plays an important role in the maintenance of overall arterial pressure and circulatory homeostasis. In terms of functional behavior, skeletal muscle is unique in the abrupt transition that occurs upon activation of the tissue. Progression from resting conditions to the active state can be accompanied by marked increases in local microvascular blood flow. For example, at rest, total skeletal muscle blood flow is approximately 1000 ml/min (20% of cardiac output), increasing to 15,000 to 25,000 ml/min (85% of cardiac output at $V_{O_2 max}$) in heavy exercise.[1] This ability to alter vascular resistance lies in (1) the microvascular anatomy of skeletal muscle, (2) maintenance of a high level of intrinsic basal tone, and (3) interactions between local and neural regulatory mechanisms.

A. VASCULAR ANATOMY OF SKELETAL MUSCLE

Recent experimental studies have demonstrated that the vasculature of individual muscles is not a simple "tree-like" branching structure, but rather is typically characterized by the existence of several large feed arterioles (approximately 100–150 μm) that supply blood into an extensive network of interconnecting and arcading arterioles (approximately 30–80 μm) (Figures 1 and 2).[2-5] Branches from the smaller arcading arterioles are referred to

0-8493-4870-6/95/$0.00+$.50

298

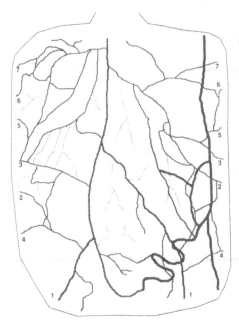

Figure 1a Arteriolar map drawn from a cremaster muscle that had been perfusion-fixed and filled with latex (Microfil). For clarity, the vasculature is presented as a flat sheet with the numbers on the left and right sides indicating *in vivo* vascular connections. These pathways are generally severed during preparation of the muscle for *in vivo* microscopy. The deferential artery (distal feed vessel) and branches that are in the mesorchial connective tissue are shown in bold. (From Hill, M. A., Trippe, K. M., Li, Q.-X., and Meininger, G. A., *Microvasc. Res.*, 44, 117, 1992.)

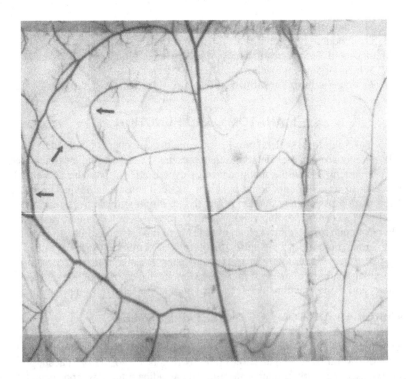

Figure 1b Photograph of a Micofil-perfused cremaster muscle preparation. The arrows indicate the presence of intramuscular arcades. (From Hill, M. A., Trippe, K. M., Li, Q.-X., and Meininger, G. A., *Microvasc. Res.*, 44, 117, 1992.)

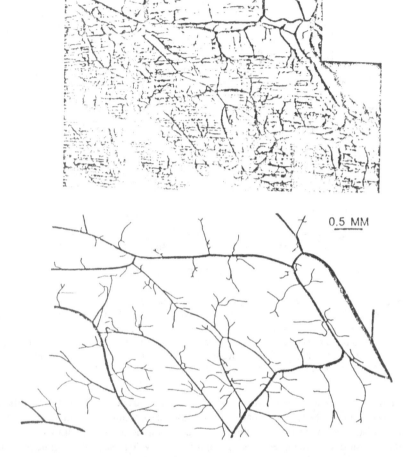

0.5 MM

Figure 2 Photographic montage of a carbon-filled rat spinotrapezius muscle microcirculatory preparation is shown in the upper panel, and a line drawing of the arcading arterial vessels is shown in the lower panel. The figure emphasizes the extensive arterial arcade network that is characteristic of skeletal muscle. (From Engelson, E. T., Schmid-Schonbein, G. W., and Zweifach, B. W., *Microvasc. Res.*, 30, 34, 1985.)

as the transverse arterioles that subsequently branch into terminal arterioles, which give rise to the capillary bed. It is thought that the function of the arteriolar arcades is to maintain a near-uniform arterial pressure down to the level of the transverse arterioles and a uniform pressure distribution across the muscle. The transverse and terminal arterioles, by virtue of a high level of basal tone, act to control blood flow and capillary perfusion at the local level, in concert with tissue metabolic demands.

The existence of the arcading arteriolar network has important implications for the microvascular pressure profile within a given skeletal muscle. Early studies indicated an approximate 50 to 60% drop in arterial pressure at the point of entry of the feed vessels into the muscle, implying that a substantial portion of vascular resistance lies upstream from the actual muscle microcirculation.[6,7] It is, however, now evident that the fraction of upstream resistance was overestimated due to surgical disruption of feed vessels that occurred during the exteriorization of tissues for *in vivo* microscopy.[3,4] A more reasonable estimate of the upstream pressure drop is 25 to 30% of mean arterial pressure. Figure 3

300

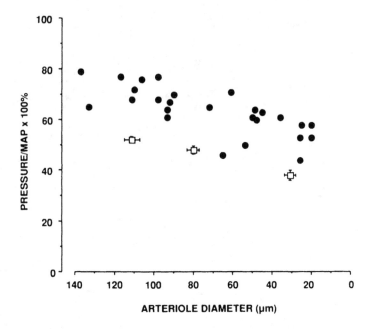

Figure 3 *Cremaster muscle arteriolar pressure profile obtained from opened preparations in which the deferential (distal) feed vessel was left intact (closed circles). For comparison, earlier results obtained using the conventional preparation (severed distal feeder) are shown (open squares). The data is presented as intravascular pressure normalized to each animal's mean arterial pressure at the time of the microvascular pressure measurement. (From Hill, M. A., Trippe, K. M., Li, Q.-X., and Meininger, G. A., Microvasc. Res., 44, 117, 1992.)*

illustrates the arteriolar pressure profile for rat cremaster muscle obtained when the major feed vessels are left intact; for comparison, intravascular pressure measurements obtained when the distal feed vessel (deferential arteriole) was ligated are also shown. It can be seen that pressure in the main feed vessel is approximately 70 to 80% of systemic pressure and that pressure is maintained at approximately 50 to 60% of systemic at the level of transverse arterioles (20–50 μm in diameter). Similar pressure profiles have been found in spinotrapezius and gracilus muscles when all feed vessels are left intact.[4]

B. MICROVASCULAR CONTROL MECHANISMS IN SKELETAL MUSCLE
1. Local Regulatory Mechanisms
Skeletal muscle exhibits a number of microvascular regulatory mechanisms that together act to match O_2 supply with metabolic demands, control local blood flow and pressure, and maintain a basal level of peripheral resistance. The three principal mechanisms of intrinsic vascular control in skeletal muscle are myogenic, metabolic, and flow-dependent regulation. These mechanisms form the basis for the physiologic events that occur during functional and reactive hyperemia and blood flow autoregulation. More in-depth discussions, including that relating to interactions between these mechanisms, can be found in reviews by Granger et al.,[8] Johnson,[9] and Meininger et al.[10]

a. Myogenic Mechanisms
An increase in intravascular pressure in skeletal muscle arterioles results in a local vasoconstriction, while a decrease in pressure elicits vasodilatation. As a consequence, myogenic vasoconstriction in response to increased arterial pressure would be expected to limit hyperperfusion and the transfer of the pressure increase to the exchange vessels. This in turn reduces the possibility of excess fluid filtration and edema. The response is

more intense in the smaller arterioles (<50 μm in diameter), based on both rate and extent of vasoconstriction, and is an inherent property of the vascular smooth muscle.[11,12]

b. Metabolic Mechanisms

Skeletal muscle arterioles have the capability of adjusting the degree of vascular tone in accordance with local metabolic conditions.[8,13,14] In response to declining oxygen levels or increasing concentrations of vasoactive products of metabolism (for example adenosine, K^+ or lactate), the terminal arterioles (<15 to 20 μm in diameter) undergo marked vasodilatation. The consequence of this response is an increased oxygen supply, together with the convective washout of parenchymal tissue metabolites that accumulate in the interstitial space. On return to basal metabolic conditions, the vasoactive stimulus is removed and vascular resistance returns toward normal.

c. Flow-Dependent Dilatation

The basis for this regulatory mechanism is that alterations in blood flow velocity can affect alterations in arteriolar diameter. Recent studies indicate that alterations in shear stress, consequent to changes in velocity, stimulate production and release of vasoactive substances from the vascular endothelium.[15] Candidate factors include nitric oxide and prostacyclin. Thus, in response to increased shear stress, the production of endothelial-derived mediators would elicit arteriolar dilatation, while at decreased shear stress levels arterioles would tend to constrict. It appears that under normal conditions, flow-dependent dilatation would function as a secondary mechanism requiring a myogenic or metabolic event for its stimulation.

d. Interactions Between Local Regulatory Mechanisms

The above mechanisms do not exist in isolation and under some circumstances may act to reinforce each other (e.g., metabolic, myogenic, and flow-dependent mechanisms under conditions of increased or decreased arterial pressure) or to oppose each other (e.g., myogenic and flow-dependent regulatory mechanisms are opposed by metabolic mechanisms during increased venous pressure). In resting skeletal muscle, it appears that myogenic mechanisms dominate local metabolic regulation as pressure-induced arteriolar vasoconstriction can be maintained despite marked decreases in blood flow and declining parenchymal oxygen levels.[11] The exact *in vivo* spatial arrangement of these regulatory mechanisms is, at present, uncertain. In one model, Granger[16] has suggested a series-coupled control scheme whereby different levels of the arteriolar vasculature are predominately associated with the different control mechanisms; terminal arterioles being responsive to metabolic factors, intermediate arterioles responding to myogenic stimuli, and the larger arterioles being sensitive to changes in shear stress. Thus, in a situation where metabolic stimuli lead to dilation of the terminal arterioles, pressure would decrease in the myogenically sensitive vessels, causing dilation of this segment. Further, the vasodilation would cause an increase in blood flow velocity and a shear stress-mediated release of vasodilator factors from the endothelium that would act to reinforce the myogenic and metabolic responses. Correction of the original metabolic stimulus would result in a return to basal in all three segments. Other models have been suggested for the coupling of local responses between vascular segments including: (1) propagated vasomotor responses (vasodilatation and vasoconstriction),[17,18] (2) series-coupling, whereby a single control modality varies in its level of responsiveness along the vasculature,[19] and (3) counter-current exchange of vasoactive substances between paired venules and arterioles.[20,21]

2. Neural Mechanisms

Skeletal muscles have been shown to possess adrenergic, cholinergic, and peptidergic innervation.[22,23] With respect to adrenergic nerves, studies using fluorescence localization techniques have demonstrated a discontinuous pattern of innervation, with a general trend for decreasing density of the nerve plexus as arteriolar diameter decreases and an absence of regular innervation of the capillaries and small venules. Saltzman et al.[24] further showed that in rat spinotrapezius muscle there is dense innervation of the transverse arterioles at the point of branching from the arcade vessels. Innervation at this site favors a role for neural mechanisms in the local control of microvascular blood flow. Functional studies of adrenergic innervation suggest that the smaller arterioles ($<50\,\mu m$) are the most sensitive to nerve stimulation and topical application of exogenous adrenergic agonists.[25] While this may appear to conflict with the described patterns of innervation, the increased responsiveness of the smaller vessels may reflect an inherent increase in contractile activity per se, more optimal physical conditions (i.e., length-tension relationship), or a more optimal smooth muscle/transmitter relationship.[26,27]

In addition to direct effects, adrenergic mechanisms also interact with the local control mechanisms described above. Examples of such interactions include (1) enhanced myogenic reactivity in the presence of adrenergic stimulation,[28,29] (2) terminal arteriole sympathetic escape, despite maintained nerve stimulation,[27] due to accumulation of vasoactive metabolites, and (3) local autoregulatory responses that occur secondarily to nerve-induced changes in local pressure and flow.[30] In studies of the *in vivo* rat cremaster muscle microcirculation Faber, and co-workers[31,32] have shown that the relative distribution of α-adrenergic receptor subtypes varies with arteriolar location within the vascular network. These authors demonstrated that first- and second-order arterioles utilize both α_1- and α_2-adrenoceptors, while the smaller third- and fourth-order vessels (transverse/terminal arterioles) predominately utilize α_2-receptors. The α_2-responses were shown to be more susceptible to inhibition by myogenic and metabolic stimuli. Faber therefore proposed a model whereby α_2-adrenergic mechanisms interact more readily with local myogenic and metabolic regulatory mechanisms to coordinate local oxygen supply/demand while α_1-mechanisms tend to preserve reflex control of resistance at upstream sites.[32]

In addition to adrenergic innervation, a number of vasoactive peptides have been shown to be associated with the perivascular nerves. In rat cremaster muscle, Fleming et al.,[23] using immunohistochemical techniques, demonstrated neuropeptide Y to be a co-transmitter with norepinephrine and further showed that substance P and calcitonin gene-related peptide (CGRP) immunoreactivity was located in periarteriolar axons. It is likely that substance P and CGRP are localized in sensory neurons and mediate vasodilatation and changes in vascular permeability. A similar distribution was also reported in rabbit tenuissimus muscle.[33]

3. Hormonal and Paracrine Mechanisms

Skeletal muscle arterioles respond vigorously to a variety of topically and systematically administered vasoactive hormones and paracrine factors. With respect to the more classical hormones, direct *in vivo* studies have shown that the transverse and terminal arterioles show marked vasoconstriction to angiotensin II,[34,35] endothelin,[36] norepinephrine,[6] and vasopressin.[37] Paracrine factors, such as nitric oxide (endothelium-derived relaxing factor, EDRF), the arachidonic acid metabolites prostacyclin and PGE_2, and possibly the yet-to-be characterized endothelium-derived hyperpolarizing factor (EDHF), are potent dilators of small skeletal muscle arterioles.[38,39] Endogenous production of EDRF has been implicated in the response to topically applied agents (e.g., acetylcholine) and to physical factors such as shear stress stimuli.[38-40] Similarly, endogenous vasodilator prostaglandin production has been demonstrated by vasoconstriction following treatment with cyclooxygenase inhibitors such as indomethacin and flufenamic acid.[34,35] In addition to these substances, it has become evident that some growth factors (e.g., platelet-derived growth factor[41]) and immunologic factors (e.g., tumor necrosis factor[42]) possess vasoreactivity; however, the physiologic significance of such effects has yet to be established.

Interactions between paracrine factors and the earlier described local control mechanisms are also evident in skeletal muscle microcirculation. For example, local inhibition of prostaglandin production by cyclooxygenase inhibitors leads to enhanced basal tone and arteriolar myogenic responsiveness to acute increases in intravascular pressure.[43]

In addition to affecting changes in vessel diameter, a number of hormonal and paracrine factors will also act to increase vascular permeability. Local application of histamine results in dilatation of skeletal muscle arterioles while also causing macromolecular leakage from the postcapillary venules.[44] Leukotriene B_4, a metabolite of arachidonic acid, similarly causes an increase in venular permeability and extravasation of leukocytes.[45]

II. PATHOLOGY

A. PATHOLOGIC PROCESSES DIRECTLY IMPACTING ON SKELETAL MUSCLE MICROCIRCULATION

While there is little information regarding disease processes specifically affecting the skeletal muscle microvasculature, a number of pathologic states that impact on a variety of tissues also have significant effects on muscle. In such cases, the effects on the skeletal muscle circulation may have a major effect on overall vascular resistance and circulatory homeostasis. The pathologic processes outlined below are listed as separate entities, but it is highly likely that a number of similar mechanisms are involved in these states.

1. Low-Flow States

The response of skeletal muscle microvasculature to hypoperfusion is an important determinant of the degree to which total peripheral resistance, and hence arterial pressure, is maintained during states of inadequate perfusion. Mild hypovolemia is associated with reflex vasoconstriction of arterioles, which acts to increase peripheral resistance and arterial pressure. Arteriolar vasoconstriction also leads to a decrease in capillary pressure, which favors absorption of fluid from the interstitium and as a consequence increased plasma volume. Mean circulatory filling pressure is, in addition, maintained by neurogenic and hormonal stimulation of capacitance vessels.

During severe prolonged hypovolemia, local regulatory mechanisms eventually dominate, with the arterioles undergoing relaxation. The exact signals that stimulate the local vasodilatation are not known, but presumably result from impaired metabolism. This paradoxical vasodilatation, which occurs despite decreased systemic pressure, has been referred to as a state of decompensation.[46] While there is escape from arteriolar constriction, venular constriction tends to be maintained. These events occur not only following hemorrhage-induced hypovolemia but also in septic shock such as that caused by administration of bacterial endotoxin. This latter condition is currently being studied at the level of the skeletal muscle microvasculature by a number of groups.[47,48]

In addition to globally reduced blood flow, impaired skeletal muscle perfusion can occur at a localized level as in the case of compartment syndrome. In this disorder, increased tissue pressure within a muscular compartment (resulting from fractures, contusions, healing burns, etc.) can lead to venous hypertension, markedly impaired capillary blood flow, and tissue necrosis.[49]

2. Inflammation

The inflammatory response in skeletal muscle represents a complex interaction between several cell types and chemical mediators (e.g., histamine, bradykinin, leukotrienes). Histamine released from mast cells has been shown to cause dilatation of precapillary arterioles and increased permeability of the postcapillary venules.[44] The formation of edema appears to be a result of the increase in permeability, rather than an increase in capillary pressure consequent to arteriolar dilatation, as the increase in venular permeability occurs at histamine levels lower than that required for an arteriolar effect.[8] The increase in permeability involves, in part, a cytoskeleton-mediated contraction of endothelial cells.[50] Inflammation in skeletal muscle is also associated with extravasation of leukocytes through the endothelial lining of small venules (see below). The process of leukocyte adhesion, diapedesis, and extravasation has been shown to be stimulated by mediators such as leukotriene B_4 and inflammatory cytokines.[45,51]

3. Reperfusion Injury

Reperfusion of tissues after an extended period of ischemia is often characterized by further deterioration of tissue function and necrosis. Despite reinstitution of blood flow, some capillaries will remain nonperfused, leading to an increase in total peripheral resistance, increased permeability, and edema. A key determinant of this response appears to involve an interaction between leukocytes, in particular neutrophils, and the postcapillary venular endothelium.[52] Normal leukocyte function (e.g., phagocytosis, emigration) requires cell-cell interaction, but in excess may represent a damaging phenomena to the microcirculation by obstruction of capillaries and production of cytotoxic free radicals. The adhesion of leukocytes to endothelial cells requires the involvement of specific glycoprotein adhesion molecules,[51,53] for example, the integrins and selections. Such molecules exist on the surface of both the leukocytes and endothelial cells, and activation or upregulation of either site may enhance adhesion.[51] Adhesion to postcapillary endothelial cells appears to be favored over that of arterial endothelium due to both hemodynamic mechanisms and inherently more optimal adhesion conditions.[52] The leukocyte contribution to reperfusion injury in skeletal muscle has been demonstrated in dog gracilis muscle by the absence of increased vascular resistance and permeability when reperfused with granulocyte-depleted blood.[54] Specific monoclonal antibodies directed at integrin adhesion molecules have also been used to protect against reperfusion injury.[55,56] Additional support for a role for leukocytes was provided by the studies of Korthuis et al.,[57] which quantitated post-ischemia accumulation of neutrophils in dog gracilis muscle by measuring an increase in the activity of the neutrophil enzyme myeloperoxidase. (For further information, see Chapter 6 of this volume.)

4. Reconstructive Surgery

Microsurgical techniques that allow the replantation of severed limbs, musculocutaneous flap transfer, and muscle transplantation are often complicated by post-operative events some of which may involve the microcirculation rather than thrombosis at the site of a vascular anastomosis. In a number of recent reports, skeletal muscle microcirculatory preparations, in experimental animals, have been used to examine the sequelae of such surgical procedures.[58,59] Barker and colleagues have used the rat cremaster muscle, isolated so as to be supplied by a single neurovascular bundle, to simulate the effect of arterial injury and repair on microemboli formation. These authors have demonstrated that the microemboli released from an iliac artery repair site cause impaired cremaster muscle capillary perfusion, as measured by a decreased number of perfused capillaries. The mechanism by which the emboli impaired perfusion was suggested to be related to the release of vasoactive mediators (e.g., platelet-derived thromboxane A_2) rather than simple mechanical obstruction. Microvascular dysfunction following surgical repair may also result from leukocyte-endothelial cell interactions similar to that described above.

As situations involving replantation and tissue repair are often associated with denervation in addition to disruption of the blood supply, experimental studies have been performed to examine the effect of acute denervation on the extent of an ischemia/reperfusion injury. Using an *in vivo* rat cremaster muscle preparation, subjected to a 3-h period of ischemia, Chen et al.[60] demonstrated that microcirculatory function was further impaired by denervation.

B. SKELETAL MUSCLE AS A "MODEL" TISSUE FOR MICROVASCULAR DYSFUNCTION IN GENERAL

Skeletal muscle has been used as a model tissue for studying the general effects of several experimental disease states on microcirculatory function and structure. Two common examples include genetic and experimentally induced models of hypertension and diabetes. In the case of experimental diabetes *in vivo*, rat and mouse cremaster muscle preparations have been used to demonstrate alterations in vasoreactivity to exogenously applied agonists (e.g. angiotensin II[35] and norepinephrine[61]), impaired myogenic reactivity,[62] the effect of the disorder on the arteriolar pressure distribution[62] and alterations in vascular permeability.[63] *In vitro* studies using isolated, cannulated, first-order cremaster muscle arterioles have been used to show that short-term experimental diabetes adversely affects the mechanical properties of these vessels.[64] In experimental hypertension, numerous studies have used skeletal muscle microcirculatory preparations to demonstrate, for example, alterations in microvascular hemodynamics,[6] vascular reactivity,[65] mechanical properties,[66] and vessel growth patterns (e.g., remodeling, rarefaction, and hypertrophy).[67]

It is likely that skeletal muscle microvascular beds will be valuable as "model tissues" for the study of cardiovascular disorders that have been engineered in transgenic animals; for example, the transgenic hypertensive rat derived via the transgenic expression of a mouse renin gene (Ren-2 gene) on the genetic background of Sprague-Dawley rats.[68] Recent studies using a mouse mutant deficient in P selectin have demonstrated the importance of this endothelial cell adhesion molecule in leukocyte rolling and extravasation.[69] Similarly, it can be advantageous to compare microcirculatory responses in different inbred strains of laboratory animals. For example, the SJL strain of mice shows a markedly enhanced histamine-induced increase in skeletal muscle microvascular permeability as compared to the BALB/c strain.[70]

III. METHODS AND TECHNIQUES TO STUDY MUSCLE MICROCIRCULATION

Skeletal muscle microcirculation has been studied using four main approaches: (1) whole intact organ, (2) exteriorized microvascular bed, (3) isolation and cannulation of microvessel segments, and (4) study of fixed tissue.

A. WHOLE-ORGAN APPROACHES

A variety of whole-organ techniques have been used for the global study of skeletal muscle microcirculation, including implanted flow probes,[71] indicator washout techniques,[72] infusion of radiolabeled microspheres,[73] microcannulation of intact muscles (e.g., cat gastrocnemius) for measurement of segmental vascular resistance,[74] and perfused hindquarter preparations.[75] Similarly, isolated limb preparations in combination with isogravimetric techniques have been used for capillary pressure, fluid filtration, and absorption measurements.[76] Whole-organ approaches have also been effectively used in combination with the *in vivo* study of exteriorized tissues (see following section). For example, implanted flow probes can be used to provide information regarding total organ blood flow while simultaneous direct studies provide data at a particular microvascular site within the tissue being studied.[77] These whole-organ techniques are necessarily indirect in that they do not provide observations on single microvessels and as such will not be detailed in this chapter. However, it should be stressed that whole-organ approaches are useful in identification of global hemodynamic events and often form the basis for the design of direct microcirculatory approaches.

B. *IN VIVO* STUDY OF EXTERIORIZED TISSUES

Exteriorized muscle preparations in combination with *in vivo* microscopic techniques gained considerable popularity in the 1970s and 1980s. A listing of commonly used preparations is

Table 1 Examples of Experimental Preparations Used for *In Vivo* Video Microscopy of Skeletal Muscle Microcirculation

Species	Muscle	Ref.[a]
Cat	Sartorius	78
	Tenuissimus	79
Rabbit	Tenuissimus	80
Rat	Cremaster	5, 81
	Spinotrapezius	4, 82
	Gracilus	4, 83
	Diaphragm	84
Mouse	Cremaster	85
Bat	Tensor plagiopatagii	86
Hamster	Cremaster	87
	Retractor	88

[a] In general, references are limited to a single example of a given preparation.

shown in Table 1. These techniques have provided direct observation of microcirculatory beds, enabled direct application of vasoactive substances, and further allowed for the study of local vasoregulatory mechanisms (e.g., metabolic and myogenic autoregulation, reactive hyperemia). With respect to hemodynamic parameters, these preparations have been used for the measurement of vessel diameter, red cell velocity, microvascular pressures, microvascular permeability, and leukocyte adhesion. This approach continues to be extremely useful; however, there are a number of factors that complicate their use. Consideration must be given to the fact that the vessels are being studied in a network situation; for example, when a vasoactive agent is applied globally to the surface of an exteriorized muscle preparation, it may affect vessels other than at the site of observation such that if a vasomotor response is elicited either up- or downstream, this may alter intravascular pressure and/or flow and result in the stimulation of local regulatory mechanisms. Conditions of the buffer used to superfuse the muscle preparation should be closely monitored and should match that found *in vivo* (e.g., pH, pO_2, pCO_2, temperature, and osmolality). These preparations require general anesthesia of the animals that may adversely affect cardiovascular and respiratory status; the reader is referred to articles by Longnecker and Seyde[89] and Bohlen[90] for specific information on appropriate anesthetic regimens. Thus, there are numerous variables that must be considered, not only in experimental design but also in interpretation of *in vivo* experimental data.

As it is beyond the scope of this brief chapter to describe the procedures for the many available *in vivo* skeletal muscle preparations, the rat exteriorized cremaster muscle is presented as a typical example. The method described is a variation on that described in 1973 by Baez.[81] This tissue provides a relatively thin sheet of skeletal muscle (200–300 μm), which is easily transilluminated (especially in younger animals; <200 g body weight) to give reasonable optical clarity. The reader is referred to the references in Table 1 for specific details of other preparations.

In our studies, rats were anesthetized with a combination of urethane (425 mg/kg) and α-chloralose (100 mg/kg) injected intramuscularly; supplementary doses of 20 to 40% were administered intraperitoneally when indicated. A tracheostomy (polythethylene tubing, Intramedic PE200-PE240) is performed to ensure a patent airway and either the femoral or carotid artery cannulated (PE50) for measurement of mean arterial pressure. A rectal temperature probe is inserted for monitoring core temperature. A longitudinal incision is made in the ventral scrotal skin to expose the right testis with its surrounding cremaster

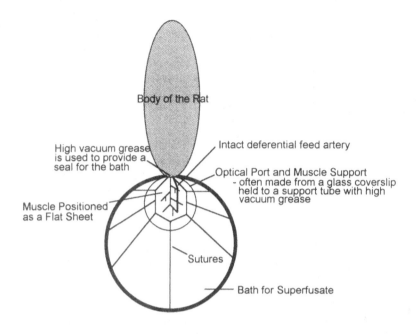

High vacuum grease is used to provide a seal for the bath

Intact deferential feed artery

Optical Port and Muscle Support - often made from a glass coverslip held to a support tube with high vacuum grease

Muscle Positioned as a Flat Sheet

Body of the Rat

Sutures

Bath for Superfusate

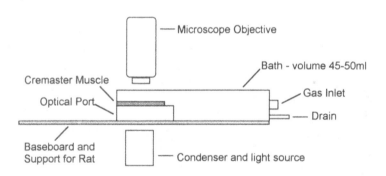

Microscope Objective

Bath - volume 45-50ml

Cremaster Muscle

Gas Inlet

Optical Port

Drain

Baseboard and Support for Rat

Condenser and light source

Figure 4 Typical set-up used for *in vivo* study of the cremaster muscle microcirculation. The upper panel shows a top view of the tissue bath, while the lower panel gives the side view and relationship to the microscope light source and objective lens.

muscle. At this stage, it is advisable to ensure that the muscle is kept moist by continually dripping warmed physiologic salt solution onto its surface. The connective tissue fascia overlying the muscle is dissected away, taking care not to damage the cremaster muscle by stretching. The cremaster muscle itself is opened using electrocautery to prevent bleeding. The line of cauterization is located on the side of the cremaster muscle opposite the major feed arteriole and should be selected so as to minimize disruption of major intramuscular vessels that are visible to the eye. At this stage, the animal is positioned so that its hind legs straddle a custom-designed plexiglass tissue bath into which the muscle can be positioned. The muscle is then secured as a flat sheet by 6-0 nylon suture; typically, seven equally spaced ties pass from the cauterized edges of the tissue and are anchored to the wall of the bath (Figure 4). The muscle is supported by an optical port, the top of which consists of a

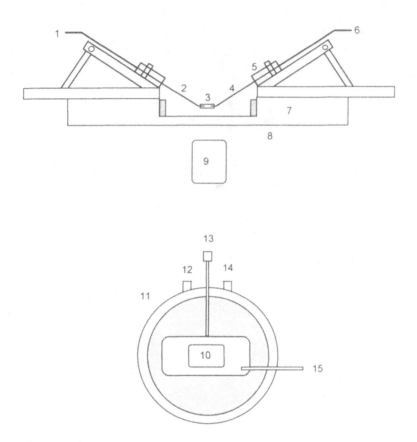

1.	to water manometer	9.	microscope objective
2.	primary pipette	10.	microvessel chamber
3.	microvessel segment	11.	temperature controlled water jacket
4.	secondary pipette	12.	water jacket inflow
5.	pipette holder	13.	suffusate inflow
6.	to stopcock	14.	water jacket outflow
7.	alumina baseplate	15.	suffusate vacuum overflow
8.	plexiglass chamber insert (see lower figure)		

Figure 4 *Continued.*

circular microscope coverslip held into position by high vacuum grease. The cauda epididymis is then dissected free of the testis, and the vessels supplying and draining the testis ligated and the testis excised.

This procedure ensures that both the distal (deferential) and proximal (external spermatic) feed vessels to the cremaster remain intact. It must however be appreciated that the preparation represents somewhat of a compromise in that a number of vascular pathways are severed when the muscle is opened in order to obtain optical clarity and accessibility to the major feed vessels. If this compromise cannot be accommodated in the experimental design, alternatives include (1) not opening the cremaster muscle[5,91,92] or (2) selection of a different preparation (Table 1).

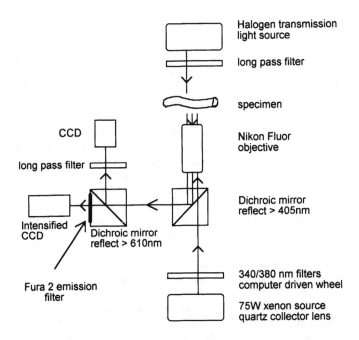

Figure 4 *Continued.*

At completion of surgery, the rat preparation is positioned on the stage of an upright microscope equipped with a transmission light source. The tissue bath is filled with a Kreb's-Ringer bicarbonate buffer maintained at physiologic conditions with respect to pH (7.35–7.45), temperature (34°C), pO_2 (<35 mmHg), and pCO_2 (40–50 mmHg). The gas tensions and pH can be controlled by directly bubbling the tissue bath with a controlled mixture of CO_2 and N_2. The bath can be static or connected to a continual superfusion system; if a static bath is chosen, it should be replaced regularly (approximately every 15 min) and be of sufficient volume (45–50 ml) that evaporative effects will be minimal. After establishing the superfusate conditions, the muscle should be examined for signs of damage; preparations showing (1) petichial hemorrhages, (2) areas of obviously sluggish blood flow or nonperfusion, or (3) adherence of white cells to venular/arteriolar endothelium should be discarded. In addition, arterioles less than 50 μm in diameter should possess significant basal tone and those less than 30 μm commonly exhibit rhythmic changes in vessel diameter (vasomotion). With respect to the extent of basal tone, the small arterioles (third and fourth branching order) will typically dilate to 150 to 175% of basal diameter in response to topically applied dilators such as adenosine ($10^{-4} M$) and papaverine ($10^{-5} M$).[93]

Consideration should be given as to the influence of neural pathways on the microcirculatory events being studied. Skeletal muscle preparations can be denervated, either chemically by topical application of appropriate antagonists (e.g., phentolamine, propranolol, etc.) or by section of the neural pathways supplying the tissue. In the case of the rat cremaster muscle preparation, Faber[31] has described a surgical denervation technique involving sectioning of the genitofemoral, iliolinguial, iliohypogastric, and lateral cutaneous nerves. If required, this procedure should be performed just prior to exteriorization of the muscle. Alternatively, the neural pathways supplying the muscle can be isolated and directly stimulated to examine the effects of innervation.[94]

As mentioned earlier in this section, *in vivo* exteriorized muscle preparations can be used for studying a number of aspects of microvascular reactivity and function. A number of methods exist for the quantitation of microvascular dimensions and hemodynamics when using *in vivo* exteriorized muscle preparations. Vessel diameters are generally measured on the monitor screen using calibrated electronic video calipers[95] or by image shearing.[96] In this latter approach, a section of the video image is displaced laterally such that one wall (e.g., left) of the vessel is aligned with its opposite (right) wall. The magnitude of the displacement can be calibrated such that it indicates vessel diameter. While these methods are somewhat subjective, given that they are manually controlled, automated measuring systems[97,98] suitable for transilluminated *in vivo* skeletal muscle preparations can be difficult to use. This is mainly due to the interference from the skeletal muscle fibers, particularly if tissue movement occurs. A number of systems exist for measurement of axial red cell velocity (e.g., image tracking, dual slit, optical grating) that have been reviewed by Johnson.[99] From measurements of vessel diameter and red cell velocity, volumetric blood flow can be estimated: Flow = $(V \times \pi r^2)/1.6$ nl/s, where V is the axial red cell velocity and r is the vessel radius. A value of 1.6 is required for conversion of the measured axial red cell velocity to average velocity across the vessel and is applicable for microvessels of diameter greater than 15 μm (for smaller vessels the correction factor approaches 1.0).[100] This calculation assumes a circular cross-section, an assumption that may not always be appropriate, particularly in venules and heavily constricted arterioles.[100,101] Intravascular micropressures can be measured in skeletal muscle preparations using the servo-null micropipette system developed from the work of Wiederhielm et al.[102] In this system, a high-resistance glass micropipette (1–2 μm tip diameter, containing 2 *M* NaCl) is introduced into the lumen of a microvessel using a micromanipulator. The pressure needed to maintain a constant resistance in the micropipette is assumed to be equivalent to that within the vessel.

For the microscopy procedures described above, transillumination using a standard tungsten halogen light source is generally adequate. In a number of situations, however, it is necessary to use an epi-illumination light source such as a xenon or a mercury lamp. This is necessary when examining thick skeletal muscle preparations or if vascular permeability is to be assessed. In this latter situation, an appropriately filtered epi-illumination source is used in combination with an infused fluorescent tracer (e.g., FITC-albumin) to detect leakage of the fluorescent molecule from the vascular space. Detection of fluorescence generally requires a video camera capable of detecting very low levels of light; for example, a silicon-intensified target (SIT) tube camera or an intensified CCD (charge-coupled device) camera. This adds considerably to the cost of an *in vivo* microscopy system.

REFERENCES

1. **Rowell, L. B.**, *Human Cardiovascular Control*, Oxford University Press, New York, 1993.
2. **Engelson, E. T., Schmid-Schonbein, G. W., and Zweifach, B. W.**, The microvasculature in skeletal muscle. II. Arteriolar network anatomy in normotensive and hypertensive rats, *Microvasc. Res.*, 30, 34, 1985.
3. **Hill, M. A., Simpson, B. E., and Meininger, G. A.**, Altered cremaster muscle hemodynamics due to disruption of the deferential feed vessels, *Microvasc. Res.*, 39, 349, 1990.
4. **DeLano, F. A., Schmid-Schonbein, G. W., Skalak, T. C., and Zweifach, B. W.**, Penetration of the systemic blood pressure into the microvasculature of rat skeletal muscle, *Microvasc. Res.*, 41, 92, 1991.
5. **Hill, M. A., Trippe, K. M., Li, Q.-X., and Meininger, G. A.**, Arteriolar arcades and pressure distribution in cremaster muscle microcirculation, *Microvasc. Res.*, 44, 117, 1992.
6. **Bohlen, H. G., Gore, R. W., and Hutchins, P. M.**, Comparison of microvascular pressures in normal and spontaneously hypertensive rats, *Microvasc. Res.*, 13, 125, 1977.
7. **Meininger, G. A., Harris, P. D., and Joshua, I. G.**, Distribution of microvascular pressure in skeletal muscle of one-kidney, one-clip, two-kidney, one-clip and deoxycorticosterone-salt hypertensive rats, *Hypertension*, 6, 27, 1984.

8. **Granger, H. J., Meininger, G. A., Borders, J. L., Morff, R. J., and Goodman, A. H.,** Microcirculation of skeletal muscle, in *The Physiology and Pharmacology of the Microcirculation, Vol. 2*, Mortillaro, N. A., Ed., Academic Press, New York, 1984, chap. 7.

9. **Johnson, P. C.,** Autoregulation of blood flow, *Circ. Res.*, 59, 483, 1986.

10. **Meininger, G. A., Falcone, J. C., and Hill, M. A.,** Autoregulation and resistance artery function, in *The Resistance Vasculature*, Bevan, J. A., Halpern, W., and Mulvany, M. J., Eds., Humana Press, New Jersey, 1991, chap. 20.

11. **Johnson, P. C.,** The myogenic response, in *Handbook of Physiology, Sect. 2, Vol. II*, Bohr, D. F., Somlyo, A. P., and Sparks, H. V., Eds., *Am. Physiol. Soc.*, Bethesda, MD, 1980, chap. 15.

12. **Meininger, G. A. and Davis, M. J.,** Cellular mechanisms involved in the vascular myogenic response, *Am. J. Physiol.*, 263, H647, 1992.

13. **Granger, H. J. and Shepherd, A. P.,** Intrinsic microvascular control of tissue oxygen delivery, *Microvasc. Res.*, 4, 49,1973.

14. **Sparks, H. V.,** Effect of local metabolic factors on vascular smooth muscle, in *Handbook of Physiology, Sect. 2, Vol. II*, Bohr, D. F., Somlyo, A. P., and Sparks, H. V., Eds., *Am. Physiol. Soc.*, Bethesda, MD, 1980, chap. 17.

15. **Koller, A. and Kaley, G.,** Endothelium regulates skeletal muscle microcirculation by a blood flow velocity-sensing mechanism, *Am. J. Physiol.*, 258, H916, 1990.

16. **Granger, H. J.,** Coordinated microvascular reactions mediated by series coupling of metabolic, myogenic and flow-sensitive resistance elements, *FASEB J.*, 3, A1387, 1989.

17. **Segal, S. S. and Duling, B. R.,** Propagation of vasodilation in resistance vessels of the hamster: Development and review of a working hypothesis, *Circ. Res.*, 61(Suppl. II), 20, 1987.

18. **Segal, S. S. and Duling, B. R.,** Flow control among microvessels coordinated by intercellular conduction, *Science*, 234, 868, 1986.

19. **Lang, D. J. and Johnson, P. C.,** Size dependence of arteriolar responses to arteriole pressure reduction, in *Microvascular Networks: Experimental and Theoretical Studies*, Popel, A. S. and Johnson, P. C., Eds., Karger, Basel, 1986, 112.

20. **Falcone, J. C. and Bohlen, H. G.,** EDRF from rat intestine and skeletal muscle venules causes dilation of arterioles, *Am. J. Physiol.*, 258, H1515, 1990.

21. **Hester, R. L.,** Venular-arteriolar diffusion of adenosine in hamster cremaster muscle microcirculation, *Am. J. Physiol.*, 258, H1918, 1990.

22. **Fuxe, K. and Sedvall, G.,** The distribution of adrenergic nerves to the blood vessels in skeletal muscle, *Acta Physiol. Scand.*, 64, 74, 1965.

23. **Fleming, B. P., Gibbins, I. L., Morris, J. L., and Gannon, B. J.,** Noradrenergic and peptidergic innervation of the extrinsic vessels and microcirculation of the rat cremaster muscle, *Microvasc. Res.*, 38, 255, 1989.

24. **Saltzman, D., DeLano, F. A., and Schmid-Schonbein, G. W.,** The microvasculature in skeletal muscle. VI. Adrenergic innervation of arterioles in normotensive and hypertensive rats, *Microvasc. Res.*, 44, 263, 1992.

25. **Marshall, J. M.,** The influence of the sympathetic nervous system on individual vessels of the microcirculation of skeletal muscle of the rat, *J. Physiol.*, 332, 169, 1982.

26. **Gore, R. W.,** Wall stress: A determinant of regional differences in response of frog microvessels to norepinephrine, *Am. J. Physiol.*, 222, 82, 1972.

27. **Boegehold, M. A. and Johnson, P.C.,** Response of arteriolar network of skeletal muscle to sympathetic nerve stimulation, *Am. J. Physiol.*, 254, H919, 1988.

28. **Faber, J. E. and Meininger, G. A.,** Selective interaction of α-adrenoceptors with myogenic regulation of microvascular smooth muscle, *Am. J. Physiol.*, 259, H1126, 1990.

29. **Liu, J., Hill, M. A., and Meininger, G. A.,** Mechanisms of myogenic enhancement by norepinephrine, *Am. J. Physiol.*, 266, H440, 1994.

30. **Meininger, G. A. and Trzeciakowski, J. P.,** Vasoconstriction is amplified by autoregulation during vasoconstrictor-induced hypertension, *Am. J. Physiol.*, 254, H709, 1988.

31. **Faber, J. E.,** *In situ* analysis of α-adrenoceptors on arteriolar and venular smooth muscle in rat skeletal muscle microcirculation, *Circ. Res.*, 62, 37, 1988.

32. **Faber, J. , Ikeoka, K., Leech, C., Nishigaki, K., Ohyanagi, M., and Ping, P.,** Vascular smooth muscle α-adrenoceptor distribution and control of resistance, terminal arteriole and capacitance vessels, in *Resistance Arteries, Structure and Function*, Mulvany, M. J., Ed., Elsevier, Amsterdam, 1991, 266.

312

33. **Ohlen, A., Thureson-Klein, A., Lindbom, L., Hokfelt, T., and Hedqvist, P.,** Substance P and NPY innervation of microvessels in the rabbit tenuissimus muscle, *Microvasc. Res.*, 36, 117, 1988.
34. **Fleming, J. T. and Joshua, I. G.,** Mechanism of the biphasic response to angiotensin II, *Am. J. Physiol.*, 247, H88, 1984.
35. **Hill, M. A. and Larkins, R. G.,** Altered microvascular reactivity in streptozotocin-induced diabetes in rats, *Am. J. Physiol.*, 257, H1438, 1989.
36. **Joshua, I. G.,** Endothelin-induced vasoconstriction of small resistance vessels in the microcirculation of the rat cremaster muscle, *Microvasc. Res.*, 40, 191, 1990.
37. **Liard, J. F., Deriaz, O., Schelling, P., and Thibonnier, M.,** Cardiac output distribution during vasopressin infusion or dehydration in conscious dogs, *Am. J. Physiol.*, 243, H663, 1982.
38. **Koller, A., Messina, E. J., Wolin, M. S., and Kaley, G.,** Endothelial impairment inhibits prostaglandin and EDRF-mediated dilation *in vivo*, *Am. J. Physiol.*, 257, H1966, 1989.
39. **Persson, M. G., Gustafsson, L. E., Wiklund, N. P., Hedqvist, P., and Moncada, S.,** Endogenous nitric oxide as a modulator of rabbit skeletal muscle microcirculation *in vivo*, *Br. J. Pharmacol.*, 100, 463, 1990.
40. **Kuo, L., Chilian, W. M., and Davis, M. J.,** Interaction of pressure- and flow-induced responses in porcine coronary resistance vessels, *Am. J. Physiol.*, 261, H1706, 1991.
41. **Berk, B. C., Alexander, R. W., Brock, T. A., Gimbrone, M. A., and Webb, R. C.,** Vasoconstriction: A new activity for platelet-derived growth factor, *Science*, 232, 87, 1986.
42. **Vicaut, E., Hou, X., Payen, D., Bousseau, A., and Tedgui, A.,** Acute effects of tumor necrosis factor on the microcirculation in rat cremaster muscle, *J. Clin. Invest.*, 87, 1537, 1991.
43. **Hill, M. A., Davis, M. J., and Meininger, G. A.,** Cyclooxygenase inhibition potentiates myogenic activity in skeletal muscle arterioles, *Am. J. Physiol.*, 258, H127, 1990.
44. **Flynn, S. B. and Owens, D. A. A.,** The effects of histamine on skeletal muscle vasculature in cats, *J. Physiol.*, 265, 795, 1977.
45. **Lindbom, L., Hedqvist, P., Dahlen, S. E., Lindgren, J. A., and Arfors, K. E.,** *Acta Physiol. Scand.*, 116, 105, 1982.
46. **Bond, R. F., Peissner, L. C., and Manning, E. S.,** Skeletal muscle decompensation in dogs subjected to prolonged hypovolemia: Neural versus humoral mechanisms, *Circ. Shock*, 4, 115, 1977.
47. **Baker, C. H. and Sutton, E. T.,** Arteriolar endothelium-dependent vasodilation occurs during endotoxin shock, *Am. J. Physiol.*, 264, H1118, 1993.
48. **Cryer, H. G., Garrison, R. N., Kaebnick, H. W., Harris, P. D., and Flint, L. M.,** Skeletal muscle microcirculatory responses to hyperdynamic *E. coli* sepsis in unanesthetized rats, *Arch. Surg.*, 122, 86, 1987.
49. **Engelund, D. and Kjersgaard, A. G.,** Acute compartment syndrome, *Ugeskr. Laeger*, 153, 1110, 1991.
50. **Alexander, J. S., Hechtman, H. B., and Shepro, D.,** Phalloidin enhances endothelial barrier function and reduces inflammatory permeability *in vitro*, *Microvasc. Res.*, 35, 308, 1988.
51. **Butcher, E. C.,** Leukocyte-endothelial cell recognition: Three (or more) steps to specificity and diversity, *Cell*, 67, 1033, 1991.
52. **Schmid-Schonbein, G. W.,** The damaging potential of leukocyte activation in the microcirculation, *Angiology*, 44, 45, 1993.
53. **Springer, T. A.,** Adhesion receptors of the immune system, *Nature*, 346, 425, 1990.
54. **Korthuis, R. J., Grisham, M. B., and Granger, D. N.,** Leukocyte depletion attenuates vascular injury in postischemic skeletal muscle, *Am. J. Physiol.*, 254, H823, 1988.
55. **Carden, D. L., Smith, J. K., and Korthuis, R. J.,** Neutrophil-mediated microvascular dysfunction in postischemic canine skeletal muscle: Role of granulocyte adherence, *Circ. Res.*, 66, 1436, 1990.
56. **Simpson, P. J., Todd, R. F., Fantone, J. C., Mickelson, J. K., Griffin, J. D., and Lucchesi, B. R.,** Reduction of experimental canine myocardial reperfusion injury by a monoclonal antibody (anti-Mo1, anti-CD11b) that inhibits leukocyte adhesion, *J. Clin. Invest.*, 81, 624, 1988.
57. **Smith, J. K., Grisham, M. B., Granger, D. N., and Korthuis, R. J.,** Free radical defense mechanisms and neutrophil infiltration in postischemic skeletal muscle, *Am. J. Physiol.*, 256, H789, 1989.
58. **Barker, J. H., Acland, R. D., Anderson, G. L., and Patel, J.,** Microcirculatory disturbances following the passage of emboli in an experimental free-flap model, *Plast. Reconstr. Surg.*, 90, 95, 1992.

59. Barker, J. H., Gu, J. M., Anderson, G. L., O'Shaughnessy, M., Pierangeli, S., Johnson, P., Galletti, G., and Ackland, R. D., The effects of heparin and dietary fish oil on embolic events and the microcirculation downstream from a small-artery repair, *Plast. Reconstr. Surg.*, 91, 335, 1993.

60. Chen, L. E., Seaber, A. V., and Urbaniak, J. R., Combined effect of acute denervation and ischemia on the microcirculation of skeletal muscle, *J. Orthop. Res.*, 10, 112, 1992.

61. Morff, R. J., Microvascular reactivity to norepinephrine at different arteriolar levels and durations of streptozotocin-induced diabetes, *Diabetes*, 39, 354, 1990.

62. Hill, M. A. and Meininger, G. A., Impaired arteriolar myogenic reactivity in early experimental diabetes, *Diabetes*, 42, 1226, 1993.

63. Beals, C. C., Bullock, J., Jauregui, E. R., and Duran, W. N., Microvascular clearance of macromolecules in skeletal muscle of spontaneously diabetic rats, *Microvasc. Res.*, 45, 11, 1993.

64. Hill, M. A. and Ege, E. A., Effect of aminoguanidine treatment on the mechanical properties of isolated arterioles from streptozotocin-induced diabetic rats, *Diabetes*, 43, 1450, 1994.

65. Bohlen, H. G., Arteriolar closure mediated by hyperresponsiveness to norepinephrine in hypertensive rats, *Am. J. Physiol.*, 236, H157, 1979.

66. Falcone, J. C., Granger, H. J., and Meininger, G. A., Enhanced myogenic activation in skeletal muscle arterioles from spontaneously hypertensive rats, *Am. J. Physiol.*, 265, H1847, 1993.

67. Prewitt, R. L., Wang, D. H., and Hill, M. A., Hypertension, in *Pathophysiology of the Microcirculation*, Mortillaro, N. A. and Taylor, A. E., Eds., CRC Press, Boca Raton, FL, 1994, p. 61.

68. Mullins, J. J., Peters, J., and Ganten, D., Fulminant hypertension in transgenic rats harboring the mouse Ren-2 gene, *Nature*, 344, 541, 1990.

69. Mayadas, T. N., Johnson, R. C., Rayburn, H., Hynes, R. O., and Wagner, D. D., Leukocyte rolling and extravasation are severely compromised in P selectin-deficient mice, *Cell*, 74, 541, 1993.

70. Yong, T., Meininger, G. A., and Linthicum, D. S., Enhancement of histamine-induced vascular leakage by pertussis toxin in SJL/J mice but not BALB/c mice, *J. Neuroimmunol.*, 45, 47, 1993.

71. Haywood, J. R., Shaffer, R. A., Fastenow, C., Fink, G. D., and Brody, M. J., Regional blood flow measurement with pulsed Doppler flowmeter in conscious rat, *Am. J. Physiol.*, 241, H273, 1981.

72. Baker, C. H., Sutton, E. T., and Davis, D. L., Microvessel mean transit time and blood flow velocity of sulfhemoglobin-RBC, *Am. J. Physiol.*, 238, H745, 1980.

73. Tuma, R. F., Vastahare, U. S., Irion, G. L., and Wiedeman, M. P., Considerations in use of microspheres for flow measurements in anesthetized rat, *Am. J. Physiol.*, 250, H137, 1986.

74. Bjornberg, J., Grande, P.-O., Maspers, M., and Mellander, S., Site of autoregulatory reactions in the vascular bed of cat skeletal muscle as determined with a new technique for segmental vascular resistance recordings, *Acta Physiol. Scand.*, 133, 199, 1988.

75. Brody, M. J., Shaffer, R. A., and Dixon, R. L., A method for the study of peripheral vascular responses in the rat, *J. Appl. Physiol.*, 18, 645, 1963.

76. Diana, J. N., Fleming, B. P., and Kinasewitz, G. T., The measurement of whole-organ capillary filtration coefficients, in *Microcirculatory Technology*, Baker, C. H. and Nastuk, W. L., Eds., Academic Press, New York, 1986, chap. 28.

77. Meininger, G. A., Lubrano, V. M., and Granger, H. J., Hemodynamic and microvascular responses in the hindquarters during the development of renal hypertension in rats, *Circ. Res.*, 55, 609, 1984.

78. House, S. D. and Johnson, P. C., Diameter and blood flow of skeletal muscle venules during local blood flow regulation, *Am. J. Physiol.*, 250, H828, 1986.

79. Eriksson, E. and Myrhage, R., Microvascular dimensions and blood flow in skeletal muscle, *Acta Physiol. Scand.*, 86, 211, 1972.

80. Reneman, R. S., Slaaf, D. W., Lindbom, L., Tangelder, G. J., and Arfors, K.-E., Muscle blood flow disturbances produced by simultaneously elevated venous and total muscle tissue pressure, *Microvasc. Res.*, 20, 307, 1980.

81. Baez, S., An open cremaster preparation for the study of blood vessels by *in vivo* microscopy, *Microvasc. Res.*, 36, 56, 1973.

82. Gray, S. D., Rat spinotrapezius muscle preparation for microscopic observation of the terminal vascular bed, *Microvasc. Res.*, 5, 395, 1973.

83. Prewitt, R. L., Chen, I. I. H., and Dowell, R. F., Microvascular alterations in the one-kidney, one-clip renal hypertensive rat, *Am. J. Physiol.*, 246, H728, 1984.

84. **Boczkowski, J., Vicaut, E., and Aubier, M.,** A preparation for *in vivo* study of the diaphragmatic microcirculation in the rat, *Microvasc. Res.*, 40, 157, 1990.

85. **Bohlen, H. G. and Niggl, B. A.,** Arteriolar anatomical and functional abnormalities in juvenile mice with genetic or streptozotocin induced diabetes mellitus, *Circ. Res.*, 45, 390, 1979.

86. **Wiederhielm, C. A. and Slaaf, D. W.,** A new skeletal muscle preparation for the study of microvascular function in intact unanesthetized animals, *Microvasc. Res.*, 33, 413, 1987.

87. **Segal, S. S. and Duling, B. R.,** Communication between feed arteries and microvessels in hamster striated muscle: Segmental vascular responses are functionally coordinated, *Circ. Res.*, 59, 283, 1986.

88. **Sullivan, S. M. and Pittman, R. N.,** Hamster retractor muscle: A new preparation for intravital microscopy, *Microvasc. Res.*, 23, 329, 1982.

89. **Longnecker, D. E. and Seyde, W. C.,** Anesthetic regimens: Advantages and disadvantages, in *Microcirculatory Technology*, Baker, C. H. and Nastuk, W. L., Eds., Academic Press, New York, 1986, chap. 22.

90. **Bohlen, H. G.,** Microvascular studies in chronic experimental hypertension and diabetes mellitus, in *Microcirculatory Technology*, Baker, C. H. and Nastuk, W. L., Eds., Academic Press, New York, 1986, chap. 8.

91. **Mohrman, D. E. and Heller, L. J.,** Effect of aminophylline on adenosine and exercise dilation of rat cremaster arterioles, *Am. J. Physiol.*, 246, H592, 1984.

92. **Vicaut, E. and Stucker, O.,** An intact cremaster muscle preparation for studying the microcirculation by *in vivo* microscopy, *Microvasc. Res.*, 39, 120, 1990.

93. **Ballard, S. T., Hill, M. A., and Meininger, G. A.,** Effect of vasodilation and vasoconstriction on microvascular pressures in skeletal muscle, *Microcirc. Endothel. Lymph.*, 7, 109, 1991.

94. **Fleming, B. P., Barron, K. W., Howes, T. W., and Smith, J. K.,** Response of the microcirculation in rat cremaster muscle to peripheral and central sympathetic stimulation, *Circ. Res.*, 61(Suppl. II), II-26, 1987.

95. **Goodman, A. H.,** Un calibreur video simple pour l'utilization en microscopie video, *Innov. Tech. Biol. Med.*, 9, 350, 1988.

96. **Intaglietta, M. and Tompkins, W. R.,** Microvascular measurements by video image shearing and splitting, *Microvasc. Res.*, 5, 309, 1973.

97. **Halpern, W., Osol, G., and Coy, G. S.,** Mechanical behavior of pressurized *in vitro* prearteriolar vessels determined with a video system, *Ann. Biomed. Eng.*, 12, 463, 1985.

98. **Magers, S. and Faber, J. E.,** Real-time measurement of microvascular dimensions using digital cross-correlation image processing, *J. Vasc. Res.*, 29, 241, 1992.

99. **Johnson, P. C.,** Flow measurement techniques in the microcirculation, in *Microcirculatory Technology*, Baker, C. H. and Nastuk, W. L., Eds., Academic Press, New York, 1986, chap. 11.

100. **Baker, M. and Wayland, H.,** On-line volume flow rate and velocity profile measurements for blood in microvessels, *Microvasc. Res.*, 7, 131, 1974.

101. **Davis, M. J.,** Determination of volumetric flow capacity in capillary tubes using an optical doppler velocimeter, *Microvasc. Res.*, 34, 223, 1987.

102. **Wiederhielm, C. A., Woodbury, J. W., Kirk, S., and Rushmer, R. F.,** Pulsatile pressures in the microcirculation of frog's mesentery, *Am. J. Physiol.*, 207, 173, 1964.

Chapter 24

Skin Microcirculation

John H. Barker and Terence J. Ryan

CONTENTS

I. ANATOMY AND FUNCTION

The skin is a fascinating organ. At once immediately private and blatantly public, skin is the interface between a fairly stable and constant internal milieu and an erratic and ever-changing external environment. As the boundary between our inside and our outside, the skin sees as much action and intrigue as any border town. It is both the window through which we feel the world and the movie screen upon which we project our personal feelings for the world to see.[56]

If one all-encompassing word could be used to describe the anatomy and function of the skin, it would be "change." There is no "standard skin." Its anatomy and function varies with age and the region of the body where it lives. It is constantly adapting to an environment that supplies repetitive physical and chemical insults.[54]

The functions of the skin are display and communication, protection and repair, thermoregulation, perception and control of its barrier properties. The latter includes water loss, sweating, and immunological surveillance. It is a rich factory of keratin's, cytokines, and many other agents such as Vitamin D and prostaglandins. If one includes the subcutaneous adipose tissue as part of the skin, then one incorporates a rich capillary bed that is luxurious in both brown and white adipose tissue, serving the functions of energy production, pressure dissipation, and insulation.

Skin failure is as great a disability as failure of any other organ when it comes to survival and achieving ones potential. "Burns" are but one example of an effect of the external environment that causes death and disfigurement. Failure of blood supply to the skin is the commonest reason for nonhealing. Leg ulcers, pressure sores, or ischemic necrosis of the peripheries, leading to amputation, are significant clinical problems. The rapid expansion of research into biology of wound healing has brought the skin into prominence and has drawn attention to its variability, ranging from the biology of fetal development through the degeneration of aging.

Because it is so accessible, there are many new ways of studying the skin. They include the laser Doppler, video TV microscopy, and various histopathologic techniques identifying the many properties of the endothelial cells. The experienced eye is marvelously subtle at recognizing minor degrees of flushing or pallor, and even the most ancient systems of medicine include the feel of the pulse and the pinkness of the tongue. In this chapter, the structure, function, pathology, and research of the skin as it relates to its microcirculation will be reviewed.

A. VASCULAR ANATOMY OF THE SKIN

Despite its rather simple appearance, skin is a remarkably complex organ. A section of skin measuring about 1.5 cm^2 and 3 mm thick contains an average of 1 m of blood vessels, 3.7 m of nerves, 100 sweat glands, and more than 3 million cells.[56]

If the skin as an organ can be characterized by change, so can the architecture of its vasculature, in particular its microvasculature. The small vessels in the skin are constantly in a state of flux, adapting to growth of the organism, the specific wear and tear to which a given region is exposed, the climatic variations of the surroundings, and finally to aging.

The skin is the largest organ of the human body (in an adult, it measures approximately 3 mm thick × 2 m^2 and weighs 2 kg) at any given time in resting, normo-thermic conditions contains 4.5% of the body's circulating blood; by comparison, this same figure for skeletal muscle is 13.2%.[58] When inflamed, it can increase blood flow many-fold and sustain this for repair. The skin microcirculation can be defined anatomically as arterioles, capillaries, venules, lymphatic capillaries, and arteriovenous anastomoses, or all vessels presenting a diameter of less than 300 µm. The larger vessels supplying the skin microcirculation can be said to arise from three separate sources: the *direct cutaneous vessels*, the *musculocutaneous perforators*, and the *fasciocutaneous perforators*.[31] The larger vessels from these three systems spread through the subcutaneous tissue, giving branches to the supplying arterioles in the overlaying dermis (Figure 1).

The "supplying arterioles" (diameter 40–60 µm) form a rich network of vessels in the deep or reticular dermis called the *reticular plexus*. This plexus gives off branches supplying the deep structures in the dermis (sweat glands, deep part of hair follicles) and feeds the terminal arterioles. The "terminal arterioles" (diameter 30–40 µm) are located in the superficial or papillary dermis and form the *papillary, superficial,* or *horizontal plexus*. As their name suggests, the terminal arterioles end in the capillaries (diameter 5–10 µm) that protrude perpendicularly from the horizontal plexus to form *papillary* or *capillary loops*. These "capillary loops" can be visualized directly, through the epidermis, using capillaroscopy[10,44,122] (see "Clinical Capillaroscopy" in this chapter and Chapter 11 in this volume). Superficial to the basal membrane zone (the barrier between the dermis

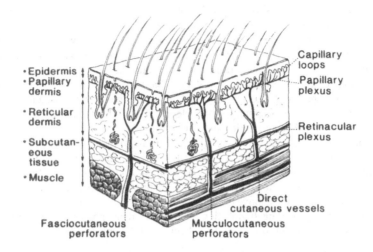

Figure 1 An artists schematic of the three principle vascular networks supplying the skin microcirculation.

and epidermis) lies the epidermis, the skin's outermost layer. The epidermis has no blood vessels, receiving its nutrition through diffusion from the underlying rich network of capillaries. The skin capillary loops vary in structure and density according to the region of the body. Where the epidermis is thin and the epithelial ridges are flattened, their density is sparse (thigh, calf, nose, forehead, and temporal region).[86]

Compared to other organs, skin is relatively poorly supplied with capillaries. Muscle may have 2000 capillaries per square millimeter of tissue,[73] myocardium 5500,[128] while skin may have only 150 capillaries per square millimeter at the surface.[86] However, comparisons can be misleading, grossly underestimating the richness of a capillary bed supporting a growing or healing epidermis, a fat lobule, a sweat gland, or a hair follicle.[111]

There is a difference between newborn skin and adult skin. Initially, the capillary bed is rich, but in the adult much of the mid and deep dermis becomes merely a system of communicating vessels connecting the richer capillary bed of the upper dermis with the sweat gland or hair follicle and the underlying adipose tissue.[109] This attenuation of blood supply during the development of the skin has been well shown in a correlation of functional and morphological parameters using isotope clearance techniques in the dermis of pig skin.[133] Pasyk et al.[98] compared facial skin with other areas of the body such as thigh and lower leg skin and noted a reduction of arteriole supply in the latter. It should be remembered that adipose tissue, with its rich capillary bed but sluggish circulation, projects upward into the dermis surrounding the sweat coils and the dermal papilla of the hair.[109] In old age, loss of the supporting adipose tissue contributes to the atrophy of the capillary bed. The lower leg of patients with peripheral vascular disease is characteristically hairless, sweatless, and devoid of fat. Wound healing is delayed in such skin, not only because of arterial perfusion but because there is no reserve of endothelium to support the angiogenesis required for granulation tissue formation. With aging, the epidermal ridges flatten,[41,100] and the larger vessels in the dermis experience changes with thinning of vessel walls and increase in vessel diameters presenting characteristic irregular aneurismal dilatation's.

Downstream from the capillaries are the "postcapillary venules" (diameter 10–30 μm), followed by the "collecting venules" (diameter 50–70 μm), and finally the larger veins (70–300 μm) that drain the skin. "Arteriovenous shunts" or "anastomoses" (AVAs) are normally occurring vessels in most tissues. They are vessels that act as bridges between the arterial and venous sides of the circulation, thus bypassing the capillaries. As such, they are very effective at diverting blood to or away from the functional capillary bed and thus the nutritional exchange they provide. The existence of these vessels in the skin is essential to its primary function of thermoregulation (see below). In skin, AVAs are found predominantly in the middle and deep dermis and present fairly constant diameters of approximately 50 μm. The number of AVAs in the skin varies greatly from region to region and from report to report, but they predominate in the head, hands, and feet. They are richly innervated and respond to both electrical and chemical stimuli, often very differently from neighboring arteries and arterioles.

"Lymphatics" of the skin can be classified according to their structure into lymphatic capillaries or "initial lymphatics," collecting lymphatics, and main lymph trunks. The lymphatic capillaries form two networks, one lying superficial immediately deep to the papillary dermis with occasional projections into papilla, and the other lying deep in the reticular dermis immediately above the adipose tissue.[106,109,110] The deep capillary lymphatics drain into the collecting lymphatics (characterized by possessing valves), which empty into the large lymph trunks in the subcutaneous lymphatics.[9]

B. MICROVASCULAR FUNCTION IN SKIN

In its role of mediating the organism's relationship with its surrounding environment, the skin's principal functions are thermoregulation, blood storage or reservoir, local defense, and nutrition. The mechanisms that regulate blood flow to the skin and thus enable it to carry out these important functions can be categorized into (1) local, (2) neural, and (3) hormonal mechanisms.

1. Local Mechanisms Regulating Skin Blood Flow

Local mechanisms are those acting in the immediate vicinity of the vessel or vessel bed and can be divided into metabolic and physical. Metabolic factors or autoregulation of blood flow in the skin is not as important as in other organs where metabolic demands are greater than that of skin. When present, the most prevalent metabolic factors that dilate skin vessels are an increase in pCO_2 (hypercapnia), a decrease in pO_2 (hypoxia), a decrease in pH (acidosis), and the presence of interstitial potassium.

Physical factors regulating skin blood flow are: increased or decreased perfusion pressures in arterioles, local temperature, and an increase in blood flow itself. Increased perfusion pressure distends the vessels and triggers a reflex vasoconstriction, which in turn increases resistance. Inversely, decreased perfusion pressure causes skin arterioles to relax and resistance to decrease. This reflex is termed the "myogenic response" and is thought to be the predominant local mechanism regulating skin blood flow. The myogenic response theory contends that these arterioles possess a basal tone that maintains them in a constant state of partial constriction. This basal tone, though influenced by neuronal, hormonal, thermal, and other local factors, persists independent of these factors and is thought to be responsible for the vessel maintaining a certain tonicity following sympathectomy. The myogenic response is also implicated in the reflex hyperemia seen following prolonged periods of ischemia and in the autoregulatory capability of the skin circulation, whereby flow is regulated locally according to local nutritional requirements.

Local temperature changes can affect blood flow in skin. A minor increase in local temperature can produce an important increase in skin blood flow that is independent of changes in nutrient flow due to increased metabolism. A drop in temperature has the opposite effect. These local changes in flow result from changes in diameters of the resistance vessels and to a lesser degree from blood viscosity changes.[116]

Another physical factor that can regulate skin blood flow is increased flow itself. Apparently, high shear stresses influence the vessel's endothelial cells, stimulating them to release vasoactive substances (Reference 57 and see Chapter 30 in this volume) that cause arteriolar dilatation.[81] Recent *in vivo* investigations have found this response to be graded according to the magnitude of flow increase, and that this mechanism is capable of inducing maximal vasodilatation.[119]

2. Neural Mechanisms Regulating Skin Blood Flow

When one sees the intensity and immediate nature of the emotional response in "blushing," it is easy to imagine that the dilatation seen in the dermal microcirculation could be mediated by neural mechanisms.[31] Neural control to the skin microcirculation is supplied by sympathetic nerves that, at the level of the skin vessels, end in α- and β-adrenergic receptors causing vasoconstriction and dilatation, respectively. Human skin vessels are assumed to be almost entirely (95%) innervated by α-(vasoconstrictor) receptors. There are no known vasodilator nerve fibers to the cutaneous vessels; thus, vasodilatation is brought about by decreasing constrictor tone.

Constriction of skin vessels is caused by noradrenaline binding to α-receptors.[93] Then, chemical reactions in which free calcium concentrations in the cytoplasm of the vascular smooth muscle cells increases causing these to constrict. Vasodilatation is produced by β-adrenergic stimulation causing relaxation of the vascular smooth muscle cells most likely through hyperpolarization, the reverse of depolarization caused by constrictor agents. A decrease in calcium concentrations in smooth muscle cells, either passively or actively by a calcium pump, could play a role in this process; however, this is still not well proven.

3. Hormonal Mechanisms Regulating Skin Blood Flow

Epinephrine and norepinephrine can both act directly on α-adrenergic receptors in the cutaneous vessels, causing vasoconstriction. Serotonin also constricts these vessels, while histamine and bradykinin are known vasodilators. Most experimental work done on the effects of norepinephrine on vessels has been done in arteries. However, in recent *in vivo* experiments, the same responses were found in the smaller arterioles (12-μm diameter). These smaller vessels have actually been found to be more sensitive to norepinephrine than the larger (330-μm diameter) resistance vessels.[52]

Several arachidonic acid metabolites, prostaglandins, and thromboxanes have opposing effects on the microcirculation. Thromboxane A2 (TXA2) and prostaglandin F2 alpha (PGF2α) are potent vasoconstrictors, while prostaglandin E1 (PGE1) and prostacyclin (PGI2) are potent vasodilators. Leukotrienes(LTC4, LTD4) have also been shown to increase blood flow in skin microcirculation.

No discussion of the effects of norepinephrine or prostaglandins on the microvascular system would be complete without reference to the advances in our understanding of neuropeptides. The complex innervation of the capillary bed of the skin includes (1) a vasoconstriction system of noradrenaline and neuropeptide Y, (2) a vasodilatory system of acetylcholine, vasoactive intestinal peptide, and peptide histamine isoleucine, and (3) an afferent system that includes substance P (SP), neurokinin A (NKA), and calcitonin gene-related peptide CGRP.

The vasoconstriction system originating in sympathetic ganglia can directly cause vasoconstriction, potentiate norepinephrine or, paradoxically, inhibit the release of norepinephrine. The parasympathetic system causes vasodilatation, employing acetylcholine, which affects smooth muscle relaxation only if the endothelium is intact. Vasoactive intestinal peptide and peptide histamine isulencine act directly on smooth muscle and do not need the endothelium as an intermediary. These various agents necessarily act on different receptors. SP and NKA are also dependent on endothelium but CGRP is not. The latter is a strong activator of adenylate cyclase and produces a prolonged erythema with an increase in blood flow without weal formation.[15] SP also induces keratinocyte-derived inflammatory mediators such as IL-1.[17]

C. THERMOREGULATORY CIRCULATION

In its role as an interface with the environment, perhaps the skin's most important function is to maintain the body's temperature at levels compatible with life. Blood flow in response to thermoregulatory stimuli can vary from 1 to as much as 150 ml/100 g skin per minute. It has been postulated that these impressive variations are possible because blood can be shunted through ASAs. At any given time in normal resting conditions, the skin is perfused with 20 to 30 times the amount of blood necessary for its minimal nutritive requirements. Besides the requirements for repair, the purpose for this constant state of overperfusion is thermoregulation.

Thermoregulatory control is mainly neuronal and chemical. The centers in the brain regulating temperature are the hypothalamic centers. The effectors in the skin are the A-V anastomoses dominated by the sympathetic vasoconstrictor fibers and the general vasoconstrictor discharges distributed in the rest of the skin vessels in the body. The latter are associated with basal tone. The AVAs are located predominantly in the face, hands, and feet. When resting at thermally comfortable levels, nearly 50% of the dermal blood flow is in the hands, feet, and head. The AVAs are more sensitive to neurogenic stimulation than are the rest of the vessels with the general vasoconstrictor discharges. Reduction of flow in these regular vessels is brought on by vasoconstrictor discharge, whereas active dilation beyond the basal level is caused exclusively by release of bradykinin, which occurs when sweat glands are excited.

Regulation of heat works as follows. In the case of an increase of ambient temperature, first the AVAs of the head and hands dilate, and this results from a general neuronal discharge (remember: AVAs are more sensitive to neuronal stimulation and therefore in a general discharge, the regions containing AVAs will be more affected). This is followed by dilation of feet AVAs and finally dilation of the rest of the vessels in other areas. If this dilation is not sufficient to restore heat balance, sweat glands become active. Like dilation, sweat gland activation is regional starting on the forehead and the arms and center of the dorsum. The loss of heat by this mechanism is through radiative conductive and evaporative pathways as the heat on the skin's surface makes contact with ambient air. In the cold the reverse order of shut down occurs. Using these mechanisms, a normal individual can regulate body temperature comfortably between 15 and 40°C.

D. NUTRITIONAL CIRCULATION TO THE SKIN

Nutritive demands of uninjured skin at rest are minimal. Healthy skin (not wounded) can withstand up to 12 h of complete ischemia and still recover. However, there are components of erector pili muscle, fat cells, or anagen hair in the skin that are more sensitive to ischemia. By comparison, muscle can only tolerate 4 to 6 h of ischemia before experiencing irreversible damage.

The average blood flow to skin is approximately 20 ml per minute per 100 g tissue (with large regional differences). Skin in the finger can withstand flows as low as 0.5 to 1.0 ml/min/100 ml tissue (cold and vasoconstricted) for prolonged periods and still recover. At maximal vasodilatation, skin has a blood flow of more than 100 ml/min/100 g tissue. The fact that skin is normally perfused with approximately 20 ml/min/100 g tissue, and yet its nutritional requirements are 15 to 30 times less than this, points to the fact that nutrition is a minor role played by skin microcirculation. For the most part, the metabolism of the skin is suppressed by habitual cooling compared to internal organs. Furthermore, much of the metabolism of the epidermis is anaerobic, the majority of supra basal cells having lost their mitochondria.

II. PATHOLOGY

A. PATHOLOGIC PROCESSES DIRECTLY IMPACTING SKIN MICROCIRCULATION

In the newborn, the blood supply to the skin is a uniform capillary bed having approximately the same density of capillaries in all areas. With growth of the skin during the first 3 months, plus its adaptation to the temperature of the environment, shunting systems and regional variations in the numbers of arterioles supplying the surface area influence the development of a capillary system so that in areas such as the hands and feet, and elbows and knees, there is a greater number of capillary vessels than in areas such as the shin, thigh, or cheek. But there are many diseases of the newborn, like strawberry hemangioma or the capillary nevus, that are aberrant patterns of angiogenesis.[108]

There are a handful of diseases involving the skin that affect billions of persons and are of concern to organizations like the World Health Organization. As part of pathogenesis, blood supply to the skin and its compromisation have to be taken into account in every case. Thus, Lepromatous leprosy creates a capillary bed that becomes phagocytic for bacilli and in which localization at sites such as the anterior nasal septum[70] or the incisors and the peripheral nerve at sites of cooling explains the ultimate vulnerability of the tissue. Leishmaniasis depends on hematogenous spread and localization in certain capillary beds for the pathogenesis of its disease.[70] Schistosomiasis is a magnificent example of a focus of a particular organism — in particular, venular beds. Diseases like schistosomiasis and malaria require penetration of the epidermis and entry into the microcirculation. The techniques whereby parasites and insects are able to do this often require fairly specific microcirculatory preferences. Elephantiasis due to microfilariasis ultimately requires that an organism preferentially seek a particular region of the lymphatics.[20] Apart from these important infective diseases, degenerative diseases, such as the leg ulcer of venous disease[127] or the decubitus of the elderly or paraplegic,[30] also have monographs devoted to them and to the role of blood supply.

Inflammatory disease of the skin, such as urticaria and vasculitis[107] require an understanding of how the microcirculation responds to pharmacological agents and how they become the focus of localization of hematogenously spread disease, such as immune complexes. The interaction of the neutrophil with the endothelium is a significant part of this and it, too, has attracted a large number of monographs.[77] Other forms of degenerative disease are sometimes modulated by endocrine factors and affect women more than men. Involvement of adipose tissue of the breast or thigh in disorders such as mastopathia or cellulite[109] cannot be understood without an assessment of the relationship of the adipose cell to its blood supply.

Any study of the skin would be incomplete without taking into account the effects of aging and exposure to UV light that may accelerate the process. Aging[112] is associated with a considerable reduction in the capillary bed and there is an association with peripheral vascular disease. Whether one is studying diabetes mellitus or hypertension, the effect on the central cardiovascular system of a gross atrophy of the capillary bed, which it supplies, must be taken into account. It is by no means certain whether the capillary bed atrophies because of peripheral vascular disease or whether peripheral vascular disease and hypertension is, in part, induced by the atrophy of the periphery. Like the age-related disorders skin cancer and melanoma, one must include in their pathogenesis the capacity for hematogenous spread or lymphatic spread. Diagnosis now includes dermatoscopy which derived from capillary microscopy. Exactly how a melanoma induces a blood supply[112] or how an abnormal cell finds its way into the lymphatics becomes of greater significance as the numbers of persons dying from these diseases increases.

There are one or two specific diseases known to dermatologists, such as psoriasis and atopic eczema, that also merit a special examination of the microcirculation. Psoriasis induces the very special anatomical pattern of upper dermal vasculature.[111] The functional responses of the skin vasculature in atopic eczema include the fact that a minor scratch produces a white reaction instead of a pink reaction, and reflexes in response to environmental temperature are altered. The alteration of itch threshold due to a rise in skin temperature and its interaction with neuropeptides, mast cells, and immunological processes all merit a literature that refers to the microcirculation.[111] With respect to responses of the skin to cooling, there is also the literature on cold-induced skin diseases such as Raynaud's phenomenon, the vibration white finger, and diseases such as acrocyanosis or scleroderma.[21] The skin being a principal organ of thermoregulation, one needs to search also the literature on hypothermia in the newborn[18] and hyperthermia[101] in order to get a comprehensive view of the role of skin blood supply in disease processes.

B. CLINICAL APPLICATION OF SKIN MICROCIRCULATION RESEARCH

The skin microcirculation is readily accessible to modern microcirculation techniques. Therefore, it is no surprise that practically all clinical microcirculation studies have been done in the skin. In spite of this, to date we have just barely scratched the surface in terms of possible applications in which skin microcirculation can be used as a window into the physiology and pathology of the circulatory system. It is not a new concept in medicine to use the skin as an indicator of systemic well-being or disease. The key is to apply modern microcirculation techniques as a tool to better observe phenomena in the skin that have been described for centuries.

The proceedings of the Asian Microcirculation Society include descriptions of the contemporary application of videomicroscopy to some of the most ancient problems in Chinese medicine.[22,132] The use of the laser Doppler to study the persisting debilitating limb pain and color change following traumatic injury in Charcot's oedéme bleu[30] or the reinterpretation of nailfold capillary morphology at birth in the light of recent observations that the developmental defects in the microcirculation *in utero* can determine adult diseases such as hypertension or cardiac infarctation[6] and the use of Fournier analysis to analyze the pulse[75] are examples of the value of microcirculation techniques.

III. METHODS AND TECHNIQUES TO STUDY SKIN MICROCIRCULATION

A. GENERAL CONSIDERATIONS FOR SKIN PREPARATIONS

Anatomical studies of skin microcirculation have been carried out using fixed histological preparations or microvascular casting/clearing techniques. Most of the techniques used to study skin microcirculation function have been techniques that indirectly measure tissue perfusion. These indirect techniques measure properties such as surface temperature, oxygen, bleeding, and color; or, by injecting substances into the skin circulation, the dispersion of these can be measured and these values are taken to indicate the location and in some cases the degree to which a region is perfused. Though these indirect methods of measuring the function of skin circulation have provided valuable information, the fact that the values they provide are indirect indicators of perfusion often leads to conflicting and confusing findings. In this final section, we will list and briefly describe the more commonly used indirect techniques and focus with more detail on the direct measurement techniques used in modern microcirculation research — specifically, intravital microscopy.

B. INDIRECT SKIN MICROCIRCULATION MEASUREMENT TECHNIQUES

1. Laser Doppler Flowmetry (LDF)

LDF has been used extensively both in the clinical setting and in experimental animals. It is based on the principal that laser light scattered on moving objects, such as red blood cells, undergoes a frequency shift according to the Doppler principle. In tissue, part of the light is absorbed and part is reflected or "scattered" back. The small portion of this back-scattered light that is Doppler-shifted is analyzed, and a signal proportional to the number of moving objects times their mean velocity is calculated and given as red blood cell (RBC) flux. In 1972, Riva et al.[105] first used the LDF technique to measure blood flow in rabbit eye retinal vessels. In 1977, Holloway and Watkins[63] developed the first LDF instrument device for clinical use.

Nilsson et al.[90] improved the original instrument by correcting the then-poor signal-to-noise ratio and this gave way to many LDF studies on various physiological and pathophysiological topics in skin.[78,82,123] The recent application of scanning technology and instruments with more controlled depth discrimination[62] have added immensely to the practicality of using this system for measuring skin circulation. The advantages of LDF are that it is noninvasive, simple to use, continuous measurements can be obtained, and measurements can be made anywhere on the skin surface. Disadvantages are that it is very sensitive to movement artifacts and cannot provide quantitative flow values, i.e., ml/100 g tissue/min.

2. Temperature Measurements

This technique can be used both clinically and in the experimental setting. Skin surface temperature is an inaccurate method of measuring skin circulation and depends on several factors, such as blood flow rate in tissues underlying the skin, activity of nearby muscles, and the rate of sweat evaporation. Temperature does not necessarily reflect blood flow in the skin microcirculation and therefore should not be used as a measure of blood flow in patients.[47] However, when heat loss from the surface temperature probe being used for measurements is controlled by insulation, heat flux measurements can measure core temperature at least over the trunk. More information can be gained, especially in the neonate, by continuously monitoring core and peripheral temperatures simultaneously.

3. Isotope Clearance

This technique is for use only in the experimental setting and is based on calculating the washout rate of injected radioactive substances in tissue sections. A variety of compounds (^{24}Na, ^{125}I, ^{99}Tc, ^{133}Xe) have been found to give reproducible and reliable data when used to study blood flow in skin flaps.[33,59,94,133] The main disadvantage of this technique is that isolated flow determinations can only be done about once daily because of the slow washout of the radioactive substance. Also, the hazards inherent in the use of radioactive materials is a consideration. ^{99}Tc has a short half-life and, when coupled to a colloid, can be used repeatedly for lymphatic studies.

4. Transcutaneous Oxygen Tension Measurements (PtcO₂)

This method is used both clinically and in the experimental setting. It can give continuous measurements and has been reported to be useful clinically for post-operative monitoring of skin flaps.[1,121] However, overall, this technique has been disappointing as an index of skin perfusion and has for the most part been abandoned. A disadvantage of note is that for proper use, its probe must be heated, which in itself can affect skin blood flow.

5. Fluorescein Diffusion Tests

This technique is used clinically and experimentally by making the plasma of the blood phosphorescent by injecting into it sodium-fluorescein. In the latter situation, fluorescein can be attached to a larger molecule such as albumen or to different molecular weight dextrans so that it remains longer within the vessel lumen. Clinically, fluorescein dye is used to visualize the extent to which a surgically lifted flap is perfused,[99] to detect aberrations in the vasculature of the eye, and to visualize discontinuities on the eye's corneal surface. To study flap perfusion, the dye is injected intravenously and a hand-held lamp (Woods lamp) that emits a specific wavelength of light in the precise area of dye stained (perfused) tissue is used to directly visualize the skin surface. Tissue without dye is nonperfused. This technique, though reported to underestimate flap survival,[80,87,118] is used extensively in flap surgery and in the hands of many is considered to give accurate postoperative predictions of skin flap necrosis.[102,104] Disadvantages of this technique include some adverse systemic side effects of the dye.[80] Furthermore, the high doses of dye used (10–15 mg/kg) make repeated measurements impossible within 12 to 18 h. This has been remedied by Silverman et al.,[118] who in 1980 introduced the use of dermofluorometry where lower doses of dye (1.5 mg/kg) can be given, allowing repeated measurements within 1 h.[125] Fluorescein measurements, performed as described above, lack the capacity to monitor dynamic blood flow continuously.

When fluorescein is used tagged to a larger molecule in combination with direct vital microscopy, it remains within the vessel (or leaks out slowly) and can be used to measure dynamic flow parameters like red blood cell velocities, vessel diameters, functional capillary densities, and macromolecular leakage (see below).

6. Photoplethysmography (PPG)

This technique is used both clinically and experimentally and is based on the principle that when the skin surface is illuminated with infrared light, the amount of reflected light varies with the content of blood in that illuminated section of tissue. As the tissue blood content varies with the pulse wave, a pulsatile signal is obtained. This method is used widely for continuous post-operative skin flap monitoring.[4,60] Disadvantages of this technique are that it requires considerable experience in deciphering the pulse curve and, since the values only indicate the presence or absence of pulse wave, they cannot be quantified.

7. Radioactive Microspheres

This technique is used only in the experimental setting and is based on the principle that small spheres, "microspheres," with uniform diameters, when injected into the circulation, will become trapped in vessels with diameters smaller than theirs. Thus spheres with a diameter of 15 μ are used to calculate the capillary blood flow, while 50-μ spheres will be trapped in both capillaries and AVAs, thus resulting in a measurement of total skin blood flow. AVA blood flow can be calculated as a difference between these two values.[95,96] After injection of the radioactively tagged spheres into the left ventricle, the portion of skin to be studied is removed and measured for radioactivity with radiometry. This method has been shown to be reliable and reproducible when used in skin flaps on pigs.[95] The main disadvantage of this technique is that only one flow value can be obtained unless different isotopes are used, since to perform the radiometric measurement, the animal must be sacrificed. There are also several technical difficulties with the technique,[95] and the hazard of working with radioactivity must be considered.

C. DIRECT SKIN MICROCIRCULATION MEASUREMENT TECHNIQUES

Vital microscopy can be performed both clinically and experimentally and consists of directly viewing the skin's microcirculation at high magnification through its surface. This is the only technique available in which continuous, quantitative measurements of dynamic microcirculatory parameters can be directly viewed and quantified: e.g., vessel diameters, RBC velocities, functional capillary densities, macromolecular leakage, white cell-endothelium interaction, vasomotion, etc. Optimal viewing of the skin microcirculation using this technique is limited to a few tissues in human subjects and in animal models. For the best images, the tissues must be thin enough (less than 400 μm) to be transilluminated. Alternatively, in the case where it is desirable to study thicker tissues, epi-illumination (light projected onto the same surface the observation is being made) can be used. However, this technique requires the aid of fluorescent dyes injected into the bloodstream, and the resolution of the microvascular field is limited by the lack of penetration, the consequence being that only a small part of the microcirculation (that which is closest to the surface; capillary loops) can be seen. In these cases, the low level of emitted light from the fluorescent emissions requires the use of very sensitive low-light-level cameras (silicone intensifier target image tube, SIT) or a high-powered light source (Argon ion laser).

When these direct microscopy techniques are applied clinically, there is no skin region on humans thin enough to be transilluminated; thus, "almost always" (see below) epi-illunination is used. The above-mentioned limitations of this technique limit clinical observations to the final tip of the microcirculation, i.e., the papillary capillary loops immediately beneath the skin surface. All studies of the arteriolar and venular sections of the microcirculation must be performed in animal preparations. In an isolated case, Branemark[16] implanted skin chambers in surgically created skinfolds in the arms of human subjects. The original report in which Branemark provides a detailed account of his direct observations and measurements of human skin microcirculation and the techniques used to obtain these is highly recommended reading.

1. Clinical Capillaroscopy

The papillary capillary loops in human skin can be viewed directly at high magnification (10–60×) and measured using ordinary light microscopy (Reference 45 and also see Chapter 11 in this volume). Optimal images are obtained by applying oil to the skin (to enhance its transparency), shining light on it at a 45° angle, and using blue or green filters interposed in the light path. This technique has been used widely for studying skin capillaries in many regions of the body. However, most of the work done has been in the nailfold. To do so, a small metal bracket attached to the microscope objective holds the finger tip still so the capillaries at high magnification (250–1000×) stay in focus and in the field of view for prolonged periods of observation. Vessel diameters, RBC velocities and, by injecting dyes, macromolecular leakage can be measured (for details see Chapter 11 in this volume).

By coupling the microscope used for these observations with a closed-circuit video and computer analysis system, the images obtained can be quantified, thus providing objective measurements of human skin capillaries. These techniques applied to clinical practice have become a science/field termed "Dynamic Videophotometric Capillaroscopy." The technique of dynamic capillaroscopy has been described in detail elsewhere (Reference 44 and Chapter 11 in this volume).

These methods have been used to study many pathologies affecting the skin circulation such as Raynaud's phenomenon,[64] arterial,[45] and venous insufficiency,[46] scleroderma,[78] and diabetes (Reference 123 and Chapters 1, 3, and 11 in this volume). Also, these techniques have been applied in patients with pathologies not directly related to skin: hypertension (Reference 48 and Chapter 4 in this volume), leukemia,[45] and polycytemia (Reference 92 and Chapter 29 in this volume). This technique has important clinical potential not only for studying the physiology and pathophysiology of skin microcirculation, but also, and perhaps more importantly, evaluating and monitoring treatments, prognosis, early detection of disease, and perhaps even prevention.

The advantages of this technique are obvious. The findings in studies performed in human subjects can be directly applied in all stages of patient care, i.e., diagnosis, prevention, treatments, prognosis, etc. This technique is noninvasive and chronic studies can be performed easily. The major disadvantage is that only the capillary section of the microcirculation can be studied.

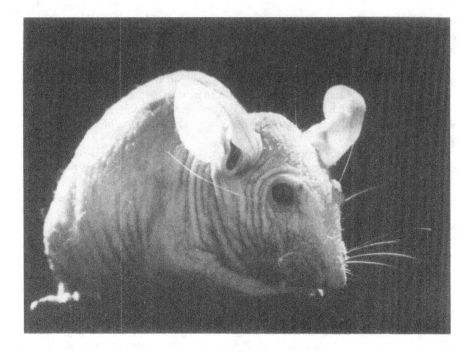

Figure 2 The Homozygous (hr/hr) hairless mouse. The relatively large size and thin structure enable easy access to the mouse ear (skin) microcirculation using direct vital microscope techniques.

2. Homozygous (hr/hr) Hairless Mouse Ear

The hairless mouse ear was first described as a model for studying skin microcirculation by Eriksson et al.[43] Their work was later expanded upon by Barker et al.[6] The hairless mouse, though in appearance, similar to the athymis nude mouse, is immunologically intact (Figure 2). Though their hairless appearance is curious and endearing "to some," the use of these animals for studying skin microcirculation has little to do with their lack of hair. Instead, the hairless mouse ear is ideal for direct viewing of skin microcirculation more because of its relatively large size, thin structure, and easy accessibility.

The ear measures approximately 13×13 mm (6% of the animals total body surface area) and consists of a central cartilage layer sandwiched between two full thickness dermal layers, giving an overall thickness of 300 μm (Figure 3). The circulation to the ear arises from three to four neurovascular bundles entering the ear at its base. At this point, the arterioles present diameters of 80 to 100 μm and, as they project radially toward the periphery of the ear, they give off descending orders of arterioles before reaching the capillaries. The capillaries (7–10 μm) form characteristic loops around empty but otherwise normal hair follicles. These drain into postcapillary venules (10–20 μm), which in turn become collecting venules and eventually larger venules (200–300 μm) that accompany larger arterioles making up the previously mentioned principal neurovascular bundles located in the base of the ear.[6,43]

To view the ear microcirculation, the animals are anesthetized (Ketamine, 50 mg/kg and Xylazine, 5 mg/kg; i.p.) and three suture (9-0 nylon) loops are placed at opposite poles around the ear's periphery for handling without disturbing its microvasculature. The animals are placed face down on a plexiglass observation platform with the ear to be studied gently extended (using the suture loops) over an elevated microscope slide incorporated into the platform (Figure 4). The animal and platform are then placed on the

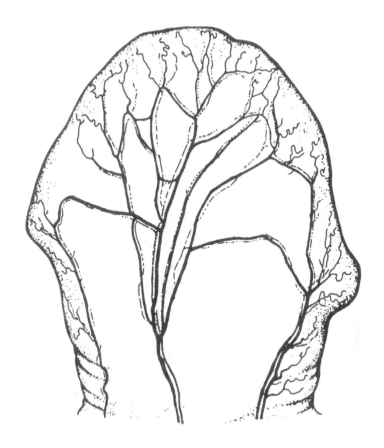

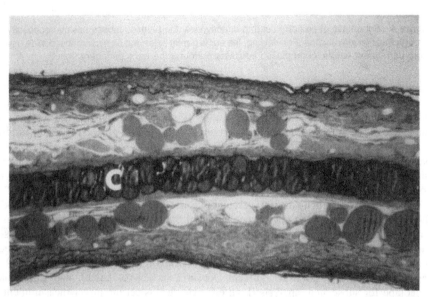

Figure 3 Schematic of hairless mouse ear (top) that receives its blood supply through three to four principal neurovascular bundles entering the ear at its base. Bottom: cross-section of mouse ear with a central cartilage "C" layer sandwiched between two full-thickness dermal layers.

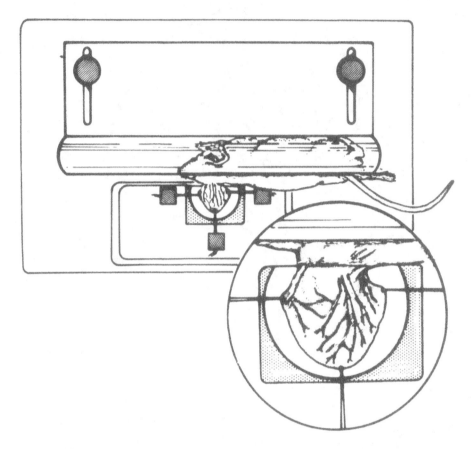

Figure 4 Schematic of platform used to directly view the hairless mouse ear microcirculation through the vital microscope. For viewing, the ear is gently extended on a microscope slide using three permanent suture loops placed equidistant around the ear's periphery (inset).

stage of a vital microscope (Ernst Leitz GmbH, Wild Wetzler, Germany), the ear is transilluminated (Xenon lamp, XBO-75, Leitz GmbH, Wild Wetzler, Germany), and its microcirculation viewed at high magnification (Figure 5). To enhance the contrast of the image of the moving blood in the microcirculation, a narrow-band (443.2 nm) filter is interposed in the path of the light transilluminating the ear. The wavelength of light passing through this filter is absorbed by the hemoglobin in the RBCs thus the final image is that of dark blood vessels contrasted against a lighter background. Image contrast enhancement can also be achieved using vital dyes introduced into the animal's bloodstream. Dyes light up the intravascular plasma, thus contrary to the above method, the image seen through the microscope is that of the blood vessels brightly lit against a darker background of the surrounding extra vascular space (Figure 6); details of these methods are provided in Chapter 10 of this volume. The microscope image is recorded with a low-light camera (NCR, Ultracon 1101, Lancaster, PA), displayed on a high-resolution monitor (VM-173U, Hitachi Denshi Ltd, Tokyo, Japan), and stored on videotape for subsequent analysis (Figure 6). Using this set-up, direct measurements (RBC velocity, vessel diameters, functional capillary density, macromolecular leakage, and white cell-endothelium interaction) can be performed from either live or recorded images. For detailed descriptions of these measuring techniques, see Chapter 10 in this volume.

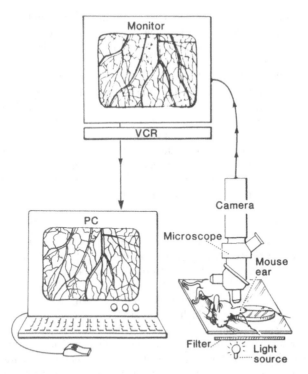

Figure 5 Computer-assisted videomicroscopic set-up used to view and quantitatively analyze hairless mouse ear microcirculation.

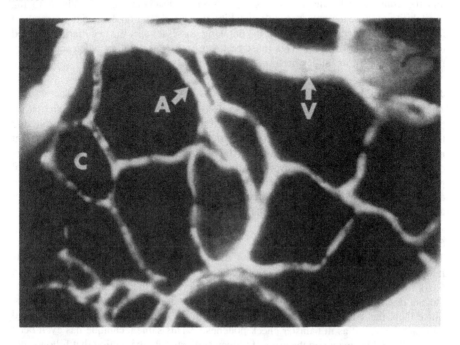

Figure 6 Hairless mouse ear microcirculation as seen at high magnification (400×) through the vital microscope. Using these techniques, arterioles "A," capillary loops "C," and venules "V" can be viewed directly in the live animal.

Using the hairless mouse ear model, various physiological[6,79] and pathophysiologic processes involving skin microcirculation have been studied; for example, scald burns,[14] vasoactive drugs,[53] reperfusion injury,[7,120] ischemia,[69,71] skin flap failure,[6,8] wound healing,[8a,12,69,72] and angiogenesis.[49]

Advantages of this model are: observations and measurements can be made in physiologically intact tissue (no surgical preparation is necessary); chronic observations are possible (repeated observations can be made indefinitely); if necessary, observations can be made in the awake animal (a restrainer can be used eliminating the need for anesthesia); the contralateral ear can be used as a control; and the ear is non-hair bearing (hair removal from ears is not necessary). Disadvantages are: when anesthesia is used during observations and measurements, it can influence measurements (anesthesia has been shown to affect microcirculatory parameters[27,29]); and obtaining optimal images is demanding, making measurements relatively difficult.

3. Bat Wing

The bat wing was first used for studying the circulation in 1852 by Jones.[65] For studying skin microcirculation per se, Nicoll and Webb[89] introduced the bat wing model. Later, Wiedeman presented a thorough description of its microvascular anatomy[128] and function.[129,130] For a review, see Reference 131.

Due to its thin structure, viewing the microcirculation in the transilluminated bat wing provides excellent images from which RBC velocity, vessel diameters and functional capillary densities can be readily measured. Using this model, physiological[13,35-38,124] and pathophysiologic microvascular mechanisms[39] have been studied. As a preparation, the bat wing has particular value for the examination of the sebaceous apparatus.

Advantages are: observations can be made in physiologically intact tissue (no surgical preparation necessary); chronic observations can be made in nonanesthetized animals; and the contralateral wing can be used as control. Disadvantages are related to the availability of these animals, particularly taking into consideration they do not reproduce in captivity. Furthermore, the skin of the bat wing possesses specific peculiarities related to its very specific function. This must be taken into consideration when interpreting results obtained from studies performed in this model.

4. Hamster Cheek Pouch

The everted hamster cheek pouch has been used extensively to study microcirculatory physiology as well as other tissues transplanted into it.[40,50,117] This is made possible due to its thin structure which, when extended and transilluminated with a common light microscope, provides excellent images of the microcirculation in which most microcirculatory parameters can be measured. Advantages of this preparation are: no surgical preparation is necessary; chronic observations can be performed; the contralateral tissue can be used as control; and its thin structure permits excellent images. Disadvantages are: anesthesia is necessary during observations.

5. Implantable Chambers

The concept of implanting a transparent chamber into the skin to directly view its microcirculation first appeared in the literature in 1928 when Sandison[114] along with Clark and Clark,[23,24] working in the same laboratory, published a remarkable series of elegant descriptions of their observations of the microcirculation in rabbit ear chambers. Since then, the same principle has been applied in the dorsal skin of mice,[2] rats,[97] and hamsters,[42] as well as in hamster cheek pouches.[113] This same technique has even been used in skinfolds created on the arms of human subjects.[16] In the section that follows, the more commonly used of these preparations will be described briefly.

a. Rabbit Ear Chamber

Sandison's[114] original description of the implantable chamber technique consisted of removing a full-thickness section of skin from the rabbit ear and replacing it with a transparent window. Through this window the microcirculation of connective tissue that grows inward to cover the glass slide could be viewed directly. Under the light microscope, the growth of new capillaries developing "buds" or "sprouts" from preexisting vessels was described. Descriptions were made of "capillaries without blood flow regressing within 24 hours," and "vessels with the greatest apparent blood flow differentiated into arteries and veins." These original descriptions of angiogenesis form the foundation on which our current understanding of vascular development rests. Since Sandison's first description of the rabbit ear chamber, this preparation has been applied extensively to study a wide variety of physiologic phenomena: angiogenesis,[39,61,74] wound healing,[61] and pathophysiologic processes, tumors,[25,115] thrombosis,[11] radiation pathology,[88] and inflammation.[134]

As can be seen by numerous studies in which this model is used to study angiogenesis, it is particularly useful for determining the number and length of new vessels over extended periods. This is due to the fact it is possible to return to precisely the same microscopic area by positioning the chamber in the same orientation on the microscope stage. Vessel diameters, RBC velocities, macromolecular leakage, functional capillary density, and the presence and dynamics of white cell-endothelium interaction can also be measured in this preparation. The advantages of this model are: chronic observations can be made in nonanesthetized animals; the images obtained are excellent; and the contralateral ear can be used as a control. A disadvantage is that maintaining the animal for long periods with an intact and usable chamber is somewhat cumbersome.

b. Hamster Skinfold Chamber

The skinfold chamber technique in the rat and mouse are identical to that in the hamster. Herein we will describe only the latter and refer the reader to the references provided for details on the former. The implantable chamber technique[42] is ideally adapted in hamsters as the chamber frames are easily implanted on their loose dorsal skin under relatively little tension. In Syrian Golden hamsters, the chamber is prepared by sandwiching the dorsal skin between two plexiglass, Teflon®-coated aluminum or titanium frames and securing it in place with suture and small screws. Prior to placing the skin between the two chamber frames, the dorsal hair is removed using common, commercially available hair removal cream. A circular section of one layer of the uplifted skinfold is dissected away, leaving a single layer to be observed. This single layer consists of depilated skin, subcutaneous fat, and paniculous carnosus muscle. The center of each frame has a round port or "window" where a removable glass coverslip is fixed in place. It is through this transparent window that the uplifted dorsal tissue is transilluminated and viewed at high magnification using light microscopy. Observations and measurements can be initiated 48 h following chamber implantation and can be performed repeatedly for up to 4 weeks.

Though this model is considered to be a skin preparation, in fact what is viewed through the microscope is the panniculus carnosus muscle, which is a very thin layer of striated muscle found immediately beneath and firmly attached to subcutaneous fat and the skin. Remnants of this muscle are found in humans. However, in loose-skinned animals, it is highly developed and its contractions permit these animals to shake off insects and debris from their fur. Through the microscope, muscle rather than skin capillaries are seen, due mainly to the significantly higher density of capillaries in the former compared to the latter (see Section I.A).

The hamster skinfold chamber model has been used extensively to study reperfusion injury,[83] hemodilution,[85] implantation of homologous tissues (see References 51 and 84, see Chapter 22 in this volume), spontaneous vasomotion,[27] shock,[28] and vasoactive drugs.[29]

Advantages of this model are: chronic observations in nonanesthetized animals are possible and the thin structure of the tissue provides excellent images of the microcirculation in which most microvascular parameters can be readily measured. Disadvantages are: surgical preparation is necessary and rather than true skin microcirculation, what is actually viewed in this preparation is the striated muscle microcirculation underlying the skin.

c. Hamster Cheek Pouch Chamber

Sanders and Shubik[113] first described applying the chamber technique in the hamster cheek pouch. They describe implanting a plexiglass chamber in the intact cheek pouch of the hamster to study the microcirculation of the tissue itself. However, most studies using this model have focused on studying transplanted homographs into the chamber, e.g., tumors,[55] cardiac,[32] renal,[26] pulmonary,[34] brain,[68] pituitary,[19] and the epidermis.[91] These different tissues can be successfully implanted into the cheek pouch without being rejected due to three unique features particular to this organ: (1) it has greatly reduced lymphatic drainage,[5] (2) it possesses an areolar tissue barrier,[103] and (3) it lacks adrenergic innervation.[66] The cheek pouch chamber technique is described elswhere in detail by Joyner and Gilmore.[67]

REFERENCES

1. **Achauer, B. M., Black, K. S., and Litke, D. K.,** Transcutaneous PO_2 in flaps: A new method of survival prediction, *Plast. Reconstr. Surg.,* 6, 738, 1980.
2. **Algire, G. H.,** An adaptation of the transparent chamber technique to the mouse, *J. Natl. Cancer Inst.,* 4, 1–11, 1943.
3. **Bader, D. L.,** *Pressure Sores: Clinical Practice and Scientific Approach,* Macmillan, London, pp. 283, 1990.
4. **Bardach, J., Voots, R. J., and McCabe, B. F.,** The role of photoplethysmography in the prediction of experimental flap survival, *Otolaryngology,* 86, 492, 1978.
5. **Barker, C. F. and Billingham, R. E.,** *Adv. Immunol.,* 25, 1–54, 1977; **Barker, D. J. P.,** Fetal and infant origins of adult disease, *Br. Med. J.,* 368, 1, 1993.
6. **Barker, J. H., Hammersen, F., Bondar, I., Uhl, E., Galla, T. J., Menger, M. D., and Messmer, K.,** The hairless mouse ear for *in vivo* studies of skin microcirculation, *Plast. Reconstr. Surg.,* 83, 948–959, 1989.
7. **Barker, J. H., Bartlett, R., Funk, W., Hammersen, F., and Messmer, K.,** The effect of superoxide dismutase on the skin microcirculation after ischemia and reperfusion, *Prog. Appl. Microcirc.,* 12, 276, 1987.
8. **Barker, J. H., Hammersen, F., Bondar, I., Galla, T. J., Menger, M. D., and Messmer, K.,** Direct monitoring of capillary perfusion following normovolemic hemodilution in an experimental skin flap model, *Plast. Reconstr. Surg.,* 86, 946–954, 1990.
8a. **Kjolseth, D., Kim, M. K., Andresen, L., Morsing, A., Frank, J. M., Schuschke, D., Anderson, G. L., Banis, J. C., Tobin, G. R., Weiner, L. J., and Barker, J. H.,** Direct visualization and measurements of wound neovascularization: Application in microsurgery research, *Microsurgery,* 15(6), 390–398, 1994.
9. **Boggon, R. P. and Palfrey, A. J.,** The microscopic anatomy of the human lymphatic trunks, *J. Anat.,* 114, 389–405, 1973.
10. **Bollinger, A., Butti, P., Barras, J. P., Trachsler, H., and Siegenthaler, W.,** Red blood cell velocity in nail fold capillaries of man measured by a television microscopy technique, *Microvasc. Res.,* 7, 61–72, 1974.
11. **Boncinelli, S., Nerucci, P., Marsili, M., Lorenzi, P., Fenati, E., De Stefano, L. C., Biagiotti, S., and Giovannoni, L.,** Experimental study of argon laser-induced microthrombosis during PG12 infusion, *Eur. Surg. Res.,* 19(3), 171–177, 1987.

12. **Bondar, I., Barker, J. H., Uhl, E., Galla, T. J., Hammersen, F., and Messmer, K.,** A new model for studying microcirculatory changes during dermal wound healing, *Eur. Surg. Res.*, 191, 379–388, 1991.

13. **Bouskela, E. and Wiederhielm, C. A.,** Distensibility of capillaries in the bat wing, *Blood Vessels*, 26(6), 325–334, 1989.

14. **Boykin, J. V. and Pittman, R. N.,** *In vivo* microcirculation of a scald burn and the progression of postburn dermal ischemia, *Plast. Reconstr. Surg.*, 66, 191–198, 1980.

15. **Brain, D. D., Tippins, J. R., Morris, H. R., McIntlyre, I., and Williams, T. J.,** Potent vasodilator activity of calcitonin gene-related peptide in human skin, *J. Invest. Dermatol.*, 87, 533–536, 1986.

16. **Branemark, P. I.,** Rheological aspects of low flow states, in *Microcirculation as Related to Shock*, Shepro, D. and Fulton, G. P., Eds., Academic Press, New York, 1968, 161.

17. **Brown, J., Perry, P., and Ansel, J.,** Substance P induction of keratinocyte cytokines, *J. Invest. Dermatol.*, 92, 407, 1989.

18. **Bruck, K.,** Neonatal thermal regulation, in *Neonatal and Fetal Medicine Physiology and Pathophysiology*, Polin, R. A. and Fox, W. N., Eds., Grune and Stratton, New York, 1993, 488.

19. **Campbell, G. T., Wagoner, J., Gregrson, K. A., and Joyner, W. L.,** Immunohistochemical visualizations of prolactin, growth hormone, and a substance resembling placental lactogen in the *in situ* and ectopic pituitary in the hamster, *Endocrinology*, 105, 905–910, 1979.

20. **Casley-Smith, J. R., Feldi, M., Fyan, T. J., Witte, M. I. I., Witte, C. L., Cluzan, R., Partsch, I. I., Jamal, S., and O'Brien, B.,** Lymphoedema, in Summary of the 10th International Congress of Lymphology Working Group Discussion and Recommendations in Adelaide, Australia (August 10–17, 1985), *Lymphology*, 18, 148–168, 1985.

21. **Champion, R. H.,** Reactions to cold, in *Textbook of Dermatology*, 5th ed., Champion, G. R. H., Burton, J. L., and Ebling, F. J. G., Eds., Blackwell Scientific, Oxford, 1992, 833–848.

22. **Chen Wen-Chich.,** Current status of studies on microcirculation in Peoples Republic of China. Abstracts of the First Asian Congress of Microcirculation, published by Japanese Society of Microcirculation, 1993.

23. **Clarck, E. R. and Clarck, E. L.,** Microscopic observations on the growth of blood capillaries in the living mammal, *Am. J. Anat.*, 64, 251–301, 1939.

24. **Clarck, E. R. and Clarck, E. L.,** Observations on changes in blood vascular endothelium in the living animal, *Am. J. Anat.*, 57, 385–438, 1935.

25. **Clauss, M. A. and Jain, R. K.,** Interstitial transport of rabbit and sheep antibodies in normal and neoplastic tissues, *Cancer Res.*, 50(12), 3487–3492, 1990.

26. **Click, R. L., Joyner, W. L., and Gilmore, J. P.,** Reactivity of glomerular afferent arterioles in renal hypertension, *Kidney Int.*, 15, 109–115, 1979.

27. **Colantuoni, A., Bertuglia, S., and Intaglietta, M.,** Quantitation of rythmic diameter changes in arterial microcirculation, *Am. J. Physiol.*, 246, H508–H517, 1984.

28. **Colantuoni, A., Bertuglia, S., and Intaglietta, M.,** Microvessel diameter changes during hermorrhagic shock in unanesthetized hamsters, *Microvasc. Res.*, 30, 133–142, 1985.

29. **Colantuoni, A., Bertuglia, S., and Intaglietta, M.,** The effects of α- or β-adrenergic receptor agonists and antagonists and calcium entry blockers on spontaneous vasomotion, *Microvasc. Res.*, 28, 143–158, 1984.

30. **Cooke, E. D., Steinberg, M. D., Pearson, R. M., Fleming, C. E., Toms, S. L., and Elusade, J. A.,** Reflex sympathetic dystrophy and repetitive strain injury: Temperature and microcirculatory changes following mild cold stress, *J. Roy. Soc. Med.*, 86, 690–693, 1993.

31. **Cormack, G. C. and Lumberly, B. G. H.,** Arterial anatomy of skin flaps, *The Microcirculation*, Churchill Livingstone, Edinburgh, 1986, 15–43.

32. **Cornish, K. G., Joyner, W. L., and Gilmore, J. P.,** Pharmacological responses of the microvasculature of transplanted cardiac tissue, *Pharmacol. Biochem. Behav.*, 17, 1285–1286, 1983.

33. **Daly, M. J. and Henry, R. E.,** Quantitative measurement of skin perfusion with Xenon-133, *J. Nucl. Med.*, 21, 156, 1980.

34. **Davis, M. J., Joyner, W. L., and Gilmore, J. P.,** Microvascular pressure distribution and responses of pulmonary allograft in cheek pouch arterioles in the hamster to oxygen, *Circ. Res.*, 49, 125–132, 1981.

35. **Davis, M. J., Shi, X., and Sikes, P. J.,** Modulation of bat wing venule contraction by transmural pressure changes, *Am. J. Physiol.*, 262(3Pt. 2), H625–H634, 1992.

36. **Davis, M. J. and Sikes, P. J.**, Myogenic responses of isolated arterioles: Test for a rate sensitive mechanism, *Am. J. Physiol.*, 259(6Pt. 2), H1890–H1900, 1990.

37. **Davis, M. J. and Sikes, P. J.**, A rate sensitive component to the myogenic response is absent from bat wing arterioles, *Am. J. Physiol.*, 256(1Pt. 2), H32–H40, 1989.

38. **Davis, M. J.**, Spontaneous contractions of isolated bat wing venules are inhibited by luminal flow, *Am. J. Physiol.*, 264(4Pt. 2), H1174–H1186, 1993.

39. **Dudar, T. E. and Jain, R. K.**, Microcirculatory flow changes during tissue growth, *Microvasc. Res.*, 25, 1–21, 1983.

40. **Duling, B. R.**, The preparation and use of the hamster cheek pouch for studies of the microcirculation, *Microvas. Res.*, 5, 423–429, 1973.

41. **Ellis, R. A.**, Aging of the human male scalp, in *The Biology of Hair Growth*, Montagna, W. and Ellis, R. A., Eds., Academic Press, New York, 1958, 469–485.

42. **Endrich, B. and Messmer, K.**, *Handbook of Microsurgery*, Vol. I, Olszewski, W. L., Ed., CRC Press, Boca Raton, FL, 1984, 79–105.

43. **Eriksson, E., Boykin, J. V., and Pittman, R. N.**, Method for *in vivo* microscopy of the cutaneous microcirculation of the hairless mouse ear, *Microvasc. Res.*, 19, 374, 1980.

44. **Fagrell, B., Frinck, A., and Intalietta, M.**, A microscope-television system for studying flow velocity in human skin capillaries, *Am. J. Physiol.*, 233, H318–H321, 1977.

45. **Fagrell, B., Tooke, J., Ostergren, J., and Miligan, D.**, *Verh. Dtsch. Ges. Inn. Med.*, 90, 250–251, 1984.

46. **Fagrell, B.**, Local microcirculation in chronic venous incompetence and leg ulcers, *Vasc. Surg.*, 13, 217–225, 1979.

47. **Fagrell, B.**, *The Physiology and Pharmacology of Microsurgery*, Vol. 2, Olszewski, W. L., Ed., Academic Press, Orlando, FL, 1984, 133–180.

48. **Fagrell, B., Lundberg, G., Olsson, A. G., and Ostergren, J.**, *VASA*, 15, 56–60, 1986.

49. **Frank, J. M., Barker, J. H., Kaneko, S., Joel, C., Ogden, L., Lane, J., Anderson, G. L., and Tobin, G. R.**, *In vivo* analysis of growth factor induced angiogenesis, (Abstract), *Eur. Surg. Res.*, 25, 44, 1993.

50. **Fulton, G. P. and Lutz, B. R.**, The use of the hamster cheek pouch and cinephotomicrography for research on the microcirculation and tumor growth and for teaching purposes, *Boston Med.*, 8, 13–19, 1957.

51. **Funk, W., Roth, H. H., Foitzik, T., and Endrich, B.**, Homologous spleen transplant: neovasculatization and angioarchitecture, *Eur. Surg. Res.*, 16, 115 (Abstr.), 1984.

52. **Furness, J. B. and Marshall, J. M.**, Correlation of the directly observed responses of mesenteric vessels of the rat nerve stimulation and noradrenaline with the distribution of adrenergic nerves, *J. Physiol.*, 239, 75–88, 1974.

53. **Galla, T. J., Saetzler, R. K., Hammersen, F., and Messmer, K.**, Increase in skin flap survival by the vasoactive drug Buflomedil, *Plast. Reconstr. Surg.*, 87, 130–138, 1991.

54. **Goldsmith, L. A.**, *Physiology, Biochemistry and Molecular Biology of the Skin*, Oxford University Press, New York, 1529, 1991.

55. **Goodall, C. M., Sanders, A. G., and Shubik, P.**, Studies of vascular patterns in living tumors with a transparent chamber inserted in a hamster cheek pouch, *J. Natl. Cancer Inst.*, 35, 497–521, 1965.

56. **Grossbart, T. A. K.**, The skin: Matters of the flesh, in *Mind Body Medicine*, Coleman, D. and Gurin, J., Eds., Consumer Reports Book, New York, chap. 8, 1993.

57. **Griffith, T. M. and Edwards, D. H.**, *Am. J. Physiol.*, 258, H1171–H1180, 1990.

58. **Grosser-Brockhoff, F. and Schoedel, W.**, Physiologie und Pathologie des Kreislaufes, in *Handbuch der Thoraxchiruegie*, Berlin, 1957.

59. **Handel, N., Zaremy, H. A., and Graham, L. S.**, Computerized determination of blood flow in pedicle flaps by clearance of epicutaneous, applied 133 Xenon, *J. Surg. Res.*, 20, 579, 1976.

60. **Harrison, D. H., Girling, M., and Mott, G.**, Experience in monitoring the circulation in free-flap transfers, *Plast. Reconstr. Surg.*, 68, 543, 1981.

61. **Hashimoto, H. and Prewitt, R. L.**, Microvascular density changes during wound healing, *Int. J. Microcirc.: Clin. Exp.*, 5, 303–310, 1987.

62. **Hirata, K., Nagasaka, T., and Noda, Y.**, Partitional measurement of capillary and arteriovenous anastomotic blood flow in the human finger by laser Doppler flowmeter, *Eur. J. Appl. Physiol.*, 57, 616–621, 1988.

63. **Holloway, G. A., Jr. and Watkins, D. W.,** Laser Doppler measurement of cutaneous blood flow, *J. Invest. Dermatol.*, 69, 306–309, 1977.

64. **Jacobs, M. J. H. M.,** Thesis, University of Linburg, Maastrich, Holland.

65. **Jones, T. W.,** *Philos. Trans. Roy. Soc. London*, 142, 131–133, 1852.

66. **Joyner, W. L., Champbell, G. T., Peterson, C., and Wagoner, J.,** Adrenergic neurons: Are they present on microvessels in cheek pouches of hamsters?, *Microvasc. Res.*, 26, 27–35, 1983.

67. **Joyner, W. L. and Gilmore, J. P.,** Tissues grafted into cheek pouch of the hamster, in *Microcirculatory Technology*, Baker, C. H. and Nastuk, W. L., Eds., Academic Press, Orlando, FL, chap. 1, 1986.

68. **Joyner, W. L., Gilmore, J. P., Young, R., and Blank, D. U.,** Microanatomy and vascular reactivity of cerebral microvessels allografted into the hamster cheek pouch, *Fed. Proc. Fed. Am. Soc. Exp. Biol.*, 44, 1009, 1985.

69. **Kamler, M., Lehr, H. A., Barker, J. H., Saetzler, R., Galla, T. J., and Mesmer, K.,** Impact of ischemia on tissue oxygenation and wound healing: Intravital microscopic studies on the hairless mouse ear model, *Eur. Surg. Res.*, 25, 30–37, 1993.

70. **Kanan, M. W. and Ryan, T. J.,** Endonasal localization of blood borne viable and non-viable particulate matter, *Br. J. Dermatol.*, 92, 475, 663–674, 1975.

71. **Kim, M. K., Ogden, L., Barker, J. H., Anderson, G. L., White, S. W., Ohl, E., Kamler, M., and Tobin, G. R.,** Basic fibroblast growth factor induces angiogenesis in ischemic tissue, *Surg. Forum*, 42, 632–635, 1991.

72. **Kjolseth, D., Frank, J. M., Barker, J. H., Rosenthal, A., Anderson, G. L., Acland, R. D., Campbell, F. R., and Tobin, G. R.,** Comparison of the effects of commonly used wound agents on epithelialization and neovascularization, *J. Am. Coll. Surg.*, 179, 305–312, 1994.

73. **Krogh, A.,** Anatone und Physiologie des Capillaren, in *Arteriendes Hundes., Anat. Anz.*, Springer, Berling, 4, 276(1889), 1929.

74. **Lebel, L. and Gerdin, B.,** Sodium hyaluronate increases vascular ingrowth in the rabbit ear chamber, *Int. J. Exp. Pathol.*, 72(2), 111–118, 1991.

75. **Lindqvist, A., Parviainen, P., Kolari, P., Tuominen, J., Valimaki, I., Antila, K., and Laitinen, L. A.,** A non-invasive method for testing neural circulatory control in man, *Cardiovasc. Res.*, 23, 262–272, 1989.

76. **Low, P. A., Neumann, C., Dyck, P. J., Fealy, R. D., and Tuck, R. R.,** *Mayo Clin. Proc.*, 58, 583–592, 1983.

77. **Mantovani, A., Bussolino, F., and Dejana, E.,** Cytokine regulation of endothelial cell function, *FASEB J.*, 6, 2591–2600, 1992.

78. **Maricg, H. R.,** *Arthritis Rheum.*, 24, M59–M65, 1981.

79. **Mayrovitz, H. N.,** Age and site variability of skin blood perfusion in the hairless mouse ear determined by laser Doppler flowmetry, *Int. J. Microcirc.: Clin. Exp.*, 11(3), 297–306, 1992.

80. **McCraw, J. B., Myers, B., and Shankli, K. D.,** The value of fluorescein in predicting the viability of arterialized flaps, *Plast. Reconstr. Surg.*, 60, 710, 1977.

81. **Melkumyants, A. M., Balashov, T. A., Smiesko, V., and Khayuntin, V. M.,** *Bull. Exp. Biol. Med.*, 101, 568–570, 1986.

82. **Menger, M. D., Barker, J. H., and Messmer, K.,** Capillary blood perfusion during post-ischemic reperfusion in striated muscle, *Plast. Reconstr. Surg.*, 89, 1104–1114, 1992.

83. **Menger, M. D., Hammersen, F., Barker, J. H., Feifel, G., and Messmer, K.,** Tissue P_{O_2} and functional capillary density in chronically ischemic skeletal muscle, *Adv. Exp. Med. Biol.*, 222, 631–636, 1987.

84. **Menger, M. D., Jaeger, S., Walter, P., Feifel, G., Hammersen, F., and Messmer, K.,** Angiogenesis and hemodynamics of the microvasculature of transplanted islets of Langerhans, *Diabetes*, 38(Suppl.), 199–201, 1989.

85. **Menger, M. D., Sack, F. U., Barker, J. H., Feifel, G., and Messmer, K.,** Quantitative analysis of microcirculatory disorders after prolonged ischemia in skeletal muscle: Therapeutic effects of prophylactic isovolemic hemodilution, *Res. Exp. Med.*, 188, 151–156, 1988.

86. **Moretti, G., Ellis, R. A., and Mescon, H.,** Vascular patterns in the skin of the face, *J. Invest. Dermatol.*, 33, 103–112, 1959.

87. **Myers, B.,** Prediction of skin slough at the time of operation with the use of fluorescein dye, *Surgery*, 51, 158, 1962.

88. **Narayan, K. and Cliff, W. J.,** Use of rabbit ear chamber and strontium-90 source to study radiation pathology *in vivo, Microvasc. Res.,* 21(3), 384–389, 1981.
89. **Nicoll, P. A. and Webb, R. L.,** Vascular patterns and active vasomotion as determinates of flow through minute vessels, *Angiology,* 6, 291–308, 1955.
90. **Nilsson, G. E., Tenland, T., and Oberg, P. A.,** Evaluation of laser Doppler flow meter for measurement of tissue blood flow, *IEEE Trans. Biomed. Eng.,* 27, 597, 1980.
91. **Nishioka, K. and Ryan, T. J.,** The influence of epidermis and other tissues on blood vessel growth in the hamster cheek pouch, *J. Invest. Dermatol.,* 58, 33–45, 1972.
92. **Ostergren, J. and Fagrell, B.,** Skin capillary blood cell velocity in patients with arterial obliterative disease and polycythemia: A disturbed reactive hyperemia response, *Clin. Physiol.,* 5, 35–43, 1985.
93. **Owen, M. P., Quinn, C., and Bevan, J. A.,** *Am. J. Physiol.,* 249, H404–H414, 1985.
94. **Palmer, B., Jurell, G., and Norberg, K. A.,** The blood flow in experimental skin flaps in rats studied by means of the 133 Xenon clearance method, *Scand. J. Plast. Reconstr. Surg.,* 6, 6, 1972.
95. **Pang, C. Y., Neligan, P., and Nakutsuka, T.,** Assessment of microsphere technique for measurement of capillary blood flow in random skin flaps in pigs, *Plast. Reconstr. Surg.,* 74, 513, 1984.
96. **Pang, C. Y., Neligan, P., Nakatsuka, T., and Sasaki, G. H.,** Assessment of the fluorescein dye test for prediction of skin flap viability in pigs, *J. Surg. Res.,* 41, 173, 1986.
97. **Papenfuss, H. D., Gross, J. F., Intagietta, M., and Treese, F. A.,** Transparent access chamber for the rat dorsal skin fold, *Microvasc. Res.,* 18, 311–318, 1979.
98. **Pasyk, K. A., Thomas, S. V., Hassett, C. A., Cherry, G. W., and Faller, R.,** Regional differences in capillary density of the normal human dermis, *Plast. Reconstr. Surg.,* 83, 939–945, 1989.
99. **Perbeck, L.,** Fluorescein flowmetry: A blood flow measurement method, Thesis, Karolinska Institute, Stockholm, Sweden, 1985.
100. **Perera, P., Kurhan, A. K., and Ryan, T. J.,** The development of the cutaneous microvascular system in the newborn, *Br. J. Dermatol.,* 82(Suppl. 5), 86–91, 1970.
101. **Porter, A. M. W.,** Sweat and thermoregulation in hominids. Comments prompted by the publications of Wheeler, P. E., 1984–1993, *J. Hum. Evol.,* 25, 417–423, 1993.
102. **Prather, A., Blackburn, J. P., Williams, T. R., and Lynn, J. A.,** Evaluation of tests for predicting the viability of axial pattern skin flaps in the pig, *Plast. Reconstr. Surg.,* 63, 250, 1979.
103. **Ramseier, H. and Billingham, R. E.,** Studies on delayed cutaneous inflammatory reactions elicited by inoculation of homologous cells into hamster's skin, *J. Exp. Med.,* 123, 629–656, 1966.
104. **Reinish, J. F.,** The pathophysiology of skin flap circulation: The delay phenomenon, *Plast. Reconstr. Surg.,* 54, 585, 1974.
105. **Riva, C., Ross, B., and Benedek, G. B.,** Laser Doppler measurements of blood flow in capillary tubes and retinal arteries, *J. Invest. Ophthalmol.,* 11, 936, 1972.
106. **Rusznyak, I., Foldi, M., and Szabo, G.,** *Lymphatics and Lymph Circulation, Physiology and Pathology,* Perganom Press, Oxford, 1967.
107. **Ryan, T. J., Ed.,** *Microvascular Injury,* Vol. 7, Major Problems in Dermatology, Lloyd Luke Medical, London, 1976.
108. **Ryan, T. J. and Cherry, G. W., Eds.,** Vascular birthmarks: Pathogenesis and management (monograph), Oxford University Press, Oxford, 1987.
109. **Ryan, T. J. and Curri, S.,** *The Cutaneous Adipose Tissue in Series: Clinics in Dermatology,* Elsevier, London, 1989.
110. **Ryan, T. J.,** Structure and function of lymphatics, *J. Invest. Dermatol.,* 93, 18S–24S, 1989.
111. **Ryan, T. J.,** Cutaneous circulation, in *Physiology, Biochemistry and Molecular Biology of the Skin,* Goldsmith, L. A., Ed., Oxford University Press, New York, 1991, 1019–1084.
112. **Ryan, T. J.,** Direct observation of capillary modifications in the aged, in *Aging Skin — Properties and Functional Changes* (Clinical Dermatology series), Leveque, J. L. and Anache, P. G., Eds., Marcel Decker, New York, 1993, 87–104.
113. **Sanders, A. G. and Shubik, P.,** A transparent window for use in the Syrian hamster, *Isr. J. Exp. Med.,* 11, 118a, 1964.
114. **Sandison, J. C.,** Observations on the growth of blood vessels as seen in the transparent chamber introduced in the rabbit's ear, *Am. J. Anat.,* 41, 475–496, 1928.
115. **Sasaki, A., Melder, R. J., Whiteside, T. L., Herberman, R. B., and Jain, R. K.,** Preferential localization of human adherent lymphokine activated killer cells in tumor microcirculation, *J. Natl. Cancer Inst.,* 83(6), 433–437, 1991.

116. **Schmid-Schonbein, H.,** Interaction of vasomotion and blood rheology in hemodynamics, in *Clinical Aspects of Blood Viscosity and Cell Deformability*, Lowe, G. D., Ed., Springer-Verlag, New York, 1981.

117. **Sewell, I. A.,** Studies of the microcirculation using transparent tissue observation chambers inserted in the hamster cheek pouch, *J. Anat.*, 100, 839–856, 1966.

118. **Silverman, D. G., La Rossa, D. D., Barlow, C. H., Bering, T. G., Popky, L. M., and Schmidt, T. C.,** Quantification of tissue fluorescein delivery and prediction of flap viability with the fiber optic demofluorometer, *Plast. Reconstr. Surg.*, 66, 545, 1980.

119. **Smiesko, V., Lang, D. J., and Johnson, P. C.,** *Am. J. Physiol.*, 157(Heart Circ. Physiol. 26), H1958–H1965, 1989.

120. **Sorrentino, E. A. and Mayrovitz, H. N.,** Skin capillary perfusion after regional ischemia, *Int. J. Microcirc.: Clin. Exp.*, 10, 103–110, 1991.

121. **Svedman, P., Jacobsson, S., Ponnert, L., and Lindell, S. E.,** Transcutaneous oxygen tension in flaps. A preliminary report, *Chir. Plast.*, 6, 201, 1982.

122. **Tooke, J. E.,** Capillary pressure and flow velocity in diabetes, *Int. J. Microcirc.: Clin. Exp.*, 3, 494, 1984.

123. **Tooke, J. E., Ostergren, J., and Fagrell, B.,** *Int. J. Microcirc.: Clin. Exp.*, 2, 277–284, 1983.

124. **Torres-Filho, I. P.,** Venular vasomotion in the bat wing, *Microvasc. Res.*, 39(2), 246–249, 1990.

125. **Vidas, M., Weisman, R. A., and Silverman, D. G.,** Serial fluorometric assessment of experimental neurovascular island flaps, *Arch. Otolaryngol.*, 109, 457, 1983.

126. **Wearn, J.,** The extent of the capillary bed of the heart, *J. Exp. Med.*, 47, 273, 1928.

127. **Westerhof, W.,** *Leg Ulcers: Diagnosis and Treatment*, Elsevier, Amsterdam, 1993, 409.

128. **Wiedeman, M. P.,** Dimensions of blood vessels from distributing artery to collecting vein, *Circ. Res.*, 12, 375–378, 1963.

129. **Wiedeman, M. P.,** Contractile activity of arterioles in the bat wing during intraluminal pressure changes, *Circ. Res.*, 19, 559–563, 1966.

130. **Wiedeman, M. P.,** *Physical Basis of Circulatory Transport: Regulation and Exchange*, Reeve, E. B. and Guyton, A. C., Eds., 1967, 307–312.

131. **Wiedeman, M. P.,** Preparation of the bat wing for *in vivo* microscopy, *Microvasc. Res.*, 5, 417–422, 1973.

132. **Xiu, Rui-Juan,** Physiology in traditional oriental medicine, *Abstracts of the First Asian Congress for Microcirculation*, Japanese Society for Microcirculation, 1993.

133. **Young, C. M. A. and Hopewell, J. W.,** The isotope clearance technique for measuring skin blood flow, *Br. J. Plast. Surg.*, 36, 222, 1983.

134. **Zarem, H. A. and Soderberg, R.,** Tissue reaction to ischemia in the rabbit ear chamber: Effect of prednisolone on inflammation and microvascular flow, *Plast. Reconstr. Surg.*, 70(6), 667–676, 1982.

Chapter 25

Spleen Microcirculation

Alan C. Groom, Eric E. Schmidt, and Ian C. MacDonald

CONTENTS

I. ANATOMY AND FUNCTION

A. VASCULAR ANATOMY OF THE SPLEEN

The spleen represents the only lymphatic tissue specialized to filter the blood, and its microcirculation is probably the most complex of any organ in the body. The normal pattern of arterioles → capillaries → venules is interrupted by a reticular meshwork (the "intermediate circulation") placed between the capillary endings and the venous vessels (Figure 1). The reticular meshwork is the site where filtration of the blood takes place (analogous to the fuel filter of a car).

Arteries and veins enter and leave the spleen along the hilus of its concave surface and pass within trabeculae into the interior of the organ (shown schematically[1] in Figure 2). Suspended within the network of trabeculae is a three-dimensional web of reticular cells and fibers housing the white pulp and red pulp. The white pulp consists of sheaths of lymphatic tissue surrounding arteries after they leave the trabeculae (periarterial lymphatic sheaths) and thickened regions forming lymphatic nodules. The red pulp, which owes its color (and name) to the high concentration of red blood cells percolating through it, occupies 75% of the volume in normal human spleen.[2] Its reticular meshwork is honeycombed by a system of interconnected venous sinuses, present in about 50% of mammalian species including humans.[3] In other mammals, the venous system begins, instead, as small fenestrated pulp venules, these spleens being designated as "nonsinusal".

The nature of microcirculatory pathways bordering the white pulp has received little attention and is not included in Figure 2 or in standard histology texts. The clearest evidence has come from microvascular corrosion casts and will be discussed here for the normal human spleen (for details see Schmidt et al., Reference 4). The interrelationship between lymphatic nodules and surrounding vascular structures may be seen in Figure 3. Directly bordering the lymphatic nodule is the marginal sinus. This consists of a series of thin anastomosing vascular spaces, receiving a plentiful blood supply from capillaries that terminate on its outward face (not visible in Figure 3). Blood flows circumferentially through the marginal sinus before moving radially outward (via apertures in its outer wall) to the surrounding marginal zone, a finely meshed reticulum up to 200 μm thick. Beyond the marginal zone lies the extensive reticular meshwork of the red pulp.

0-8493-4870-6/95/$0.00+$.50

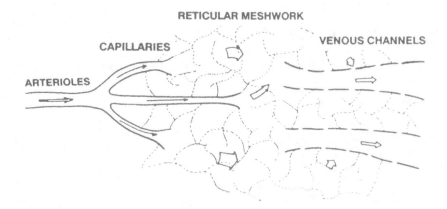

Figure 1 Simplified schematic diagram showing the unique arrangement of the splenic micro-circulation. Much of the blood percolates through a reticular meshwork interposed between capillary endings and the start of the venous channels. This meshwork presents an enormous contact surface area for blood cells and particulate material, and its large total cross-sectional area for flow results in very low blood velocities. (From MacDonald, I. C., Schmidt, E. E., and Groom, A. C., *Microvasc. Res.*, 42, 60, 1991.)

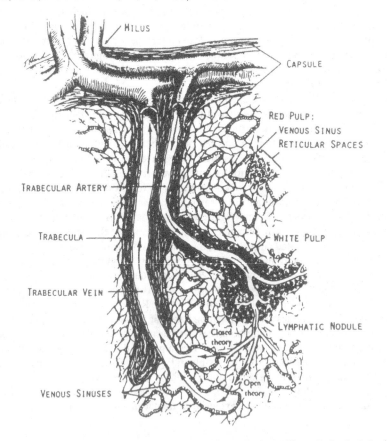

Figure 2 Schematic diagram showing structure of sinusal spleen. (From Bellanti, J. A., *Immunology: Basic Processes*, W. B. Saunders, Philadelphia, 1979.)

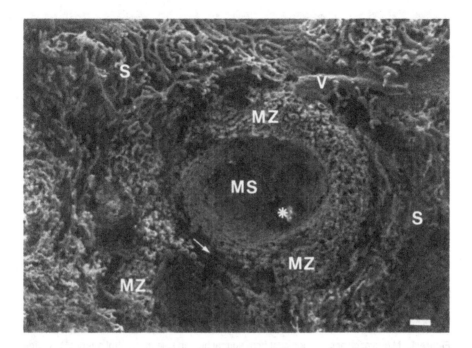

Figure 3 Microvascular corrosion cast from normal human spleen, viewed by scanning electron microscopy, showing interrelationship between lymphatic nodules (white pulp corroded away), marginal sinus (MS), marginal zone (MZ), and venous sinus (S) network in red pulp. The opening in MS (*) is the site where central artery (cast accidentally broken off) entered nodule. In the region where two nodules are close together, MZ is narrow (arrow). A collecting vein (V) has begun to fill, but the reticular meshwork of the red pulp is unfilled due to minimal amount of casting material injected (see Section III.B). Bar = 100 μm. (From Schmidt, E. E., MacDonald, I. C., and Groom, A. C., *Am. J. Anat.*, 181, 253, 1988.)

After leaving the white pulp, numerous arterioles curve circumferentially within the marginal zone, terminating as capillaries at the marginal sinus or within the marginal zone itself (Figure 4). Other vessels extend out into the red pulp, the great majority terminating within the reticular meshwork (i.e., "open" circulation), although a small number form direct connections with venous sinuses ("closed" circulation[4]). A large proportion of the flow enters the venous system via open-ended venous sinuses continuous with the marginal sinus or marginal zone (Figure 5), bypassing the reticular meshwork of the red pulp. Blood that reaches this reticular meshwork, via capillary terminations or flow outward from the marginal zone, has to enter venous sinuses via narrow interendothelial slits in sinus walls (see Section III.C, Figure 9). The walls of venous sinuses consist of long spindle-shaped endothelial cells aligned parallel to the axis of the vessel[5] (Figure 6). These cells are held in position by the processes of reticular cells, which form "hoops" around the abluminal surface of the sinus. Between adjacent hoops regions of the endothelial wall are left exposed, allowing blood to enter venous sinuses through slit-like gaps between endothelial cells. The anastomosing system of venous sinuses drains into collecting veins and, ultimately, into trabecular veins leading to the hilus.

B. MICROVASCULAR FUNCTIONS OF THE SPLEEN
Unlike other organs studied from a microcirculatory standpoint, the spleen is not concerned with transcapillary exchange in relation to metabolism. Its two primary functions

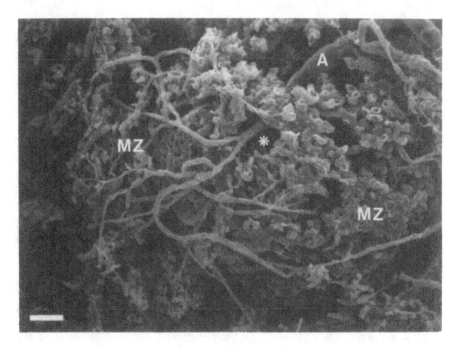

Figure 4 Microvascular corrosion cast from normal human spleen. Central artery (A) emerges from lymphatic nodule into marginal zone (MZ), and there (*) gives rise to numerous circumferentially directed arterioles and capillaries, most of which terminate in the MZ. Reticular meshwork of the red pulp is unfilled due to minimal amount of casting material injected. Bar = 50 μm. (From Schmidt, E. E., MacDonald, I. C., and Groom, A. C., *Am. J. Anat.,* 181, 253, 1988.)

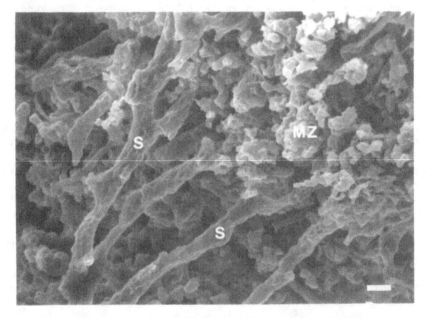

Figure 5 Microvascular corrosion cast from normal human spleen, showing many venous sinuses (S) originating via open ends in the marginal zone (MZ) bordering a lymphatic nodule. Reticular meshwork of the red pulp is unfilled due to minimal injection technique. Bar = 20 μm. (From Groom, A. C., Schmidt, E. E., and MacDonald, I. C., *Scanning Microsc.,* 5, 159, 1991.)

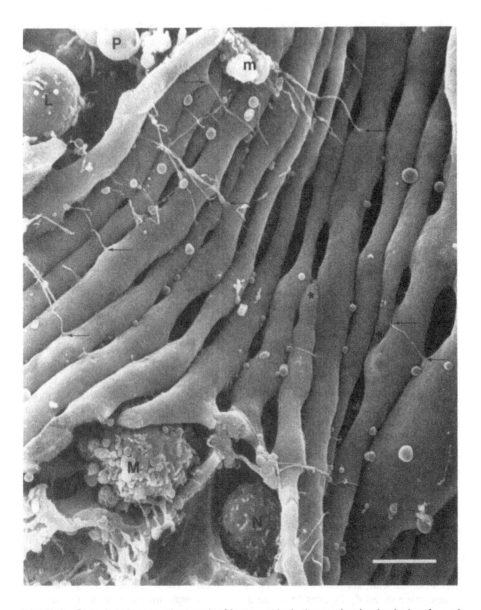

Figure 6 Scanning electron micrograph of human splenic tissue, showing luminal surface of venous sinus. Long spindle-shaped endothelial cells lie side by side with slit-like gaps between them; a few cells terminate in tapered end (*). Threadlike processes (arrow) extend from endothelial cells. Some threads may belong to macrophage (M) processes (m). L, lymphocyte; N, neutrophil; P, platelet. Bar = 5 µm. (From Fujita, T., *Archivum Histologicum Japonicum*, 37, 187, 1974.)

concern immunologic reactions and the filtration of cells and particulate matter from the blood. It has long been recognized that the spleen concentrates normal blood cells to twice arterial hematocrit, and harbors more than 30% of all circulating platelets in the body. Why this should be so has been unclear.

The importance of the spleen to the immune system was underestimated until recently. However, this organ provides a unique microenvironment for the removal of antigens from the blood, and for the cell-antigen and cell-cell interactions necessary for the development of immune responses. The spleen contains high concentrations of lymphocytes and macrophages, especially in the marginal zone, including a unique population of macrophages that ingest polysaccharide-encapsulated bacteria (which are principally responsible for post-splenectomy sepsis). Furthermore, the predominant role of the spleen in lymphocyte recirculation is now recognized, the daily traffic of lymphocytes through this organ (4×10^{11} cells) far exceeding the combined traffic through all lymph nodes (3×10^9 cells, Pabst[6]). The large cross-sectional area for flow presented by the reticular meshwork of the marginal zone and red pulp causes a marked reduction in blood flow velocity, leading to low shear rates and enhanced interaction of antigens with immunocompetent cells. Activated B and T lymphocytes migrate to their respective compartments in the white pulp, for antibody production, proliferation, and differentiation into effector cells. B lymphocytes migrate to lymphatic nodules and T lymphocytes to the periarterial lymphatic sheath.

The filtration of blood by the spleen includes the removal of particulate material and of blood cells unsuitable for continued circulation. This function has been studied principally with respect to red blood cells (RBCs). Three microcirculatory structures unique to the spleen underlie the filtration capabilities of this organ. First, the reticular meshwork presents an enormous surface area to which cells and particulate material may adhere, and produces low shear rates that promote such interactions. Thereby, the reticular meshwork provides a mechanism for filtration based on surface interactions rather than on size restriction (its channels generally being several RBC diameters wide). The reticular meshwork is common to all spleens, sinusal or nonsinusal, and provides the primary mechanism for filtration of the blood.

A second mechanism of filtration is present in sinusal spleens (e.g., human), in that blood leaving the reticular meshwork of the red pulp must enter the venous system by passing through narrow interendothelial slits (IES) in walls of venous sinuses (Section III.C, Figure 9). This process requires blood cells to undergo considerable deformation, since each IES is well below 1 μm in width *in vivo* (below the limit of resolution of the light microscope). In this way, cells that are not sufficiently deformable are filtered out from the blood and retained within the reticular meshwork for phagocytosis. In nonsinusal spleens, the pulp venules lack such IES but receive flow freely through open ends and rounded fenestrations in their walls; the sizes of the fenestrations are mostly large enough to allow unimpeded entry of RBCs into the venule.[7]

A third mechanism for blood filtration is present in spleens of some species, whether sinusal or nonsinusal. Small ellipsoidal sheaths, consisting of finely meshed reticulum filled with macrophages, surround many arterial capillaries a short distance before their termination in either the marginal zone or the red pulp. The capillary within each sheath has a porous wall, allowing blood to enter the sheath. These ellipsoids (or periarterial macrophage sheaths[8]) are sites for clearance of particulate matter from the blood. The human spleen possesses both venous sinuses and ellipsoids, in addition to the reticular meshwork, giving it every advantage for its task of filtering the blood.

The spleen carries out several different functions with respect to RBCs filtered out of the bloodstream, including destruction, repair, or maturation. Abnormal or senescent RBCs are selectively retained within the reticular meshwork and destroyed by phagocytic cells.[9] RBCs containing inclusion bodies are subjected to a "pitting" process at IES in sinusal spleens[10]: most of the cell squeezes through the IES, leaving a small portion containing the nondeformable inclusion bodies trailing behind on the reticular meshwork side of the IES. This situation persists until the trailing portion is phagocytosed, the membrane reseals, and the "repaired" cell is once again free to circulate. Reticulocytes released from the bone marrow are sequestered in the reticular meshwork for a 1- to 2-day period of maturation, and are then returned to the circulation; these reticulocytes amount to 8% of all splenic RBCs.[11] There is evidence that splenic macrophages serve as "nurse" cells, assisting in the maturation of such immature RBCs.[12]

Although the primary functions of the spleen are immunologic reactions and blood filtration, the organ also has an intriguing ability to concentrate blood cells within the red pulp. The intrasplenic hematocrit is twice that of arterial blood. Spleens of such species as horse, goat, dog, and cat are very contractile and serve as a reservoir of RBCs for use during emergencies, analogous to "blood doping" in athletes. However, in humans and many other mammalian species, the spleen exhibits little contractility and this reservoir function appears to be lacking, leaving the high intrasplenic hematocrit unexploited.

What is the origin of this high hematocrit? Various possibilities have been suggested, the most well known being that hemoconcentration is carried out within venous sinuses under the control of afferent and efferent sphincters.[13] However, other investigators have not been able to confirm such a mechanism. Furthermore, nonsinusal spleens concentrate RBCs to an equally high hematocrit within the reticular meshwork.[14] Recently, it has been shown that hemoconcentration is a rheological consequence of RBC flow through the reticular meshwork.[15] The very low shear rates and enormous surface area for RBC interactions with the reticular meshwork not only provide an environment ideally suited for trapping abnormal RBCs, but also cause normal RBCs to be delayed, transiently but repeatedly, as they pass through the meshwork. Since the plasma flows on freely, the mean RBC velocity is reduced below that of plasma, and intrasplenic hematocrit must rise in consequence. This follows from the law of conservation of mass, and is the inverse of the "Fahraeus effect" observed when RBCs move faster than plasma in blood flowing through narrow tubes.

It has been known for many years that pooling of platelets also occurs in the spleen. Young platelets are preferentially retained (humans[16]) and probably undergo late maturation, analogous to that shown to occur for reticulocytes. The exchangeable platelet pool in human spleen has been calculated to be about one third of the total number of circulating platelets in the body.[17] How this high concentration of platelets comes about has not been explained. It may well be that transient but repeated surface interactions with the reticular meshwork cause platelets to move more slowly than plasma, giving rise to an inverse Fahraeus effect similar to that observed for RBCs. Thus, the high intrasplenic hematocrit and the high platelet concentration may be considered as merely side effects of the filtration mechanism for abnormal or immature blood cells, provided by the reticular meshwork.

II. PATHOLOGY

The spleen is rarely the primary site of disease, but is affected by a wide range of disease processes originating elsewhere in the body. Consequently, it has been difficult to study the pathology of the spleen per se, and most textbooks provide little information on this organ. There are two gross indicators of pathology of the spleen: a change in its size, usually enlargement (splenomegaly), or a change in its activity (hypo- or hypersplenism). Little is known about changes in splenic microcirculatory blood flow in disease.

Splenomegaly can arise from a variety of causes, including obstruction of the venous outflow (locally or downstream at the liver), hematological disorders, infections, or neoplasms.[18] Studies of two types of congestive splenomegaly, "Banti's syndrome" with or without liver cirrhosis,[19,20] have demonstrated similar morphological changes from normal spleen: a 10- to 13-fold increase in total volume of red pulp, a marked increase in the number of venous sinuses and an almost twofold reduction in their diameter, and a decreased thickness of reticular meshwork between adjacent sinuses. Blood cell storage within the organ is greatly increased under these conditions. Although it is difficult to develop a chronic animal model of congestive splenomegaly, much can be learned from acute experiments in which splenic venous pressure is elevated to 25 cm H_2O.[21] Under these conditions, the cat spleen dilated and its RBC content rose from the normal 26% to a value 51% of the total RBC mass of the body. Blood flow through the fast splenic pathway was reduced to zero, the entire inflow passing via slow routes within the reticular meshwork (see Section III).

Splenomegaly may occur secondarily in hematological disorders, including hereditary spherocytosis, thalassemia, and sickle cell anemia.[22,23] The reticular meshwork of the red pulp becomes chronically congested with the abnormal RBCs because their decreased deformability restricts passage through interendothelial slits into venous sinuses (e.g., hereditary spherocytosis[24]). However, adhesion of such cells to the reticular meshwork must also play an important role, as indicated by acute experiments in the nonsinusal spleen of cat. Following injection into the bloodstream of a small volume of autologous RBCs rendered spherocytic by heat treatment, one half of the RBC mass in the red pulp of the spleen was immobilized.[25] Since the large fenestrations in walls of pulp venules do not restrict entry of RBCs, surface interactions of heat-treated RBCs with the reticular meshwork must have caused the congestion of the red pulp. In splenomegaly, increased pooling of platelets also occurs, probably due to the increase in total mass of the spleen and surface interactions between platelets and the reticular meshwork.[26]

Increased activity of the spleen with normal organ size is seen in immune thrombocytopenia (ITP). In this condition, the spleen produces large quantities of antiplatelet antibodies, leading to accelerated phagocytosis of platelets by splenic macrophages. In chronic ITP, lymphoid hyperplasia is often found, characterized by large numbers of lymphatic nodules containing active germinal centers.[27] Changes in splenic microcirculatory pathways in patients with chronic ITP have recently been described,[28] based on the study of microvascular corrosion casts (see Section III). First, a striking proliferation of arterioles and capillaries is found in the white pulp and marginal zone, seen as extensive vascularization in 92.3% of lymphatic nodules vs. 0.6% in normal spleens. Second, there is an absence of the marginal sinus in 89.4% of lymphatic nodules vs. 4.9% in normal spleens. These changes may not be specific to ITP alone, but could be a reflection of lymphoid hyperplasia, which occurs in other disorders as well.

III. MODELS AND TECHNIQUES

Three different experimental approaches have been used to gain new insights regarding microcirculatory blood flow through the spleen.

A. ISOLATED SPLEEN PREPARATION

Intact spleens are essential for these studies, effectively ruling out human spleens since tissue samples will have been removed by the pathologist. The organ is treated as a "black box" and information is obtained by examining input-output relationships. Two quite different experimental approaches may be used: (1) kinetics of RBC and plasma washout during Ringer perfusion, and (2) splenic drainage with the inflow occluded. The first approach yields quantitative data on splenic blood compartments (Figure 7) and transit times,[14,29,30] together with reticulocyte sequestration.[11,31] The second approach makes it possible to sample selectively (and anaerobically) blood from the reticular meshwork of the red pulp, leading to analysis of the metabolic microenvironment for RBCs sequestered in the organ under various experimental conditions.[32,33] A combination of both approaches provides a powerful tool for studying in animal models (e.g., dog, cat, rat) the role of the spleen as a microvascular filter for immature, abnormal, and senescent RBCs from the blood, and splenic microvascular perfusion and function under abnormal conditions. (For details see References 21 and 34.)

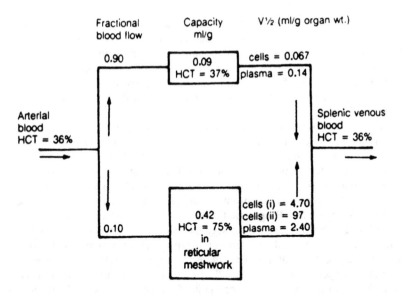

Figure 7 Compartmental model for distribution of blood in cat spleen. Nine tenths of splenic arterial blood passes through the smaller compartment ("fast") that contains blood of similar hematocrit (37%). One tenth of total blood flow passes through the reticular meshwork of the red pulp (the major compartment: "slow", combining two compartments for RBCs and one for plasma) that contains blood of hematocrit 75%. (From Levesque, M. J. and Groom, A. C., *Am. J. Physiol.*, 231, 1665, 1976.)

Intrasplenic blood flow distribution in a chronic animal model of congestive splenomegaly needs to be examined using the isolated spleen preparation. Acute experiments have shown dramatic changes in intrasplenic flow distribution when splenic venous pressure is elevated to 25 cm H_2O, corresponding to a complete shunting of blood to the slow pathway.[21] Whether a similar situation also prevails under the chronic conditions encountered clinically is unknown. Also of interest is intrasplenic flow distribution during hematological disorders. This can be mimicked in an acute animal model by injecting damaged RBCs into the circulation and, after equilibration (1 h), studying the kinetics of RBC washout from the isolated, Ringer-perfused spleen.[25] Autologous RBCs rendered spherocytic by heat treatment, or damaged with glutaraldehyde, neuraminidase, N-ethylmaleimide, etc., may be used.[21,25,34]

The causes of RBC deterioration during prolonged transit through the splenic red pulp remain unknown, although we now know that low values of pH, O_2 tension, or glucose concentration are not responsible.[32,33] Other parameters can be examined by means of the splenic drainage procedure. Finally, accurate information regarding the exchangeable platelet pool of the spleen may be obtained from the kinetics of platelet washout in isolated, Ringer-perfused spleens.

B. "MINIMAL INJECTION" MICROVASCULAR CORROSION CASTING

By means of this technique, a plastic replica of microcirculatory pathways is obtained, which may be examined by scanning electron microscopy (SEM). However, a modified approach is necessary for the spleen. Since the fractional blood volume of this organ is so high (0.5 ml/g in cat), filling the entire microvasculature with casting material produces dense casts in which individual flow pathways cannot be followed. The RBC washout studies (Section III.A) showed that 90% of the inflow travels to the splenic vein via fast pathways that occupy only 18% of the total blood space. This suggested that injection of minimal quantities of casting material would selectively yield a corrosion cast of the fast pathways. Extensive filling of the slower routes through the reticular meshwork would thereby be avoided, leaving an open view of blood vessels and their connections. By varying the volume of material injected in successive experiments, one can gain information regarding the morphological counterparts of fast vs. slow pathways and their sequence of filling.

Microvascular corrosion casting may be applied to spleens of humans as well as laboratory animals. Normal human spleens are available from transplant donors, but a large portion of the organ is used for tissue typing; with surgically removed spleens from various disease states, samples are first taken by the pathologist. In either case, it is possible to obtain a cast from a portion of the organ. In brief, the procedure is as follows. A major arterial branch, distant from any incision, is cannulated and the spleen is perfused with ~1 liter of heparinized Ringer solution at 100 cm H_2O pressure, resulting in washout of most of the RBCs from the perfused segment. A low-viscosity methacrylate resin, e.g., modified Batson's compound[35] or Mercox (Dainippon Ink and Chemicals, Tokyo), is then injected at a rate of 2 to 4 ml/min. The volume of compound used varies according to the amount of tissue perfused, but is generally 1 to 5 ml for a "minimal-injection" cast. The organ is then left undisturbed for several hours for polymerization of the resin to occur. Pieces of tissue ~1 cm^2 are cut from the filled segment and the tissue is corroded away from these samples with 40% KOH at 60°C for 5 to 6 days. The vascular casts are then carefully rinsed in distilled water, air-dried, mounted on SEM stubs, and sputter-coated with gold for examination by SEM. (For full details, see Reference 4.)

The fact that a limited region of the organ is perfused from the arterial branch cannulated gives rise to a "natural dissection" in the cast, at the boundary between the filled segment and the adjacent unperfused tissue. No cutting is necessary on this face of the cast and, thereby, fragmentation of the replicas of fine vascular paths can be avoided. At this "natural" boundary, vascular pathways in the interior of the spleen can be followed without interruption.

Examination of such "minimal injection" casts yields views such as those shown in Figures 3 to 5, which clarify the nature of microcirculatory pathways in normal human spleen[4] and show differences from other mammalian spleens.[21,34,36-39] In addition, changes in microcirculatory pathways with disease may be studied. One example of this, in chronic ITP, is the striking proliferation of arterioles and capillaries in the white pulp and marginal zone (Figure 8). The consistency of such changes has been verified by examination of casts of seven ITP and eight normal human spleens, for a total of 415 lymphatic nodules studied[28] (see Section II). Possibilities for future work include studying whether the changes seen in ITP are specific to this disease or merely reflect follicular hyperplasia, which occurs in several disorders. There is need to study splenic microcirculatory flow paths in congestive splenomegaly, and also in hematological disorders.

C. VIDEOMICROSCOPY OF TRANSILLUMINATED SPLEENS *IN VIVO*

Microvascular corrosion casts make it possible to identify the flow pathways of the splenic microcirculation, whereas *in vivo* microscopy makes it possible to visualize and describe quantitatively the movement of blood through these pathways. However, *in vivo* microscopy is restricted to animal spleens that are sufficiently thin to be transilluminated (e.g., rat, mouse). The spleen must be stabilized so that the viewed surface does not undergo respiratory movement, but remains within the plane of focus. This is difficult to achieve using an upright microscope, but with an inverted microscope the spleen rests on a coverslip window above the objective lens and the stationary lower surface of the organ is examined. Objective lenses of high magnification (up to 100×) and short working distance can then be used over a large working area.

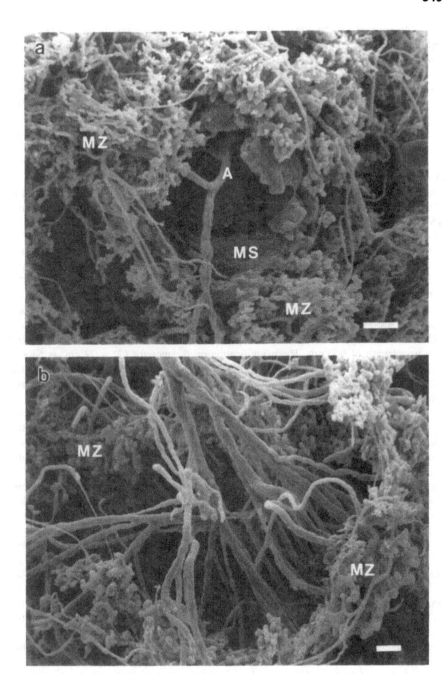

Figure 8 (a) Microvascular corrosion cast from normal human spleen, showing relationship between the arterial tree (A), a lymphatic nodule (white pulp corroded away), and the surrounding marginal sinus (MS) and marginal zone (MZ). Note the sparsity of vessels within the nodule, typical of normal spleens. Bar = 50 μm. (b) Cast from human spleen in chronic immune thrombocytopenia, showing great proliferation of arterioles and capillaries within a lymphatic nodule. Most of these vessels pass out into the surrounding marginal zone (MZ). The marginal sinus is absent. Bar = 50 μm. (From Schmidt, E. E., MacDonald, I. C., and Groom, A. C., *Blood*, 78, 1485, 1991.)

Image contrast can be enhanced considerably by using oblique lighting (fiber optic light guide at ~45°) rather than conventional illumination. Under these conditions, more light is reflected from one side of each structure than the other, resulting in shadowing that imparts a three-dimensional quality to the image. The hemoglobin within the organ acts as a red filter and there is no color contrast in the image. However, the use of a black and white video camera with extended red sensitivity (Newvicon, Panasonic WV-1550) results in excellent image contrast, far superior to that seen through the eyepieces of the microscope. A limitation of *in vivo* microscopy is that one can only observe a layer of tissue up to ~50 μm thick at the surface of the organ.

In brief, the technique is as follows. The animal is anesthetized and maintained at 37°C. A small incision is made in the abdominal wall and the tip of the spleen is withdrawn by gentle traction on the fat and pancreatic tissue adhering to the hilar side. The animal is placed on an acrylic platform on the stage of the inverted microscope (e.g., Nikon, Diaphot TMD), with the tip of the spleen resting on a coverslip window above the objective lens. The spleen is superfused with saline at 37°C, and is covered by transparent Saran® film that holds it down gently, restricting lateral and vertical motion at the plane of focus. The image obtained by oblique transillumination is monitored with the video camera (see above), and a character generator is used to add stopwatch information to the video signal. The combined signal is recorded on an SVHS videocassette recorder with slow-motion replay capability. Photographs can be taken from the monitor by means of a 35-mm camera, using normal or slow-motion replay such that each image is averaged from several successive video fields. The optical resolution of our system for a 100× objective is 0.46 μm, calculated at a wavelength of 600 nm. The magnification on the monitor (21 × 27 cm) is 5300×, corresponding to 0.07 μm per video line. Thus, an RBC 6 μm in diameter produces an image 32 mm in width, easily measurable with a millimeter scale. Calibration is done using a stage micrometer. (For full details, see Reference 40.)

The power of this technique cannot fully be appreciated except by viewing microcirculatory events in real time from the video monitor. However, by viewing sequential photographs taken from the monitor, one can gain an impression of the dynamic events recorded. Figure 9 presents a series of such images showing an RBC squeezing through an interendothelial slit (IES) in a venous sinus wall of rat spleen (see Section I.A). The direction of blood flow was invariably from the reticular meshwork into venous sinuses, not the reverse as some have suggested. The IES itself cannot be seen in the pictures, but the position and shape of the RBC within it reveal its location. The RBC has begun to enter the lumen of the venous sinus in Figure 9a, and is shown at the half-way point in its passage through the IES in Figure 9b. In the subsequent views, the RBC passes further into the lumen until it is tethered by a long "tail" that remains momentarily trapped by the IES (Figure 9f). Finally, the RBC escapes completely (not shown) and is swept away by the rapid flow within the lumen. An appreciation of the timing of these events can be gained from the stopwatch readings in each view. The flow of RBCs through IES occurs in brief discontinuous bursts, separated by periods of zero, or near zero, flow. From the video recordings, quantitative information may be obtained, e.g., in normal rats the maximum instantaneous rate of RBC flow per IES is 10 cells/s and the RBC transit times range from 0.02 to 60.5 s.[40]

An important feature of the technique is that oblique illumination gives enhanced image contrast even in solid organs where no color contrast exists. Consequently, one can also obtain excellent images of leukocytes or platelets within the microcirculation. Figure 10 shows marginated lymphocytes within a venule in mouse spleen. RBCs and platelets can be distinguished in the image during periods when the flow velocity is momentarily zero (Figure 10a), but appear blurred when flow resumes (Figure 10b). Marginated lymphocytes can either roll along the wall, at mean speeds of 11 to 20 μm/s, or remain stationary for periods up to >400 s.[41] A different type of interaction of lymphocytes with

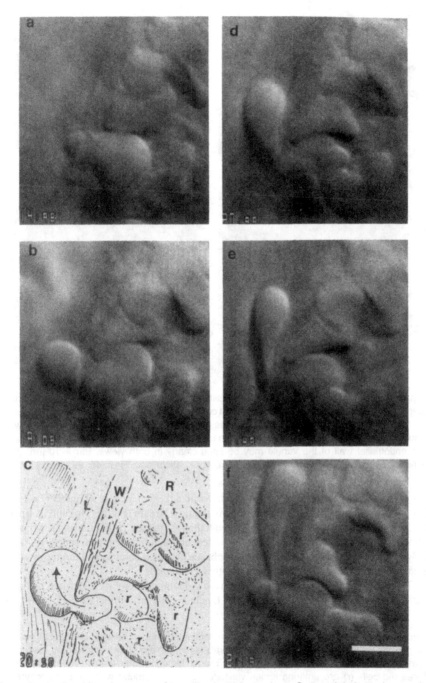

Figure 9 *In vivo* videomicroscopy of transilluminated rat spleen. Sequential photomicrographs of a red cell passing from the reticular meshwork into a venous sinus, via an interendothelial slit in the vessel wall. The venous sinus (diameter 17 μm) runs vertically at left of photos and is only partially shown. Numbers in bottom left corners give time in seconds and hundredths of a second. The schematic (Figure 9c) shows the locations of the sinus lumen (L), sinus wall (W), and numerous red cells (r) within the reticular meshwork of the red pulp (R). Bar = 5 μm. (From MacDonald, I. C., Ragan, D. M., Schmidt, E. E., and Groom, A. C., *Microvasc. Res.*, 33, 118, 1987.)

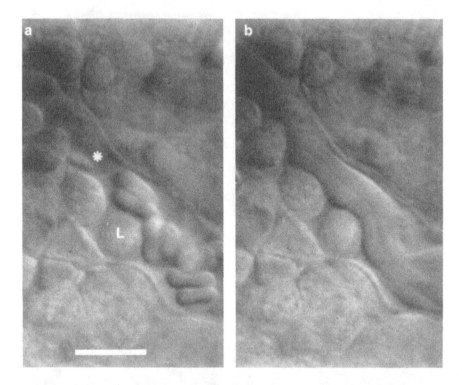

Figure 10 *In vivo* videomicroscopy of transilluminated mouse spleen, showing marginated lymphocytes within a venule. (a) Individual red cells and a platelet (*) can be distinguished when the flow is momentarily zero. Four lymphocytes (L) adhere to the vessel wall. (b) Blood flow has resumed, giving blurred images except for the marginated lymphocytes which are stationary. The endothelial wall of the venule may be seen clearly in both views. Bar = 10 μm. (From Schmidt, E. E., MacDonald, I. C., and Groom, A. C., *Microvasc. Res.*, 40, 99, 1990.)

vessel walls may also be seen in which focal adhesion occurs (Figure 11a–f), the lymphocyte adopting a hand mirror shape in the flow stream (Figure 11c) and its tip then proceeding to migrate slowly over the endothelial surface (Figure 11d–f). Migration occurs in random directions at speeds two orders of magnitude less than speeds of rolling. Polymorphonuclear leukocytes and macrophages may also be observed migrating slowly along vessel walls, and interacting with other blood cells.[41]

The possibilities for application of *in vivo* videomicroscopy in spleen are many and varied, especially when fluorescently labeled cells are injected and viewed by

Figure 11 *In vivo* videomicroscopy of transilluminated mouse spleen. Sequential views of lymphocyte within venule. Elapsed time intervals (seconds) are shown in lower left corners. (a) Lymphocyte (L) carried by the flow, squeezes through lumen towards bulging endothelial cell (*). Three red cells (r) are entering lumen via fenestrations in venular wall. (b) Lymphocyte has arrested in contact with endothelial cell. Blood flow continues through lumen (left to right), the moving cells giving blurred images: RBC velocity 294 μm/sec ± 87 (SD). (c) Lymphocyte has changed shape and remains attached to wall by narrow pseudopod. (d) Pseudopod has increased its width and developed a ragged-edged tip. (e) Point of attachment of psedopod to endothelial surface has shifted upstream ~2 μm. (f) Tip of pseudopod has migrated 5 μm over endothelial surface and now attaches to opposite side of vessel. One minute later lymphocyte became detached, carried away by flow (not shown). Bar = 10 μm. (From Schmidt, E. E., MacDonald, I. C., and Groom, A. C., *Microvasc. Res.*, 40, 99, 1990.)

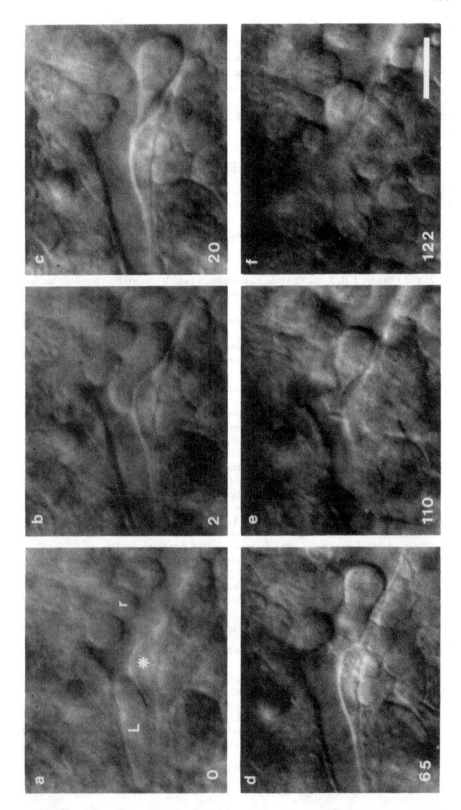

epifluorescent- and transillumination simultaneously. The detailed mechanisms for trapping abnormal or senescent RBCs, in the reticular meshwork or at IES, and the nature and time course of cellular destruction by macrophages can be observed and quantified. Whether platelets are concentrated within the reticular meshwork by a similar mechanism to that responsible for the high hematocrit[15] can now be addressed. Many immune related cell-cell interactions are amenable to study, as well as lymphocyte traffic. The exciting possibility exists of studying the time course and routes of migration of different lymphocyte subsets through the spleen.

ACKNOWLEDGMENTS

We thank Mrs. Barbara Anderson for typing this manuscript. Our own research reported here was supported by a grant to A.C.G. from the Medical Research Council of Canada.

REFERENCES

1. **Bellanti, J. A.,** *Immunology: Basic Processes,* W. B. Saunders, Philadelphia, 1979.
2. **Van Krieken, J. H. J. M., Te Velde, J., Hermans, J., and Welvaart, K.,** The splenic red pulp; a histomorphometrical study in splenectomy specimens embedded in methylmethacrylate, *Histopathology,* 9, 401, 1985.
3. **Snook, T.,** A comparative study of the vascular arrangements in mammalian spleens, *Am. J. Anat.,* 87, 31, 1950.
4. **Schmidt, E. E., MacDonald, I. C., and Groom, A. C.,** Microcirculatory pathways in normal human spleen, demonstrated by scanning electron microscopy of corrosion casts, *Am. J. Anat.,* 181, 253, 1988.
5. **Fujita, T.,** A scanning electron microscopy study of the human spleen, *Arch. Histol. Jpn.,* 37, 187, 1974.
6. **Pabst, R.,** The role of the spleen in lymphocyte migration, in *Migration and Homing of Lymphoid Cells,* Vol. 1, Husband, A. J., Ed., CRC Press, Boca Raton, FL, 1988, 63.
7. **Blue, J. and Weiss, L.,** Vascular pathways in nonsinusal red pulp: An electron microscope study of the cat spleen, *Am. J. Anat.,* 161, 135, 1981.
8. **Blue, J. and Weiss, L.,** Periarterial macrophage sheaths (ellipsoids) in cat spleen: An electron microscope study, *Am. J. Anat.,* 161, 115, 1981.
9. **Weiss, L.,** New trends in spleen research: Reticuloendothelial basis of the clearance of blood by the spleen, in *Disorders of the Spleen: Pathophysiology and Management,* Pochedly, C., Sills, R. H., and Schwartz, A. D., Eds., Marcel Dekker, New York, 1989, chap. 14.
10. **Koyama, S., Aoki, S., and Deguchi, K.,** Electron microscopic observations of the splenic red pulp with special reference to the pitting function, *Mie Med. J.,* 14, 143, 1964.
11. **Song, S. H. and Groom, A. C.,** Sequestration and possible maturation of reticulocytes in the normal spleen, *Can. J. Physiol. Pharmacol.,* 50, 400, 1972.
12. **Pictet, C. L., Orci, L., Forssmann, W. G., and Girardier, L.,** An electron microscopic study of the perfusion-fixed spleen. II. Nurse cells and erythrophagocytosis, *Z. Zellforsch. Mikrosk. Anat.,* 96, 400, 1969.
13. **Knisely, M. H.,** Spleen studies. I. Microscopic observations of the circulatory system of living, unstimulated mammalian spleens, *Anat. Rec.,* 65, 23, 1936.
14. **Levesque, M. J. and Groom, A. C.,** Washout kinetics of red cells and plasma from the spleen, *Am. J. Physiol.,* 231, 1665, 1976.
15. **MacDonald, I. C., Schmidt, E. E., and Groom, A. C.,** The high splenic hematocrit: A rheological consequence of red cell flow through the reticular meshwork, *Microvasc. Res.,* 42, 60, 1991.
16. **Watson, H. H. K. and Ludlam, C. A.,** Survival of 111-Indium platelet subpopulations of varying density in normal and postsplenectomized subjects, *Br. J. Haematol.,* 62, 117, 1986.
17. **Shulman, N. R. and Jordan, J. V., Jr.,** Platelet kinetics, in *Hemostasis and Thrombosis,* 2nd ed., Colman, R. W., Hirsch, J., Marder, V. J., and Salzman, E. W., Eds., Lippincott, Philadelphia, 1987, 431.

18. **Chandor, S. B.**, The pathology of the spleen, in *The Spleen: Structure, Function, and Clinical Significance*, Bowdler, A. J., Ed., Chapman and Hall, London, 1990, chap. 7.

19. **Suzuki, T.**, Application of scanning electron microscopy in the study of the human spleen: Three-dimensional fine structure of the normal red pulp and its changes as seen in splenomegalias associated with Banti's syndrome and cirrhosis of the liver, *Acta Haem. Jpn.*, 35, 506, 1972.

20. **Yamamoto, K.**, Morphological studies of the spleen in splenomegalic liver cirrhosis comparing with the spleen in idiopathic portal hypertension (so-called Banti's syndrome without liver cirrhosis), *Acta Path. Jpn.*, 28, 891, 1978.

21. **Groom, A. C. and Schmidt, E. E.**, Microcirculatory blood flow through the spleen, in *The Spleen: Structure, Function, and Clinical Significance*, Bowdler, A. J., Ed., Chapman and Hall, London, 1990, chap. 4.

22. **Anderson, D. R. and Kelton, J. G.**, Hemolysis, thrombocytopenia and the spleen, in *The Spleen: Structure, Function, and Clinical Significance*, Bowdler, A. J., Ed., Chapman and Hall, London, 1990, chap. 13.

23. **Serjeant, G. R.**, The spleen in sickle cell disease, in *The Spleen: Structure, Function, and Clinical Significance*, Bowdler, A. J., Ed., Chapman and Hall, London, 1990, chap. 16.

24. **Suzuki, T., Hataba, Y., and Sasaki, H.**, Fine architecture of the splenic terminal vascular bed as revealed by arterial and venous pressure-loading perfusion fixation, *J. Electron Microsc. Tech.*, 12, 132, 1989.

25. **Levesque, M. J. and Groom, A. C.**, Sequestration of heat-treated autologous red cells in the spleen, *J. Lab. Clin. Med.*, 90, 666, 1977.

26. **Bowdler, A. J. and Videbaek, A.**, Splenic pooling and the survival of blood cells, in *The Spleen: Structure, Function, and Clinical Significance*, Bowdler, A. J., Ed., Chapman and Hall, London, 1990, chap. 8.

27. **Tavassoli, M. and McMillan, R.**, Structure of the spleen in idiopathic thrombocytopenic purpura, *Am. J. Clin. Pathol.*, 64, 180, 1975.

28. **Schmidt, E. E., MacDonald, I. C., and Groom, A. C.**, Changes in splenic microcirculatory pathways in chronic idiopathic thrombocytopenic purpura, *Blood*, 78, 1485, 1991.

29. **Song, S. H. and Groom, A. C.**, Storage of blood cells in spleen of the cat, *Am. J. Physiol.*, 220, 779, 1971.

30. **Cilento, E. V., McCuskey, R. S., Reilly, F. D., and Meineke, H. A.**, Compartmental analysis of circulation of erythrocytes through the rat spleen, *Am. J. Physiol.*, 239 (*Heart Circ. Physiol.*, 8), H272, 1980.

31. **Song, S. H. and Groom, A. C.**, The distribution of red cells in the spleen, *Can. J. Physiol. Pharmacol.*, 49, 734, 1971.

32. **Groom, A. C., Levesque, M. J., and Bruckschweiger, D.**, Flow stasis, blood gases and glucose levels in the red pulp of the spleen, *Adv. Exp. Med. Biol.*, 94, 567, 1977.

33. **Groom, A. C., Levesque, M. J., Nealon, S., and Basrur, S.**, Does an unfavorable environment for red cells develop within the cat spleen when abnormal cells become trapped?, *J. Lab. Clin. Med.*, 105, 209, 1985.

34. **Groom, A. C., Schmidt, E. E., and MacDonald, I. C.**, Microcirculatory pathways and blood flow in spleen: New insights from washout kinetics, corrosion casts, and quantitative intravital microscopy, *Scanning Microsc.*, 5, 159, 1991.

35. **Nopanitaya, W., Aghajanian, J. G., and Gray, L. D.**, An improved plastic mixture for corrosion casting of the gastrointestinal microvascular system, in *Scanning Electron Microscopy, Part III*, Becker, R. P. and Johari, O., Eds., SEM Inc., Illinois, 1979, 751.

36. **Schmidt, E. E., MacDonald, I. C., and Groom, A. C.**, Circulatory pathways in the sinusal spleen of the dog, studied by scanning electron microscopy of microcorrosion casts, *J. Morphol.*, 178, 111, 1983.

37. **Schmidt, E. E., MacDonald, I. C., and Groom, A. C.**, The intermediate circulation in the nonsinusal spleen of the cat, studied by scanning electron microscopy of microcorrosion casts, *J. Morphol.*, 178, 125, 1983.

38. **Schmidt, E. E., MacDonald, I. C., and Groom, A. C.**, Microcirculation in rat spleen (sinusal), studied by means of corrosion casts, with particular reference to intermediate pathways, *J. Morphol.*, 186, 1, 1985.

39. **Schmidt, E. E., MacDonald, I. C., and Groom, A. C.,** Microcirculation in mouse spleen (nonsinusal) studied by means of corrosion casts, *J. Morphol.,* 186, 17, 1985.
40. **MacDonald, I. C., Ragan, D. M., Schmidt, E. E., and Groom, A. C.,** Kinetics of red blood cell passage through interendothelial slits into venous sinuses in rat spleen, analyzed by *in vivo* microscopy, *Microvasc. Res.,* 33, 118, 1987.
41. **Schmidt, E. E., MacDonald, I. C., and Groom, A. C.,** Interactions of leukocytes with vessel walls and with other blood cells, studied by high resolution intravital videomicroscopy of spleen, *Microvasc. Res.,* 40, 99, 1990.

Chapter 26

Thyroid Microcirculation

Linda J. Huffman and George A. Hedge

CONTENTS

I. ANATOMY AND FUNCTION

A. VASCULAR ANATOMY OF THE THYROID

Each thyroid lobe is supplied by arterial blood from two primary sources.[1,2] A superior thyroid artery, arising principally from the external carotid artery, supplies blood to the rostral area of the thyroid lobe. An inferior thyroid artery, deriving most often from the thyrocervical trunk, supplies blood to the caudal areas of the thyroid lobe. In addition to these bilateral arterial inputs to the thyroid, a thyroid ima artery may be located anterior to the trachea and, when present, provides blood to the inferior portion of the gland. This accessory artery appears to arise most often from the brachiocephalic artery, the right common carotid artery, or the aortic arch. Significant anastomoses among the arterial inputs to the thyroid gland occur, with the superior thyroid artery uniting with the contralateral artery in the isthmus area and with the inferior thyroid artery on the posterior and anterior surface of the thyroid gland. Anastomoses between thyroid arteries and the tracheal arterial supply (e.g., inferior laryngeal artery and tracheoesophageal artery) also exist.

The venous efflux from the thyroid drains into bilateral superior, middle, or inferior thyroid veins.[1,2] The superior thyroid veins lie in close proximity to the superior thyroid arteries and empty into the internal jugular vein. A middle thyroid vein may, or may not, be present, or may occur in parallel. These also empty into the internal jugular veins. The inferior thyroid veins often anastomose and form a venous plexus below the thyroid before emptying into the right or left brachiocephalic vein.

One of the most striking features of the vascular anatomy of the thyroid gland is the complex network of blood capillaries that encapsulate each follicle.[3-5] These basket-like capillary networks, deriving from interlobular and interfollicular arteries, are relatively independent from follicle to follicle and are sinusoidal in nature. An intriguing aspect of thyroid cell physiology is that not all epithelial cells and follicular units function at identical rates. Rather, an intercellular heterogeneity exists that encompasses such processes as growth, thyroglobulin synthesis, iodination, and endocytosis.[6] Since each follicle is enclosed in a relatively distinct capillary network, such an arrangement would permit a parallel heterogeneity in the local control of the thyroid vasculature to occur within this gland.[7]

B. MICROVASCULAR FUNCTIONS OF THE THYROID

It has been noted by a number of researchers that the thyroid gland, per unit weight, has among the highest rates of blood flow in the body.[8,9] Studies in humans have reported that this rate, under resting conditions, may range from 2.5 to 5.6 ml/min · g.[10] Furthermore, it has been estimated that the thyroid gland receives approximately 1.5% of the cardiac output in both sexes, whereas the weight of the thyroid comprises only 0.03% of the total body weight.[10] Such a high rate of blood flow to the thyroid may subserve a number of important functions of this endocrine organ.

1. Delivery Functions of Thyroid Blood Flow

As for any organ, the blood flow to the thyroid provides oxygen and energy sources necessary to support the ongoing activity of cells within the gland. However, it was noted as early as 1836 that this did not appear to be the sole function of the thyroidal vasculature.[11] It is now generally accepted that a primary function of blood flow to the thyroid is to provide sufficient quantities of iodine, a necessary substrate for thyroid hormone biosynthesis. The relationship between thyroid blood flow and iodide uptake was recognized in an elegant mathematical model by Riggs[12] and has empirical, correlative support.[13,14] Although a causal link between iodide uptake and thyroid blood flow has not been proved, it is tempting to speculate that blood flow to this gland may be one of the autoregulatory mechanisms operating within the thyroid to maintain adequate iodide uptake during dietary iodine deficiency.[15]

In addition to an important role in the thyroidal iodide presentation rate, thyroid blood flow would also serve to deliver thyrotropin (thyroid stimulating hormone) to this gland. As the name implies, thyrotropin is an important regulator of thyroid follicular cell function and virtually all of the activities of thyroid follicular cells can be affected by this pituitary hormone. The presentation rates of tropic hormones to other endocrine organs (e.g., the ovary and adrenal) have been postulated to be one mechanism whereby glandular function is modulated.[16-18] However, to date it is unresolved whether such a phenomenon occurs in the thyroid gland. Observations that the exogenous administration of vasoactive peptides, at doses known to affect thyroid blood flow, do not appear to alter thyrotropin-induced responses do not support this possibility.[19,20]

2. Exchange Functions of Thyroid Blood Flow

Thyroxine and triiodothyronine are hormones synthesized by follicular cells within the thyroid. By definition, hormones are substances secreted by an endocrine organ and transported in the bloodstream to specific target organs. Therefore, an important function of thyroid blood flow is to transport hormones produced by this gland from the site of synthesis to distant targets via the generalized circulation. In addition, the export of calcitonin, a hormone produced by parafollicular cells within the gland, is also dependent upon blood flow from the thyroid. An interesting issue, however, is whether hormone output from the thyroid is directly dependent upon thyroid blood flow. This does not seem to be the case. Rather, thyrotropin appears to be the primary determinant of thyroid hormone secretion.[21] Furthermore, the increases in thyroid blood flow that occur following increases in circulating thyrotropin may only reflect the increased metabolic demands of thyroidal follicular cells and may not be directly related to the increase in thyroid hormone secretion induced by thyrotropin.[9,22] The lack of concordance between thyroid hormone secretion and thyroid blood flow is perhaps not too surprising. The thyroid gland is unique in that it can store large amounts of thyroxine and triiodothyronine. Furthermore, the half-lifes and actions of thyroid hormones in the body are relatively long in duration. The minute-to-minute regulation of the hormonal output of the thyroid that potentially could be affected by alterations in blood flow would therefore be less important for this glandular organ.

II. PATHOLOGY

Under normal conditions, thyroid blood flow appears to be relatively labile. A two- to threefold range of values can be observed among resting individuals or even in experimental animals.[9,10,21,23] This variability may be the result of influences from baroreceptor reflexes, neural stimuli, or seasonality.[9,21,24] However, independent of these fluctuations in basal blood flow, certain pathological states do appear to alter thyroid blood flow in a consistent manner across experimental species and man.

A. CONDITIONS KNOWN OR THOUGHT TO AFFECT THE THYROID MICROCIRCULATION

Patients with Graves' disease (toxic diffuse goiter) or overactive thyroids may exhibit marked increases in thyroid blood flow when compared to thyroid blood flow in individuals without any overt thyroid dysfunction.[25-29] The pronounced thyroidal vascularity in Graves' disease can often be discerned by an audible bruit upon auscultation of the thyroid gland area and may present a surgical problem.[30]

Treatment with Lugol's iodine has been recommended as a palliative measure to decrease thyroid blood flow in patients with Graves' disease and the rationale for such treatment has received empirical support.[31-34] However, this does not appear to be a unique thyroidal response in Graves' disease since normal individuals or experimental animals with increased iodine intake also show reductions in thyroid blood flow during this treatment regimen.[35-37] The prolonged administration of thyroid hormones can also decrease thyroid blood flow in experimental animals.[38]

Intake of a diet low in iodine for 2 weeks by normal humans, as well as rats, is associated with increases in thyroid blood flow.[35,37] The increase in thyroid blood flow seen in this condition is not associated with an alteration in plasma thyrotropin levels and, thus, appears primarily to involve an autonomous intrathyroidal adjustment to iodine deficiency. However, a change in the sensitivity of the thyroid gland to thyrotropin stimulation cannot be excluded and this possibility has received experimental support.[39]

Drugs or ingested substances associated with increases in thyrotropin levels may also increase thyroid blood flow. The thioureas are especially effective in this regard. However, it has been documented that thyrotropin per se may or may not acutely increase thyroid blood flow in man or experimental animals.[9,22] Any thyrotropin-induced increases in thyroid blood flow are primarily observed when the intracellular stores of iodine or of thyroid hormones are compromised.[38,40] A parallel phenomenon may occur in man. Graves' disease patients may be rendered euthyroid with antithyroid drug treatment. However, overtreatment with antithyroid drugs may result in elevated thyrotropin levels and the maintenance of increased thyroidal vascularity in such individuals.[33]

Another situation in which thyroid blood flow may be altered is following surgical removal of a portion of the gland. Subtotal thyroidectomy in rats results in compensatory alterations that include increases in blood flow per mass of the remaining thyroid remnant.[41] This phenomenon would be of adaptive significance in maintaining and supporting thyroid hormone synthesis in the face of a reduction in total functional organ mass.

B. CLINICAL APPLICATIONS OF THYROID MICROCIRCULATORY STUDIES

Evaluation of the thyroid microcirculation or of blood flow in thyroid arteries has a number of potentially valuable clinical applications. Assessment of thyroidal vascularity may assist in the diagnosis of solitary thyroid nodules, especially in cases of nonpalpable metastases.[42-45] Such evaluations may be most useful in the preoperative assessment of the extent of thyroid carcinoma as well as post-operative evaluation of the success of thyroid resection of carcinoid masses.[43] The differential diagnosis of an agenetic thyroid lobe vs. that of a suppressed thyroid lobe due to an autonomous functioning thyroid nodule has been made using angiographic techniques.[46] In addition, some distinction between thyroid and parathyroid lesions appears possible using thyroid blood flow-imaging procedures.[47]

The assessment of thyroid blood flow can also be used to detect overactive thyroid glands, e.g., in patients with Graves' disease or the occurrence of thyroid storm.[26-29,48,49] Furthermore, such monitoring may be useful in indexing the response of Graves' disease patients to radioactive iodine therapy or preoperative iodine treatment.[32-34,50]

Endemic goiter, as a result of iodine deficiency, is not as common now because of iodide supplementation of salt and bread. However, there are still areas of the world where iodine intake is low or marginal. Pregnant women appear to be especially suscep-tible to goitrogenesis, as indexed by an increase in thyroid volume and biochemical analyses, when iodine intake is restricted.[51,52] Furthermore, iodoprophylaxis can prevent such goitrogenic alterations during pregnancy.[51] As previously discussed, thyroid blood flow is inversely correlated with iodine intake and appears to be a sensitive index of iodine status. The use of currently available noninvasive procedures to assess both thyroid volume and blood flow may, therefore, be very useful in monitoring maternal thyroid function during pregnancy.

III. MODELS AND TECHNIQUES

A number of experimental and clinical approaches to the measurement of thyroid blood flow have been reported in the literature. In general, all of the animal models that have been used to study the thyroid circulation respond similarly to specific stimuli and, when evaluated, parallel alterations in thyroid blood flow are seen in humans. Therefore, important information concerning the thyroid microcirculation can be derived from studies using experimental animal models that should have direct clinical relevance. However, in this section, we will limit our focus to approaches that have been used to evaluate thyroid vascularity in humans. It should be noted that, although vital microscopic techniques have been used successfully in other vascular beds, these direct techniques have not been applied clinically or in experimental animals in studies of the thyroid microcirculation.

Electromagnetic blood flowmetry is a technique that has been used to index thyroid artery blood flow in humans.[22,25] In this case, the transducer of an electromagnetic blood flowmeter is positioned around the thyroid artery during surgical intervention; thus, this procedure requires vessel dissection and manipulation. A magnetic field is produced across the artery and the motion of blood through this field generates an induced voltage that is proportional to velocity.[53] Using this approach, absolute blood flow measurements in milliliters per minute are possible. However, the calibration procedure requires brief occlusions of the artery that may, by itself, affect vascular reactivity. In addition, the effects of general anesthesia on the thyroid vasculature must be considered. Although such monitoring of thyroid artery blood flow does not specifically index microcirculatory changes within the gland, valuable information concerning overall blood flow to the thyroid has been obtained using this approach.[22,25]

Angiography of the thyroid gland has also been used clinically to evaluate the thyroid vasculature. This procedure is somewhat invasive in that injection catheters must be inserted. Therefore, light sedation and local anesthesia at the site of arterial catheter insertion are usually required. A femoral or axillary approach is usually undertaken and the contrast medium injected most often into the subclavian artery, brachiocephalic trunk, or selectively into a thyroid artery.[42,43,54] For evaluation, a series of stereoscopic films are rapidly obtained following the start of the contrast media injection. A background exposure is usually obtained just before injection of the contrast medium and used in an electronic subtraction imaging technique.[55] Complications of a cerebral or spinal nature or hematomas at the site of catheter insertion have been noted in 5% of patients undergoing this procedure.[43] In addition, the thyroid is exposed to a radiation dose from the contrast media.

Radionuclide thyroid angiography, using intravenously injected technetium-99m, has also been performed clinically.[31,34,46,48,49] Although technetium-99m, like iodide, is taken up and trapped within the thyroid gland, the amount of this material appearing immediately following injection appears primarily to be related to the blood flow within the thyroid.[56] It has been suggested that scintigrams which are obtained during the first 30 s after visualization of the carotid artery can be used clinically to evaluate thyroid vascularity.[49] The rapidity with which results can be obtained suggest that this approach may be of use in some clinical settings, i.e., the evaluation of thyroid storm.[48] Although absolute quantification of blood flow is not possible using this technique, qualitative evaluation of the thyroid scintigrams is possible, e.g., expressed as percent of dose above neck level.[31,49] It is also possible to calculate a "thyroid vascularity index" that is independent of cardiac output. This "index" is calculated by comparing the areas under normalized thyroid and carotid artery curves up to the time of the peak for the arterial curve, which reflects the first passage of the radioactive bolus.[34]

The use of technetium-99m in thyroid angiography is one example of the assessment of thyroid vascularity by the fractional distribution of an indicator. Radiolabeled iodine clearance has also been used in attempts to measure thyroid blood flow in experimental animals and humans.[13,57] While the use of iodine clearance techniques to index thyroid blood flow is theoretically possible,[12] iodide is also trapped within the thyroid gland and this process, as well as thyroid blood flow, contributes to the overall thyroidal uptake of this substance. In most circumstances, it is not possible to separate out these phenomena. Therefore, tests involving iodide uptake are useful in the assessment of overall thyroid activity, but not specifically that of thyroid blood flow.

Thallium-201 is another indicator that has been used to assess thyroid vascularity in humans.[32] Unlike iodine and technetium-99m, the thyroidal concentration of thallium-201 is not affected by perchlorate.[58-60] However, the presence of this substance in the thyroid, at least after the initial few seconds, probably reflects processes in addition to blood flow, e.g., activation of ATP-ase dependent sodium-potassium pumps.[58-60] Timing is therefore the most important consideration regarding the assessment of thyroid blood flow using fractional indicators. Evaluation of the distribution of these indicators within the first few seconds after entry into an organ appears to provide a reasonable index of blood flow.[61] However, attempts to evaluate vascularity using indicators after recirculation or after the activation of tissue-specific uptake mechanisms are fraught with error.

Doppler flowmeters and imaging systems use ultrasound methods to assess vascular function. Since the use of ultrasound methods is truly noninvasive, this approach holds great clinical promise. Recently, Doppler-based ultrasound procedures have been used in a number of studies to evaluate thyroid blood flow in humans.[26-29,33,36,37,44,47,50,62] The theoretical basis for this approach has been well described.[63] Briefly, when ultrasound is reflected by moving red blood cells, there is a velocity-dependent Doppler shift in frequency that can be measured by commercially available instruments. Ultrasound duplex scanning, which is a combination of two-dimensional imaging of internal structures and a pulsed Doppler flowmeter, has been used to obtain blood flow information from thyroid arteries.[26,27,29,33,50] The flow direction in the superior thyroid artery is opposite to that of the external carotid, and this artery can be easily located using ultrasound duplex scanning. Using this technique, the diameter of the superior thyroid artery as well as the time-averaged velocity in centimeters per second and actual blood volume flow in milliliters per minute can be assessed.[33] The values obtained with this approach seem fairly reproducible and intraartery coefficients of variation of approximately 7% for diameter, 9% for time-averaged velocity, and 18% for volume flow have been reported in euthyroid patients.[27,33] It should be noted that, although absolute values can obtained, the fact that changes in thyroid artery flow for a given patient can be monitored and alterations from normal values can be detected may be of most relevance for clinical and diagnostic applications.[64] Although cardiac output cannot be indexed, flow in the carotid artery can easily be obtained using Doppler blood flowmetry. Patients with diffuse toxic goiter have increased flow velocity in both the superior thyroid artery and common carotid artery, presumably due to the systemic consequences of the hyperthyroid state.[29] Therefore, concomitant analysis of flow velocity in the superior thyroid artery and common carotid artery may aid in the diagnosis of hyperthyroidism vs. other non-thyroidal causes for increases in common carotid arterial blood flow.[29]

Color flow Doppler ultrasonography is a tool that has been introduced recently and used in vascular diagnoses.[65] This approach has also been used to assess the vascularity of the thyroid gland itself.[28,29,36,44,47,62] Although intrathyroidal blood vessels are too small to be visualized, blood motion within areas of the thyroid can be indexed.[44] Qualitative evaluations of thyroid vascularity obtained using this procedure appear to be reproducible[44] and a semiquantitative index can be obtained using visual color grading.[36] Increases in intrathyroidal blood flow in focal areas associated with nodules, masses, and follicular adenoma have been detected using this approach.[28,29,47,62] A color flow Doppler pattern characteristic of patients with Graves' disease has been called a "thyroid inferno" and consists of a pulsatile pattern of multiple small areas of flow throughout the gland.[28] In addition to providing information regarding intrathyroidal vascularity and morphology, the color-coded duplex ultrasonographic approach can also be used to index flow in thyroid and carotid arteries.[29,37] As with most procedures, some assumptions and potential sources of variability are inherent in the use of Doppler ultrasound approaches in the evaluation of the thyroidal circulation.[37,63] In studies evaluating treatment effects on thyroid blood flow, the potential for subjective bias has been noted.[28] Therefore, video-tape analysis of the Doppler signal by clinicians or researchers naive to the patient's condition or diagnosis have often been employed in studies evaluating treatment effects on thyroid blood flow.[33,36,37,50]

Magnetic resonance phase velocity mapping is a recent advancement that may have application in the clinical assessment of regional vascular perfusion.[66] This approach is noninvasive and may permit more precise quantitation of blood flow than that which can be obtained using Doppler ultrasound techniques.[66] One recent report suggests that this approach may be of use in the evaluation of thyroid vascular function.[67]

In summary, the development of truly noninvasive procedures, i.e., Doppler ultrasound, to monitor regional blood flows has greatly assisted investigations of the human thyroid vasculature. The fact that this information can be obtained in minutes and stored on videotape for subsequent evaluation is also advantageous.[44] The ability to combine such clinically relevant information with that obtained from more rigorous, quantitative experimental studies suggests that our knowledge and appreciation of the role of the thyroid microcirculation in health and disease will expand significantly in the very near future.

REFERENCES

1. **Sloan, L. W.**, Surgical anatomy of the thyroid, in *The Thyroid*, 3rd ed., Werner, S. C. and Ingbar, S. H., Eds., Harper & Row, New York, 1971, 323.
2. **Tzinas, S., Droulias, C., Harlaftis, N., Akin, J. T. Jr., Gray, S. W., and Skandalakis, J. E.**, Vascular patterns of the thyroid gland, *Am. Surg.*, 42, 639, 1976.

3. **Hansen, J. and Skaaring, P.,** Scanning electron microscopy of normal rat thyroid, *Anatomischer Anzeiger,* 134, 177, 1973.

4. **Fujita, H. and Murakami, T.,** Scanning electron microscopy on the distribution of the minute blood vessels in the thyroid gland of the dog, rat, and rhesus monkey, *Archivum Histologicum Japonicum,* 36, 181, 1974.

5. **Fujita, H.,** Fine structure of the thyroid gland, *Int. Rev. Cytol.,* 40, 197, 1975.

6. **Studer, H., Peter, H. J., and Gerber, H.,** Natural heterogeneity of thyroid cells: The basis for understanding thyroid function and nodular goiter growth, *Endocr. Rev.,* 10, 125, 1989.

7. **Fujita, H.,** Functional morphology of the thyroid, *Int. Rev. Cytol.,* 113, 145, 1988.

8. **Söderberg, U.,** Temporal characteristics of thyroid activity, *Physiolog. Rev.,* 39, 777, 1959.

9. **Kapitola, J.,** Contemporary notions on the blood flow through the thyroid gland, *Endocrinologia Experimentalis,* 7, 147, 1973.

10. **Williams, L. R. and Leggett, R. W.,** Reference values for resting blood flow to organs of man, *Clin. Phys. Physiolog. Measurement,* 10, 187, 1989.

11. **King, T. W.,** Observations on the thyroid gland, *Guy's Hospital Rep.,* 1, 429, 1836.

12. **Riggs, D. S.,** Quantitative aspects of iodine metabolism in man, *Pharmacolog. Rev.,* 4, 284, 1952.

13. **Pochin, E. E.,** Investigation of thyroid function and disease with radioactive iodine, *Lancet,* 2, 41, 1950.

14. **Söderberg, U.,** The regulation between activity and blood flow in the thyroid gland, *Experientia,* 14, 229, 1958.

15. **Michalkiewicz, M., Connors, J. M., Huffman, L. J., Pietrzyk, Z., and Hedge, G. A.,** Is thyroid blood flow a limiting factor for thyroid iodine supply?, in *The Thyroid Gland, Environment, and Autoimmunity,* Drexhage, H. A., de Vijlder, J. J. M., and Wiersinga, W. M., Eds., Excerpta Medica, Amsterdam, 1990, 129.

16. **Porter, J. C. and Klaiber, M. S.,** Corticosterone secretion in rats as a function of ACTH input and adrenal blood flow, *Am. J. Physiol.,* 209, 811, 1965.

17. **Urquhart, J. and Li, C. C.,** Dynamic testing and modeling of adrenocortical secretory function, *Ann. N.Y. Acad. Sci.,* 156, 756, 1969.

18. **Niswender, G. D., Reimers, T. J., Diekman, M. A., and Nett, T. M.,** Blood flow: A mediator of ovarian function, *Biol. Reprod.,* 14, 64, 1976.

19. **Huffman, L. J., Connors, J. M., White, B. H., and Hedge, G. A.,** Vasoactive intestinal peptide treatment that increases thyroid blood flow fails to alter plasma T_3 or T_4 levels in the rat, *Neuroendocrinology,* 47, 567, 1988.

20. **Pietrzyk, Z., Michalkiewicz, M., Huffman, L. J., and Hedge, G. A.,** Vasoactive intestinal peptide enhances thyroidal iodide uptake during dietary iodine deficiency, *Endocr. Res.,* 18, 213, 1992.

21. **Söderberg, U.,** Short-term reactions in the thyroid gland, *Acta Physiolog. Scand.,* 42(Suppl. 147), 1, 1958.

22. **Tegler, L., Gillquist, J., Anderberg, B., Jacobson, G., Lundström, B., and Roos, P.,** Human thyroid blood flow response to endogenous, exogenous human, and bovine thyrotrophin measured by electromagnetic flowmetry, *Acta Endocrinologica,* 98, 540, 1981.

23. **Bouder, T. G., Huffman, L. J., and Hedge, G. A.,** Effects of vasoactive intestinal peptide on vascular conductance are unaffected by anesthesia, *Am. J. Physiol.,* 255, R968, 1988.

24. **Rein, H., Liebermeister K., and Schneider, D.,** Schilddrüse und carotissinus als funktionelle einheit, *Klin. Wochenschr.,* 2, 1636, 1932.

25. **Tegler, L., Gillquist, J., Anderberg, B., Lundström, B., and Johansson, H.,** Thyroid blood flow rate in man. Electromagnetic flowmetry during operation in euthyroid normal gland, nontoxic goiter, and hyperthyroidism, *J. Endocrinolog. Invest.,* 4, 335, 1981.

26. **Woodcock, J. P., Owen, G. M., Shedden, E. J., Hodgson, K. J., MacGregor, A., and Srivastava, A.,** Duplex scanning of the thyroid, *Ultrasound in Medicine and Biology,* 11, 659, 1985.

27. **Hodgson, K. J., Lazarus, J. H., Wheeler, M. H., Woodcock, J. P., Owen, G. M., McGregor, A. M., and Hall, R.,** Duplex scan-derived thyroid blood flow in euthyroid and hyperthyroid patients, *World J. Surg.,* 12, 470, 1988.

28. **Ralls, P. W., Mayekawa, D. S., Lee, K. P., Colletti, P. M., Radin, D. R., Boswell, W. D., and Halls, J. M.,** Color-flow Doppler sonography in Graves' disease: "thyroid inferno", *Am. J. Roentgenol.,* 150, 781, 1988.

29. **Wu, C.-C. and Torng, J.-K.,** The peak systolic velocity of the common carotid artery and superior thyroid artery as an indicator of thyroid function, *Kaohsiung J. Med. Sci.,* 7, 492, 1991.

30. **Kaplan, E. L.,** Thyroid and parathyroid, in *Principles of Surgery*, 4th ed., Schwartz, S. I., Shires, G. T., Spencer, F. C., and Storer, E. H., Eds., McGraw Hill, New York, 1984, chap. 38.

31. **Brownlie, B. E. W., Turner, J. G., Ellwood, M. A., Rogers, T. G. H., and Armstrong, D. I.,** Thyroid vascularity — documentation of the iodide effect in thyrotoxicosis, *Acta Endocrinologica*, 86, 317, 1977.

32. **Marigold, J. H., Morgan, A. K., Earle, D. J., Young, A. E., and Croft, D. N.,** Lugol's iodine: Its effect on thyroid blood flow in patients with thyrotoxicosis, *Br. J. Surg.*, 72, 45, 1985.

33. **Chang, D. C. S., Wheeler, M. H., Woodcock, J. P., Curley, I., Lazarus, J. R., Fung, H., John, R., Hall, R., and McGregor, A. M.,** The effect of preoperative Lugol's iodine on thyroid blood flow in patients with Graves' hyperthyroidism, *Surgery*, 102, 1055, 1987.

34. **Rangaswamy, M., Padhy, A. K., Gopinath, P. G., Shukla, N. K., Gupta, K., and Kapoor, M. M.,** Effect of Lugol's iodine on the vascularity of thyroid gland in hyperthyroidism, *Nucl. Med. Commun.*, 10, 679, 1989.

35. **Michalkiewicz, M., Huffman, L. J., Connors, J. M., and Hedge, G. A.,** Alterations in thyroid blood flow induced by varying levels of iodine intake in the rat, *Endocrinology*, 125, 54, 1989.

36. **Weissel, M., Hübsch, P., Kurtaran, A., Kainz, H., Frühwald, F.,** *In vivo* evidence for iodine-induced decrease of thyroid blood flow by color-coded Doppler sonography in normal human thyroid glands, *Acta Medica Austriaca*, 17(Suppl. 1), 64, 1990.

37. **Arntzenius, A. B., Smit, L. J., Schipper, J., van der Heide, D., and Meinders, A. E.,** Inverse relation between iodine intake and thyroid blood flow: Color Doppler flow imaging in euthyroid humans, *J. Clin. Endocrinol. Metab.*, 73, 1051, 1991.

38. **Connors, J. M., Huffman, L. J., and Hedge, G. A.,** Effects of thyrotropin on the vascular conductance of the thyroid gland, *Endocrinology*, 122, 921, 1988.

39. **Bray, G. A.,** Increased sensitivity of the thyroid in iodine-depleted rats to the goitrogenic effects of thyrotropin, *J. Clin. Invest.*, 47, 1640, 1968.

40. **Connors, J. M., Huffman, L. J., Michalkiewicz, M., Chang, B. S. H., Dey, R. D., and Hedge, G. A.,** Thyroid vascular conductance: Differential effects of elevated plasma thyrotropin (TSH) induced by treatment with thioamides or TSH-releasing hormone, *Endocrinology*, 129, 117, 1991.

41. **Michalkiewicz, M., Connors, J. M., Huffman, L. J., and Hedge, G. A.,** Increases in thyroid gland blood flow after hemithyroidectomy in the rat, *Endocrinology*, 124, 1118, 1989.

42. **Mojab, K. and Ghosh, B. C.,** Thyroid angiography, *Am. J. Surg.*, 132, 620, 1976.

43. **Zachrisson, B. F.,** Thyroid angiography, *Acta Radiologica*, Suppl. 350, 1, 1976.

44. **Fobbe, F., Finke, R., Reichenstein, E., Schleusener, H., and Wolf, K.-J.,** Appearance of thyroid diseases using colour-coded duplex sonography, *Eur. J. Radiol.*, 9, 29, 1989.

45. **Prakash, R., Jayaram, G., and Singh, R. P.,** Follicular thyroid carcinoma masquerading as subacute thyroiditis. Diagnosis using ultrasonography and radionuclide thyroid angiography, *Austr. Radiol.*, 35, 174, 1991.

46. **Prakash, R., Narayanan, R. V., and Chakravarty, J. K.,** Differentiation between suppressed thyroid tissue and thyroid hemiagenesis with Tc-99m pertechnetate radionuclide angiography, *Clin. Nucl. Med.*, 15, 605, 1990.

47. **Gooding, G. A. W. and Clark, O. H.,** Use of color Doppler imaging in the distinction between thyroid and parathyroid lesions, *Am. J. Surg.*, 164, 51, 1992.

48. **Goldfarb, C. R., Varma, C., and Roginsky, M. S.,** Diagnosis in delirium: Prompt confirmation of thyroid storm, *Clin. Nucl. Med.*, 5, 66, 1980.

49. **Lee, V. W., Welji, A. N., Shapiro, J. H., and Angtuaco, E.,** Radionuclide angiography for assessment of hyperthyroidism, *Radiology*, 142, 237, 1982.

50. **Chang, D. C. S., Woodcock, J. P., Shedden, E. J., Lazarus, J. H., Wheeler, M. H., and McGregor, A. M.,** Normalization of thyroid blood flow in Graves' hyperthyroidism following radioactive iodine therapy, *Clin. Endocrinol.*, 32, 599, 1990.

51. **Romano, R., Jannini, E. A., Pepe, M., Grimaldi, A., Oliveri, M., Spennati, P., Cappa, F., and D'Armiento, M.,** The effects of iodoprophylaxis on thyroid size during pregnancy, *Am. J. Obstet. Gynecol.*, 164, 482, 1991.

52. **Glinoer, D. and Lemone, M.,** Goiter and pregnancy: A new insight into an old problem, *Thyroid*, 2, 65, 1992.

53. **AbuRahma, A. F.,** Noninvasive techniques in peripheral arterial diseases, in *Current Noninvasive Vascular Diagnosis*, AbuRahma, A. F. and Diethrich, E. B., Eds., PSG Publishing, Littleton, Massachusetts, 1988, chap. 12.

54. **Wickbom, I., Zachrisson, B. F., and Heimann, P.,** Thyroid angiography, *Acta Radiologica*, 6, 497, 1967.

55. **Brennecke, R., Hahne, H.-J., Bürsch, J. H., and Heintzen, P. H.,** Digital videodensitometry: Some approaches to radiographic image restoration and analysis, in *Radiological Functional Analysis of the Vascular System*, Heuck, F. H. W., Ed., Springer-Verlag, Berlin, 1983, 79.

56. **Armstrong, D. I., Rodgers, T. G. H., Brownlie, B. E. W., and Turner, J. G.,** Thyroid vascularity and trapping function: Analysis of very early thryoidal technetium "uptake", *Int. J. Nucl. Med. Biol.*, 3, 65, 1976.

57. **Monkus, E. F. and Reineke, E. P.,** Thyroid circulation in the rabbit including arteriovenous difference, *Am. J. Physiol.*, 192, 268, 1958.

58. **Oster, Z. H., Strauss, H. W., Harrison, K., Burns, H. D., and Pitt, B.,** Thallium-201 distribution in the thyroid: Relationship to thyroidal trapping function, *Radiology*, 126, 733, 1978.

59. **Maayan, M. L., Volpert, E. M., Fine, E. J., Eisenberg, J., Lopez, E. M., and Dawry, F. P.,** Thyroid uptake of [201]Thallium and its control by TSH, *Acta Endocrinologica*, 97, 461, 1981.

60. **Civelek, A. C., Durski, K., Shafique, I., Matsumura, K., Sostre, S., Wagner, H. N., Jr., and Ladenson, P. W.,** Failure of perchlorate to inhibit Tc-99m isonitrile binding by the thyroid during myocardial perfusion studies, *Clin. Nucl. Med.*, 16, 358, 1991.

61. **Sapirstein, L. A.,** Regional blood flow by fractional distribution of indicators, *Am. J. Physiol.*, 193, 161, 1958.

62. **Barreda, R., Kaude, J. V., Fagien, M., and Drane, W. E.,** Hypervascularity of nontoxic goiter as shown by color-coded Doppler sonography, *Am. J. Roetgenol.*, 156, 199, 1991.

63. **Gill, R. W.,** Measurement of blood flow by ultrasound: Accuracy and sources of error, *Ultrasound Med. Biol.*, 11, 625, 1985.

64. **Kaplan, E. L.,** Invited commentary, *World J. Surg.*, 12, 475, 1988.

65. **Cape, E. G., Sung, H.-W., and Yoganathan, A. P.,** Basics of color Doppler imaging, in *Vascular Imaging by Color Doppler and Magnetic Resonance*, Lanzer, P. and Yoganathan, A. P., Eds., Springer-Verlag, Berlin, 1991, chap. 3.

66. **Maier, S. E. and Boesiger, P.,** Quantitative *in vivo* blood flow measurements with magnetic resonance imaging, in *Vascular Imaging by Color Doppler and Magnetic Resonance*, Lanzer, P. and Yoganathan, A. P., Eds., Springer-Verlag, Berlin, 1991, chap. 13.

67. **Feinberg, D. A. and Jakab, P. D.,** Tissue perfusion in humans studied by Fourier velocity distribution, line scan, and echo-planar imaging, *Magnetic Resonance Med.*, 16, 280, 1990.

Chapter 27

Urinary Bladder Microcirculation

Dale A. Schuschke and James I. Harty

CONTENTS

I. ANATOMY AND FUNCTION

A. VASCULAR ANATOMY OF THE URINARY BLADDER

There are several arteries that supply blood to various regions of the human urinary bladder. Usually, two or three superior vesical arteries originate from the patent part of the umbilical artery as it runs anterolateral to the apex and the upper part of the body of the bladder. The inferior part of the bladder, including the vesical neck, is supplied by the inferior vesical artery. The inferior vesical artery arises from the internal iliac artery and runs through the connective tissue close to the floor of the pelvis before distributing to the bladder. In the male, the base of the bladder is supplied by the artery of the ductus deferens. In the female, the base is supplied by the inferior vesical and vaginal arteries.

There are no veins accompanying the umbilical arteries. The veins of the bladder converge toward the neck of this organ. Close to the neck, the veins form the vesical plexus. The venous drainage from this plexus is lateral and posterior along the inferior arteries into the internal iliac veins. There is usually also some venous drainage anterolaterally into the lower ends of the external iliac veins.

The lymphatic drainage from the superior and inferolateral surfaces of the bladder pass to the external iliac nodes. The lymph vessels from the base drain into the external and internal iliac nodes. The vessels from the neck pass to the sacral and common iliac nodes.

The wall of the urinary bladder is composed of three distinct layers: the mucosa, submucosa, and muscularis. Most of the microvasculature is located in the subendothelial region of the mucosa, with a few vessels interspersed throughout the three layers of the muscularis. When the bladder is empty, few vessels are visible under microscopy and they have tortuous outlines. As the organ distends, large numbers of small vessels come into view and their outlines become straightened.

The superficial cells of the transitional epithelium are responsible for the osmotic barrier between urine and tissue fluids. This blood-urine barrier assures that the interchange of fluid and solutes into and out of the bladder microcirculation is between the blood and interstitial fluid compartments and does not include exchange with solutes in the urine.

0-8493-4870-6/95/$0.00+$.50

B. MICROVASCULAR FUNCTIONS OF THE URINARY BLADDER

Experimental studies of bladder microcirculation include the three general topics of blood flow, vasoreactivity, and macromolecular permeability. Several investigators have reported measuring blood flow in the urinary bladder during different states of distension. This is of particular interest since the urinary bladder is repeatedly distended and relaxed during the voiding cycle, thus exposing the bladder microvessels to large changes in bladder wall tension. Dunn[1] reported that the blood flow through the rabbit bladder is reduced to half that of a resting bladder when the bladder is distended to 20 mmHg. It is further reduced to a quarter of resting flow at a bladder pressure of 40 mmHg and reduced to 5% of normal when the bladder pressure is raised to 80 mmHg. Mehrota[2] observed in the rat urinary bladder, that there was little or no change in blood flow during intravesicular pressures less than 40 cm H_2O, but that pressures above 40 cm H_2O decreased blood flow until cessation occurred at 150 cm H_2O. Blood flow studies in the bladders of cats[3] and dogs[4] have also demonstrated reduced flow during bladder distension.

In addition to changes in intravesicular filling pressure, there are interstitial pressure fluctuations associated with peristaltic waves of contraction that also affect bladder blood flow. Like the heart during systole, during strong contractions of the bladder, the circulation comes to a standstill in most of the vessels but is rapidly resumed when the wave of contraction is over.

The rat urinary bladder microcirculation responds to topical norepinephrine by vasoconstricting[5,6] in a manner similar to that seen in other microvascular beds (rat cremaster,[7] hamster cheek pouch,[8] and rat mesentery[9]). The bladder microcirculation also responds to sodium nitroprusside with the same vasodilator response[5] seen in rat cremaster arterioles.[10] However, the threshold to both norepinephrine and nitroprusside is higher in the bladder microvessels when compared with similar-sized vessels in the rat cremaster.[7,10]

The vasomotor actions of histamine, acetylcholine, and serotonin have also been characterized in the rat bladder microcirculation. Serotonin causes constriction of the arterioles,[6] though it is less potent than norepinephrine. Histamine and acetylcholine cause the microvessels to dilate.[6]

In most cases, topical administration of prostaglandins results in dose-related arteriolar dilation; PGE_1, and PGE_2 are the most potent dilators. An exception is $PGF_{2\alpha}$ which is a potent constrictor.[6] Indomethacin significantly reduces vasodilation induced by bladder filling[3] and PGE_1 has an inhibitory effect on the action of norepinephrine and $PGF_{2\alpha}$.[6] These results imply that prostaglandins play a role in local blood flow regulation, perhaps to support the changing metabolic needs of the urinary bladder wall.

The normal microvascular endothelium in the urinary bladder seems relatively impermeable to macromolecules. In the rat, there is no spontaneous extravasation of either the plasma protein dye Evan's blue[11,12] or serum albumin (MW 69,000).[5] Capsaicin, substance P, histamine, and compound 48/80 have all been shown to induce leakage of either Evan's blue or albumin from the intact bladder microcirculation.[2,5,11,12] Histamine and 48/80-induced macromolecular leakage have been localized to the postcapillary venules.[5]

II. PATHOLOGY

A. DISEASES THAT AFFECT THE MICROCIRCULATION OF THE BLADDER

1. Cystitis

    a. **Bacterial, fungal, or viral cystitis** results in an acute inflammatory response that is usually limited to the mucosal and submucosal layers of the bladder. Microscopically, there is edema and polymorphonuclear leukocyte infiltration of these layers.

Cystoscopically, the bladder mucosa is reddened secondary to dilatation and destruction of the microvasculature. The amount of bleeding varies between slight discoloration to gross hematuria.

b. **Radiation-induced cystitis** may occur early or late in patients who have received radiation therapy to pelvic viscera.[13] Microscopically, there is mucosal edema, vascular telangiectasia, and submucosal hemorrhages. The most damaging effect in the long term is the development of an obstructive endarteritis, which results in chronic ischemia of the bladder wall. This, in turn, results in a diminished bladder capacity.

c. **Photodynamic-induced cystitis** may occur in patients who have received photodynamic therapy to treat transitional cell carcinoma of the bladder. Histologically, the changes seen are similar to radiation cystitis. These patients have hematuria acutely and some have developed a reduction of bladder capacity.[14]

d. **Chemotherapy-induced cystitis** is most commonly seen in patients on high-dose cyclophosphamide (Cytoxan).[15] Microscopic changes are similar to those seen in radiation and photodynamic-induced cystitis. However, the hematuria may be severe and even life-threatening.

e. **Interstitial cystitis** is a poorly understood, often misdiagnosed condition of the bladder.[16] Many theories have been proposed to explain its etiology, including mastocytosis (increased number of mast cells) of the bladder, an autoimmune disease, or defects in mucopolysaccharides thought to be a protective coating on the bladder mucosa. Histologically, the picture is that of a nonspecific inflammatory infiltrate. Mast cells may be seen, but are not always present. Some patients have ulcers in the bladder wall. Hematuria, if present, is usually mild and rarely life-threatening.

2. Neoplasms

a. **Papillary transitional cell carcinoma** is the most common type of bladder tumor. These tumors are characterized by an increase in the number of cells in the mucosal layer, followed by the formation of epithelial buds that protrude into the lumen of the bladder. These buds carry with them a stalk that contains supporting connective tissue and blood vessels. These papillary tumors can outgrow their blood supply and result in hematuria.

b. **Bladder hemangiomas** are rather rare lesions. They consist of clusters of blood vessels in the bladder mucosa that tend to rupture and bleed spontaneously. They are best managed by neodymium:YAG laser.

B. CLINICAL APPLICATION OF MICROCIRCULATORY STUDIES

Certain compounds that tend to concentrate in vascular stroma neoplasms emit fluorescence when exposed to an appropriate wavelength of light. Detection of this fluorescence can identify cancers that cannot be seen with the naked eye. Dihematoporphyrin ether is one such agent that has been used *in situ* to diagnose carcinoma of the bladder.[17]

III. MODELS AND TECHNIQUES

A. BLOOD FLOW

Urinary bladder blood flow has been studied in several animal models using a variety of techniques for quantitative measurements. Nemeth et al.[4] used radioisotope-labeled microspheres in dog bladders. Dunn[1] studied blood flow in the rabbit bladder with technetium-99m as the marker. Andersson et al.[3] quantitated the venous effluent from cat bladder by diverting the blood through a photoelectric drop-counter before returning the blood via the right jugular vein. In the only report of blood flow in the microcirculation of the bladder, Mehrota[2] made qualitative assessments about flow while making observations with a transilluminating microscope.

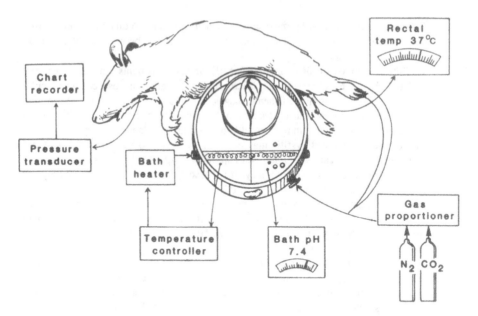

Figure 1   A schematic of the *in vivo* microscopy rat urinary bladder preparation. (From Schuschke, D. A., Reed, M. W. R., Wingren, U. F., and Miller, F. N., The rat urinary bladder: vasoactivity and macromolecular leakage in a new model, *Microvasc. Res.*, 38, 23–35, 1989.)

B. *IN VIVO* MICROSCOPY

Reports of *in vivo* microscopy studies of the urinary bladder microcirculation appear to be limited to use of the rat animal model.[2,5,6] In general, the rats are anesthetized with intraperitoneal injections of sodium pentobarbital (50 mg/kg). The animals are maintained at a rectal temperature of 36 to 37°C by placing them on a heating pad. A PE 50 cannula is placed in the left carotid artery and connected to a Statham pressure transducer to measure blood pressure. The heart rate is calculated from the pulse pressure. An indwelling bladder cannula may be placed via the urethra. The cannula is then connected to a statham low-pressure transducer to cystometrically monitor intrabladder pressures.[5,6] A lower midline laparotomy is done to expose the urinary bladder. The peritoneal reflection is then divided enabling the bladder to be exteriorized and positioned by a single seromuscular suture (5-0) in a plexiglass tissue bath with the animal lying on its right side (Figure 1). Nerves and blood vessels from the animal to the bladder remain intact. The tissue bath contains a modified Kreb's solution (NaCl, 113 mM; NaHCO$_3$, 25 mM; Dextrose, 11.6 mM; KCl, 4.7 mM; CaCl$_2$ · 2H$_2$O, 2.5 mM; MgSO$_4$ · 7H$_2$O, 1.2 mM; and KH$_2$PO$_4$, 1.2 mM). The Kreb's solution is replaced every 15 min and maintained at pH 7.4 ± 0.05 by bubbling nitrogen and carbon dioxide into the bath that sets up an equilibrium for bath PCO$_2$ and pO$_2$. A negative feedback system connected to an indwelling heater coil is used to maintain the bath temperature at 36 ± 0.5°C.

An alternative to positioning the bladder in the tissue bath is to leave it in a more *in situ* position. This is done by placing the animal on its back and retracting the abdominal wall and viscera to the sides to expose the bladder. The bladder is then kept warm and moist by a superfusate of buffer solution dripped onto the surface of the bladder.[2,6] The advantage of the *in situ* positioning is that there is less surgical intervention, thus there is less opportunity to compromise the integrity of the bladder. However, this advantage of reduced surgical handling may not be particularly significant since there was no evidence of spontaneous extravasation of albumin nor any increase in mast cell disruption when the bladder was positioned by a stay-suture in the tissue bath.[5] The advantage of maintaining the bladder in a tissue bath is that there is better control of environmental parameters like temperature and pH. An even greater advantage is that drugs topically applied in the bath are of known and constant molar concentration.

After the surgical preparation, the animal is positioned on a microscope stage for observation of the microcirculation. Illumination of the bladder is possible by both transillumination and epi-illumination. Transmitted light for the *in situ*-positioned bladder is delivered by quartz[2] or borosilicate glass rods[6] positioned under the posterior surface of the bladder. In the exteriorized bladder model, the plexiglass tissue bath has an optic port fitted with a coverslip that allows transmitted light from the microscope base to illuminate the bladder. Transillumination may also be achieved by passing an optic fiber via a urethral cannula into the bladder. Light distribution within the bladder can then be regulated by positioning of the fiber and by use of a diffusion bulb at the tip of the fiber.

Epi-illumination is done by passing light through the microscope objective onto the surface of the bladder. In the case of using epi-illumination of fluorescent tagged albumin,[5] a 100-W mercury arc lamp is used to provide the excitation light (450–490 nm). The fluorescent emission (515–535 nm) is then detected by a low-light sensitive SIT (silicon-intensified tube) camera.

Whether transmitted or epi-illumination is used as the light source, a closed-circuit television system is used to monitor the experiments and record them on videotape for off-line analysis. Since the bladder wall has rhythmic peristaltic-like waves of contraction, off-line analysis allows for freeze-frame analysis when the image is in focus. Computer-assisted off-line analysis is necessary for quantitation of leakage of fluorescent-tagged albumin.

For analysis of macromolecular leakage, a videotaped image of a region directly adjacent to a post-capillary venule is digitized and an average interstitial fluorescence of the area is determined using commercial video analysis software (Image Pro Plus). As leakage occurs, the average interstitial fluorescence increases and this change in light intensity provides an index of albumin extravasation.[10]

REFERENCES

1. **Dunn, M.,** A study of the bladder blood flow during distension in rabbits, *Br. J. Urol.,* 46, 67, 1974.
2. **Mehrota, R. M. L.,** An experimental study of the vesical circulation during distension and in cystitis, *J. Pathol. Bacteriol.,* 66, 78, 1953.
3. **Andersson, P.-O., Bloom, S. R., Mattiasson, A., and Uvelius, B.,** Changes in vascular resistance in the feline urinary bladder in response to bladder filing, *J. Urol.,* 134, 1041, 1985.
4. **Nemeth, C. J., Kahn, R. M., Kirchner, P., and Adams, R.,** Changes in canine bladder perfusion with distension, *Invest. Urol.,* 15, 149, 1977.
5. **Schuschke, D. A., Reed, M. W. R., Wingren, U. F., and Miller, F. N.,** The rat urinary bladder: Vasoactivity and macromolecular leakage in a new model, *Microvasc. Res.,* 38, 23, 1989.
6. **Young, W. F., Jr., Dey, R. D., and Echt, R.,** Comparisons of prostaglandin vasoactive effects and interactions in the *in vivo* microcirculation of the rat urinary bladder, *Microvasc. Res.,* 17, 1, 1979.
7. **Joshua, I. G., Wiegman, D. L., Harris, P. D., and Miller, F. N.,** Progressive microvascular alterations with the development of renovascular hypertension, *Hypertension,* 6, 61, 1984.
8. **Click, R. L., Gilmore, J. P., and Joyner, W. L.,** Differential response of hamster cheek pouch microvessels to vasoactive stimuli during the early development of hypertension, *Circ. Res.,* 44, 512, 1979.
9. **Collis, M. G. and Alps, B. J.,** Vascular reactivity to noradrenaline, potassium chloride, and angiotensin II in the rat perfused mesenteric vasculature preparation, during the development of renal hypertension, *Cardiovasc. Res.,* 9, 118, 1975.
10. **Miller, F. N., Joshua, I. G., and Anderson, G. L.,** Quantitation of vasodilator-induced macromolecular leakage by *in vivo* fluorescent microscopy, *Microvasc. Res.,* 24, 56, 1982.

11. **Maggi, C. A., Santicioli, P., Abelli, L., Parlani, M., Capasso, M., Conte, B., Giulani, S., and Meli, A.,** Regional differences in the effects of capsaicin and tachykinins on motor activity and vascular permeability of the rat lower urinary tract, *Naunyn-Schmiedeberg's Arch. Pharmacol.,* 335, 636, 1987.
12. **Saria, A., Hua, X., Skofitsch, G., and Lungberg, J. M.,** Inhibition of compound 48/80-induced vascular protein leakage by pretreatment with capsaicin and a substance P antagonist, *Naunyn-Schmiedeberg's Arch. Pharmacol.,* 328, 9, 1984.
13. **DeVries, C. R. and Freiha, F. S.,** Hemorrhagic cystitis: A review, *J. Urol.,* 143, 1, 1990.
14. **Harty, J. I., Amin, M., Wieman, J. T., et al.,** Complications of whole bladder dihematoporphyrin ether photodynamic therapy, *J. Urol.,* 141, 1341, 1989.
15. **Levine, L. A. and Richie, J. P.,** Urological complications of cyclophosphamide, *J. Urol.,* 141, 1063, 1989.
16. **Gillenwater, J. Y. and Wein, A. J.,** Summary of the National Institute of Arthritis, Diabetes, Digestive and Kidney Diseases Workshop on interstitial cystitis. National Institutes of Health, Bethesda, MD, August 28–29, 1987, *J. Urol.,* 140, 203, 1988.
17. **Benson, R. C., Jr., Farrow, G. M., Kinsey, J. H., et al.,** Detection and localization of *in situ* carcinoma of the bladder with hematoporphyrin derivative, *Mayo Clin. Proc.,* 57, 548, 1982.

Section V

Functional Components of the Microcirculation

Chapter 28

Angiogenesis

Johannes M. Frank

CONTENTS

I. PHYSIOLOGY OF ANGIOGENESIS

A. MECHANISMS OF ANGIOGENESIS

Angiogenesis is the process of new capillary formation. It is involved in various physiological, regenerative, and pathological processes (e.g., embryogenesis, endometrium regeneration, wound healing, tumor growth). There are malignant and benign tissues known to be a source of factors that stimulate vessel growth. Tissues that contain a high level of these factors include lymphatic tissue, retina, salivary glands, thyroid and kidney.[1-3] The cellular origin of these factors are mainly cells involved in inflammatory responses: lymphocytes, neutrophils, platelets, and macrophages.[4,5] Other cells, like mast cells, seem to potentiate angiogenesis by releasing heparin and other substances (histamine, different proteases).[6] Endothelial cells by themselves are able to stimulate angiogenesis in an autoregulating manner,[7] and tumor cells contain angiogenic factors that stimulate vessel growth.[8] The blood vessels that respond to an angiogenic stimulus are the venules. The morphological changes involved in the formation of new blood vessels are as described below and shown in Figure 1.[9,10]

1. Vessel dilation and increase in permeability
2. Activation of proteases causing a dissolution of the basement membrane of the venule at the side facing the angiogenic stimulus
3. Migration of endothelial cells toward the angiogenic stimulus
4. Proliferation of endothelial cells
5. Capillary tube and loop formation

0-8493-4870-6/95/$0.00+$.50

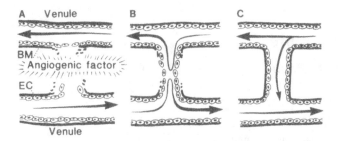

Figure 1 A: After activation of the endothelial cells (EC) by an angiogenic factor, the basement membrane (BM) is degraded and the EC start migrating through the gap. B: Soon the EC proliferate and form a new capillary tube. C: With canalization and blood flow, the new basement membrane is synthesized.

6. Canalization and synthesis of the new basement membrane
7. Association with pericytes and fibroblasts

It is a rapid process, in which endothelial cells start migrating after 24 h and new vessels can cross a wound edge after only 3 days.[11] These changes include a close functional relationship between certain cell functions and matrix components. The response of the vasculature to an angiogenic stimulus is affected by the extracellular matrix (ECM). For example, culturing endothelial cells on a matrix composed of collagen I and III enhances endothelial proliferation and migration, whereas culturing these cells on type IV and V collagen inhibits proliferation but stimulates the formation of tube-like structures.[12] The ECM can be a source of growth factors (e.g., bFGF), that are probably responsible for the mitogenic properties observed in this process.

Fibrin/fibronectin are involved in the early stages of coagulation. Together, they form with soluble growth factors, released by thrombocytes and leukocytes, an environment into which endothelial cells readily migrate.[13] There are also endothelial receptors (integrin type and non-integrin laminin-binding protein) that mediate attachment, cell migration, and spreading.[14,15]

Mechanical factors like blood pressure and flow seem to be important in the development of new capillaries. Capillaries with poor blood flow can actually regress, whereas those with high flow maintain or even expand into larger vessels.[16,17] Exercise and vasodilators induce increased flow and subsequent vessel growth.[18,19]

Another important factor in the regulation of angiogenesis is tissue oxygen tension. Hypoxia stimulates, while hyperoxia inhibits angiogenesis.[20] The stimulus seems to be the oxygen gradient; if the gradient disappears, capillary growth ceases.[21] Macrophages express angiogenic factors in a hypoxic environment and probably mediate this response.[22]

B. ANGIOGENIC FACTORS

1. Stimulators of Angiogenesis

A number of factors have been purified that stimulate angiogenesis (Table 1). These factors include peptides and non-peptides. Their mechanisms are very different and not yet fully understood. In general, they are classified as direct and indirect angiogenic factors. Direct angiogenic factors affect endothelial cells *in vitro*. In most literature, this group includes factors that have a direct mitogenic effect on endothelial cells. There also exist factors that are not mitogenic but instead induce chemotaxis of endothelial cells (e.g., tumor necrosis factor-α, Angiotropin). Indirect factors stimulate angiogenesis by accumulating other cells that release direct angiogenic factors.

Table 1 Stimulators of Angiogenesis: Mitogenic and Nonmitogenic Factors for Endothelial Cells

Mitogenic Factors	Nonmitogenic Factors
Fibroblast Growth Factor (FGF)	Tumor Necrosis Factor-alpha (TNF-α)
Vascular Endothelial Growth Factor (VEGF)	
Platelet-Derived Endothelial Cell Growth Factor (PD-ECGF)	Transforming Growth Factor-beta (TGF-β)
Epidermal Growth Factor (EGF)	Angiotropin
	Angiogenin
Transforming Growth Factor-alpha (TGF-α)	Insulin-Like Growth Factor I
Amphiregulin	
Vaccinia Growth Factor (VGF)	

a. Mitogenic Factors

Endothelial cell growth factors that bind to heparin include basic fibroblast growth factor (bFGF or FGF-2), acidic fibroblast growth factor (aFGF or FGF-1), and vascular endothelial growth factor (VEGF). The discovery of heparin affinity was an important step towards the isolation of angiogenic factors from many tissues.[23] A lot of these factors were named by their source but have since been shown to be equivalent to FGF. These factors stimulate mitogenesis, chemotaxis, differentiation, and angiogenesis. Acidic FGF (polypeptide with 140 amino acids, 18 kDa) is found primarily in neural tissue, b-FGF (polypeptide, 146 amino acids, 18 kDa) is widely distributed in normal and neoplastic tissue.[24] Endothelial cells synthesize bFGF; however, the mechanism by which it is released by these cells is not known. A possibility is that bFGF is a component of the extracellular matrix in association with heparin-like molecules that might keep it inactive until it is released by cell lysis and/or by heparinases and proteases.[13] Vascular endothelial growth factor (VEGF) is a member of the platelet-derived growth factor (PDGF) family and is a secreted protein (48 kDa). It is a specific mitogen for capillary and human umbilical vein endothelial cells.[25]

Platelet-derived endothelial cell growth factor (PD-ECGF) is a polypeptide (45 kDa) that does not bind to heparin. It is not secreted, but is sequestered intracellularly and is a specific endothelial cell mitogen.[26]

Epidermal growth factor (EGF), a polypeptide (6 kDa), is found in the mouse salivary gland and in biological fluids. EGF has a sequence homology with transforming growth factor-alpha (TGF-α), which also binds to EGF receptors. Both factors are mitogens for different cell types (e.g., keratinocytes, fibroblasts).[27,28]

TGF-α is secreted by a variety of tumor cells and normal cells (e.g., macrophages) and might be an important mediator in tumor angiogenesis. This family of angiogenic factors also includes the proteins vaccinia growth factor and amphiregulin.[29,30]

b. Nonmitogenic Factors

Tumor necrosis factor-alpha (TNF-α) is a multifunctional polypeptide (17 kDa) with mediator functions in inflammation and immunity. TNF-α inhibits endothelial cell proliferation, but influences angiogenesis by matrix and tube formation.[31] It is produced in activated macrophages and seems to be an important mediator of angiogenesis induced by these cells.[32] It is interesting to note that TNF-α given intravasculary causes coagulation, hemorrhage, and necrosis.[33] The location of release is an important factor influencing the effect TNF-α has on tissue. Angiotropin is a copper-containing polyribonucleopolypeptide (4,5 kDa) and was purified from activated monocytes. It is not a mitogen but specifically stimulates endothelial cell migration.[34] After injection, angiotropin induces vascular dilation, angiogenesis, and morphological changes in endothelial cells.

Table 2 Inhibitors of Angiogenesis

Protamine
Angiostatic steroids
Thrombospondin
Platelet factor IV
γ-Interferon
Interferon α, β
Inhibitors of metalloproteinases (TIMP-1, TIMP-2)
D-Penicillamine
Vitamin D₃ analogs
Minocycline
Fumigallin (and derivatives)
Retinoids

Angiogenin (polypeptide, 14,1 kDa, 22-24 AA) is a potent stimulator of angiogenesis, but has neither a mitogenic effect nor does it stimulate migration of endothelial cells. Angiogenin might stimulate other endothelial cell functions that are important in the development of new blood vessels or perhaps may act as an indirect factor. It is related to pancreatic RNAse and its ribonucleolytic activity appears to be important for its angiogenic activity since RNAse inhibitor also inhibits this activity.[35] Transforming growth factor-beta (TGF-β) is a homodimer with 112 amino acids per chain (25 kDa), it is synthesized and secreted in most tissues as a latent biologically inactive complex that can be activated by heat, acidification, and proteases.[36] TGF-β plays an important role in tissue regeneration of different organs (bone, eye, liver, heart, skin, etc.), embryogenesis, and acts on specific cell types (lymphocytes, macrophages, synovial cells, and epidermis cells).[37] TGF-β is not an endothelial cell mitogen, it blocks endothelial proliferation and motility *in vitro*, but stimulates angiogenesis *in vivo*.[38,39] Its *in vivo* activity might be due to a differentiating effect that TGF-β has on endothelial cells to induce extracellular matrix synthesis. This factor is extremely chemotactic for monocytes that could infiltrate and produce mitogenic factors.[40]

Insulin-like growth factor I (IGF-I) promotes chemotaxis of endothelial cells and there is evidence supporting its role in retinal neovascularization.[41] A number of low molecular weight angiogenic factors (0.2 to 1 kDa) have been isolated from different sources (e.g., tumors, macrophages, serum, adipocytes).[42-44] Prostaglandins are also able to stimulate angiogenesis and, furthermore, there seems to be a relation between copper ions and angiogenesis.[45,46] Recently, it has been shown that macrophage colony-stimulating factor (M-CSF, 45–100 kDa) induces angiogenesis *in vivo*.[47]

2. Inhibitors of Angiogenesis

During the last years, many anti-angiogenic factors have been described (Table 2). In the beginning, experiments on the chorioallantoic membrane and the promotion of angiogenesis with heparin and inhibition with protamine led to the discovery that a combination of heparin and cortisone could prevent angiogenesis. It was shown that this effect was not related to heparin's anticoagulant activity, nor to glucocorticoid and mineralocorticoid activity.[48] The mechanism of action could be by inducing the breakdown of the basement membrane, which in turn leads to capillary regression. This theory is supported by the fact that proline analogs and proline hydroxylase inhibitors induce regression of growing capillaries.[49]

Thrombospondin (160 kDa, glycoprotein) is found in platelet α-granules. It is homologous to Gp140 (140 kDa, glycoprotein), which is promoted by an active cancer suppressor gene. Both inhibit migration of endothelial cells and neovascularization.[50] Another factor found in platelet α-granules, which is anti-angiogenic, is platelet factor IV (28 kDa).[51] This protein is able to block growth factor-dependent endothelial cell stimulation. This effect can be blocked by readdition of growth factor. Perhaps in this case there exists a balance of platelet proteins which control angiogenesis, since they also contain an angiogenic factor (PD-ECGF).[50]

Gamma-interferon (50 kDa, glycoprotein) is a strong growth inhibitor for a variety of normal and transformed cells. The inhibition of capillary formation and endothelial cell proliferation seems to be mediated by an effect on the FGF receptor. Other interferons (α and β) are also known to be inhibitors of angiogenesis.[52]

Another source for anti-angiogenic factors includes certain tissues and cells. The vitreous, lens, aorta, smooth muscle cells, and kidney have been shown to contain anti-angiogenic factors.[53,54] Pericytes have been shown to be able to suppress endothelial cell growth.[55] The resistance of cartilage to tumor invasion led to the finding that cartilage is a major source for anti-angiogenic factors, e.g., two tissue inhibitors of metalloproteinases, TIMP-1 and TIMP-2.[56-58] Both the isolation of an anti-angiogenic collagenase inhibitor from cartilage,[59] and the fact that medroxyprogesterone (a substance that reduces the release of collagenase) inhibits vascularization, indicate the role for collagenase in angiogenesis.[60] Furthermore, D-penicillamine, Vitamin D_3 analogs, retinoids, Minocycline, fumigallin (and derivatives) are all anti-angiogenic. Perhaps even radical scavengers play a role in the inhibition of vessel growth.[61,62]

II. ROLE OF ANGIOGENESIS — CLINICAL ASPECTS

A. WOUND HEALING

Initiated by an injury, wound healing involves different processes that lead to tissue regeneration. These steps are coagulation, inflammation, proliferation, and remodeling.[63] Tissue disruption leads to hemorrhage, coagulation, and accumulation of platelets. Platelets release factors (e.g., TGF-β, PDGF) that attract inflammatory cells like polymorphonuclear cells and macrophages. Many of these factors and the role they play in wound healing have been investigated. Numerous studies have been done to manipulate healing with such factors.[64-71] Some of these growth factors are already used to promote healing in humans.[72,73] Their beneficial effect on healing is due to the influence they have on components of healing (e.g., matrix deposition, fibroblast proliferation, angiogenesis, epithelialization). Especially in the regulation of wound angiogenesis, macrophages and their released cytokines appear to be of great importance.[74] Angiogenesis starts about 2 days after injury and becomes prominent at 4 days.[63] About about 50 years ago, Sandison and Clark described the vessel ingrowth in the rabbit ear chamber.[16,17] These newly formed vessels are an important part in granulation tissue formation and in re-establishing tissue integrity.

B. ANGIOGENIC DISEASE

Angiogenesis appears in physiological and regenerative processes, it is also an important factor in pathological processes (Table 3). In diabetes, it is found in diabetic angiopathies especially in the retina, but also in the kidney and heart.[75,76] The reasons for this increased angiogenesis might be due to a thickening of the basement membrane followed by an impaired oxygen release in the tissue, or a lack of glycogen synthesis and storage.[77] Also, the disappearance of cells that inhibit vessel growth might be a relevant factor.[75,78]

Psoriasis is an inflammatory disease with increased epidermal proliferation and vascular abnormalities. The microvascular changes include new blood vessel formation, increased permeability, hemoconcentration, and rouleaux formation. These result in vessel obstruction and tissue hypoxia. The cutaneous angiogenesis seen in psoriasis might also depend on angiogenic factors produced by peripheral blood cells or psoriatic plaques.[79,80] Another inflammatory disease with a well-documented angiogenic component is rheumatoid arthritis.[81]

Table 3 Pathological and
Physiological Processes Where
Angiogenesis Is an Important
Factor

Pathological Angiogenesis	Physiological Angiogenesis
Diabetes	
Psoriasis	Embryogenesis
Rheumatoid arthritis	Development
Retrolental fibroplasia	
Hypertension	Endometrium regeneration
Atherosclerosis	
Tumor growth	Wound healing

Other diseases that involve angiogenesis are retrolental fibroplasia, hypertension, and atherosclerosis. Retrolental fibroplasia is a disorder with excessive vessel growth in the retina, probably in response to high oxygen tension and is mostly seen in prematurely born babies.

Antiangiogenic substances are becoming increasingly important for therapy. Preliminary results of some drugs already in use are beginning to clarify the mechanisms of the disease and the drugs themselves. For example, D-penicillaminine is successfully used in rheumatoid arthritis and is a potent inhibitor of angiogenesis.[61] Retinoids are effective in psoriasis, possibly through their effect on neovascularization.[77,82] Antineoplastic agents suppress endothelial cell growth. Methotrexate, an antineoplastic agent, is effective for both psoriasis and inflammatory arthritis.[83,84]

C. TUMOR GROWTH

Virchow in 1863 was one of the first to point out the relation between vessels and tumors.[85] In 1945, Algire et al. concluded from their experiments, using the Sandison-Clark chamber, that fast tumor growth is dependent on an adequate vascular supply and that an important feature of a growing tumor is that endothelial cell growth must be stimulated continuously.[86] Greenblatt and Shubic (1968) were able to demonstrate this vasoproliferative effect. Vessel growth was induced in the hamster cheek pouch by a melanoma that was isolated from the tissue using a filter.[8] Folkman established the hypotheses that solid tumors are angiogenesis dependent. His group was able to isolate a "tumor angiogenic factor (TAF)". They also demonstrated that tumors stopped growing at a size of 1 to 2 mm^2 if they were isolated from their vascular bed.[6] During the following years, many angiogenic factors have been isolated from tumors.[23,42,87-89] The dependency of tumors on vessel growth and the discovery of antiangiogenic substances have increased the efforts toward developing antiangiogenic substances for tumor therapy. Protamine has been used to reduce lung metastasis in mice. The combination of cortisone injections and heparin (oral administration) was shown to cause tumor regression in mice.[90] The attempt to develop a more specific antiangiogenic therapy against tumor growth led to experimental investigations of an antiserum against tumor angiogenesis factor.[91] The inhibition of growth factors that stimulate angiogenesis in tumors might also improve tumor therapy.[92,93] Hemangiomas have been successfully treated by the angiostatic property of α-interferon, and potent angiogenesis inhibitors are being prepared for clinical trials.[92,94]

Tumor angiogenesis is not characteristic of malignant tumors; it also appears in nonmalignant tumors. But the onset of angiogenesis in malignant tumors increases the

Table 4   *In Vivo* Models To Study Angiogenesis

In Vivo **Models**
Chick chorioallantoic membrane (CAM)
Rabbit cornea pocket
Hamster cheek pouch
Hamster dorsal skinfold chamber
Kidney capsule
Optic tectum
Bone chamber
Eye
Nailfold
Mouse abdominal skin flap
Hairless mouse ear
Rat sponge model
Alginate intradermal injection

number of tumor cells released in the circulation and thereby metastasis. In human breast cancer, the angiogenic potency of this tumor can be used as a prognostic marker.[95]

III. MODELS AND TECHNIQUES FOR INVESTIGATIONS

A. MODELS TO STUDY ANGIOGENESIS
1. *In Vivo* Models
There are several models to study vessel growth *in vivo* (Table 4). The rabbit ear chamber is useful to observe vessel development over a period of time and to perform measurements of the microvasculature.[16,17] This chamber was modified and also used to study angiogenesis in the dorsal subcutaneous tissue of the mouse and the hamster cheek pouch.[96,97] The rabbit cornea pocket is an *in vivo* assay to determine whether a factor is angiogenic. On the normally avascular cornea, the outgrowth of newly formed vessels from the limbus is easy to see following the application of a substance to be tested. However, it is difficult to perform quantitative measurements of this new vessel growth.[98] A widely used model is the chick chorioallantoic membrane (CAM). The problem with the CAM is that it is very sensitive to inflammation and a relatively large number of vessels grow due to the development of the CAM. This condition, on the other hand, makes the model useful to test antiangiogenic agents that, if effective, leave an avascular zone.[20,99,100] The fact that the cornea is normally avascular, and the CAM undergoes rapid vascular growth, might not represent naturally occurring angiogenesis (e.g., wound healing). There are still other useful models that allow long-term observations of vessel growth. These include the dorsal skinfold of the hamster, which is used for different studies in microcirculation, the kidney capsule, the optic tectum of xenopus laevis, and a bone chamber.[101-104] The eye, a model that needs no preparation, can be used even in humans, as can the nailfold. Intradermal assays like the triangular abdominal skin flap in mice and the homozygous hairless (hr/hr) mouse ear are good models used for direct intravital observations of angiogenesis (Figure 2).[105,106] Other *in vivo* models allow indirect measurements of angiogenesis. These include the rat sponge model or use of intradermal injections of alginate pellets.[107,108] A common problem of all these models dealing with angiogenesis is the discrimination between direct and indirect angiogenesis. Substances applied can induce inflammation and cell infiltration, which then release factors that can induce angiogenesis.

2. *In Vitro* Models
In vitro models provide methods to investigate mechanisms involved in regulating vessel growth. In these models, it is possible to study what effects different substances have on

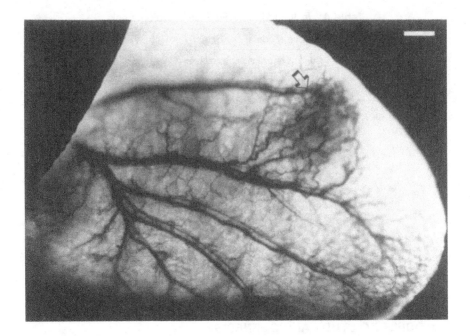

Figure 2 Intravital microscopy showing angiogenesis in the homozygous hairless (hr/hr) mouse. The arrow indicates newly formed vessels after growth factor (bFGF) injection. White bar indicates 1 mm.

cell migration, proliferation, and tube formation.[109-111] Venule endothelial cells are optimal for these assays because, *in vivo*, the capillary endothelium from venules are the cells that respond to angiogenic stimuli. Studies using endothelial cells from other sources (e.g., aortic endothelium, large vein endothelium) could lead to very different results. Not all angiogenic factors affect the endothelial cells in the same way, some have no proliferative effect and are still angiogenic, while others have no effect on endothelial cells but instead induce other cells to release angiogenic factors. Furthermore, this kind of assay allows for the isolation of substances or enzymes released by endothelial cells, which may be important for the angiogenic response (e.g., collagenase, plasminogen).[112]

B. TECHNIQUES FOR OBSERVATION AND MEASUREMENTS

1. Intravital Microscopy

A number of the previously described *in vivo* models are especially designed for intravital microscopy, which allows direct continuous observation of vessel growth. The chamber techniques or the hairless mouse ear model allow transmitted light microscopy. In models where transillumination is not possible, it may be necessary to use epi-illumination. Epi-illumination, together with fluorescence microscopy, is commonly used. By injecting a fluorochrome coupled to a plasma protein (e.g., albumin) or high molecular weight dextran, the magnified image of the vessels is clearly seen. This enhanced image of the vessels can be used to study the microvasculature in thicker tissues otherwise impossible to transilluminate.

2. Histology

Conventional histology is widely used to quantitatively analyze angiogenesis. To visualize the vessels, different approaches can be used to prepare the tissue. There are basically

Table 5 Parameters for Quantitative
Measurements of Angiogenesis

Vessel length density (mm/mm^2)
Vessel density index (intersections/mm^2)
Vessel endpoint density (number/mm^2)
Vessel segments (number/mm^2)
Vessel diameter
Blood flow
Diffusion distance

two methods. There are injection techniques where the vessels are filled with a substance (e.g., India ink, plastic resins, radio-opaque suspensions for radioautography, fluorescent marker). Alternatively, blood cells can be stained and the vessel lumen marked. The pitfall of such techniques is that there is a risk of not filling all the capillaries. This is particularly problematic considering the abundance of capillary sprouts that are often missed when using these casting methods. Histochemical staining of the basement membrane helps to reveal capillaries in histological sections. The problem here is that the basement membrane is not fully developed and thereby not all vessels stain. Also, the staining of glycosaminoglycans is not specific, and other tissue components (e.g., glycogen) are stained. Enzyme histochemistry is another possibility for detecting capillaries for investigations using alkaline phosphatase or peroxidase staining. Hematoxlin-eosin or Masson's trichrome are also used by staining the red blood cells and using these as markers of the vessels. Electron microscopy is a technique that can be used to investigate ultrastructure of the newly forming vessels. Together with immunocytochemical methods, substances can be identified that are responsible for vessel growth.[8,113-116]

3. Quantitative Measurement Systems

Important in angiogenesis research, especially in studies investigating the angiogenic response to a substance, is a way of quantitatively analyzing vessel growth. How this can be done depends on the model system being used. In histological sections, the capillaries in a defined field can be counted and the values expressed as capillary density (capillaries per square millimeter tissue). If radiolabeled substances (microspheres, ^{133}Xenon, ^{51}CR-RBC) are used with injection techniques (*in vivo* or histology), angiogenesis can be determined by gamma-counting. This method is used in *in vitro* and *in vivo* models.[107,108] In the *in vitro* models, endothelial proliferation is measured with ^{3}H-thymidine incorporation or cell counts, and cell migration is measured using modified Boyden chamber assays.[34,110,117] Tube formation and cell shape analysis of the endothelial cell are also important for a basic understanding of the different mechanisms.[111]

There is an increasing effort to develop *in vivo* analyzing systems for studying dynamic parameters at the microcirculatory level. An easy way to quantify angiogenesis is by counting the newly formed vessels or by classifying the response using a scaling system (e.g., 0 = no new vessels, 4 = many new tortuous vessels and hemorrhage).[105,118] An exact analysis of the vascular pattern is difficult and time-consuming. There are several ways to determine parameters closely related to angiogenesis (Table 5).[20] Therefore, it is necessary to trace the individual vessels to get an overview of the changes that occur during vessel growth. Recently, digital image processing has been used to expedite analysis.[119,120] This modern method allows one to automate the measurements using the images recorded with intravital videomicroscopy or from tissue prepared by injection techniques. For example, together with the hairless mouse ear model, a computer system was developed that allows one to put high-magnification images of angiogenesis together in a montage (Figure 3). This montage gives an overview of the whole vascular network

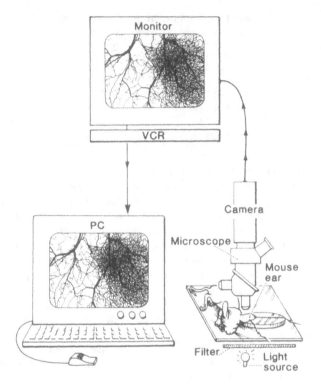

Figure 3 Experimental set-ups for intravital microscopy and computer-assisted analysis of angiogenesis.

of the organ studied and enables the investigator to perform measurements of the developing vessels. This new technique will be very helpful to evaluate quantitatively the different changes that occur during angiogenesis.

REFERENCES

1. **Auerbach, R., Kubai, L., and Sidky, Y.,** Angiogenesis induction by tumors, embryonic tissue, and lymphocytes, *Cancer Res.,* 36, 3435, 1976.
2. **Federman, J. L., Brown, G. C., Felberg, N. T., and Felton, S. M.,** Experimental ocular angiogenesis, *Am. J. Ophthalmol.,* 89, 231, 1980.
3. **Hoffman, J., McAuslan, B., Robertson, D., and Burnett, E.,** An endothelial growth stimulating factor from salivary glands, *Exp. Cell. Res.,* 102, 269, 1976.
4. **Fromer, C. H. and Klintworth, G. K.,** An evaluation of the role of leukocyte in the pathogenesis of experimentally induced corneal vascularization. III. Studies related to the vasoproliferative capability of polymorphonuclear leukocytes and lymphocytes, *Am. J. Pathol.,* 82, 157, 1976.
5. **Polverini, P. J., Cotran, R. S., Gimbrone, M. A., and Unanue, E. R.,** Activated macrophages induce vascular proliferation, *Nature,* 269, 804, 1977.
6. **Folkman, J.,** Toward an understanding of angiogenesis: Search and discovery, *Perspect. Biol. Med.,* 29, 10, 1985.
7. **Schweigerer, L., Neufeld, G., Friedman, J., Abraham, J. A., Fiddes, J. C., and Gospodarowicz, D.,** Capillary endothelial cells express basic fibroblast growth factor, a mitogen that promotes their own growth, *Nature,* 325, 257, 1987.
8. **Greenblatt, M. and Shubik, P.,** Tumor angiogenesis: Transfilter diffusion studies in the hamster by transparent chamber technique, *J. Natl. Cancer Inst.,* 41, 111, 1968.

9. **Folkman, J. and Klagsbrun, M.,** A family of angiogenic peptides, *Nature,* 329, 671, 1987.

10. **Risau, W.,** Angiogenic growth factors, *Prog. Growth Factor Res.,* 2, 71, 1990.

11. **Jonsson, K., Hunt, T. K., Brennan, S. S., and Mathes, S. J.,** Tissue oxygen measurements in delayed skin flaps: a reconsideration of the mechanisms of the delay phenomenon, *Plast. Reconstr. Surg.,* 82, 328, 1988.

12. **Madri, J. A. and Pratt, B. M.,** Endothelial cell-matrix interactions: *In vitro* models of angiogenesis, *J. Histochem. Cytochem.,* 34, 85, 1986.

13. **Vlodavsky, I., Fuks, Z., Ishai-Michaeli, R., Bashkin, P., Levi, E., Korner, G., Bar-Shavit, R., and Klagsbrun, M.,** Extracellular matrix-resident basic fibroblast growth factor: Implication for the control of angiogenesis, *J. Cell. Biochem.,* 45, 167, 1991.

14. **Basson, C. T., Knowles, W. J., Bell, L., Albelda, S. M., Castronovo, V., Liotta, L. A., and Madri, J. A.,** Spatiotemporal segregation of endothelial cell integrin and nonintegrin extracellular matrix-binding proteins during adhesion events, *J. Cell Biol.,* 110, 789, 1990.

15. **Yannariello Brown, J., Wewer, U., Liotta, L., and Madri, J. A.,** Distribution of a 69-kD laminin-binding protein in aortic and microvascular endothelial cells: Modulation during cell attachment, spreading, and migration, *J. Cell Biol.,* 106, 1773, 1988.

16. **Sandison, J. C.,** Observations on the growth of blood vessels as seen in the transparent chamber introduced in the rabbit's ear, *Am. J. Anat.,* 41, 475, 1928.

17. **Clark, E. R. and Clark, E. L.,** Observations on changes in blood vascular endothelium in the living animal, *Am. J. Anat.,* 57, 385, 1935.

18. **Waxman, A. M.,** Blood vessel growth as a problem in morphogenesis: A physical theory, *Microvasc. Res.,* 22, 32, 1981.

19. **Hudlicka, O. and Tyler, K. R.,** Factors involved in the growth of vessels, in *Angiogenesis. The Growth of the Vascular System,* Hudlicka, O. and Tyler, K. R., Eds., Academic Press, New York, 1986, 7.

20. **Strick, D. M., Waycaster, R. L., Montani, J. P., Gay, W. J., and Adair, T. H.,** Morphometric measurements of chorioallantoic membrane vascularity: Effects of hypoxia and hyperoxia, *Am. J. Physiol.,* 260, H1385, 1991.

21. **Knighton, D. R., Silver, I. A., and Hunt, T. K.,** Regulation of wound-healing angiogenesis — Effect of oxygen gradients and inspired oxygen concentration, *Surgery,* 90, 262, 1981.

22. **Knighton, D. R., Hunt, T. K., Scheuenstuhl, H., Halliday, B. J., Werb, Z., and Banda, M. J.,** Oxygen tension regulates the expression of angiogenesis factor by macrophages, *Science,* 221, 1283, 1983.

23. **Shing, Y., Folkman, J., Sullivan, R., Butterfield, C., Murray, J., and Klagsbrun, M.,** Heparin affinity: Purification of a tumor-derived capillary endothelial cell growth factor, *Science,* 223, 1296, 1984.

24. **Gospodarowicz, D., Neufeld, G., and Schweigerer, L.,** Fibroblast growth factor: Structural and biological properties, *J. Cell Physiol. Suppl.,* Suppl 5, 15, 1987.

25. **Gospodarowicz, D., Abraham, J. A., and Schilling, J.,** Isolation and characterization of a vascular endothelial cell mitogen produced by pituitary-derived folliculo stellate cells, *Proc. Natl. Acad. Sci. U.S.A.,* 86, 7311, 1989.

26. **Miyazono, K., Okabe, T., Urabe, A., Takaku, F., and Heldin, C. H.,** Purification and properties of an endothelial cell growth factor from human platelets, *J. Biol. Chem.,* 262, 4098, 1987.

27. **Carpenter, G. and Cohen, S.,** Epidermal growth factor, *Annu. Rev. Biochem.,* 48, 193, 1979.

28. **Klagsbrun, M. and D'Amore, P. A.,** Regulators of angiogenesis, *Annu. Rev. Physiol.,* 53, 217, 1991.

29. **Brown, J. P., Twardzik, D. R., Marquardt, H., and Todaro, G. J.,** Vaccinia virus encodes a polypeptide homologous to epidermal growth factor and transforming growth factor, *Nature,* 313, 491, 1985.

30. **Shoyab, M., Plowman, G. D., McDonald, V. L., Bradley, J. G., and Todaro, G. J.,** Structure and function of human amphiregulin: a member of the epidermal growth factor family, *Science,* 243, 1074, 1989.

31. **Frater-Schröder, M., Risau, W., Hallmann, R., Gautschi, P., and Böhlen, P.,** Tumor necrosis factor type a, a potent inhibitor of endothelial cell growth *in vitro,* is angiogenic *in vivo, Proc. Natl. Acad. Sci. U.S.A.,* 84, 5277, 1987.

32. **Leibovich, S. J., Polverini, P. J., Shepard, H. M., Wiseman, D. M., Shively, V., and Nuseir, N.,** Macrophage-induced angiogenesis is mediated by tumor necrosis factor-α, *Nature,* 329, 630, 1987.

33. **Nawroth, P. P. and Stern, D. M.,** Modulation of endothelial cell hemostatic properties by tumor necrosis factor, *J. Exp. Med.,* 163, 740, 1986.
34. **Hockel, M., Sasse, J., and Wissler, J. H.,** Purified monocyte-derived angiogenic substance (angiotropin) stimulates migration, phenotypic changes, and "tube formation" but not proliferation of capillary endothelial cells *in vitro, J. Cell Physiol.,* 133, 1, 1987.
35. **Strydom, D. J., Fett, J. W., and Riordan, J. F.,** The odyssey of angiogenin: A protein that induces blood vessel growth, *Anal. Chem.,* 61, 1173A, 1989.
36. **Massague, J.,** The transforming growth factor-beta family, *Annu. Rev. Cell Biol.,* 6, 597, 1990.
37. **Roberts, A. B., Flanders, K. C., Kondaiah, P., Thompson, N. L., Van Obberghen-Schilling, E., Wakefield, L., Rossi, P., de Crombrugghe, B., Heine, U., and Sporn, M. B.,** Transforming growth factor beta: Biochemistry and roles in embryogenesis, tissue repair and remodeling, and carcinogenesis, *Rec. Prog. Horm. Res.,* 44, 157, 1988.
38. **Muller, G., Behrens, J., Nussbaumer, U., Bohlen, P., and Birchmeier, W.,** Inhibitory action of transforming growth factor beta on endothelial cells, *Proc. Natl. Acad. Sci. U.S.A.,* 84, 5600, 1987.
39. **Roberts, A. B., Sporn, M. B., Assoian, R. K., Smith, J. M., Roche, N. S., Wakefield, L. M., Heine, U. I., Liotta, L. A., Falanga, V., Kehrl, J. H., and Fauci, A. S.,** Transforming growth factor type beta: Rapid induction of fibrosis and angiogenesis *in vivo* and stimulation of collagen formation *in vitro, Proc. Natl. Acad. Sci. U.S.A.,* 83, 4167, 1986.
40. **Wahl, S. M., Hunt, D. A., Wakefield, L. M., McCartney-Francis, N., Wahl, L. M., Roberts, A. B., and Sporn, M. B.,** Transforming growth factor type beta induces monocyte chemotaxis and growth factor production, *Proc. Natl. Acad. Sci. U.S.A.,* 84, 5788, 1987.
41. **Merimee, T. J., Zapf, J., and Froesch, E. R.,** Insulin-like growth factors. Studies in diabetics with and without retinopathy, *N. Engl. J. Med.,* 309, 527, 1983.
42. **Fenselau, A., Watt, S., and Mello, R. J.,** Tumor angiogenic factor. Purification from the Walker 256 rat tumor, *J. Biol. Chem.,* 256, 9605, 1981.
43. **Banda, M. J., Knighton, D. R., Hunt, T. K., and Werb, Z.,** Isolation of a nonmitogenic angiogenesis factor from wound fluid, *Proc. Natl. Acad. Sci. U.S.A.,* 79, 7773, 1982.
44. **Goldsmith, H. S., Griffith, A. L., Kupferman, A., and Catsimpoolas, N.,** Lipid angiogenic factor from omentum, *JAMA,* 252, 2034, 1984.
45. **Ziche, M., Ruggiero, M., Pasquali, F., and Chiarugi, V. P.,** Effects of cortisone with and without heparin on angiogenesis induced by prostaglandin E1 and by S180 cells, and on growth of murine transplantable tumours, *Int. J. Cancer,* 35, 549, 1985.
46. **Raju, K. S., Alessandri, G., Ziche, M., and Gullino, P. M.,** Ceruloplasmin, copper ions, and angiogenesis, *J. Natl. Cancer Inst.,* 69, 1183, 1982.
47. **Phillips, G. D., Aukerman, S. L., Whitehead, R. A., and Knighton, D. R.,** Macrophage colony-stimulating factor induces indirect angiogenesis *in vivo, Wound Rep. Reg.,* 1, 3, 1993.
48. **Folkman, J. and Ingber, D. E.,** Angiostatic steroids. Method of discovery and mechanism of action, *Ann. Surg.,* 206, 374, 1987.
49. **Ingber, D. E., Madri, J. A., and Folkman, J.,** A possible mechanism for inhibition of angiogenesis by angiostatic steroids: Induction of capillary basement membrane dissolution, *Endocrinology,* 119, 1768, 1986.
50. **Maione, T. E., Gray, G. S., Petro, J., Hunt, A. J., Donner, A. L., Bauer, S. I., Carson, H. F., and Sharpe, R. J.,** Inhibition of angiogenesis by recombinant human platelet factor-4 and related peptides, *Science,* 247, 77, 1990.
51. **Walz, D. A. and Hung, G. L.,** *In vivo* studies on the binding of heparin and its fractions with platelet factor 4, *Semin. Thromb. Hemost.,* 11, 40, 1985.
52. **Tsuruoka, N., Sugiyama, M., Tawaragi, Y., Tsujimoto, M., Nishihara, T., Goto, T., and Sato, N.,** Inhibition of *in vitro* angiogenesis by lymphotoxin and interferon-gamma, *Biochem. Biophys. Res. Commun.,* 155, 429, 1988.
53. **Preis, I., Langer, R., Brem, H., and Folkman, J.,** Inhibition of neovascularization by an extract derived from vitreous, *Am. J. Ophthalmol.,* 84, 323, 1977.
54. **Schumacher, B. L., Grant, D., and Eisenstein, R.,** Smooth muscle cells produce an inhibitor of endothelial cell growth, *Arteriosclerosis,* 5, 110, 1985.
55. **Antonelli-Orlidge, A., Smith, S. R., and D'Amore, P. A.,** Influence of pericytes on capillary endothelial cell growth, *Am. Rev. Respir. Dis.,* 140, 1129, 1989.
56. **Brem, H. and Folkman, J.,** Inhibition of tumor angiogenesis mediated by cartilage, *J. Exp. Med.,* 141, 427, 1975.

57. **Langer, R., Brem, H., Falterman, K., Klein, M., and Folkman, J.,** Isolation of a cartilage factor that inhibits tumor neovascularization, *Science,* 193, 70, 1976.

58. **Sorgente, N. and Dorey, C. K.,** Inhibition of endothelial cell growth by a factor isolated from cartilage, *Exp. Cell Res.,* 128, 63, 1980.

59. **Moses, M. A., Sudhalter, J., and Langer, R.,** Identification of an inhibitor of neovascularization from cartilage, *Science,* 248, 1408, 1990.

60. **Gross, J., Azizkhan, R. G., Biswas, C., Bruns, R. R., Hsieh, D. S., and Folkman, J.,** Inhibition of tumor growth, vascularization, and collagenolysis in the rabbit cornea by medroxyprogesterone, *Proc. Natl. Acad. Sci. U.S.A.,* 78, 1176, 1981.

61. **Matsubara, T., Saura, R., Hirohata, K., and Ziff, M.,** Inhibition of human endothelial cell proliferation *in vitro* and neovascularization *in vivo* by D-penicillamine, *J. Clin. Invest.,* 83, 158, 1989.

62. **Maciag, T.,** Molecular and cellular mechanisms of angiogenesis, *Important Adv. Oncol.,* 85, 1990.

63. **Hunt, T. K.,** The physiology of wound healing, *Ann. Emerg. Med.,* 17, 1265, 1988.

64. **McGee, G. S., Davidson, J. M., Buckley, A., Sommer, A., Woodward, S. C., Aquino, A. M., Barbour, R., and Demetriou, A. A.,** Recombinant basic fibroblast growth factor accelerates wound healing, *J. Surg. Res.,* 45, 145, 1988.

65. **Schultz, G., Rotatori, D. S., and Clark, W.,** EGF and TGF-α in wound healing and repair, *J. Cell. Biochem.,* 45, 346, 1991.

66. **Mertz, P. M., Sauder, D. L., Davis, S. C., Kilian, L., Herron, A. J., and Eaglstein, W. H.,** Il-1 as a potent inducer of wound re-epithelization, *Prog. Clin. Biol. Res.,* 365, 473, 1991.

67. **Klingbeil, C. K., Cesar, L. B., and Fiddes, J. C.,** Basic fibroblast growth factor accelerates tissue repair in models of impaired wound healing, *Prog. Clin. Biol. Res.,* 365, 443, 1991.

68. **Joyce, M. E., Jingushi, S., Scully, S. P., and Bolander, M. E.,** Role of growth factors in fracture healing, *Prog. Clin. Biol. Res.,* 365, 391, 1991.

69. **King, S. R., Hickerson, W. L., and Proctor, K. G.,** Beneficial actions of exogenous hyaluronic acid on wound healing, *Surgery,* 109, 76, 1991.

70. **Davidson, J., Buckley, A., Woodward, S., Nichols, W., McGee, G., and Demetriou, A.,** Mechanisms of accelerated wound repair using epidermal growth factor and basic fibroblast growth factor, *Prog. Clin. Biol. Res.,* 266, 63, 1998.

71. **Davidson, J. M. and Broadley, K. N.,** Manipulation of the wound-healing process with basic fibroblast growth factor, *Ann. N.Y. Acad. Sci.,* 638, 306, 1991.

72. **Robson, M. C., Phillips, L. G., Heggers, J. P., McPherson, M. A., and Heiner, L. S.,** Clinical studies on growth factors in pressure sores: preliminary report, *Prog. Clin. Biol. Res.,* 365, 95, 1991.

73. **Brown, G. L., Nanney, L. B., Griffen, J., Cramer, A. B., Yancey, J. M., Curtsinger, L. J., Holtzin, L., Schultz, G. S., Jurkiewicz, M. J., and Lynch, J. B.,** Enhancement of wound healing by topical treatment with epidermal growth factor, *N. Engl. J. Med.,* 321, 76, 1989.

74. **Cromack, D. T., Porras-Reyes, B., and Mustoe, T. A.,** Current concepts in wound healing: Growth factor and macrophage interaction, *J. Trauma,* 30, S129, 1990.

75. **Merimee, T. J.,** Diabetic retinopathy a synthesis of perspectives, *N. Engl. J. Med.,* 322, 978, 1990.

76. **Factor, S. M., Okun, E. M., and Minase, T.,** Capillary microaneurysms in the human diabetic heart, *N. Engl. J. Med.,* 302, 384, 1980.

77. **Quabbe, H. J., Schenk, K. E., Schneider, H., Semrau, M., and Hovener, G.,** Absence of muscle capillary basement membrane thickening and retinopathy in patients with myocardial infarction and impaired i.v. glucose tolerance, *Acta Diabetol. Lat.,* 20, 321, 1983.

78. **Ditzel, J.,** The problem of tissue oxygenation in diabetes mellitus as related to the development of diabetic angiopathy, in *Microcirculation 2,* Gregson, J. and Ziuff, W., Eds., Plenum Press, New York, 1976,

79. **Majewski, S., Tigalonowa, M., Jablonska, S., Polakowski, I., and Janczura, E.,** Serum samples from patients with active psoriasis enhance lymphocyte-induced angiogenesis and modulate endothelial cell proliferation, *Arch. Dermatol.,* 123, 221, 1987.

80. **Braverman, I. M. and Sibley, J.,** Role of the microcirculation in the treatment and pathogenesis of psoriasis, *J. Invest. Dermatol.,* 78, 12, 1982.

81. **Zvaifler, N. J.,** The immunopathology of joint inflammation in rheumatoid arthritis, *Adv. Immunol.,* 16, 265, 1973.

82. **Oikawa, T., Hirotani, K., Nakamura, O., Shudo, K., Hiragun, A., and Iwaguchi, T.,** A highly potent antiangiogenic activity of retinoids, *Cancer Lett.,* 48, 157, 1989.

388

83. **Hoffmeister, R. T.,** Methotrexate therapy in rheumatoid arthritis: 15 years experience, *Am. J. Med.,* 75, 69, 1983.

84. **Rees, R. B.,** Methotrexate for psoriasis: 1981, *Cutis.,* 28, 166, 1981.

85. **Virchow, R.,** *Die krankhaften Geschwülste,* Verlag August Hirschwald, Berlin, 1863,

86. **Algire, G. H., Chalkley, H. W., Legallais, F. Y., and Park, J. D.,** Vascular reactions of normal and malignant tissue *in vivo.* 1. Vascular reactions of mice to wounds and to normal and neoplastic transplants, *J. Natl. Cancer Inst.,* 6, 73, 1945.

87. **Tolbert, W. R., Kuo, M. J., and Feder, J.,** Production of tumor angiogenesis factor (TAF) by human tumor cell lines, *In Vitro,* 17, 259, 1981.

88. **Matsuno, H.,** Tumor angiogenesis factor (TAF) in cultured cells derived from central nervous system tumors in humans, *Neurol. Med. Chir.,* 21, 765, 1981.

89. **Vallee, B. L., Riordan, J. F., Lobb, R. R., Higachi, N., Fett, J. W., Crossley, G., Buhler, R., Budzik, G., Breddam, K., Bethune, J. L., and Alderman, E. M.,** Tumor-derived angiogenesis factor from rat Walker 256 carcinoma: An experimental investigation and review, *Experientia,* 41, 1, 1985.

90. **Folkman, J.,** How is blood vessel growth regulated in normal and neoplastic tissue?, *Cancer Res.,* 46, 467, 1986.

91. **Battiwalla, Z. F. and Shethna, Y. I.,** An antiserum to tumour angiogenesis factor: Therapeutic approach to solid tumours, *Anticancer Res.,* 9, 1809, 1989.

92. **Kim, K. J., Li, B., Winer, J., Armanini, M., Gillett, N., Phillips, H. S., and Ferrara, N.,** Inhibition of vascular endothelial growth factor-induced angiogenesis suppresses tumour growth *in vivo, Nature,* 362, 841, 1993.

93. **Baird, A., Mormede, L., and Bohlen, P.,** Immunoreactive fibroblast growth factor (FGF) in transplantable chondrosarcoma: Inhibition of tumor growth by antibodies to FGF, in *Perspectives in Inflammation, Neoplasia and Vascular Cell Biology,* Eddington, T. S., Kess, R., and Silverstein, S. C., Eds., Liss, New York, 1987.

94. **Ingber, D., Fujita, T., Kishimoto, S., Sudo, K., Kanamaru, T., Brem, H., and Folkman, J.,** Synthetic analogues of fumagillin that inhibit angiogenesis and suppress tumour growth, *Nature,* 348, 555, 1990.

95. **Weidner, N., Semple, J. P., Welch, W. R., and Folkman, J.,** Tumor angiogenesis and metastasis-correlation in invasive breast carcinoma, *N. Engl. J. Med.,* 324, 2, 1991.

96. **Algire, G. H.,** An adaptation of the transparent chamber technique to the mouse, *J. Natl. Cancer Inst.,* 4, 1, 1943.

97. **Goodall, C. M., Sanders, A. G., and Shubik, P.,** Studies of vascular patterns in living tumors with a transparent chamber inserted in a hamster cheek pouch, *J. Natl. Cancer Inst.,* 35, 497, 1965.

98. **Gimbrone, M. A., Jr., Cotran, R. S., Leapman, S. B., and Folkman, J.,** Tumor growth and neovascularization: An experimental model using the rabbit cornea, *J. Natl. Cancer Inst.,* 52, 413, 1974.

99. **Knighton, D. R., Fiegel, V. D., and Phillips, G. D.,** The assay of angiogenesis, *Prog. Clin. Biol. Res.,* 365, 291, 1991.

100. **Wilting, J., Christ, B., and Bokeloh, M.,** A modified chorioallantoic membrane (CAM) assay for qualitative and quantitative study of growth factors. Studies on the effects of carriers, PBS, angiogenin, and bFGF, *Anat. Embryol. Berl.,* 183, 259, 1991.

101. **Hayek, A., Culler, F. L., Beattie, G. M., Lopez, A. D., Cuevas, P., and Baird, A.,** An *in vivo* model for study of the angiogenic effects of basic fibroblast growth factor, *Biochem. Biophys. Res. Commun.,* 147, 876, 1987.

102. **Endrich, B., Asaishi, K., Gotz, A., and Messmer, K.,** Technical report — A new chamber technique for microvascular studies in unanesthetized hamsters, *Res. Exp. Med. Berl.,* 177, 125, 1980.

103. **Tiedeken, J. J. and Rovainen, C. M.,** Fluorescent imaging *in vivo* of developing blood vessels on the optic tectum of Xenopus laevis, *Microvasc. Res.,* 41, 376, 1991.

104. **Albrektsson, T.,** Repair of bone grafts. A vital microscopic and histological investigation in the rabbit, *Scand. J. Plast. Reconstr. Surg.,* 14, 1, 1980.

105. **Runkel, S., Hunter, N., and Milas, L.,** An intradermal assay for quantification and kinetics studies of tumor angiogenesis in mice, *Radiat. Res.,* 126, 237, 1991.

106. **Frank, J., Barker, J. H., Kaneko, S., Joels, C., Ogden, L., Lane, J., Anderson, G. L., and Tobin, G. R.,** *In vivo* analysis of growth factor induced angiogenesis, *Eur. Surg. Res.,* 25, S26, 1993.

107. **Andrade, S. P., Fan, T. P., and Lewis, G. P.,** Quantitative *in vivo* studies on angiogenesis in a rat sponge model, *Br. J. Exp. Pathol.,* 68, 755, 1987.
108. **Robertson, N. E., Discafani, C. M., Downs, E. C., Hailey, J. A., Sarre, O., Runkle, R. L., Jr., Popper, T. L., and Plunkett, M. L.,** A quantitative *in vivo* mouse model used to assay inhibitors of tumor-induced angiogenesis, *Cancer Res.,* 51, 1339, 1991.
109. **Folkman, J. and Haudenschild, C. C.,** Angiogenesis *in vitro, Nature,* 288, 551, 1982.
110. **Ishiwata, I., Ishiwata, C., Soma, M., Naik, D. R., Hashimoto, H., Sudo, T., and Ishikawa, H.,** Effect of tumour angiogenesis factor on proliferation of endothelial cell and tube formation, *Virchows Arch. A. Pathol. Anat. Histopathol.,* 417, 473, 1990.
111. **Kanayasu, T., Morita, I., Nakao-Hayashi, J., Asuwa, N., Fujisawa, C., Ishii, T., Ito, H., and Murota, S.,** Eicosapentaenoic acid inhibits tube formation of vascular endothelial cells *in vitro, Lipids,* 26, 271, 1991.
112. **Moscatelli, D., Flaumenhaft, R., and Saksela, O.,** Interaction of basic fibroblast growth factor with extracellular matrix and receptors, *Ann. N.Y. Acad. Sci.,* 638, 177, 1991.
113. **Tannock, I. F. and Steel, G. G.,** Quantitative techniques for study of the anatomy and function of small blood vessels in tumors, *J. Natl. Cancer Inst.,* 42, 771, 1969.
114. **Meyer, G. T. and McGeachie, J. K.,** Angiogenesis in the developing corpus luteum of pregnant rats: A stereologic and autoradiographic study, *Anat. Rec.,* 222, 18, 1988.
115. **Kaidoh, T., Yasugi, T., and Uehara, Y.,** The microvasculature of the 7,12-dimethylbenz(a)anthracene (DMBA)-induced rat mammary tumour. I. Vascular patterns as visualized by scanning electron microscopy of corrosion casts, *Virchows Arch. A. Pathol. Anat. Histopathol.,* 418, 111, 1991.
116. **Nicosia, R. F., Tchao, R., and Leighton, J.,** Histotypic angiogenesis *in vitro*: Light microscopic, ultrastructural, and radioautographic studies, *In Vitro,* 18, 538, 1982.
117. **Boyden, S. V.,** The chemotactic effect of mixtures of antibody and antigen on polymorphonuclear leukocytes, *J. Exp. Med.,* 115, 453, 1962.
118. **Folkman, J.,** Angiogenesis, in *Thrombosis and Haemostasis*, Verstraete, M., Vermylen, J., Lijnan, R., and Arnout, J., Eds., Leuven University Press, Leuven, 1987.
119. **Hayek, A., Beattie, G. M., Lopez, A. D., and Chen, P.,** The use of digital image processing to quantitate angiogenesis induced by basic fibroblast growth factor and transplanted pancreatic islets, *Microvasc. Res.,* 41, 203, 1991.
120. **Chen, P. C., Kovalcheck, S. W., and Zweifach, B. W.,** Analysis of microvascular network in bulbar conjunctiva by image processing, *Int. J. Microcirc. Clin. Exp.,* 6, 245, 1987.

Chapter 29

Blood Cells and Rheology

Dick W. Slaaf, Geert Jan Tangelder, Mirjam G. A. oude Egbrink, and Robert S. Reneman

CONTENTS

I. INTRODUCTION

Intravital microscopic observation of human skin reveals some characteristics of blood flow in the microcirculation during health and disease. In healthy humans, the capillary diameter in the skin of the nailfold is about 8 μm. Blood flow varies considerably with time and between the various capillaries. Usually, individual red blood cells (RBCs) cannot be seen. In patients with secondary Raynaud's disease, the capillary diameter is dramatically increased (to about 30–60 μm) and blood flow has become so sluggish that aggregates of RBCs can be seen. In some patients with occlusive arterial disease, blood flow has become slow, while the capillary diameter has not changed.[9]

In anesthetized animals, tissues can be transilluminated and higher magnifications used, resulting in better contrast and resolution.[61] Preparations like the tenuissimus muscle, the mesentery, or the cremaster muscle of small animals allow more detailed observation of rheological properties of blood flowing in the microcirculation. Individual RBCs can be seen to deform while passing through the capillaries. One wonders to what extent the presence of cells in blood causes an increase in the resistance to flow in the microcirculation, and whether the properties of the blood itself are constant or dependent on local conditions.

Theoretically, blood flow in the microcirculation differs considerably from blood flow in large vessels, where velocities are high and flow profiles are flattened due to the interaction between pulsatility of flow and inertia. Moreover, in the microcirculation, the entrance length for complete development of the flow profile is never met. In the microcirculation, vessel diameters are small, while blood flow velocities are relatively low and inertial forces are of minor importance.[20] Flow is governed by viscous stresses and pressure gradients. Due to the presence of blood cells, blood can no longer be treated as a Newtonian fluid, i.e., as a fluid with constant, homogeneously distributed properties that are independent of the applied forces and the size of the vessel. In the microcirculation, the non-Newtonian character of blood must be taken into account.

0-8493-4870-6/95/$0.00+$.50

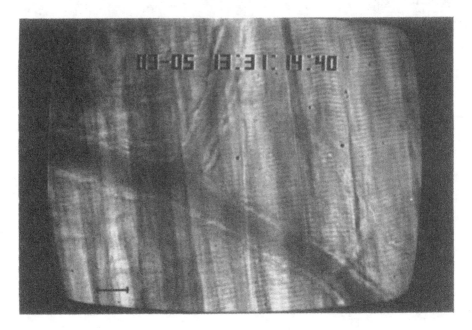

Figure 1 Transverse arteriole (flowing from left to right) of rabbit tenuissimus muscle with major side-branch. Skeletal muscle fibers run from top to bottom and the cross striations of these muscle fibers are clearly visible. Bar represents 20 µm. Recording was made using a saltwater immersion objective (magnification, 25×; numerical aperture, 0.60). Picture taken from video monitor.

Blood is a viscous fluid composed of deformable cells suspended in plasma that contains various proteins and other solutes. RBCs constitute more than 99% of the total volume of cells in blood; white blood cells (WBCs; leukocytes) make up less than 1%, and platelets (thrombocytes) make up even less of the cell volume. Normally, WBCs and platelets exert little effect on the bulk flow properties of blood.

In this chapter, we will describe general flow patterns in the microcirculation and how they may be changed by altered rheological conditions. Properties of the various blood constituents will be discussed in relation to their function and rheology. Finally, we will review several methods to measure rheological properties of blood and blood cells *in vitro*.

II. MICROCIRCULATION

Microvessels are structurally and functionally part of the tissue they supply. Arterioles (small ramifications of the feeding arteries) feed a fine network of capillaries, which are drained by venules. Depending on the requirements of the tissue, different types of networks develop. A "typical" microvascular bed does not really exist.[80] At every arteriolar bifurcation, flow is divided. At these bifurcations, however, the various blood cells are not distributed proportional to flow. Since the RBCs preferentially flow in the center of an arteriole, plasma and platelets are present at higher concentrations near the vessel wall.[67,85] Plasma may preferentially enter oblique side branches (plasma skimming). This results in considerable heterogeneity of the local microvessel hematocrit.[56,86] A similar (screening) effect has been observed for platelets.[42]

Flow in arterioles is usually so fast that the individual blood cells cannot be seen with continuous illumination. The blood presents itself as relatively transparent with streaks (Figure 1). At the level of precapillary arterioles and capillaries, blood flow velocity has

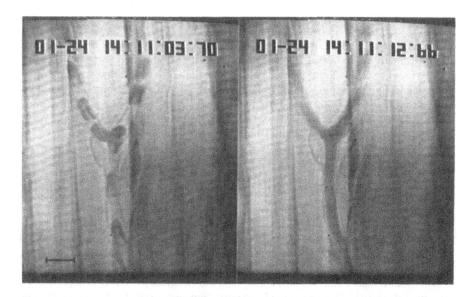

Figure 2 Bifurcating capillary of rabbit tenuissimus muscle during low flow (left) and high flow (right). Note the various shapes of RBCs (left). Bar represents 10 μm. Recording was made using a saltwater immersion objective (magnification, 50×; numerical aperture, 1.00). Pictures taken from video monitor. Time elapsed between both pictures is almost 9 s.

slowed down to about 1 mm/s or less. Individual RBCs can be observed to deform while flowing through the capillary network (Figure 2). In the draining venules, the flow patterns of the various collected streams of blood can be observed to be maintained for quite a distance. Mixing of the bloodstreams does not occur rapidly. WBCs can be observed rolling along the endothelium of venules, a phenomenon not observed in arterioles under control conditions.

Intravital microscopic observation of the circulation in human skin capillaries also reveals some of the dynamics of the microcirculation: capillary perfusion is usually not stationary, but varies with time. Even capillary hematocrit is time dependent due to the varying diameter of the terminal arterioles.[16] The phenomenon of rhythmic variations in perfusion of the terminal vascular bed has been studied extensively in rabbit tenuissimus muscle.[38,47,48,62] Rhythmic changes in diameter (vasomotion) of the feeding and terminal arterioles lead to variations in capillary perfusion (flowmotion) with cycle lengths of 2 to 30 s. The presence or absence of flowmotion can also be studied in humans using laser Doppler flowmetry, a method to assess perfusion in a small sampling volume of tissue usually of about 1 mm^3, but it can be smaller with special probes. The temporal variations in the flow patterns can be analyzed and related to various stages of diseases.[9]

High pressures are required at the input of an organ to supply it with sufficient amounts of blood. Capillary pressure, however, has to be relatively low to protect the thin capillary walls and prevent excessive fluid filtration. The arterioles are the so-called *resistance vessels*: they function as separators of the high- and low-pressure parts of the circulation and regulate the actual perfusion pressure levels in the local tissue. The point at which the steepest drop in pressure occurs, varies with the type of tissue. The use of small glass micropipettes and a servo-nulling technique allows measurement of microvascular pressures.[81] Even in the capillaries, micropressures exhibit heart synchronous pressure pulsations, albeit attenuated due to frictional resistance. In addition, pressure fluctuations due to vasomotion may be found.

III. RHEOLOGY

The energy required to make a fluid flow through a vessel segment does not only depend on the geometry of the vessel, but also on the resistance of the fluid to shearing, i.e., on its (dynamic) viscosity. In the case of a Newtonian fluid, such as plasma, the viscosity is not dependent on the applied forces or the size of the vessel. For a Newtonian fluid, the relationship between steady flow F through a vessel segment of length l and uniform diameter D and the pressure drop ΔP over that segment is given by the Hagen-Poiseuille Law (or more commonly, Poiseuille's Law):

$$F = \frac{\pi D^4 \Delta P}{128 \mu l}$$

where μ is the coefficient of dynamic viscosity of the fluid. Viscosity is defined as the ratio of shear stress (tangential force in the direction of flow per unit of sheared area) and shear rate (velocity gradient between adjacent laminae of flow streams). When in a fluid, the viscosity is independent of the actual values of shear stress and shear rate, the fluid is called Newtonian. For a non-Newtonian fluid such as blood, viscosity is dependent on the actual shear rates. For such a fluid, the term "apparent viscosity" is used to describe the ratio between shear stress and shear rate.

Bifurcations in a blood vessel disturb the local velocity profiles. How fast a velocity profile is restored (fully developed) after the site of disturbance depends on the Reynolds number (N_R) of the flow. The Reynolds number is the ratio of the inertia force and viscous force in the flow, i.e., $N_R = VD\rho/\mu$, where V is average speed of flow, D is vessel diameter, and ρ is density of fluid. In the *macro*circulation, the Reynolds numbers are relatively high.[20] Flattening of the profiles occurs due to nonsteadiness (pulsatility) of flow. Moreover, after disturbances at bifurcations, the velocity profiles never fully develop and this contributes to more pronounced flattening of the profile: the entrance length (the length required for a profile to develop fully) is longer than the distance between bifurcations. Even without disturbances at bifurcations, a fully developed profile is not necessarily a parabola. In the *micro*circulation, the Reynolds numbers are far below unity.[63] The fluid tends to flow in layers (laminae) following smooth streamlines. Within the distance of one vessel diameter, the flow profile of a Newtonian fluid becomes fully developed in small glass tubes.[10] For blood, however, this may not be the case. In the microcirculation, the influence of the pulsatility of flow (although present even in capillaries) is negligible. Flattening of the profiles occurs due to the nonuniform behavior of viscosity. In venules, where flow converges, the profile may not develop as quickly as in arterioles, if flows with different hematocrits merge, since mixing of these flows occurs relatively slowly. The low Reynolds numbers also imply that turbulence cannot occur in the microcirculation.

For a Newtonian fluid, the fully developed stationary profile is parabolic. Velocity is maximal in the center and zero at the wall, satisfying the no-slip condition at the wall. Usually, velocity profiles in the microcirculation are treated as parabolic, since one assumes that the profiles restore within a short distance after a disturbance. The actual profile is almost never assessed, since accurate measurement of the profiles is time-consuming and not always possible. However, in the microcirculation, blood cannot be treated as a Newtonian fluid. Viscosity is not constant, but increases as shear stress and shear rate are reduced, implying that the profile becomes flattened in the center of a vessel and steeper near the wall. Although pulsatile pressures are also present in the microcirculation, this pulsatility does not contribute to the flattening of the profile, since its

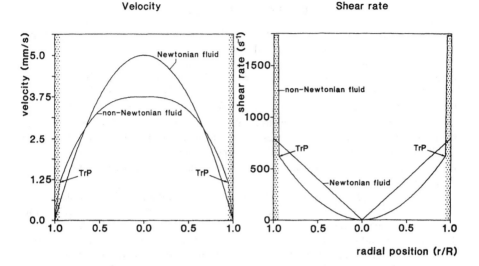

Figure 3 Left: Velocity profile for a Newtonian fluid is parabolic. The profile resulting from an actual fit is flattened as compared with a parabola. The lubricating layer (hatched areas) is present between the transition points (TrP) and the wall. Right: The shear rate is the derivative of velocity. The step at the site of the transition point is in reality a smooth transition. (From Slaaf, D. W., Tangelder, G. J., and Reneman, R. S., Physics of the microcirculation, in *Physics of the Circulation*, Strackee, J. and Westerhof, N., Eds., Springer, Heidelberg, 1993, 387–419.)

influence has become negligible compared with the viscous forces; the Reynolds number is low! Using labeled platelets as markers of flow, Tangelder and co-workers[68] were able to assess actual arteriolar velocity profiles in detail. Their findings indicate the existence of a thin lubricating layer (thickness 0.5–1.3 μm) of near-plasma viscosity at the wall (Figure 3, left). Flow velocity in this layer drops to zero at the wall. The profile in the core appears to be flattened as compared to a parabola.

Blood cells are dispersed in proportion to the velocity differences (gradient; shear rate) across the microvessel. Shear rate depends on the actual velocity profile, and is lowest in the center and highest near the wall (Figure 3, right). Endothelial cell function is influenced by the level of shear rate present at the wall, which governs the actual wear and tear exerted on these cells. Tangelder and colleagues[69] estimated in arterioles the wall shear rate from the fitted velocity profiles and obtained values that were at least 2.1 times higher than expected on the basis of a parabolic profile.

By applying Poiseuille's Law to experimental data of blood, one may obtain the apparent blood viscosity, i.e., a viscosity value assuming that blood actually behaves as a Newtonian fluid. Lipowsky and Zweifach[35] measured pressure gradient, volume flow, vascular diameter, and segment length in cat mesenteric arterioles with a diameter of 24 to 47 μm. The computed apparent viscosity ranged from 1.3 to 4 mPa.s, whereas plasma viscosity was 1.3 mPa.s. Apparent viscosity relative to plasma viscosity ranged from 1 to 3, with a median value of 2.4. Apparent viscosity is lowest in vessels of about 10 μm in diameter.[86] Apparent viscosity may also be derived from measured velocity profiles.[69] The relative apparent viscosity obtained in that way in arterioles (median: 2.12) compares well with the values obtained using micropressure measurements. The actual contribution of the RBCs to apparent viscosity depends on their distribution across the microvessel, their aggregation tendency, and deformability.

IV. RED BLOOD CELLS

Systemic hematocrit, which in practice is the relative volume of RBCs, varies in humans usually between 35 and 45%. The actual shape of RBCs depends on the forces exerted on them. When unstressed, for instance after sedimentation in a counting chamber, normal human RBCs are biconcave disks with approximately a diameter of 8 μm, and a thickness of 2 μm at the thickest point and 1 μm at the thinnest point. While passing through capillaries, RBCs can change their shape remarkably well. The RBCs flow through the capillaries in an asymmetric way. The membrane of the RBC often rotates relatively quickly around the cytoplasm (tank treading motion[18]) due to asymmetric distribution of shear stresses on the cell. This optimal adaptation to local flow conditions is combined with simultaneous mixing of the intracellular oxygenated and deoxygenated hemoglobin.

Due to an excess surface area in relation to its volume, the RBC is like a plastic bag that can be deformed in almost any shape. The mean surface area of human RBCs is 140 μm^2 and encloses the mean corpuscular volume of 90 μm^3, which is 42% less than the 156 μm^3 that could be enclosed if the RBC were a sphere.[13] The combination of excess surface area, high fluidity of its contents, and a high deformability of its cell membrane makes the RBC so highly deformable. As can be observed *in vivo*, for example in the spleen,[57] an RBC can pass through short, tiny pores of less than 1 μm in diameter because enough membrane surface area is available to allow for all required folds on either side of the pore to transport its content. When an RBC passes through a capillary, however, the volume-to-surface area ratio can still become a limiting factor. Moving through a small, tapering glass capillary, the length of an RBC will increase until the RBC becomes completely cylindrical with the same diameter as the tube. The membrane of the RBC is then completely stretched without folds. One can calculate that a human RBC cannot pass through capillaries smaller in diameter than 2.7 μm,[11] because the membrane area can hardly expand after the excess membrane has been used.[14]

When RBCs flow through capillaries, one observes strong deformations of RBCs at bifurcations. Deformability is an important rheological parameter for capillary flow. When the surface-to-volume ratio is decreased (for instance, due to osmotic swelling), the resistance to flow at the level of the smallest vessels will be increased. If the viscosity of the internal fluid of an RBC increases, due to an increase in mean corpuscular hemoglobin concentration or an alteration in the rheological properties of the hemoglobin (e.g., deoxygenation of sickle cell hemoglobin), RBC deformability decreases. Also, changes in the membrane properties itself may lead to a reduction in RBC deformability (e.g., RBC shape changes as in echinocytes). Several methods have been developed to measure RBC deformability *in vitro* (see below).

The velocity gradients present in the microcirculation disperse the RBCs. At low shear rates, the RBCs have the tendency to form aggregates: at low perfusion pressures, one can observe rouleaux of RBCs as they progress through the microvessels. Bridging between adjacent cells is caused by fibrinogen, globulins, or other macromolecules. Aggregation represents a minimization of energy at the cell surface; the macromolecular bridging energy is counterbalanced by the electrostatic repulsive energy of the negatively charged sialic acid on the RBC membranes and the work done by shear stress during flow. At very low shear rates, normal RBCs do not differ from hardened RBCs with respect to aggregate formation. A small shear rate may enhance RBC aggregation by promoting cell-cell contact. Increases in shear stress successively cause rouleaux disaggregation, deformation of the dispersed RBCs, and alignment of their major axes with the direction of flow. Several *in vitro* methods have been developed to measure RBC aggregation tendency (see below).

RBCs are not uniformly distributed across a microvessel. The concentration is greatest in the center and relatively low near the wall. Since RBCs flow preferentially in areas with the higher flow velocities, mean RBC velocity is higher than mean plasma velocity. As a consequence, mean local RBC concentration is reduced, since otherwise accumulation of RBCs would occur in the microcirculation. This so-called Fåhraeus effect is strongest in microvessels of about 10–15 µm in diameter. Plasma skimming and interactions between vessels in a network also contributes to the Fåhraeus effect.[51]

V. LEUKOCYTES

Leukocytes make up less than 1% of the total blood cell volume in humans. The diameter of a WBC floating in plasma varies from 6 to 7.5 µm. In blood smears, after settling on a glass surface, leukocytes are flattened; they have a pancake-like appearance and their apparent diameters have increased to 10 to 15 µm. The membrane surface area of leukocytes is 80 to 130% larger than required to enclose their volume. However, leukocytes are less deformable than RBCs that have an excess surface area of only 44%. In case large deformations are needed, the WBC's nucleus may become an important limiting factor.[11] Leukocytes exert little influence on bulk rheological properties of normal blood in large vessels. However, leukocytes may plug capillaries shortly or for longer periods of time during low perfusion states. The transportation of leukocytes through organs is facilitated by the presence of shunt vessels in some organs; here, leukocytes tend to bypass the true capillaries where they might have difficulties passing and thus might hamper flow. In arterioles, leukocytes preferentially flow in the center; at bifurcations, they tend to enter the vessels with the highest flow velocity.[33]

When flow in a tube is rapid, leukocytes flow close to the central part of the stream due to their size.[76] At low flow rates, the leukocytes flow mainly in the marginal stream due to the formation of RBC aggregates. This margination of leukocytes during low-flow states would increase their chances of entering and blocking side-branches at the level of the capillaries. Under control conditions, however, leukocyte plugging is a rare phenomenon and of too short a duration to compromise tissue perfusion.[6] In leukemia, however, the increased number of leukocytes and their increased rigidity may lead to significant disturbances of capillary perfusion.[34] In hemorrhagic shock, the reduction in driving pressure leads to a large increase in the number of leukocytes trapped in alveolar capillaries in the lungs of cat and dog.[37] Moreover, the number of leukocytes adhering to the endothelium in arterioles and venules is increased, as observed in histologic sections.[82,83] Intravital microscopic observations have indeed demonstrated that hemorrhagic shock produces adherence to vessel walls and blocking of capillaries in skeletal muscle.[6] Leukocytes contribute approximately 20% to the resistance to blood flow in rat gracilis muscle.[64] An increase in leukocyte count of 100%, as has been found in mature spontaneously hypertensive rats, might significantly contribute to the elevated blood pressure of these rats.[59]

In venules, leukocytes may be observed rolling along the endothelium (Figure 4). In this situation, they move with a distinctly lower velocity than the other blood cells. Rolling is considered to be the first step in their interaction with the vessel wall during inflammatory processes,[77] preceding prolonged adhesion, diapedesis, and extravascular migration. In arterioles, leukocyte rolling is usually not observed,[46,71] but it can be induced in these vessels, for example, by exposing the experimental animals to cigarette smoke.[32] In skin, leukocyte rolling can be observed under physiological conditions.[36] This may indicate a constant vigilance of the host defense mechanisms in the skin. Rolling of leukocytes in the skin is increased under unphysiological conditions. In deeper tissues such as the mesentery, leukocyte rolling might be absent under normal circumstances.[17] However, exteriorization induces rolling in this tissue. In exteriorized mesentery, almost all rolling leukocytes are granulocytes.[72] In spleen, rolling of lymphocytes also has been observed.[57] Which subtypes of leukocytes actually roll in skin is as yet unknown.

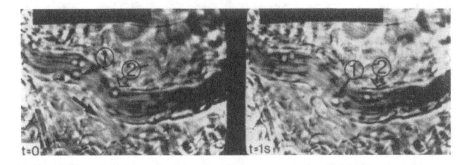

Figure 4 Venule (32–33 µm diameter) with rolling WBCs in rabbit mesentery. Bar represents 50 µm. In 1 s, leukocytes marked 1 and 2 moved less than 50 µm. Direction of flow is indicated by arrow. (From Tangelder, G. J. and Arfors, K.-E., *Blood*, 77, 1565–1571, 1991.)

Rolling leukocytes usually do not exert an appreciable influence on local resistance to flow. However, in the presence of a prominent inflammatory response, rolling and firm adhesion of leukocytes may indeed substantially increase local resistance.[28]

VI. PLATELETS

Platelets are the smallest cellular elements in the blood. In mammals, they are cytoplasmic fragments, originating from megakaryocytes in bone marrow and lung.[49] Nonactivated platelets are disk-shaped, with an average diameter of about 3 µm and a thickness of 0.6 to 1.0 µm. They constitute even less of the cellular blood volume than leukocytes.

Under normal conditions, circulating platelets come frequently close to and in apparent contact with the arteriolar vessel wall,[67,68] but do not stick to the endothelium. When a vessel is damaged, however, platelets are rapidly activated. They immediately adhere to the injured vessel wall (adhesion) and to each other (aggregation), forming a plug or thrombus, which stops bleeding. The activated platelets lose their discoid shape and form pseudopods (shape change), secrete to a varying degree the contents of their secretory vesicles (release), and promote blood coagulation at their surface (procoagulant activity). This sequence of events has been reviewed by several authors (e.g., see References 70 and 84). Although free flowing platelets have little influence on flow .esistance, formation of a thrombus might create a stenosis of such a magnitude that resistance to flow is severely increased.[19,44]

The knowledge of platelet behavior in flowing blood was until recently almost exclusively based on findings from theoretical models and *in vitro* experiments, the latter employing rigid spheres and disks. An inward radial migration was predicted for the flexible RBCs flowing in tubes.[21,23] Blood platelets, by contrast, would exhibit this effect considerably less.[22] Because of the RBC crowding in the center of the tube, it was assumed that the lighter platelets would be dispersed from the center of the vessel and this would result in higher platelet concentrations near the wall. Studies performed in perfusion chambers have shown that platelet deposition on subendothelium increases with hematocrit.[75] In a perfusion chamber, both an increase in RBC size and a decrease in RBC deformability[1,2] enhance platelet transport toward the wall.

Platelet behavior *in vivo* could be studied after development of a method to visualize them individually while they flow in a microvessel amid the excess of RBCs; to this end, the platelets were labeled *in vivo* with a fluorescent dye and observed with fluorescence microscopy.[65,66] Although in arterioles, platelets can be seen tumbling, especially near the vessel wall,[69] they tend to align with flow. This tendency is strongest near the wall.[73] Toward the center of the arteriole, their orientation is more random. Since shear rate increases from the center of the vessel toward the wall, this finding implies that in arterioles the tendency to align with flow increases with shear rate.

Interestingly, subsequent studies with fluorescently labeled platelets indicate that platelet distribution greatly differs in arterioles and venules.[85] In the vessel center, the relative platelet concentration is significantly lower in arterioles than in venules. Near the wall, the relative platelet concentration is higher in arterioles than in venules, while in the venules, a partial exclusion of platelets close to the wall could be observed. This effect is not due to leukocyte rolling.

In arterioles, where the concentration of the platelets is about two times higher near the wall than in the center of the vessel,[67] about 70% of the platelets are within the high shear domain near the wall. Hence, in case of injury, a relatively high percentage of platelets, which at the same time have a relatively low velocity, will come into contact with activating agents released from the damaged arteriolar wall or from the activated platelets themselves. Moreover, the wall shear rates will even be higher in case of bleeding or intravascular stenosis caused by a thrombus.[58] High shear rates, up to a value of $10,000$ s^{-1}, have been reported to stimulate in vitro the release reaction and aggregation of platelets.[5,74] However, such in vitro experiments do not take into account the fact that high levels of shear rate also influence endothelial functions: they stimulate the endothelial production of the platelet-inhibiting agents prostacyclin and nitric oxide.[55] This may explain why in vivo, at a site of wall injury in microvessels, no relation is found between the level of wall shear rate, which may be as high as $16,000$ s^{-1} in a stenosed vessel segment on the one hand, and the number of emboli produced, which is a measure of platelet aggregation, on the other.[45]

Various methods have been developed to study platelet-vessel wall interactions following vessel wall injury in vivo by direct observation. The use of the thermal energy of a laser to induce platelet-vessel wall interactions has been claimed to be the most accurate and standardized method. The laser beam, which can traverse the optical system of the intravital microscope, is focused inside the vessel close to the wall.[4,60,78] Proper positioning appears to be critical. It is questionable to which degree vessel wall damage is actually induced in this way; ultrastructural and functional studies suggest that intravascular platelet reactions might primarily be caused by adenosine diphosphate (ADP) released from heat-coagulated RBCs.[29,80]

A different kind of platelet-vessel wall interaction can be induced by mechanical injury. Puncture of an arteriolar or venular vessel wall with a glass micropipette results in a short bleeding and induction of a thromboembolic reaction.[43] Within 1 s after puncture, a thrombus is formed, which is stationary and consists of tightly packed platelets that are probably strongly activated. Subsequently, newly passing platelets are still activated, although more weakly. They adhere to the thrombus and form a loosely packed mass on its downstream side. From time to time, this downstream part embolizes, leaving the shape of the original thrombus virtually unchanged. This process of embolization lasts significantly longer in arterioles than in venules of the mesentery, suggesting different endothelial functioning in both vessel types. No direct relationship has been found between any of the thromboembolic parameters and wall shear rate in both arterioles and venules.[43,44]

A similar kind of thromboembolic reaction is evoked by microsurgery of small arteries. In fact, thromboembolism is considered to be the primary cause of early failure of microsurgical procedures. Emboli, released from an arterial repair site, enter the microcirculation[3] and, during the first hour, significantly decrease perfusion of the capillary bed in the affected tissue,[7] either by direct obstruction of arterioles or capillaries, or by the release of vasoconstricting agents. However, emboli often break apart after a short period of time, causing restoration of flow. This suggests that in an embolus, the aggregation forces between adjacent platelets are rather weak and easily disrupted; it is not clear which mechanism is responsible for this disruption.

VII. CLINICAL RHEOLOGY

Organ perfusion is not only determined by the condition of the vasculature, but also by the properties of the blood itself. Several methods have been developed to measure various properties of blood and its constituents. Any reduction in deformability of RBCs results in an increase in resistance to flow. A good review of methods and applications is found in Reference 12. The clinical importance of RBC deformability has been reviewed by Mokken and colleagues.[41] In this section, a short overview is given.

A. PLASMA VISCOSITY

Blood plasma is a Newtonian fluid. In humans, its viscosity is 1.2 to 1.3 mPa.s at 37°C. Plasma viscosity is mainly a function of the concentration of large proteins like fibrinogen and some of the globulins. Plasma viscosity is usually calculated from the time that a fluid needs to travel through a standardized capillary over a certain distance at a given driving pressure.[27] Reference fluids with known viscosity are used to calibrate the instrument. Temperature control is essential and should be set at body temperature. Reproducibility of the method is excellent (CV < 1%). Plasma should be stored at room temperature in closed containers and not be frozen, since precipitation of proteins may occur. In some cases, differences in plasma viscosity between patients and healthy controls may be significant; but in terms of circulatory consequences, the question is whether the obtained differences are sufficiently important as compared to changes in other parameters, e.g., related to the vascular network.

B. BLOOD VISCOSITY

Blood is a non-Newtonian fluid, which means that its viscosity depends on the actual shear rates, which in a microvessel vary from center to wall. The average viscosity of blood flowing through a microvessel is called its *apparent viscosity*. Measurement of whole blood viscosity should be performed if possible at several standardized shear rates. No reference method for its measurement exists. In rotational viscometers, a cone is rotated on top of a stationary plate or a cylinder is rotated within a cylinder. In both cases, a thin layer of blood is sheared. In the first apparatus, the resulting shear rates are homogeneous; in the second machine, the variation in shear rate is limited. Shear rate is determined by geometry and by the rate of rotation. Shear stress is calculated from torque and geometry.[12] Measurements show that at a given temperature, viscosity is a function of shear rate, plasma viscosity, and the concentration, deformability, and aggregation tendency of the RBCs. Relative apparent viscosity (relative to plasma viscosity) increases exponentially with increasing hematocrit, especially for hematocrits above 45%. Standardization can be achieved by providing data at native hematocrit and at 45%. The variation of blood viscosity with shear rate at a given hematocrit and plasma viscosity is attributable to shear-dependent changes in cell deformation. Whole blood viscosity data actually represent the integrated effects of these factors and do not allow for a more detailed interpretation.

C. RED BLOOD CELL AGGREGATION

Aggregation between RBCs occurs under conditions with low shear rate or stasis. A finite yield stress has to be overcome before flow will occur.[52] Optical density of blood depends on flow.[31] This principle is applied in the Myrenne optical aggregometer. Light transmission is measured during shearing of 20 µl blood at 600 s^{-1} in a cone-and-plate device, and subsequently during aggregation when rotation has been reduced to 5 s^{-1} or has stopped. Aggregation is measured as the area under the curve during the first 10 s of the aggregation process. One test takes about half a minute. The data cannot be calibrated since no suspension standards of know aggregation are available.

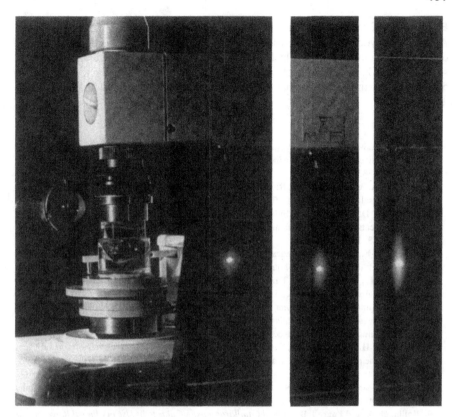

Figure 5 Composite picture showing details of laser extension mounted on viscometer. The diffraction patterns of cells at rest, and under medium and high shear stress (from left to right), are also shown. Note that while the elongation of the RBCs occurs in the horizontal plane, the elongation of the diffraction pattern is vertically oriented. (From Hardeman, M. R., Goedhart, P., and Breederveld, D., *Clin. Chim. Acta*, 165, 227–234, 1987.)

D. BLOOD FILTRATION AND RBC DEFORMABILITY

RBC deformability can be measured by driving an RBC suspension through a filter and calculating the flow properties from the pressure-flow data.[53,54] The shear stresses exerted on the RBCs are determined by the driving pressure. Since filters are not uniform, each filter has to be calibrated, for instance, by measuring the flow of the suspending fluid alone. At a hematocrit of more than 25%, cell-cell interactions influence the outcome.[12] At a hematocrit of less than 15%, the individual RBC deformability is the major determinant.

Various methods are available to measure deformability of individual RBCs. One way to measure its deformability is to aspirate an RBC by a micropipette.[15] The negative pressure required to suck part of the RBC into a micropipette is evaluated. Deformability can also be assessed with the single erythrocyte rigidometer. The passage time of RBCs through a small pore under a shear stress of about 3 Pa is determined.[30] The result is given as a histogram of passage times. Using a counter-rotating cone-plate Rheoscope, the deformations of individual RBCs can be observed directly.[50] When a rotational viscometer is combined with laser diffraction ellipsometry, the average deformability of a sample of RBCs can be assessed from the ratio of the long and short axis of the resulting diffraction pattern[8,24,25] (see Figure 5). The same instrument also may be modified to assess RBC aggregation.[26]

E. PHOTOHEMOLYSIS

A microhemolytic assay may be used to detect differences in composition and strength of the RBC membrane.[39,40] Light activation of a photoactive compound present in a solution of RBCs produces hemolysis. Differences in rate of hemolysis and time to reach 50% of the maximal response may be used to characterize alterations in RBCs.

REFERENCES

1. **Aarts, P. A. M. M., Bolhuis, P. A., Sakariassen, K. S., Heethaar, R. M., and Sixma, J. J.,** Red blood cell size is important for adherence of blood platelets to artery subendothelium, *Blood*, 62, 214–220, 1983.
2. **Aarts, P. A. M. M., Heethaar, R. M., and Sixma, J. J.,** Red blood cell deformability influences platelet-vessel wall interaction in flowing blood, *Blood*, 64, 1228–1233, 1984.
3. **Acland, R. D., Anderson, G., Siemionow, M., and McCabe, S.,** Direct *in vivo* observations of embolic events in the microcirculation distal to a small-vessel anastomosis, *Plast. Reconstr. Surg.*, 84, 280–288, 1989.
4. **Arfors, K.-E., Dhall, D. P., Engeset, J., Hint, H., Matheson, N. A., and Tangen, O.,** Biolaser endothelial trauma as a means of quantifying platelet activity *in vivo*, *Nature*, 218, 887–888, 1968.
5. **Badimon, L., Badimon, J. J., Turitto, V. T., and Fuster, V.,** Thrombosis: Studies under flow conditions, *Ann. N.Y. Acad. Sci.*, 516, 527–540, 1987.
6. **Bagge, U. and Braide, M.,** Leukocyte plugging of capillaries *in vivo*, in *White Blood Cells. Morphology and Rheology as Related to Function*, Bagge, U., Born, G. V. R., and Gaehtgens, P., Eds., Martinus Nijhoff, The Hague, 1982, 89–102.
7. **Barker, J. H., Acland, R. D., Anderson, G. L., and Patel, J.,** Microcirculatory disturbances following the passage of emboli in an experimental free-flap model, *Plast. Reconstr. Surg.*, 90, 95–102, 1992.
8. **Bessis, M. and Mohandas, N.,** A diffractiometric method for the measurement of cellular deformability, *Blood Cells*, 1, 307–313, 1975.
9. **Bollinger, A. and Fagrell, B.,** *Cinical Capillaroscopy. A Guide to its Use in Clinical Research and Practice*, Hogrefe and Huber, Toronto, 1990.
10. **Caro, C. G., Pedley, T. J., Schroter, R. C., and Seed, W. A.,** *The Mechanics of the Circulation*, Oxford University Press, Oxford, 1978.
11. **Chien, S., Usami, S., and Skalak, R.,** Blood flow in small tubes, in *Handbook of Physiology*, Sect. 2, The Cardiovascular System, Vol. 4, Microcirculation, Part 1, chap. 6, Renkin, E. M. and Michel, C. C., Eds., American Physiological Society, Bethesda, MD, 1984, 217–249.
12. **Chien, S., Dormandy, J., Ernst, E., and Matrai, A.,** *Clinical Hemorheology. Applications in Cardiovascular and Hematological Disease, Diabetes, Surgery and Gynecology*, Martinus Nijhoff, Dordrecht, 1987.
13. **Evans, E. A. and Fung, Y. C.,** Improved measurements of the erythrocyte geometry, *Microvasc. Res.*, 4, 335–347, 1972.
14. **Evans, E. A., Waugh, R., and Melnik, L.,** Elastic area compressibility modulus of red cell membrane, *Biophys. J.*, 16, 585–595, 1976.
15. **Evans, E. A. and Skalak, R.,** *Mechanics and Thermodynamics of Biomembranes*, CRC Press, Boca Raton, FL, 1980.
16. **Fagrell, B., Intaglietta, M., and Östergren, J.,** Relative hematocrit in human skin capillaries and its relation to capillary blood flow velocity, *Microvasc. Res.*, 20, 327–335, 1980.
17. **Fiebig, E., Ley, K., and Arfors, K.-E.,** Rapid leukocyte accumulation by "spontaneous" rolling and adhesion in the exteriorized rabbit mesentery, *Int. J. Microcirc. Clin. Exp.*, 10, 127–144, 1991.
18. **Fischer, T. M., Stoehr-Liesen, M., and Schmid-Schonbein, H.,** The red cell as a fluid droplet: Tank tread-like motion of human erythrocyte membrane in shear flow, *Science*, 202, 894–896, 1978.
19. **Folts, J. D., Gallagher, K., and Roew, G. G.,** Blood flow reductions in stenosed canine coronary arteries: Vasospasm or platelet aggregation?, *Circulation*, 65, 248–255, 1982.
20. **Fung, Y. C.,** Biodynamics, *Circulation*, Springer, New York, 1984.
21. **Goldsmith, H. L.,** Red cell motions and wall interactions in tube flow, *Fed. Proc.*, 30, 1578–1588, 1971.

22. **Goldsmith, H. L.,** The flow of model particles and blood cells and its relation to thrombogenesis, in *Progress in Hemostasis and Thrombosis,* Vol. 1, Spaet, T. H., Ed., Grune and Stratton, New York, 1972, 97–139.

23. **Goldsmith, H. L.,** The microrheology of human erythrocyte suspensions. Applied mechanics, *Proc. 13th Int. Congr. Theoret. Appl. Mech.,* Beeker, E. and Mikhailov, G. K., Eds., Springer, Berlin, 1973, 85–103.

24. **Groner, W., Mohandas, N., and Bessis, M.,** New optical technique for measuring erythrocyte deformability with the ektacytometer, *Clin. Chem.,* 26(10), 1435–1442, 1980.

25. **Hardeman, M. R., Goedhart, P., and Breederveld, D.,** Laser diffraction ellipsometry of erythrocytes under controlled shear stress using a rotational viscometer, *Clin. Chim. Acta.,* 165, 227–234, 1987.

26. **Hardeman, M. R., Bauersachs, R. M., and Meiselman, H. J.,** RBC laser diffractometry and RBC aggregometry with a rotational viscometer: Comparison with rheoscope and Myrenne aggregometer, *Clin. Hemorheol.,* 8, 581–593, 1988.

27. **Harkness, J.,** A new instrument for the measurement of plasma viscosity, *Lancet,* 2, 280–284, 1963.

28. **House, S. D. and Lipowsky, H. H.,** Leukocyte-endothelium adhesion: Microhemodynamics in mesentery of the cat, *Microvasc. Res.,* 34, 363–379, 1987.

29. **Hovig, T., McKenzie, F. N., and Arfors, K.-E.,** Measurement of the platelet response to laser-induced microvascular injury. Ultrastructural studies, *Thromb. Diath. Haemorrh.,* 32, 695–703, 1974.

30. **Kiesewetter, H., Dauer, U., Teitel, P., Schmid-Schönbein, H., and Trapp, R.,** The single erythrocyte rigidometer (SER) as a reference for RBC deformability, *Biorheology,* 19, 737–753, 1982.

31. **Klose, H. J., Volger, E., Brechtelsbauer, H., Heinich, L., and Schmid-Schönbein, H.,** Microrheology and light transmission of blood. I. The photometric effects of red cell aggregation and cell orientation, *Pflügers Arch.,* 333, 126–139, 1972.

32. **Lehr, H. A., Kress, E., and Menger, M. D.,** Involvement of 5-lipoxygenase products in cigarette smoke-induced leukocyte/endothelium interaction in hamsters, *Int. J. Microcirc. Clin. Exp.,* 12, 61–73, 1993.

33. **Ley, K., Pries, A. R., and Gaehtgens, P.,** Preferential distribution of leukocytes in rat mesentery microvessel networks, *Eur. J. Physiol. (Pflügers Arch.),* 412, 93–100, 1988.

34. **Lichtman, M. A.,** Rheology of leukocytes, leukocyte suspensions and blood in leukemia, *J. Clin. Invest.,* 52, 350–358, 1973.

35. **Lipowsky, H. H. and Zweifach, B. W.,** Methods for the simultaneous measurement of pressure differentials and flow in single unbranched vessels of the microcirculation for rheological studies, *Microvasc. Res.,* 14, 345–361, 1977.

36. **Mayrovitz, H.,** Leukocyte rolling: A prominent feature of venules in intact skin of anesthetized hairless mice, *Am. J. Physiol.,* 262, H157–H161, 1992.

37. **Mellander, S. and Lewis, D. H.,** Effect of hemorrhagic shock on the reactivity of resistance and capacitance vessels and on capillary filtration transfer in cat skeletal muscle, *Circ. Res.,* 13, 105–118, 1963.

38. **Meyer, J. U., Lindbom, L., and Intaglietta, M.,** Coordinated diameter oscillations at arteriolar bifurcations in skeletal muscle, *Am. J. Physiol.,* 253, H568–H573, 1987.

39. **Miller, F. N., Tangelder, G. J., Slaaf, D. W., and Reneman, R. S.,** Use of microphotohemolysis to distinguish differences in erythrocyte treatments, *Blood Cells,* 17, 555–566, 1991.

40. **Miller, F. N., Tangelder, G. J., Slaaf, D. W., and Reneman, R. S.,** Quantitation of erythrocyte photohemolysis by light microscopy, *Blood Cells,* 17, 567–579, 1991.

41. **Mokken, F. Ch., Kedaria, M., Henny, Ch. P., Hardeman, M. R., and Gelb, A. W.,** The clinical importance of erythrocyte deformability, a hemorrheological parameter, *Ann. Hematol.,* 64, 113–122, 1992.

42. **Öfjord, E. S. and Clausen, G.,** Relative flow of blood cells, platelets and microspheres in outer and inner renal cortex, *Am. J. Physiol.,* 251, H242–H246, 1986.

43. **oude Egbrink, M. G. A., Tangelder, G. J., Slaaf, D. W., and Reneman, R. S.,** Thromboembolic reaction following wall puncture in arterioles and venules of the rabbit mesentery, *Thromb. Haemost.,* 59, 23–28, 1988.

44. **oude Egbrink, M. G. A., Tangelder, G. J., Slaaf, D. W., and Reneman, R. S.,** Fluid dynamics and the thromboembolic reaction in mesenteric arterioles and venules, *Am. J. Physiol.,* 260, H1826–H1833, 1991.

45. **oude Egbrink, M. G. A., Tangelder, G. J., Slaaf, D. W., and Reneman, R. S.,** Wall shear rate and blood cell vessel wall interactions in microvessels, *Rev. Port. Hemorreol.,* 5(Suppl. 2), 133–139, 1991.

46. **oude Egbrink, M. G. A., Tangelder, G. J., Slaaf, D. W., and Reneman, R. S.,** Influence of platelet-vessel wall interactions on leukocyte rolling *in vivo, Circ. Res.,* 70, 355–363, 1992.

47. **Oude Vrielink, H. H. E., Slaaf, D. W., Tangelder, G. J., and Reneman, R. S.,** Changes in vasomotion pattern and local arteriolar resistance during stepwise pressure reduction, *Pflügers Arch. (Eur. J. Physiol.),* 414, 571–578, 1989.

48. **Oude Vrielink, H. H. E., Slaaf, D. W., Tangelder, G. J., Weijmer-van Velzen, S., and Reneman, R. S.,** Analysis of vasomotion waveform changes during pressure reduction and adenosine application, *Am. J. Physiol.,* 258, H29–H37, 1990.

49. **Pennington, D. G.,** Thrombopoiesis, in *Haemostasis and Thrombosis,* Bloom, A. L. and Thomas, D. P., Eds., Churchill Livingstone, Edinburgh, 1987, 1–19.

50. **Pfafferott, C., Nash, G. B., and Meiselman, H. J.,** Red blood cell deformability in shear flow, *Biophys. J.,* 47, 695–704, 1985.

51. **Pries, A. R., Ley, K., and Gaehtgens, P.,** Generalization of the Fåhraeus principle for microvascular networks, *Am. J. Physiol.,* 251, H1324–H1332, 1986.

52. **Rampling, M. W.,** Red cell aggregation and yield stress, in *Clinical Blood Rheology,* Vol. 1, Lowe, G. D. O., Ed., CRC Press, Boca Raton, FL, 1988, 43–64.

53. **Reid, H. L., Barnes, A. J., Lock, P. J., Dormandy, J. A., Dormandy, T. L.,** A simple method for measuring erythrocyte deformability, *J. Clin. Pharmacol.,* 29, 855–858, 1976.

54. **Reinhart, W. H., Usami, S., Schmalzer, E. A., Lee, M. M. L., and Chien, S.,** Evaluation of red blood cell filterability test: Influences of pore size, hematocrit level, and flow rate, *J. Lab. Clin. Med.,* 104, 501–516, 1984.

55. **Rubanyi, G. M., Romero, J. C., and Vanhoutte, P. M.,** Flow-induced release of endothelium-derived relaxing factor, *Am. J. Physiol.,* 250, H1145–H1149, 1986.

56. **Sarelius, I. H. and Duling, B. R.,** Direct measurement of microvessel hematocrit, red cell flux, velocity, and transit time, *Am. J. Physiol.,* 243, H1018–1026, 1982

57. **Schmidt, E. E., MacDonald, I. C., and Groom, A. C.,** Interactions of leukocytes with vessel walls and with other blood cells, studied by high-resolution intravital videomicroscopy of spleen, *Microvasc. Res.,* 40, 99–117, 1990.

58. **Schmid-Schönbein, H., Rieger, H., and Fischer, T.,** Fluid-dynamic boundary conditions for thrombotic processes in high shear environments *in vivo,* in *Blood Vessels: Problems Arising at the Border of Natural and Artificial Vessels,* Effert, S. and Meyer-Erkelenz, J. D., Eds., Springer, Berlin, 1976, 57–63.

59. **Schmid-Schönbein, G. W., Seiffge, D., DeLano, F. A., Shen, K., and Zweifach, B. W.,** Leukocyte counts and activation in spontaneously hypertensive and normotensive rats, *Hypertension,* 17, 323–330, 1991.

60. **Seiffge, D. and Kremer, E.,** Influence of ADP, blood flow velocity, and vessel diameter on the laser-induced thrombus formation, *Thromb. Res.,* 42, 331–341, 1986.

61. **Slaaf, D. W., Jongsma, F. H. M., Tangelder, G. J., and Reneman, R. S.,** Characteristics of optical systems for intravital microscopy, in *Microcirculatory Technology,* Baker, C. H. and Nastuk, W. L., Eds., Academic Press, Orlando, 1986, 211–228.

62. **Slaaf, D. W., Oude Vrielink, H. H. E., Tangelder, G. J., and Reneman, R. S.,** Vasomotion under altered perfusion conditions, *Prog. Appl. Microcirc.,* 15, 75–86, 1989.

63. **Slaaf, D. W., Tangelder, G. J., and Reneman, R. S.,** Physics of the microcirculation, in *Physics of the Circulation,* Strackee, J. and Westerhof, N., Eds., Springer, Heidelberg, 1993, 387–419.

64. **Sutton, D. W. and Schmid-Schönbein, G. W.,** Elevation of organ resistance due to leukocyte perfusion, *Am. J. Physiol.,* 262, H1646–H1650, 1992.

65. **Tangelder, G. J., Slaaf, D. W., and Reneman, R. S.,** Fluorescent labelling of blood platelets *in vivo, Thromb. Res.,* 28, 803–820, 1982.

66. **Tangelder, G. J., Slaaf, D. W., and Reneman, R. S.,** Localization within a thin optical section of fluorescent blood platelets flowing in a microvessel, *Microvasc. Res.,* 23, 214–230, 1982.

67. **Tangelder, G. J., Slaaf, D. W., Teirlinck, H. C., and Reneman, R. S.,** Distribution of blood platelets flowing in arterioles, *Am. J. Physiol.*, 248, H318–H323, 1985.
68. **Tangelder, G. J., Slaaf, D. W., Muijtjens, A. M. M., Arts, T., oude Egbrink, M. G. A., and Reneman, R. S.,** Velocity profiles of blood platelets and red blood cells flowing in arterioles of the rabbit mesentery, *Circ. Res.*, 59, 505–514, 1986.
69. **Tangelder, G. J., Slaaf, D. W., Arts, T., and Reneman, R. S.,** Wall shear rate in arterioles *in vivo*: Least estimates from platelet velocity profiles, *Am. J. Physiol.*, 254, H1059–H1064, 1988.
70. **Tangelder, G. J., oude Egbrink, M. G. A., Slaaf, D. W., and Reneman, R. S.,** Blood platelets: An overview, *J. Reconstruc. Microsurg.*, 5, 167–171, 1989.
71. **Tangelder, G. J. and Arfors, K.-E.,** Inhibition of leukocyte rolling in venules by protamine and sulphated polysaccharides, *Blood*, 77, 1565–1571, 1991.
72. **Tangelder, G. J., oude Egbrink, M. G. A., Arfors, K.-E., Slaaf, D. W., and Reneman, R. S.,** Interactions between marginated granulocytes, platelets and venular endothelium *in vivo*, in *Vascular Medicine*, Boccalon, H., Ed., Elsevier Amsterdam, 1993, 353–357.
73. **Teirlinck, H. C., Tangelder, G. J., Slaaf, D. W., Muijtjens, A. M. M., Arts, T., and Reneman, R. S.,** Orientation and diameter distributions of rabbit blood platelets flowing in small arterioles, *Biorheology*, 21, 317–331, 1984.
74. **Turritto, V. T. and Baumgartner, H. R.,** Platelet interaction with subendothelium in flowing rabbit blood: Effect of blood shear-rate, *Microvasc. Res.*, 17, 38–54, 1979.
75. **Turritto, V. T. and Weiss, H. J.,** Red blood cells: Their dual role in thrombus formation, *Science*, 207, 541–543, 1980.
76. **Vejlens, G.,** The distribution of leukocytes in the vascular system, *Acta Pathol. Microbiol. Scand. Suppl.*, 33, 11–239, 1938.
77. **von Andrian, U. H., Chambers, J. D., McEvoy, L. M., Bargatze, R. F., Arfors, K.-E., and Butcher, E. C.,** Two step model of leukocyte-endothelial cell inflammation: Distinct roles for LECAM-1 and the leukocyte (β) 2 integrins *in vivo*, *Proc. Natl. Acad. Sci. U.S.A.*, 88, 7538–7542, 1992.
78. **Weichert, W., Pauliks, V., and Breddin, H. K.,** Laser-induced thrombi in rat mesenteric vessels and antithrombotic drugs, *Haemostasis*, 13, 61–71, 1983.
79. **Wiedeman, M. P.,** Vascular reactions to laser *in vivo*, *Microvasc. Res.*, 8, 132–138, 1974.
80. **Wiedeman, M. P.,** Architecture, in *Handbook of Physiology*, Sect. 2, The Cardiovascular System, Vol. 4, Microcirculation, Part 1, chap. 2, Renkin, E. M. and Michel, C. C., Eds., American Physiological Society, Bethesda, MD, 1984, 11–40.
81. **Wiederhielm, C. A., Woodbury, J. W., Kirk, S., and Rushmer, R. F.,** Pulsatile pressures in the microcirculation of frog's mesentery, *Am. J. Physiol.*, 207, 173–176, 1964.
82. **Wilson, J. W., Ratliff, N. B., and Hackel, D. B.,** The lung in hemorrhagic shock. I. *In vivo* observations of pulmonary microcirculation in cats, *Am. J. Pathol.*, 58, 337–353, 1970.
83. **Wilson, J. W.,** Leukocyte sequestration and morphologic augmentation in the pulmonary network following hemorrhagic shock and related forms of stress, *Adv. Microcirc.*, 4, 197–232, 1972.
84. **White, J. G.,** Platelet structural physiology: The ultrastructure of adhesion, secretion and aggregation in arterial thrombosis, *Cardiovasc. Clin.*, 18, 13–33, 1987.
85. **Woldhuis, B., Tangelder, G. J., Slaaf, D. W., and Reneman, R. S.,** Concentration profile of blood platelets differs in arterioles and venules, *Am. J. Physiol.*, 262, H1217–H1223, 1992.
86. **Zweifach, B. W. and Lipowsky, H. H.,** Pressure-flow relations in blood and lymph microcirculation, in *Handbook of Physiology*, Sect. 2, The Cardiovascular System, Vol. 4, Microcirculation, Part 1, chap. 7, Renkin, E. M. and Michel, C. C., Eds., American Physiological Society, Bethesda, MD, 1984, 251–307.

Chapter 30

Endothelial Cells

Una S. Ryan

CONTENTS

I. INTRODUCTION

The endothelium is a complex, unique organ with a vast surface area and an aggregate mass equal to that of the liver. In cross-sections of the arterial wall, the endothelium appears as a thin and insignificant layer that belies its importance and significance in homeostasis.[1] It is at the level of the microvasculature that the extreme thinness of the endothelium is particularly evident in cross-sections (Figure 1).

Resulting from its strategic interposition between the blood and all other tissues in the body, the endothelium has many diverse functions and provides a dynamic interface for interaction with cells and molecules arriving via the blood or from the tissue side.[2] For example, endothelial cells (ECs), particularly those of the pulmonary capillaries, are capable of converting angiotensin I to angiotensin II and of degrading bradykinin.[3] Thus, the endothelium can regulate blood pressure by inactivating a substance that lowers blood pressure (bradykinin) and by causing the delivery of a potent hypertensive substance (angiotensin II) directly into the circulation.[4] Both of these effects are achieved by interaction of circulating substances with an enzyme, angiotensin-converting enzyme, kinase II localized on the surface of endothelial cells *in situ* and in culture.[3] Localization of angiotensin-converting enzyme (ACE) on endothelial cells was the first of many findings that led to the recognition of a number of processing, or "metabolic", functions of endothelium.[1] The endothelial disposition of ACE also led to the development of assays useful for the identification of endothelial cells in culture and to the development of orally effective antihypertensive drugs that target ACE.

Subsequent studies of EC properties have received much impetus from the development of techniques for the isolation, characterization, and culture of ECs.[5] ECs from a wide variety of species and vessel origins, including the microvasculature, can now be grown reproducibly in culture.

In the quiescent state, the endothelium acts to maintain the blood's fluidity and resists thrombosis, but thrombotic functions take over when the cells are perturbed. The endothelium also acts as a selective barrier between the elements in the blood and the extravascular space and serves to convey signals between the tissues and the circulating elements. During infection or when activated by cytokines or components of the coagulation or complement systems, the endothelium functions to attract leukocytes, allowing their emigration to sites of inflammation. The endothelium also has local regulatory

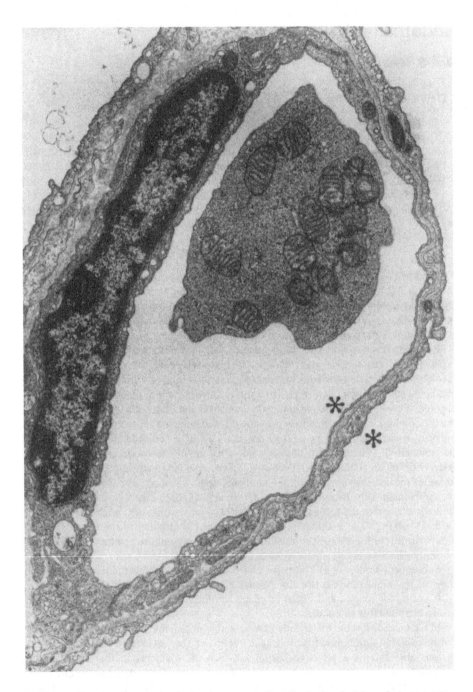

Figure 1 Electron micrograph of rat pulmonary capillary illustrating that (e.g., between aster-isks) the endothelial cell is extremely thin, little more than two apposing plasma membranes. (From Ryan, U. S. and Ryan, J. W., *Metabolic Functions of the Lung*, Bakhle, Y. S. and Vane, J. R., Eds., *Vol. 4 of Lung Biology in Health and Disease*, Lenfant, C., Ed., Marcel Dekker, New York, 1977, chap. 7, 197–232.)

functions, being a key controller of vascular tone as well as an important modulator of vascular remodeling through its influence on the growth of the underlying vascular smooth muscle cells and by secretion of extracellular matrix components. Toward all these functions, the endothelium synthesizes a diverse armament of hormones, mediators, and growth modulators, some of which are expressed constitutively and others which are only induced in response to various stimuli. However, the same anatomic location that makes the microvascular endothelium so unique and diverse in its biologic functions, makes it an immediate target of vascular injury and an ideal candidate to initiate events leading both to local and systemic damage.

II. ENDOTHELIAL BARRIER AND TRANSDUCING FUNCTIONS

The interactions between neighboring ECs serve to maintain vascular integrity, regulate vascular permeability, and control leukocyte traffic. The junctions between ECs vary in different parts of the circulation and in different organs. In much of the vasculature, where ECs form a continuous monolayer, gap junctions predominate.[6] A decrease in both gap junctions and tight junctions is seen in areas of regenerating endothelium.[7] In contrast, in the brain and retina where the development of edema can be dangerous, tight (occluding) junctions predominate. While the blood-brain barrier is recognized to be a highly selective anatomic and physiological barrier that regulates the entry and exit of cerebral nutrients and biologically important substances necessary for the maintenance of cerebral metabolism and neuronal activity, the endothelium of all organs serves to mediate the passage of solutes, nutrients, lipids, and hormones to the interstitium, often involving a complex system of membrane receptors and transporters. In addition to endothelial-endothelial cell interactions, endothelial smooth-muscle cell interactions occur primarily via gap junctions where cytoplasmic bridges of smooth muscle cells extend through fenestrations in the internal elastic lamina to contact the endothelium.[8] Gap junctions provide a pathway for the transportation of ions and small molecules and could provide a route of entry of mediators from endothelium to smooth muscle and vice versa. In addition, some endothelium-derived factors are freely diffusible and penetrate smooth muscle cells directly, independent of gap junctions. Others bind to receptors on the surface of the smooth muscle cell and elicit responses through second messengers.

The endothelium and smooth muscle cells form an integrated alliance; the close association of these two cell types allows for the efficacy of the most influential of the endothelium-derived vasomodulating factors, endothelium-derived relaxing factor/nitric oxide (EDRF/NO) and demonstrates the transducing role of the endothelium. A blood-borne agonist interacting with receptors on the ECs leads to release of a mediator that modulates smooth muscle relaxation.

III. ENDOTHELIAL HEMOSTATIC FUNCTIONS

ECs have both thrombotic and thrombo-resistant properties. In the quiescent state, they are antithrombotic, but can be induced to become procoagulant. ECs inhibit thrombus formation by interfering with the coagulation cascade, inhibiting platelet adhesion/aggregation, and activating fibrinolytic pathways. The luminal surface of the EC contains anionic heparin-like glycosaminoglycans that are synthesized by the ECs and bind thrombin, the key enzyme of blood coagulation, and antithrombin III, a serum protein that binds and inactivates thrombin. In the presence of ECs, thrombin reacts primarily with antithrombin III, resulting in rapid inactivation of the enzyme. Thrombin also interacts with thrombomodulin on the EC surface. Thrombomodulin binds both thrombin and protein C, and the thrombin-thrombomodulin-protein C complex markedly accelerates the activation of protein C.[9] Protein C, with the intermediary protein S, inhibits factor Va and factor XIII in the coagulation cascade.[10,11] ECs are also thought to produce a lipoprotein-associated inhibitor of coagulation known as TFPI (tissue factor pathway inhibitor) or LACI (lipoprotein-associated coagulation inhibitor).[12] This factor is a potent inhibitor of factor Xa the factor VIIa/TF-complex.[13] Although there is no direct evidence of its being made in ECs, it is currently hypothesized that the heparin-releasable form is associated with endothelial glycosaminoglycans.[14] ECs also synthesize prostacyclin (PGI_2), a potent inhibitor of platelet aggregation.[15] Other products released by ECs that prevent platelet adhesion/aggregation include adenosine and nitric oxide (NO). Moreover, there is clear synergism between the antiaggregatory effect of PGI_2 and the effect of NO at subthreshold levels.[16]

Clot dissolution through enhancement of the fibrinolytic system is another EC anticoagulant defense mechanism. ECs synthesize both tissue-type plasminogen activators (t-PA) as well as urokinase-type plasminogen (u-PA) activators.[17] The synthesis and release of plasminogen activators by ECs is stimulated by thrombin, activated protein C, epinephrine, vasopressin, and bradykinin.

In contrast to the anticoagulant mechanisms described above, the EC, when perturbed mechanically or exposed to bacterial endotoxin, thrombin, tumor necrosis factor, or interleukin-1, can interact with blood components to promote coagulation.[18-20] The procoagulant activity is the result of increased production of tissue factor (thromboplastin), von Willebrand factor (factor VII_{vw}), plasminogen activator inhibitor, platelet-activating factor, and extracellular matrix components. Tissue factor, released by damaged cells, functions with factor VII in activating factor X, initiating the "extrinsic pathway" of coagulation and potentiates the cleavage of factor IX (activating the "intrinsic pathway" as well). In the presence of factor VIII_{vw}, activated factor IX further activates factor X. The activated factor X, formed via either pathway, then converts prothrombin to thrombin in a reaction that requires factor V. Thrombin converts soluble fibrinogen to insoluble fibrin, activates platelets, and inhibits vessel-wall fibrinolytic activity. The factor VIII_{vw} synthesized by ECs is also bound by collagen types I, III, IV, and V and helps mediate platelet adhesion to the subendothelium through a specific glycoprotein receptor on the platelet surface, glycoprotein IIb/IIIa (which also serves as a receptor for fibrinogen).[21] The importance of factor-VIII_{vw} in platelet adhesion to the subendothelium and subsequent thrombosis is evidenced by the fact that in von Willebrand's disease, there is a marked decrease in platelet adhesion that can be reversed by administration of f-VIII_{vw}.[22] ECs also synthesize other proteins that stimulate the coagulation cascade (although this may not be the primary function of these proteins) including thrombospondin, collagens, and fibronectin. Procoagulant activity also involves alterations in fibrinolysis through the regulated expression of t-PA and specific plasminogen activator inhibitors. In fact, the activity of t-PA in plasma is based on the amount of t-PA released as well as on the level of PAI present.[23,24]

Thus, the hemostatic potential of the endothelium results from a complex balance between active factors that have opposing biological actions and between active factors and specific inhibitors. Upset of this balance could lead to conditions predisposing both to local and widespread embolic and thrombolic responses.

IV. ENDOTHELIAL CONTROL OF VASCULAR WALL FUNCTION

ECs play a key role in modulating vasomotor tone. Many substances produced by ECs affect local vasomotor tone and a complex interaction exists between those elements that control hemostasis: vascular modeling and vasomotor reactivity. The fact that ACE is localized on ECs established a role for endothelium in the control of blood pressure.[3] The renin-angiotensin system is now also known to play a role in vascular remodeling.[25]

Abluminally released PGI_2 is a potent vasodilator and antiaggregant. PGI_2 released by ECs can be stimulated by pulsatile pressure and so can the endogenous mediators thrombin, bradykinin, angiotensin II, histamine, platelet-derived growth factor (PDGF), IL-1, and adenine nucleotides.[26-28] The effects of PGI_2 are opposed by thromboxane, a prostanoid produced by activated platelets, and its effects include causing platelet aggregation and vasoconstriction.[29] Aspirin, an irreversible inhibitor of cyclooxygenase, owes its efficacy to the EC's ability to synthesize cyclooxygenase continuously, while the platelet cannot. This leads to cumulative inhibition of thromboxane A_2 formation, while the ECs continue to produce PGI_2.[30]

EDRF was first described by Furchgott and Zawadzki who demonstrated that the relaxation of the rabbit aorta by acetylcholine depended on the presence of an endothelial lining and was the results of a non-prostanoid diffusible substance.[31] Subsequently, it was suggested that EDRF may be NO or a related oxide species.[32,33] This has since been confirmed by Moncada and colleagues.[34,35]

NO is synthesized from the amino acid L-arginine by the enzyme NO synthase (NOS) and its actions are mediated by increases in cellular cGMP.[36-38] Arginine analogs (such as L-NG-monomethyl arginine) are potent inhibitors of NO production and their effects can be reversed by arginine. Blockade of NO synthesis in animals results in marked increases in blood pressure underlying the importance of NO release in maintaining resting blood pressure.[39,40] Several isozymes of NOS exist. The constitutive enzyme is Ca^{2+}/calmodulin dependent and releases picomolar concentrations of NO. In several cell types, a second form of Ca^{2+}-independent NOS can be induced by inflammatory mediators.[41,42] The inducible NOS produces NO at the nanomolar level and its induction can be prevented by pretreatment with glucocorticoids. NO, in addition to mediating vasodilation, inhibits platelet adhesion and aggregation as previously described. It also limits SMC proliferation and inhibits leukocyte-EC interactions. After reperfusion injury, sodium nitrite prevents leukocytes from adhering and infiltrating into the vessel wall,[43] perhaps by an effect of NO on EC adhesion molecule expression.

More than 30 substances have been shown to elicit endothelium-dependent relaxations of isolated blood vessels, including acetylcholine, the calcium ionophore A23187, bradykinin, thrombin, and endothelin, indicating the importance of this factor in local autoregulation of vascular tone. Defects in EC production of EDRF/NO have been seen in a number of disease states, including atherosclerosis, hypertension, and diabetes, and may contribute to their pathogenesis.[44,45] There is mounting evidence to suggest that mild trauma to microvessels is sufficient to impair temporarily the dilating responses of microvessels without irreversible injury to the vessels.

In addition to the vasodilators PGI_2 and NO, the endothelium also releases vasoconstrictor substances in response to a variety of stimuli.[46] In 1988, Yanagisawa et al. identified endothelin, a linear 21-amino acid peptide secreted by ECs.[47] Endothelin is the most potent vasoconstrictor substance yet discovered, with a potency 10 times that of angiotensin II. Intense vasoconstriction and decreased blood flow have been seen in multiple species in which ET-1 has been infused, although it is rapidly removed from the bloodstream, suggesting a local vasoregulatory role.[48,49] Three pharmacologically separate endothelin isopeptides have been identified in mammalian species, namely endothelin-1 (ET-1), endothelin-2, and endothelin-3. ET-1 is the only one known to be made by ECs.

Many substances, including thrombin, epinephrine, transforming growth factor-β, and the Ca^{2+} ionophore A23187, increase preproendothelin mRNA as well as increase the release of vasoactive ET-1 from ECs.[47] The release of ET-1 is slow, consistent with the fact that it requires new synthesis. The fact that ET-1 is secreted by numerous cell types and that receptors are widely distributed among many tissues, including blood vessels, brain, lungs, kidneys, adrenal glands, spleen, and intestines, suggests that endothelin has multiple biologic roles.

In addition to its long-acting vasoconstrictor and pressor actions, ET-1 has numerous biologic activities, including mitogenicity for cultured mesangial cells, Swiss 3T3 cells, capillary ECs, and SMCs. Elevated levels of ET-1 have been detected in patients who have suffered a myocardial infarction as well as in acute renal failure, acute ischemic stroke, and hypertensive states; however, it is unclear as to whether the elevated ET-1 levels actually contribute to the pathogenesis of these diseases or are the result of concurrent disease processes.[50,51] We have demonstrated in a rat model of arterial injury that high levels of ET-1 worsen post-angioplasty restenosis and may act through a direct mitogenic effect on the underlying SMCs.[52]

V. LEUKOCYTE/ENDOTHELIAL CELL ADHESIVE INTERACTIONS

Interaction of leukocytes with the endothelium is a routine physiologic function. Under normal circumstances, over 75% of granulocytes are adherent to the endothelium where they remain ready for release by specific stimuli to join the circulating pool. Lymphocytes, on the other hand, circulate through the plasma and, as part of their normal course, emigrate through specialized post-capillary venules in lymphoid tissues, returning to the plasma after a few hours. When this delicate system is upset by an inflammatory process, changes occur in the endothelium that allow not only adhesion but emigration of leukocytes to the site. These interactions of leukocytes with the endothelium are carefully controlled by specific adhesion molecules. At present, three different groups of adhesive receptors/ligands are known to participate in leukocyte adhesion. These include proteins of the integrin family or LEU-CAMS (leukocyte cellular adhesion molecules),[53,54] members of the immunoglobulin-related molecules or ICAMs (intercellular adhesion molecules),[55] and carbohydrate binding proteins called selectins or LEC-CAMs (lectin-epidermal growth factor-complement cell adhesion molecule).[56,57]

The most important integrins present on leukocytes belong to the β1 (CD11/CD18) and β2 (VLA-4, CD49d/CD29) subfamilies.[6,58] Although integrins are constitutively expressed on the surface of leukocytes, they are normally in a functionally inactive state. Conversion to the active state is rapid in response to chemotactic factors, cytokines, antigens, or mitogens. The importance of leukocyte integrins to immunologic defense against inflammatory processes is demonstrated in the human disease leukocyte adhesion deficiency (LAD). Neutrophils from patients with LAD lack expression of leukocyte integrins and exhibit defective leukocyte-EC adhesion in *in vitro* assays correlating with the absence of these cells at sites of inflammation.[59]

ECs possess at least three adhesive receptors in the immunoglobulin family, namely ICAM-1, ICAM-2, and VCAM (INCAM-110), which serve as counter receptors for the leukocyte integrins.[60-62] They are single-chain N-glycosylated polypeptides. ICAM-1 contains five immunoglobulin domains. It is not only present on ECs, but is present on a variety of other cells including leukocytes. ECs constitutively express ICAM-1 in low amounts, but increased levels are easily induced by a variety of cytokines including interferon-γ, IL-1, and TNF-α.[63] Following stimulation, increased expression can be detected within 4 h and expression is maintained for over 24 h. ICAM-2 is similar to ICAM-1 but contains only two immunoglobulin domains. ICAM-2 is constitutively expressed by ECs and is not increased after cytokine activation.[64] This may indicate more of a role for ICAM-2 in routine EC-leukocyte interactions, whereas ICAM-1 becomes more important in activated ECs. VCAM-1 is also expressed following endothelial activation by cytokines.[65] VCAM-1 selectively binds mononuclear cells such as lymphocytes and monocytes and is the counter-receptor for the β2 integrin VLA4.[66] VCAM-1 has been found at sites of chronic inflammation but its expression is not restricted to ECs. Macrophages and fibroblast-like cells also appear to express VCAM-1.[67]

Three members of the selectin family currently exist: L-selectin (LEC-CAM-1, LAM-1, Leu 8, and TQ-1), E-selectin (LEC-CAM-2, ELAM-1, endothelial-leukocyte adhesion molecule), and P-selectin (LEC-CAM-3 PADGEM, platelet-activation-dependent-granulocyte-external-membrane protein, GMP-140, CD62).[68-73] L-selectin is confined to leukocytes and is involved in leukocyte homing. E-selectin is found on ECs, and P-selectin is found on both ECs and platelets. These molecules are transmembrane glycoproteins that contain an amino-terminal lectin domain, followed by an epidermal growth factor-like domain, and a varying number of complement-like consensus repeats. P- and E-selectin bind sialyated Lewis X (SleX) carbohydrates, which are commonly found on glycoproteins and glycolipids of myeloid cells. The natural ligand for L-selectin remains elusive.

E-selectin is an adhesion protein for monocytes and neutrophils, but not lymphocytes. It is expressed on the EC surface 4 to 6 h after stimulation by cytokines, and is downregulated by 24 h.[74] It is not contained within the cytoplasm of cells, and requires new protein synthesis for expression.[69] E-selectin has been shown to be expressed transiently on microvascular endothelium in certain pathologic settings, particularly acute and chronic inflammatory processes in which cytokine generation is thought to occur.[75] P-selectin is present in both platelets and ECs, although the endothelial protein is primarily found in postcapillary venules.[76] Endothelial P-selectin is expressed constitutively and is located in membranes of Weibel-Palade bodies, the secretory granules of endothelium in which large multimers of factor-VIII$_{vw}$ are stored.[72,77,78] Following stimulation with agonists such as thrombin or histamine, P-selectin is rapidly distributed to the cell surface where it binds neutrophils, monocytes, and platelets.[79] In stimulated cultured endothelium, surface expression of P-selectin is rapid, within 10 min. Downregulation then occurs over the next 30 min. Exposure of ECs to oxidants results in prolonged expression of P-selectin on their surface and thus may provide a direct role for oxygen radicals in neutrophil adhesion.[80] P-selectin is an excellent candidate for directing the initial adherence of unstimulated neutrophils and monocytes to sites of inflammation. Progression of the inflammatory stimulus can then activate other adhesive receptors on both cells, thus stimulating leukocyte emigration to the site of tissue damage.[81] P-selectin's presence on platelets and its localization with factor-VIII$_{vw}$ also suggest a role for this molecule in hemostasis. Stimulated platelets expressing P-selectin may then recruit neutrophils and monocytes to the thrombus. The activated monocyte with its procoagulant surface could then amplify thrombin generation and clot formation.

Clearly, the identification and characterization of these adhesive molecules have provided new insights into the increasingly complex interactions of ECs, platelets, and leukocytes.[82] Current investigation has focused on the exploitation of this knowledge to identify paths for therapeutic intervention.

VI. ENDOTHELIAL CELLS IN ISCHEMIA/REPERFUSION

Ischemic injury to the heart or brain is twofold. The initial insult results in tissue hypoxia with its associated cellular alterations, whereas the second insult occurs after reperfusion with the generation of toxic oxygen radicals.

The initial hypoxic episode results in specific alterations in cellular metabolism as the oxygen-deprived cell switches from aerobic metabolism to anaerobic metabolism, decreasing the cellular pH concurrent with a build-up in metabolites such as lactate. Cells starved of oxygen for too long eventually die; however, a number of cells can survive the initial hypoxic episode quite well. A hypoxic environment is not necessarily toxic to ECs; however, the hypoxic state does induce multiple reversible changes in endothelial pathology,[83] one of which is a switch from the normal anticoagulant state of the EC to one that promotes clot formation. Hypoxia induces thrombomodulin activity on the EC cell surface, resulting in activation of factor X as well as inhibition of EC fibrinolytic activity. Hypoxia also results in an inhibition of the barrier function of the endothelium and, since the production of EDRF requires oxygen, the hypoxia and ischemia result in vasospasm. Clearly, the initial hypoxic insult sets the stage for continued thrombosis and contributes to the pathology seen in ischemic injury. For instance, the loss of barrier function in areas of ischemic vascular injury is a direct result of injury to the endothelium.

Adhesion of neutrophils to vascular endothelium is an early event in their recruitment into acute inflammatory or ischemic regions. It is important to recognize that endothelial-neutrophil adhesive mechanisms occur very rapidly following injury, and that the specificity of the reaction resides with the altered endothelium and does not occur randomly as would be the case if activation of the neutrophils were to activate adhesion. The complement system is known to be involved in inflammatory[84] and ischemic[85] injury. Complement fixation has recently been shown to provide a potent and rapid stimulus for neutrophil adhesion.[86]

VII. CONCLUSION

Thus, despite their deceptive thinness in transverse section, ECs are highly active and responsive cells. It is clear from the foregoing discussion that ECs perform a multitude of functions, some constitutively and some that are induced following activation. It is not yet known whether all aspects of endothelial activation occur concomitantly; nevertheless, they share some common mechanisms of cellular signal transduction.

Pathological and pathophysiological conditions would be expected to involve a number of situations that would alter the normal interactions of ECs with blood-borne molecules, and to alter the communication systems between endothelium and other cell types. Thus, conditions that do not necessarily involve loss or death of ECs may set the stage for later irreversible endothelial damage. Studies of the mechanisms underlying regulation of EC activation and interaction of ECs with inflammatory, immune, and complement systems should lead to improved understanding of modulations of EC structure, function, and behavior during a wide variety of diseases.

REFERENCES

1. **Ryan, U. S.,** Structural basis for metabolic activity, *Annu. Rev. Physiol.,* 44, 223, 1982.
2. **Ryan, U. S.,** Pulmonary endothelium: A dynamic interface, *Clin. Invest. Med.,* 9, 124, 1986.
3. **Ryan, U. S., Ryan, J. W., Whitaker, C., and Chiu, A.,** Localization of angiotensin converting enzyme (kininase II): Immunocytochemistry and immunofluorescence, *Tissue Cell,* 8, 125, 1976.
4. **Ryan, U. S.,** Processing of angiotension and other peptides by the lungs, in *Handbook of Physiology — The Respiratory System, 1,* Fishman, A. P. and Fisher, A. B., Eds., Am. Physiol. Soc., Bethesda, MD, 1985, 351.
5. **Ryan, U. S. and Maxwell, G.,** Isolation, culture and subculture of bovine pulmonary artery endothelial cells: Mechanical methods, *J. Tiss. Cult. Meth.,* 10, 3, 1986.
6. **Larson, R. S. and Springer, T. A.,** Structure and function of leukocyte integrins, *Immunol. Rev.,* 114, 181, 1990.
7. **Spagnoli, L. G., Pietra, G. C., Villaschi, S., and Jones, L. W.,** Morphometric analysis of gap junctions in regenerating endothelium, *Lab. Invest.,* 46, 139, 1982.
8. **Ryan, U. S. and Ryan, J. W.,** Vital functions and activities of endothelial cells, in *The Biology of the Endothelial Cell,* Nossel, H. L. and Vogel, H. J., Eds., Academic Press, New York, 1982, 301.
9. **Esmon, N. L., Owen, W. G., and Esmon, C. T.,** Isolation of a membrane bound cofactor for thrombin-catalyzed activation of protein C, *J. Biol. Chem.,* 257, 859, 1982.

10. **Walker, F. J., Secton, P. W., and Esmon, C. T.,** The inhibition of blood coagulation by activated protein C through the selective inactivation of activated factor V, *Biochim. Biophys. Acta,* 571, 333, 1979.

11. **Stern, D. M., Nawroth, P. P., Harris, K., and Esmon, C. T.,** Cultured bovine aortic endothelial cells promote activated protein C-protein S-mediated inactivation of factor Va, *J. Biol. Chem.,* 261, 713, 1986.

12. **Broze, G. J., Jr.,** The role of tissue factor pathway inhibitor in a revised coagulation cascade, *Semin. Hematol.,* 29, 159, 1992.

13. **Broze, G. J., Jr., Warren, L. A., Novotny, W. F., Higuchi, D. A., Girard, J. J., and Miletich, J. P.,** The lipoprotein-associated coagulation inhibitor that inhibits the factor VII-tissue factor complex also inhibits factor Xa: Insight into its possible mechanism of action, *Blood,* 71, 335, 1988.

14. **Sandset, P. M., Abildgaard, U., and Larsen, M. L.,** Heparin induces release of extrinsic pathway inhibitor, *Throm. Res.,* 50, 803, 1988.

15. **Weksler, B. B., Marcus, A. J., and Jaffe, E. A.,** Synthesis of prostaglandin I_2 (prostacyclin) by cultured human and bovine endothelial cells, *Proc. Natl. Acad. Sci, U.S.A.,* 126, 365, 1977.

16. **Radomski, M. W., Palmer, R. M., and Moncada, S.,** The anti-aggregating properties of the vascular endothelium: Interactions between prostacyclin and nitric oxide, *Br. J. Pharmacol.,* 92, 6539, 1987.

17. **Levin, E. and Loskutoff, D. J.,** Cultured bovine endothelial cells produce both urokinase and tissue-type plasminogen activators, *J. Cell. Biol.,* 94, 631, 1982.

18. **Colucci, M., Balcon, G. I., Lorenzet, R., et al.,** Cultured human endothelial cells generate tissue factor in response to endotoxin, *J. Clin. Invest.,* 71, 1893, 1983.

19. **Bevilacqua, M. P., Pober, J. S., Majeau, G. R., Fiers, W., Cotran, R. S., and Gimbrone, M. A., Jr.,** Recombinant tumor necrosis factor induces procoagulant activity in cultured human vascular endothelium: Characterization and comprison with the actions of interleukin 1, *Proc. Natl. Acad. Sci. U.S.A.,* 83, 4533, 1986.

20. **Nawroth, P. P. and Stern, D. M.,** Modulation of endothelial cell hemostatic properties by tumor necrosis factor, *J. Exp. Med.,* 163, 740, 1986.

21. **Sakariassen, K. S., Nievelstein, P. F. E. M., Coller, B. A., and Sixma, J. J.,** The role of glycoprotein 1b and 11b-111a in platelet adherence to human artery subendothelium, *Br. J. Haematol.,* 63, 681, 1986.

22. **Weiss, H. J., Baumgartner, H. R., Tchopp, T. B., Turitto, V. T., and Cohen, D.,** Correction by factor VIII of the impaired platelet adhesion to subendothelium in von Willebrand's disease, *Blood,* 51, 267, 1978.

23. **Brommer, E. J. P., Verheijen, J. H., Chang, G. T. G., and Rijken, D. C.,** Masking of fibrinolytic response to stimulation by an inhibitor of tissue-type plasminogen activator in plasma, *Thromb. Haemost.,* 52, 154, 1984.

24. **Nilsson, I. M., Ljungèr, H., and Tengborn, L.,** Two different mechanisms in patients with venous thrombosis and defective fibrinolysis: Low concentration of plasminogen activator or increased concentration of plasminogen activator inhibitor, *Br. Med. J.,* 290, 1453, 1985.

25. **Powell, J. S., Rouge, M., Muller, R. K., and Baumgartner, H. R.,** Cilazapril suppresses myointimal proliferation after vascular injury: Effects on growth factor induction in vascular smooth muscle cells, *Basic Res. Cardiol.,* 86, 65, 1991.

26. **Bhagyalakshmi, A. and Frangos, J. A.,** Mechanism of shear-induced prostacyclin production in endothelial cells, *Biochem. Biophys. Res. Commun.,* 158, 31, 1989.

27. **Baenziger, N. L., Fogerty, F. J., Mertz, L. F., and Chernuta, L. F.,** Regulation of histamine-mediated prostacyclin synthesis in cultured human vascular endothelial cells, *Cell,* 24, 915, 1981.

28. **Crutchley, D. J., Ryan, J. W., Ryan, U. S., and Fischer, G. H.,** Bradykinin-induced release of prostacyclin and thromboxanes from bovine pulmonary artery endothelial cells, *Biochim. Biophys. Acta,* 751, 99, 1983.

29. **Hamberg, M., Svensson, J., and Samuelson, G.,** Thromboxanes: A new group of biologically active compounds derived from prostaglandin endoperoxides, *Proc. Natl. Acad. Sci. U.S.A.,* 72, 2994, 1975.

30. **Fitzgerald, G. A., Oates, J. A., Hawiger, J., et al.,** Endogenous biosynthesis of prostacyclin and thromboxane and platelet function during chronic administration of aspirin in man, *J. Clin. Invest.,* 71, 676, 1983.

416

31. **Furchgott, R. F. and Zawadzki, J. V.,** The obligatory role of endothelial cells in the relaxation of arterial smooth muscle by acetylcholine, *Nature,* 373, 299, 1980.
32. **Khan, M. T. and Furchgott, R. F.,** Similarities of behavior of (NO) and endothelium-derived relaxing factor in perfusion cascade bioassay system, *Fed. Proc.,* 46, 385, 1987.
33. **Ignarro, L. J., Byrns, R. E., Buga, G. M., and Wood, K. S.,** Endothelium-derived relaxing factor (EDRF) released from artery and vein appears to be nitric oxide (NO) or a closely related radical species, *Fed. Proc.,* 46, 644, 1987.
34. **Palmer, R. M., Ferrige, A. G., and Moncada, S.,** Nitric oxide release accounts for the biological activity of endothelium-derived relaxing factor, *Nature,* 327, 524, 1987.
35. **Hutchinson, P. J., Palmer, R. M., and Moncada, S.,** Comparative pharmacology of EDRF and nitric oxide on vascular strips, *Eur. J. Pharmacol.,* 141, 445, 1987.
36. **Moncada, S., Palmer, R. M. J., and Higgs, E. A.,** Biosynthesis and endogenous roles of nitric oxide, *Pharmacol. Rev.,* 43, 109, 1991.
37. **Palmer, R. M., Ashton, D. S., and Moncada S.,** Vascular endothelial cells synthesize nitric oxide from L-arginine, *Nature,* 333, 664, 1988.
38. **Rapoport, R. M. and Murad, F.,** Agonist induced endothelium-dependent relaxation in rat thoracic aorta may be mediated through cyclic GMP, *Circ. Res.,* 52, 352, 1983.
39. **Rees, D. D., Palmer, R. M. J., and Moncada, S.,** Role of endothelium-derived nitric oxide in the regulation of blood pressure, *Proc. Natl. Acad. Sci. U.S.A.,* 86, 3375, 1989.
40. **Aisaka, K., Gross, S. S., Griffith, O. W., and Levi, R.,** NG-Methylarginine, an inhibitor of endothelium-derived nitric oxide synthesis, is a potent pressor agent in the guinea pig: Does nitric oxide regulate blood pressure *in vivo*?, *Biochim. Biophys. Acta,* 160, 881, 1989.
41. **Knowles, R. G., Merrett, M., Salter, M., and Moncada, S.,** Differential induction of brain, lung and liver nitric oxide synthase by endotoxin in the rat, *Biochem. J.,* 270, 833, 1990.
42. **Busse, R. and Mulch, A.,** Induction of nitric oxide synthase by cytokines in vascular smooth muscle cells, *FEBS Lett.,* 275, 87, 1990.
43. **Johnson, G. P. S., Tsao, D., Malloy, D., and Leffer, A. M.,** Cardioprotective effects of acidified sodium nitrite in myocardial ischemia with reperfusion, *J. Pharmacol. Exp. Ther.,* 252, 35, 1990.
44. **Gryglewski, R. J., Botting, R. M., and Vane, J. R.,** Mediators produced by the endothelial cell, *Hypertension,* 12, 530, 1988.
45. **Flavahan, N. A.,** Atherosclerosis or lipoprotein-induced endothelial dysfunction. Potential mechanisms underlying reduction in EDRF/nitric oxide activity, *Circulation,* 85, 1927, 1992.
46. **Rubanyi, G. M. and Vanhoutte, P. M.,** Hypoxia releases a vsoconstrictor substance from the canine vascular endothelium, *J. Physiol.,* 364, 45, 1985.
47. **Yanagisawa, M., Kurihara, H., Kimura, S., et al.,** A novel potent vasoconstrictor peptide produced by vascular endothelial cells, *Nature,* 332, 411, 1988.
48. **Goetz, K. L., Wang, B. C., Madwed, J. B., Zhu, J. L., and Leadley, R. J., Jr.,** Cardiovascular, renal, and endocrine responses to intravenous endothelin in conscious dogs, *Am. J. Physiol.,* 255, R1604, 1988.
49. **DeNucci, G., Thomas, R., D'Orleans-Juste, P., et al.,** Pressor effects of circulating endothelin are limited by its removal in the pulmonary circulation and by the release of prostacyclin and endothelium-derived relaxing factor, *Proc. Natl. Acad. Sci. U.S.A.,* 85, 9797, 1988.
50. **Miyauchi, T., Yanagisawa, M., Tomizawa, T., et al.,** Increased plasma concentrations of endothelin-1 and big endothelin-1 in acute myocardial infarction [letter], *Lancet,* 2, 53, 1989.
51. **Tomita, K., Ujiie, K., Nakanishi, T., et al.,** Plasma endothelin levels in patients with acute renal failure, *N. Engl. J. Med.,* 321, 1127, 1989.
52. **Trachtenberg, J. D., McGraw, D., Sun, S., et al.,** The effect of ET-1 infusion on the development of intimal hyperplasia following balloon catheter injury, *J. Cardiovasc. Physiol.,* (Suppl. 8) S355–S359, 1993.
53. **Hynes, R. O.,** Integrins: A family of cell surface receptors, *Cell,* 48, 549, 1986.
54. **Ruoslahi, E.,** Integrins, *J. Clin. Invest.,* 87, 1, 1991.
55. **Williams, A. F. and Barclay, A. N.,** The immunoglobulin superfamily — domains for cell surface recognition, *Annu. Rev. Immunol.,* 6, 381, 1988.
56. **Brandley, B. K., Swiedler, S. J., and Robbins, P. W.,** Carbohydrate ligands of the LEC cell adhesion molecules, *Cell,* 63, 861, 1990.
57. **Springer, T. A. and Lasky, L. A.,** Sticky sugars for selectins, *Nature,* 349, 196, 1991.

58. **Arnout, M. A.,** The structure and function of the leukocyte adhesion molecules, CD11/CD18, *Blood,* 75, 1037, 1990.

59. **Kishimoto, T. K., Larson, R. S., Corbi, A. L., Dustin, M. L., Staunton, D. E., and Springer, T. A.,** The leukocyte integrins, *Adv. Immunol.,* 46, 149, 1991.

60. **Marlin, S. D. and Springer, T. A.,** Purified intercellular adhesion molecule-1 (ICAM-1) is a ligand for lymphocyte function-associated antigen 1 (LFA-1), *Cell,* 51, 813, 1987.

61. **Gahmberg, C. G., Nortamo, P., Zimmermann, D., and Ruoslahti, E.,** The human leukocyte-adhesion ligand, intercellular-adhesion molecule 2. Expression and characterization of the protein, *Eur. J. Biochem.,* 195, 177, 1991.

62. **Springer, T. A.,** Adhesion receptors of the immune system, *Nature,* 346, 425, 1990.

63. **Dustin, M. L., Rothlein, R., Bhan, A. K., Dinarello, C. A., and Springer, T. A.,** Induction by IL-1 and interferon-gamma: Tissue distribution, biochemistry, and function of a natural adherence molecule (ICAM-1), *J. Immunol.,* 137, 245, 1986.

64. **Nortamo, P., Li, R., Renkonen, R., et al.,** The expression of human leukocyte adhesion molecular intercellular adhesion molecule-2 is refractory to inflammatory cytokines, *Eur. J. Immunol.,* 21, 2629, 1991.

65. **Carlos, T. M., Schwartz, B. R., Kovach, N. L., et al.,** Vascular cell adhesion molecule-1 mediates lymphocyte adherence to cytokine-activated cultured human endothelial cells, *Blood,* 76, 965, 1990.

66. **Elices, M. J., Osborn, L., Takada, Y., et al.,** VCAM-1 on activated endothelium interacts with the leukocyte integrin VLA4 at a site distinct from the VLA4/fibronectin binding site, *Cell,* 60, 577, 1990.

67. **Koch, A. E., Burrows, J. C., Haines, G. K., Carlos, T. M., Harlan, J. M., and Leibovich, S. J.,** Immunolocalization of endothelial and leukocyte adhesion molecules in human rheumatoid and osteoarthritic synovial tissues, *Lab. Invest.,* 64, 313, 1991.

68. **Bevilacqua, M., Butcher, E., Furie, B., et al.,** Selectins: A family of adhesion receptors, *Cell,* 67, 233, 1991.

69. **Bevilacqua, M. P., Stengelin, S., Gimbrone, M. A., Jr., and Seed, B.,** Endothelial leukocyte adhesion molecule 1: An inducible receptor for neutrophils related to complement regulatory proteins and lectins, *Science,* 243, 1160, 1989.

70. **Kansas, G. S.,** Structure and function of L-selectin, *APMIS,* 100, 287, 1992.

71. **Michl, J., Qiu, Q. Y., and Kuerer, H. M.,** Homing receptors and addressins, *Curr. Opin. Immunol.,* 3, 373, 1991.

72. **McEver, R. P., Beckstead, J. H., Moore, K. L., Marshall-Carlson, L., and Bainton, D. F.,** GMP-140, a platelet alpha-granule membrane protein, is also synthesized by vascular endothelial cells and is localized in Weibel-Palade bodies, *J. Clin. Invest.,* 84, 92, 1989.

73. **Lasky, L. A.,** Lectin cell adhesion molecules (LEC-CAMs): A new family of cell adhesion proteins involved with inflammation, *J. Cell. Biochem.,* 45, 139, 1991.

74. **Pober, J. S., Bevilacqua, M. P., Mendrick, D. L., Lapierre, L. A., Fiers, W., and Gimbrone, M. A., Jr.,** Two distinct monokines, interleukin 1 and tumor necrosis factor, each independently induce biosynthesis and transient expression of the same antigen on the surface of cultured human vascular endothelial cells, *J. Immunol.,* 136, 1680, 1986.

75. **Cotran, R. S., Gimbrone, M. A., Jr., Bevilacqua, M. P., Mendrick, D. L., and Pober, J. S.,** Induction and detection of a human endothelial activation antigen *in vivo, J. Exp. Med.,* 164, 661, 1986.

76. **McEver, R. P.,** GMP-140: A receptor for neutrophils and monocytes on activated platelets and endothelium, *J. Cell. Biochem.,* 45, 156, 1991.

77. **Hattori, R., Hamilton, K. K., Fugate, R. D., McEver, R. P., and Sims, P. J.,** Stimulated secretion of endothelial von Willebrand factor is accompanied by rapid redistribution to the cell surface of the intracellular granule membrane protein GMP-140, *J. Biol. Chem.,* 264, 7768, 1989.

78. **Bonfanti, R., Furie, B. C., Furie, B., and Wagner, D. D.,** PADGEM (GMP140) is a component of Weibel-Palade bodies of human endothelial cells, *Blood,* 73, 1109, 1989.

79. **Geng, J. G., Bevilacqua, M. P., Moore, K. L., et al.,** Rapid neutrophil adhesion to activated endothelium mediated by GMP-140, *Nature,* 343, 757, 1990.

80. **Patel, K. D., Zimmerman, G. A., Prescott, S. M., and McIntyre, T. M.,** Oxygen radicals induce human endothelial cells to express GMP-140 and bind neutrophils, *J. Cell. Biol.,* 112, 749, 1991.

81. **Lo, S. K., Van Seventer, G. A., Levin, S. M., and Wright, S. D.,** Two leukocyte receptors (CD11a/CD18 and CD11b/CD18) mediate transient adhesion to endothelium by binding to different ligands, *J. Immunol.*, 143, 3325, 1989.

82. **Ryan, U. S. and Worthington, R. E.,** Cell-Cell contact mechanisms, *Curr. Opin. Immunol.*, 4, 33, 1992.

83. **Ogawa, S., Gerlach, H., Esposito, C., Pasagian-Macaulay, A., Brett, J., and Stern, D.,** Hypoxia modulates the barrier and coagulant function of cultured bovine endothelium, *J. Clin. Invest.*, 85, 1090, 1990.

84. **Mulligan, M. S., Yeh, C. G., Rudolph, A. R., and Ward, P. A.,** Protective effects of soluble CR1 in complement- and neutrophil-mediated tissue injury, *J. Immunol.*, 148, 1479, 1992.

85. **Hill, J., Lindsay, T. D., Oritz, F., Yeh, C. G., Hechtman, H. B., and Moore, F. D.,** Soluble complement receptor Type 1 ameliorates the local and remote organ injury after intestinal ischemia-reperfusion in the rat, *J. Immunol.*, 149, 1723, 1992.

86. **Marks, R. M., Todd, R. F., III, and Ward, P. A.,** Rapid induction of neutrophil-endothelial adhesion by endothelial complement fixation, *Nature*, 339, 314, 1989.

Chapter 31

Interstitium and Lymphatics

John R. Casley-Smith

CONTENTS

I. THE INTERSTITIUM

The interstitium (connective tissue) has two basic components. (1) The gel-phase: structural members (various cells, collagen, elastic tissue, hyaluronic acid, etc. — which will not be further discussed here, although the "collagen diseases" often have microcirculatory components). (2) The sol-phase: spaces, filled with water, between these solid elements. This water contains the usual plasma crystalloids and the plasma proteins that leak out (concentrations differ from in the blood because of varying amounts of filtration and removal). To these are added any products (useful or waste) of the local cells.

Normally, the interstitial water is in equilibrium. Each solute is added at the same rate as it is removed, but the rates differ for the different solutes. However, the interstitium is far from homogeneous. There are many and different sources (blood and cells) and sinks (blood, cells, and lymphatics) for its different components (Figure 1). Also, the larger molecules are excluded from those parts of it that contain much proteoglycan (hyaluronic acid), etc. Details can be found in References 1, 32, 37, and 45.

A. TISSUE CHANNELS

Tissue channels are present in all tissues and form a continuous system, from the top of the head to the big toe. They can be demonstrated by filling them with plastic or highly-charged ferrocyanide ions, which are repelled from the gel-phase.[3-5,14] The channels can vary widely in both size and number. Normally, they are some 100 nm in diameter and occupy about 1% of the volume of the interstitial tissues that have so far been studied (granulation tissue, joint capsules, subcutaneous tissue, and cerebral cortex). They form randomly connected channels, but this randomness is only local. The tissue channels are

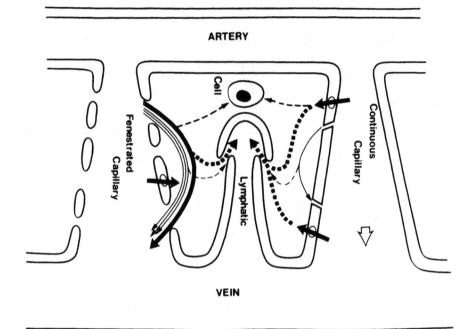

Figure 1 A diagram of the microcirculation, showing the two kinds of blood capillaries. Water and crystalloids (fine arrows) pass out at the arterial ends (via interendothelial junctions or fenestrae) and re-enter at the venous ends, but some passes to the lymphatics (fine broken arrows). In regions with continuous capillaries, plasma protein (thick arrows) leaks to the tissues via vesicles and is removed by the lymphatics and proteolytic cells (broken thick arrows). In fenestrated regions, the same occurs except that much protein exits via the fenestrae and most re-enters via them.

more frequent around blood capillaries, and alter in size and number according to the volume of fluid flowing through the tissues.

Tissue channels are usually relatively short. While they form a continuous system throughout the body, any fluid that enters them usually passes to a blood capillary or an initial lymphatic after only a few microns. However, in some regions (e.g., muscles) where the initial lymphatics only occur at the periphery (in the perimysium), the fluid has to flow for some millimeters or centimeters before it leaves the system of tissue channels. In yet other regions, where the initial lymphatics are completely absent (e.g., the brain and inner eye), fluid must travel many centimeters before it eventually enters the initial lymphatics. In these tissues, the channels in which it flows occur (among other places) along the basement membranes of the cerebral and retinal blood capillaries (Virchow-Robin spaces). They connect with others in the adventitia of the arteries of the brain and the Circle of Willis. They finally empty into the true lymphatics in the adventitia of the internal carotid artery in the neck — outside the skull, and into true initial lymphatics in other similar regions (Figure 2) — cribriform plate, spinal and cranial nerves, inner ear.[5,22,28,34,47] Some of the Virchow-Robin spaces also drain into the cerebrospinal fluid and then into arachnoid villi draining into initial lymphatics as well as into the blood.

While it is considered, quite correctly, that true (endothelialized) lymphatics do not exist in the brain and inner eye, this does not mean that these structures do not need, and do not have, a lymphatic drainage. Occlusion of the lymphatics in the neck induces a

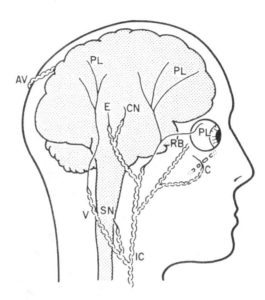

Figure 2 A diagram of the lymphatic drainage of the brain and eye. This is all via prelymphatics (PL). Apart from true lymphatics in the retrobulbar region (RB), the sclera and the most anterior part of the eye. The prelymphatics of the brain start in the Virchow-Robin spaces; those in the eye around the retinal and other vessels. These connect with prelymphatics in the adventitia of larger vessels that discharge into true, endothelialized, initial lymphatics (outside the skull) in the adventitia of the internal carotid (IC) and (probably, but not studied) of the vertebral arteries (V). Other drainage is via other prelymphatics draining into the subarachnoid space, which is drained by arachnoid villi (AV), into both the blood and the lymphatic system, and into lymphatics at the cribriform plate (C), cranial nerves (CN), spinal nerves (SN), and the inner ear (E).

lymphedema of the brain and retina, just as it does in the facial regions, whose true lymphatics also drain by this path. For this reason, such an important system of well-ordered tissue channels, which acts like (and empties into) true lymphatics, is often called "the prelymphatic system."

Edema increases the numbers and dimensions of the tissue channels[15,16] (Figure 3). This is only to be expected since edema involves the presence of excessive amounts of water in the tissues, and since (presumably) the gel-phase of the interstitial tissue has as much water adsorbed to it as is possible before any excess is present in tissue channels. There is, however, always an equilibrium between the various forces and the amounts of fluid in the two phases.

Tissue channels enlarge rapidly as edema tears the tissues apart. Once the edema ceases, while they shrink rapidly initially, they remain slightly abnormal for many months. Thus, after a simple incised wound, the volumes of the channels increased by some 400 times after 1 week[15] (Figure 3). The channels remained greater than normal for 6 months — some 4 to 5 months after the wound had completely disappeared clinically! All sizes of channels increased in numbers, and many were found to be much larger than those normally seen. As the condition healed, the largest channels disappeared first, presumably by becoming smaller ones. The calculated hydraulic conductivity was increased by 10^5 times at the time of maximal edema (at 1 week), the same increase as was observed by Guyton et al.[29] in a simple low-protein edema.

In acute lymphedema of rats' skin or brain, the tissue channels increase in volume 20 times, by 3 days after the operation[16] (Table 1). The numbers of both the large and small channels increase greatly, as do the diameters of the largest channels.

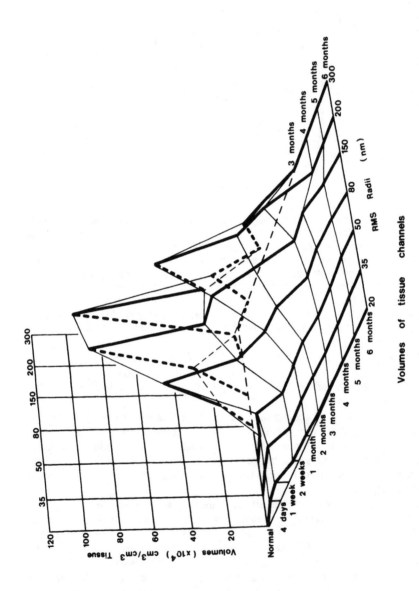

Figure 3 How the volumes of tissue channels, of various root-mean-square (RMS) radii, vary after a simple incised wound. The scale does not allow it to be shown here, but the numbers and volumes only returned to normal after 6 months, long after the wound has completely invisible and, apparently, healed. (From Casley-Smith, J. R. and Vincent, A. H., *Tissue Cell*, 12, 761–771, 1980.)

Table 1 Tissue Channel Alterations in Lymphoedema

Diameters (nm)	Normal Skin and Brain	Lymphedema Skin Acute	Skin Chronic	Brain Acute	Brain Chronic
		No. of Channels/100 μ^2			
6–33	11	113	59	253	141
33–47	1.8	40	13	33	21
47–66	1.5	28	8.8	19	12
66–120	1.6	17	9.8	15	14
120–210	0.15	4.8	5.0	5.0	3.2
210–290	0	0.75	1.7	0.71	0.89
290–420	0	0.65	0.72	0.89	0.47
Volumes of channels (ml $\times$ 10^{-4}/ml tissue)	16	313	245	334	234
Hydraulic conductivity (cm^4 $\times$ 10^{-12}/dyne s)	1.6	110	140	130	88
Diffusional conductivity (cm^2 $\times$ 10^{-4}/D)	11	200	160	220	150

Note: Adapted from Reference 16. The normal values for the skin and the brain were not significantly different and are combined; other differences were mostly significant at the 0.1% level.

The interstitial tissue becomes much more permeable to all kinds of molecules and particles during edema.[6,30,31,33,35,36] This is obviously the effect of the great increases in the tissue channels. Indeed, injected dyes, or those leaving the blood vessels, form large lakes of color instead of just fine streamers.

B. PROTEOLYSIS IN THE TISSUES

Tissue proteolysis, while not strictly speaking part of the microcirculation, is intimately related to it. A number of cells in the tissues lyse proteins, e.g., macrophages, basal epithelial cells, fibroblasts, etc.[9,25] The macrophages in particular have a very important role in reducing chronic high-protein edemas by this mechanism. This is, of course, only their physiological role; in inflammation and other pathological conditions, they act both in an immunological way and in the lysis of excess proteins, dead cells, and bacteria, etc. These cells are normally very numerous in the tissues.[13] Very approximate calculations[5] indicated that macrophages may remove about 30% of the protein that reaches the tissues from the blood capillaries. However, a model implies their normal role may be much less than this (Table 5), while they have a considerable effect in limiting high-protein edemas.[8] This activity can be much increased by the benzopyrone drugs.

II. THE STRUCTURE AND FUNCTIONING OF LYMPHATICS

The lymphatics are far more numerous than is usually realized. They are about as numerous as the blood vessels — omitting the arteries, arterioles, and the arterial side of the capillaries. Each lymphatic is usually larger than its corresponding venous vessel.

A. THE INITIAL LYMPHATICS

These are also known as lymphatic capillaries or terminal lymphatics. They are arranged differently in different tissues, but often occur in plexuses, especially in the skin. Even just beneath every square centimeter of the capsule of most organs, there is some 70 cm of these vessels.[3]

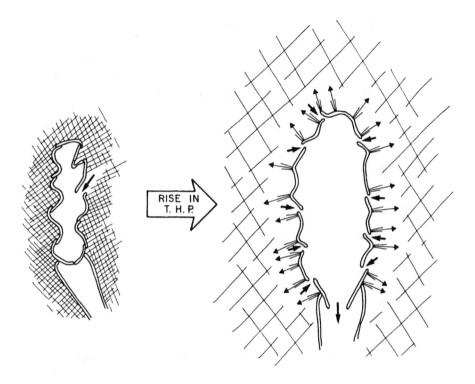

Figure 4 A diagram of the effects of elevated tissue hydrostatic pressure (THP) on initial lymphatic functioning. Provided the tissue is somewhat edematous (as it will speedily become with such a THP), the swollen interstitial tissue pulls on the anchoring filaments (thin arrows) that hold the initial lymphatics open; they also hold many junctions slightly open, allowing fluid to enter. Hence, in place of a few widely open junctions, there are many slightly open ones, through which fluid is forced (thicker arrows) down a hydrostatic pressure gradient.

Essentially, the only major structural difference between the initial lymphatics and the venous blood capillaries is that the lymphatics have many openable junctions (Figure 4). This ability of the junctions to be opened is probably caused by the relative lack of adhesion devices between the endothelial cells, by the tenuous basement membranes, and by the attachment of fibrils (anchoring filaments) to the exteriors of the endothelium — joining this to the interstitial tissue so that its swelling or movements will tug on the lymphatic endothelium. (For other details of the fine structure of the initial lymphatics, see References 4, 5, and 47).

During edema, the swollen tissues pull on the fibrils, dilating the initial lymphatics and separating the endothelial cells, thus opening the junctions (Figure 4). This does not occur in normal tissue, except when large movements of the tissues also pull on these fibrils. Normally, the junctions are opened during the filling of the initial lymphatics because the inflow of fluid pushes the cells apart. The openings range from 30 nm to many micrometers. They are relatively rare (1–2%) in inactive, quiescent, regions; in the intestinal villi, some 6% of the junctions are open. During injury and edema, they come to number some 50% of the junctional sections. Fluid, macromolecules, particles, cells, etc. enter mainly via the open junctions.

There are also many small vesicles in the lymphatic endothelium. Since these can only allow material to pass down concentration gradients, they do not usually contribute to the net proteins (or fluids) entering the initial lymphatics. Vacuoles can carry chylomicra

Table 2 Characteristics of Initial Lymphatic Functioning under Various Conditions

	Most of the Body	Most of the Body in Edema	Kidney and ? Other Regions	Brain and Eye[a]
Tissue hydrostatic pressure	Negative	Positive	Positive	Positive
Total tissue pressure[b]	Variable	"Constant"	"Constant"	"Constant"
Lymph flow during anesthesia	Much reduced	"Normal"	"Normal"	"Normal"
Protein to lymph via small vesicles	"None"	"Occurs"	Occurs	—
Junctions under normal conditions	A few open widely	Many open widely	Many open slightly	—
Mode of initial lymphatic functioning	Force pump	Conduit[c]	Conduit	Conduit

Note: From Reference 9. Quotation marks indicate that the statement is only approximate.

[a] While the brain and inner eye have only nonendothelialized prelymphatics, these are included here to emphasize the similarity between their role and that of the initial lymphatics when they are acting as conduits.

[b] While the total tissue pressure does vary considerably with the pulse, it appears that this is too rapid to allow the initial lymphatics to function as force pumps[4]; lower frequencies (respiration, muscle contractions, etc.) permit this to occur.

[c] If total tissue pressure varies here, force pump activity is usually added to the conduit mode.

across the initial lymphatic endothelium. This is useful in the small intestine during a fatty meal if there is little fluid to wash them through the initial lymphatic junctions.

The junctions open during the filling-phase, when the total tissue pressure is low; they close during the emptying-phase, when this pressure is high — during compression of the tissues. Thus, the junctions act as inlet valves, preventing the escape of macromolecules during compression of the initial lymphatics. At this time, much of the water is probably regurgitated into the tissues (thus concentrating the protein in the lymph). Simultaneously, whole lymph is forced on into the collecting lymphatics and thus eventually reaches the blood. While some workers disagree,[1,41,42,44] the lymph (at least in the initial lymphatics) is probably normally more concentrated than the tissue fluid (reviewed in References 4, 5, and 7). While the forces causing the formation of lymph are fascinating and have caused much argument (*loc. cit.*), they are not really relevant here and will not be mentioned further.

What is important is that the initial lymphatics function as millions of little force pumps, and that these are powered by varying total tissue pressures. The openable junctions act as inlet valves; the intralymphatic valves of the collecting lymphatics (and probably the protruding nuclei of the endothelial cells of the initial lymphatics) act as outlet valves. These force pumps are powered by variations in total tissue pressure, which are caused by muscular contraction, movements, respiration, and variations in external pressure (changing position, massage, etc.). Without these *variations* in total tissue pressure, the pumps cannot function[5,7]; then fluid, etc., accumulates in the interstitial tissue.

If however the tissue hydrostatic pressure is greater than the intralymphatic hydrostatic pressure, the initial lymphatics can still drain the tissues without such variations in total tissue pressure.[4,7] Such a downhill flow can occur only in tissues that normally have a positive tissue hydrostatic pressure (kidney, liver, etc.) or when it is elevated during edema.

Thus, the initial lymphatics can act in two ways (Table 2). In most normal tissues (where the tissue hydrostatic pressure is less than that in the initial lymphatics), they act as force pumps, with the junctions opening and closing as the total tissue pressure varies. In the few regions with normally positive tissue hydrostatic pressures, and in edema, they act as conduits. Flow then occurs along a continually decreasing hydrostatic pressure gradient, although no doubt any pumping assists it.

B. THE COLLECTING LYMPHATICS

There is no sharp division between the initial lymphatics, where uptake occurs, and the true collecting lymphatics, which are entirely specialized for transporting the lymph. As one moves centrally, open junctions gradually become fewer and fewer, the vessels get larger and their walls more muscular, and the intralymphatic valves become more frequent. Even the efferent collecting lymphatics leaving the more peripheral lymph nodes may have some open junctions, and thus can be considered as lymphatic exchange vessels. The larger lymphatics can be seen individually, visually, or by lymphangiography, and can be operated on using microsurgery. Vessels of this size, or larger, are sometimes referred to as "lymphatic trunks." Their anatomy and histology have recently been excellently reviewed.[26] There are many separate lymphatic drainage areas (lymphotomes) whose drainage all ultimately passes into the same collecting lymphatic. These regions are separated by "lymphatic watersheds" (on each side of which the lymph drains into different collectors).

The musculature of the walls of collecting lymphatics is never very great — rather less than in the equivalent veins. However, it performs a useful function. Together with the many intralymphatic valves, it transforms the whole vessel into a series of pumps.[38] These intrinsic contractions do not, however, provide the only force that propels the lymph. The intralymphatic valves permit any variation in total tissue pressure (e.g., from the contractions of adjacent muscles, respiration, movement, and massage) to force the lymph in one direction only, i.e., centrally. It should be emphasized that, while the intrinsic contractions of the collecting lymphatics can propel the lymph in them, such contracting muscle does not occur in the initial lymphatics, except in the wings of a few species of bats!

Most of the resistance to lymph flow occurs, not in the collecting lymphatics, but in the lymph nodes. This is particularly so if they are inflamed as a result of disease in the region they drain, or if they have become chronically fibrosed. The nodes are frequently discussed, and will not be mentioned further.

The main sites where lymph is returned to the blood are the unions of the thoracic duct, and of the right lymph duct, with the great veins in the neck. However, there are many other places where such communications exist. It is not certain to what extent they are normally patent, although it is well known that much more lymph is formed in the periphery than ever reaches the main lymph ducts.[33] Such additional communications open when the intralymphatic pressures rise high enough — and thus help to prevent lymphedema.

III. REGULATION OF TISSUE VOLUME

The amount of fluid in the tissues (V_I) is regulated by many factors. Some *Safety Factors against Edema* have been known for a long time and have been measured in various conditions[30,31,42] (Table 3). These are actually equally *safety factors against dehydration*. They might just be called *Factors Affecting Fluid Volume* (or *Factors*). Those usually discussed are: interstitial hydrostatic pressure (P_I), interstitial colloidal osmotic pressure (Π_I), and lymphatic uptake (J_{VL}), which is the only one the body can control. This uptake is greater if there is edema or if protein concentrations are high in the tissues.[7,43]

However, there are many more factors than just these, some 15 in all.[8] These often influence V_I because, via Π_I, this is affected by the tissue protein concentration (C_I), which in turn is affected by the total tissue protein (q_I) and also, in a negative-feedback

Table 3 Ultimate Safety Factors Against Edema and Dehydration

1. Tissue Hydrostatic Pressure (P_I) — ↑ in edema
   Rises ↑↑ in extreme edema; *ultimately the only one still rising in severe edema*
2. Tissue Colloidal Osmotic Pressure (Π_I) — ↓ in edema
   Varies with: Tissue protein conc., i.e., with V_I and protein flux: from blood, to lymph and proteolysis
3. Lymph Flow (J_{VL}) — ↑ in edema
   Rises ↑↑ in moderate edema; ↓ in extreme edema (lymphatics collapse)
   ↑↑↑ if protein concentration is high in tissues (EDLF)[a]

Note: As noted in the text, these are only the final results of some 15 factors, arranged in a variety of hierarchies. Some of these factors have opposite effects in different hierarchies.

[a] From Taylor, A. E., *Lymphology*, 23, 111–123, 1990.

loop, by V_I. V_I is constant only if q_I is also constant. Protein leakage from the blood (J_{PC}) adds to q_I; it is reduced by protein removal via the lymphatics (J_{PL}) and via proteolysis in the tissues (J_{PM}). Factors are often in hierarchies. Some are in many, sometimes with opposite actions in each hierarchy.

When fluid inflow and outflow are equal, a steady state is present. A steady state is caused by the balance of all the negative feedbacks of all the factors, acting through their various hierarchies. Steady states occur not only normally but also in the various edemas (Table 4). In edema, they are largely unrecognized, but in fact are extremely important. For example, a lymphedematous limb can be relatively constant in size for years, in spite of considerable variations in many of the forces affecting it.

The relative importance of the various factors alter from the normal to an edematous condition, and indeed can be quite different from one edema to another.[8] Thus, J_{VL} and J_{PL} decrease to 0 in lymphedema. Proteolysis (J_{PM}) has very little effect on the normal state and has little effect on trauma, but when it is stimulated by benzopyrones, its effect on V_I is quite remarkable (Table 5), although the actual value of J_{PM} has only increased four times. The effect of no proteolysis on V_I in lymphedema is also marked, as is its increase by benzopyrones — although J_{PM} is only mildly greater.

The ultimate factors (PI, Π_I, and J_{VL}) are shown in Table 5, calculated from a model[8] for: the normal condition, various edemas, and some variations in these. Consistent units are used so that their effects may be compared. Apart from the lymphedematous conditions, the edemas are all relatively mild. The wide variations in V_I and q_I are evident; yet each of the rows represent steady states in which V_I and q_I both tend to the limits shown. In normal and lymphedema, P_I has a similar effect to that of Π_I; in the other edemas (except in trauma with the lymphatics obstructed), its effect is much greater than that of Π_I or J_{VL}. When V_I tend toward extremes, P_I is the only factor that can continue to increase — effectively without limit. Its role becomes more and more important, until it far

Table 4 Normal and Edematous Steady States

Normal Conditions
   Tissue fluid volume (V_I) and total protein content (q_I) are constant
   (Because if protein varies, so does Π_I and therefore V_I)
Edematous Conditions (after time)
   V_I and q_I are again constant; i.e., there is a new steady state
   (Because if protein varies, so does Π_I and therefore V_I)
   Importance of factors varies with condition
   In very severe edema, all factors → maxima, and have no increasing effect **except** the tissue hydrostatic pressure (P_I);
   P_I can increase without limit and is the ultimate Safety Factor in severe edema!

Table 5 Tissue Fluid Volume (V_I) and Total Protein Content (q_i) — per 100 g Normal Tissue Effects of the Final Factors Are Shown, Expressed as ml/min Alterations in V_I

	V_I (ml)	q_i (g)	$-(P_I + 10)$ (ml/min)	Π_I (ml/min)	$-J_{VL}$ (ml/min)
Normal	15	2.1	0.14	≈0.12	>>0.01
Venous edema	21	1.4	0.22	>>0.05	≈0.05
Low plasma proteins	76	0.7	0.40	>>>0.00	<<<0.13
Trauma	114	94	1.33	>>0.75	>>>0.14
Trauma, no lymphatics	140	172	1.78	>1.26	>>>0.00
Trauma, no proteolysis	118	99	1.34	>>0.77	>>0.15
Trauma treated by benzopyrones	68	51	1.25	>>0.68	>>0.13
Lymphedema	51	12	0.19	≈0.22	>>>0.00
Lymphedema, no proteolysis	143	53	0.39	≈0.39	>>>0.00
Lymphedema treated by benzopyrones	24	4.3	0.13	≈0.16	>>>0.00
Lymphedema — raised external pressure	14	11	0.90	≈0.92	>>>0.00

Note: From a computer model, based on 100 g tissue (Reference 8). P_I and J_{VL} are shown as negative since increases in these reduce V_I; $-(P_I + 10)$ mmHg is used to avoid problems caused by P_I changing sign. Note the huge variations in V_I (tissue fluid volume) in the various edemas, and how the various factors change in importance. Note also that removing the effect of proteolysis hardly increases V_I very much in trauma, but increasing it has a very considerable effect. On the other hand, removing the effect of proteolysis causes a very great increase in lymphedema. Increasing proteolysis, or greatly raising the external pressure, reduces lymphedema greatly.

outweighs those of all the other factors. It is the ultimate reason why a severe edema does not expand to fill the known universe! Excess fibrous tissue (which is such a feature of chronic inflammation) causes P_I to increase much more rapidly as V_I increases (it decreases tissue compliance). Hence, excess fibrosis is beneficial in limiting chronic edema, however disadvantageous it may be in other ways.

IV. DISEASES INVOLVING THE INTERSTITIUM AND LYMPHATICS

It is almost impossible to think of any disease process that does not involve the interstitium to some extent and thus affect the lymphatics. Even many psychiatric conditions are known to be associated with physical alterations in the brain! However, this generalization, while many agree with its truth, has so far had little impact in practice. This is because the most usual alteration to the interstitium is edema, which is so common that it is largely ignored. Yet edema, by itself, has many deleterious effects.

A. THE DELETERIOUS EFFECTS OF EDEMAS

These are many (reviewed in Reference 9, Chapter 3). Some are common to all edemas. Swelling is the most obvious. Any swelling, if it occurs rapidly, causes pain. Loss of function may be present at both the tissue and cellular levels. At the tissue level, this is caused by added bulk or edema of joints; at the cellular level, it is caused by poor oxygen transport, which also results in poor wound healing. Reduced oxygenation is produced because the swollen tissues cause cells to lose membrane-to-membrane contacts that are so important for the transmission of this, lipid-soluble, gas.

High-protein edemas (i.e., with protein concentrations of 1 g/100 ml or more) have all the effects of low-protein ones, plus others caused by the excessive amounts of protein in the tissues. Willoughby and Di Rosa[46] postulated that altered native proteins may be basic mediators for both acute and chronic edema. This hypothesis has been verified by chronically injecting rats with their own plasma.[13] After a few weeks, this caused chronic inflammation. Blood vessels and lymphatics were damaged and their numbers increased. There were considerable alterations in the interstitial tissue. Fibroblast numbers increased 125 times and collagen fibers echoed these alterations. (It is of no little interest that the benzopyrones greatly reduced all these pathological changes.) These alterations in the tissues, produced by simple injections of protein, are almost identical with those of subacute and chronic lymphedema [reviewed in References 6 and 9 (Chapter 3)]. That is, increased fibroblasts and macrophages numbers, fibrosis, mild small-lymphocytosis, increases in numbers of blood capillaries and initial lymphatics, and the alterations to their morphology.

It is evident that edema has many deleterious effects and should always be reduced, if possible. To do this effectively, it is necessary to understand its causes. Edema can only occur[23,24] when the *lymphatic load* (i.e., the fluid or plasma protein needing to be removed by the lymphatic system) exceeds the *lymphatic transport capacity* (i.e., the ability of the lymphatic system to remove it). Protein is as important as fluid (see above). However, protein is removed by proteolysis in the tissues as well as by the lymphatics, so for protein it is the *lymphatic transport and proteolysis capacity* that is important.

The lymphatics are one of the most important defense mechanisms against edema. The lymph flow lets us classify the various forms of edema in a useful manner into *high-* and *low-flow* edemas [reviewed in References 9 (Chapter 2), 23, and 24]. These are again subdivided into "*high-protein*" and "*low-protein*," with an arbitrary dividing line of 1 g/ 100 ml protein concentration in the edema fluid. A fifth class also occurs, with devastating effects, when a high load and a low transport capacity occur together — *safety-valve edema*. Separating these categories is essential since they distinguish between edemas with widely different causes, effects, and (to some extent) treatments.

B. HIGH-FLOW, LOW-PROTEIN EDEMAS

These occur because excess fluid leaves essentially normal blood vessels. This may be because of raised venous pressure (e.g., in late congestive cardiac failure) or low blood colloidal osmotic pressure (e.g., nephrosis). It used to be thought that hunger edema was caused by the latter, but it now seems that this is produced by weakening of the interstitial tissue and the low tissue hydrostatic pressures caused by high tissue compliance. Edema of the lower legs in the aged is also often caused in this way because the skin and connective tissue stretch easily, keeping the tissue hydrostatic pressure low.

C. HIGH-FLOW, HIGH-PROTEIN EDEMAS

In most of the body, this is caused by injured blood vessels (burns, other mediators of acute inflammation, trauma, avitaminosis). However, in regions with fenestrated capillaries (e.g., the liver), simply raising the venous hydrostatic pressure will produce it.

D. LOW-FLOW, HIGH-PROTEIN EDEMAS (LYMPHEDEMA)

This has many causes [References 9 (Chapter 2) and 24], from poorly developed or functioning lymphatics, to their removal or blocking by surgery, radiation, filariae, etc. It is far more common than is usually realized. Over 20 million women suffer from post-mastectomy lymphedema alone; filariasis causes some 90 million cases. Chronic venous insufficiency, while venous in etiology, almost always has a lymphedema component because the lymphatic collectors run parallel to the veins and are involved in their diseases. The total is some 400 million cases.

V. TREATMENTS OF DISEASES INVOLVING THE INTERSTITIUM AND LYMPHATICS

Naturally, if possible, treatment is always directed toward the original cause of the disease. Because of the deleterious effects of edema, treating this as well often assists healing. Depending on the disease, such treatments have some features in common; others often differ considerably.

A. HIGH-FLOW, LOW-PROTEIN EDEMAS

Treating the underlying cause is essential, but sometimes the edema is quite localized and can easily be reduced by compression stockings. Diuretics are excellent in some cases, but quite unnecessary in others (e.g., in ankle edema of the aged caused by lax tissues). Improving lymphatic functioning (e.g., by complex physical therapy — see below) is often helpful.

B. HIGH-FLOW, HIGH-PROTEIN EDEMAS

Again, treating the cause is of primary importance, but complex physical therapy is often helpful; so is increasing tissue proteolysis by macrophages via the benzopyrones.

C. LOW-FLOW, HIGH-PROTEIN EDEMAS (LYMPHEDEMA)

Diuretics are quite useless, except briefly in emergencies. Surgery is occasionally successful, but is usually a failure.[26] This is because lymphovenous anastomoses tend to thrombose and reduction operations often have late results that are worse than the disease. Two methods of treatment are very helpful: complex physical therapy (C.P.T.) and the benzopyrone drugs.

C.P.T. is a daily regime of specialized massage, compression bandaging (followed by a compression garment when the course is ended), special exercises, and skin care.[10,26,27,39] It is based upon the emptying of the normal lymphotomes adjacent to the blocked ones and causing lymph to cross the watersheds into the normally drained lymphotomes. This increases the numbers and sizes of the collateral lymphatics joining the lymphotomes, providing an alternative pathway. Typical results give a mean reduction of half of the edema over a 4-week course (loc. cit.; Figure 5). This is followed by a much lesser, but significant reduction over the next 6 to 12 months (the intermediate phase) while the body remodels. A further 4-week course removes about half of the remaining edema. Recent lymphedemas, with little fibrosis, may even be completely reduced by the first course of C.P.T.

The benzopyrone group of drugs have many actions, but they all reduce all forms of both acute and chronic high-protein edema in animals and man (reviewed Reference 9, Chapters 6, 7, and 8). All those studied have been shown to do this by increasing both the numbers of macrophages and their normal proteolysis per cell. These drugs thereby provide another path by which protein, and its osmotically held water, can be removed from the tissues. Removing the excess protein also reduces the chronic inflammation, which results from the simple chronic accumulation of excess plasma proteins and the consequent excess fibrosis.[13]

Widely differing benzopyrones have been shown to reduce human post-mastectomy, primary and other lymphedemas [References 2, 9 (Chapter 8), 11, 17, 20, 21, and 40]. They even reduce the lymphedema and elephantiasis caused by filariasis[18,19] (Figure 6). The results obtained with C.P.T. are improved a further 25% by these drugs.[12] They also decrease the incidence of secondary acute inflammation by removing the "incubation medium" for bacteria. Unlike C.P.T., they reduce lymphedema slowly — over months to years; however, no compression garments are needed since the body can remodel over this period.

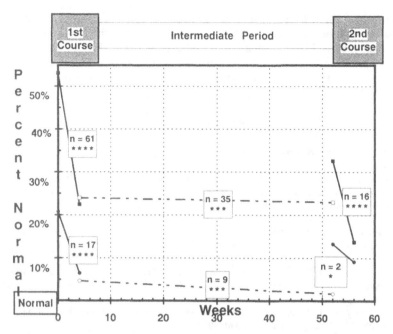

Figure 5 Mean reductions for lymphedema of the arm treated with Complex Physical Therapy. The top set of lines are Grade 2, the lower set are Grade 1. Patient numbers are shown for each period, together with the significances of the alterations in edema. Fewer patients were in each succeeding group, so their initial values differ from the final ones of the preceding group. Well over half of the initial edema was lost in the first course. This loss was not only maintained but slightly increased during the intermediate period (–··–··–). About half of the remainder was again lost during the second course. (From Morgan, R. G., Casley-Smith, J. R., Mason, M. R., and Casley-Smith, J. R., *J. Hand Surg. — British*, 4, 437–492, 1992.)

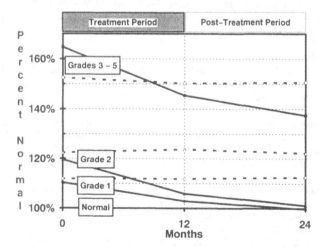

Figure 6 Filaritic lymphedema and elephantiasis treated with 5,6 benzo-α-pyrone for one year and followed for another year. The amounts of edema are shown as percentages of normal, calculated from the mean individual values for the regression lines. Reductions by the active drug (—) were very significant for all grades during treatment (*left*). After treatment ceased, the reductions were not only maintained, but even significantly increased still more (*right*). The placebo groups (– – –) were unchanged. (From Casley-Smith, J. R., Wang, C. T., Casley-Smith, J. R., and Cui Zi-hai, *Br. Med. J.*, 307, 1037–1041, 1993.)

Because benzopyrones provide an alternative path for protein removal, these drugs can reduce any high-protein edema. Clinical trials have shown their effectiveness in many such conditions, including trauma (accidental and surgical), chronic venous diseases, chronic hepatitis, pancreatitis, ionizing radiation, etc. (reviewed in Reference 9, Chapters 8 and 11). They do not treat the underlying condition, but remove much of the edema, thus improving healing.

REFERENCES

1. **Aukland, K. and Nicolaysen, G.,** Interstitial fluid volume: Local regulatory mechanisms, *Physiol. Rev.*, 61, 556–643, 1981.
2. **Braun, H. D., Becker, T., and Meyer, U.,** Behandlung von Stauungserscheinungen nach Ablatio mammae und Bestrahlung, *München medicinische Wissenschaft*, 113, 1630–1633, 1971.
3. **Casley-Smith, J. R.,** Efficiencies of the initial lymphatics, *Z. Lymphologie (J. Lymphol.)*, 2, 24–29, 1978.
4. **Casley-Smith, J. R.,** Mechanisms in the formation of lymph, *Int. Rev. Physiol., Cardiovasc. Physiol.*, Guyton, A. C. and Hall, J. E., Eds., University Park Press, Baltimore, MD, 1982, 147–187.
5. **Casley-Smith, J. R.,** The structure and functioning of the blood vessels, interstitial tissues, and lymphatics, in *Lymphangiology*, Földi, M. and Casley-Smith, J. R., Eds., Schattauer, Stuttgart, 1983, 27–164.
6. **Casley-Smith, J. R.,** Injury and the lymphatic system, in *Lymphangiology*, Földi, M. and Casley-Smith, J. R., Eds., Schattauer, Stuttgart, 1983, 335–372.
7. **Casley-Smith, J. R.,** The effect of variations in tissue protein concentration and tissue hydrostatic pressure on fluid and protein uptake by the initial lymphatics, and the action of calcium dobesilate, *Microcirc. Endoth. Lymph.*, 2, 385–416, 1985.
8a. **Casley-Smith, J. R.,** A model of the factors affecting interstitial volume in oedema; Part I: Hierarchies, some new factors and their equations, *Biorheology*, 29, 535–548, 1992.
8b. **Casley-Smith, J. R.,** A model of the factors affecting interstitial volume in oedema; Part II: Their effects at various abnormal steady-states, *Biorheology*, 30, 9–30, 1993.
8c. **Casley-Smith, J. R.,** A model of the factors affecting interstitial volume in oedema; Part III: Partial derivatives and integrals at various volumes, *Biorheology*, 30, 93–106, 1993.
9. **Casley-Smith, J. R. and Casley-Smith, J. R.,** *High-Protein Oedemas and the Benzo-Pyrones*, Lippincott, Sydney, (Copies: J. R. Casley-Smith, Uni. Adel., GPO Box 498, SA 5001, Australia).
10. **Casley-Smith, J. R. and Casley-Smith, J. R.,** Modern treatment of lymphoedema. I. Complex physical therapy: The first 200 Australian limbs, *Australas. J. Dermatol.*, 33, 61–68, 1992.
11. **Casley-Smith, J. R. and Casley-Smith, J. R.,** Modern treatment of lymphoedema. II. The benzopyrones, *Australas. J. Dermatol.*, 33, 69–74, 1992.
12. **Casley-Smith, J. R. and Casley-Smith, J. R.,** Effects of various combinations of complex physical therapy, benzo-pyrones and Mercury compression on lymphoedema, which combination works best?, in *Progress in Lymphology XIII*, Cluzan, R. V., Pecking, A. P., and Lokiec, F. M., Eds., Excerpta Med. Int. Cong. Series, 994, Elsevier, Amsterdam, 1992, 537–538.
13. **Casley-Smith, J. R. and Gaffney, R. M.,** Excess plasma proteins as a cuase of chronic inflammation and lymphoedema, *J. Pathol.*, 133, 243–272, 1981.
14. **Casley-Smith, J. R. and Vincent, A. H.,** The quantitative morphology of interstitial channels in some tissues of the rat and rabbit, *Tissue Cell*, 10, 571–584, 1978.
15. **Casley-Smith, J. R. and Vincent, A. H.,** Variations in the numbers and dimensions of tissue channels after injury, *Tissue Cell*, 12, 761–771, 1980.
16. **Casley-Smith, J. R., Földi-Börcsök, E., and Földi, M.,** Fine structural study of the tissue channels' numbers and dimensions in normal and lymphoedematous tissues, *Z. Lymphol.*, 3, 49–58, 1979.
17. **Casley-Smith, J. R., Morgan, R. G., and Piller, N. B.,** Treatment of lymphoedema of the arms and legs with 5,6-benzo-α-pyrone, *N. Engl. J. Med.*, 329, 1158–1163, 1993.

18. **Casley-Smith, J. R., Jamal, S., and Casley-Smith, Judith R.,** Reduction of filaritic lymphoedema and elephantiasis by 5,6-benzo-α-pyrone (coumarin) and the effects of diethylcarbamazine (DEC), *Ann. Trop. Med. Parasitol.*, 87, 247–258, 1993.

19. **Casley-Smith, J. R., Wang, C. T., Casley-Smith, Judith R., and Cui Zi-hai,** Treatment of filaritic lymphoedema and elephantiasis with 5,6-benzo-[α]-pyrone (coumarin), *Br. Med. J.*, 307, 1037–1041, 1993.

20. **Clodius, L. and Piller, N. B.,** The conservative treatment of post-mastectomy lymphoedema, in *Advances in Lymphology*, Bartos, V. and Davidson, J. W., Eds., Prague, Avicenum, 1982, 471–474.

21. **Cluzan, R. and Pecking, A.,** Benzopyrone (Lysedem) double blind crossing over study in patients with secondary upper limb edemas, in *Progress in Lymphology XII*, Nishi, M., Uchino, S., and Yabuki, S., Eds., Excerpta Med. Int. Cong. Ser. 887, Elsevier, Amsterdam, 1990, 453–454.

22. **Csanda, E. and Obál, F., Jr.,** Central nervous system and lymphatic system, in *Lymphangiology*, Földi, M. and Casley-Smith, J. R., Eds., Stuttgart, Schattauer, 1983, 475–508.

23. **Földi, M.,** The lymphatic system. A review, *Z. Lymphologie* (J. Lymphology), 1, 16–19 and 44–56, 1977.

24. **Földi, M.,** Insufficiency of lymph flow, in *Lymphangiology*, Földi, M. and Casley-Smith, J. R., Eds., Stuttgart, Schattauer, 1983, 195–214.

25. **Földi, M. and Casley-Smith, J. R.,** The roles of the lymphatics and the cells in high protein oedemas, *Mol. Aspects Med.*, 2, 77–146, 1978.

26. **Földi, M. and Kubik, S.,** Lehrbuch der Lymphologie für Mediziner und Physiotherapeuter, mit Anhang, Praktisch hinweise für die Physiotherapie, Gustav Fischer, Stuttgart, 1989.

27. **Földi, E., Földi, M., and Clodius, L.,** The lymphedema chaos; a lancet, *Ann. Plastic Surg.*, 22, 505–515, 1989.

28. **Grüntzig, J.,** The eye and the lymphatic system, in *Lymphangiology*, Földi, M. and Casley-Smith, J. R., Eds., Schattauer, Stuttgart, 1983, 535–556.

29. **Guyton, A. C., Scheel, K., and Murphree, D.,** Interstitial fluid pressure. III. Its effect on resistance to tissue fluid mobility, *Circ. Res.*, 19, 412–414, 1966.

30. **Guyton, A. C., Granger, H. J., and Taylor, A. E.,** Interstitial fluid pressure, *Physiol. Rev.*, 51, 527–563, 1971.

31. **Guyton, A. C., Barber, B. J., and Moffatt, D. S.,** Theory of interstitial pressures, in *Tissue Fluid Pressure and Composition*, Hargens, A. R., Ed., Williams & Wilkins, Baltimore, MD, 1981, 11–19.

32. **Haljamäe, H.,** Anatomy of the interstitial tissue, *Lymphology*, 11, 128–132, 1978.

33. **Hauck, G.,** Vital microscopic results of the substance transport in the extravascular space and quantitative aspects of the video analysis, in *Ergebnisse der Angiologie*, Földi, M., Ed., Schattauer, Stuttgart, 12, 51–60, 1976.

34. **Magari, S.,** The spinal chord and the lymphatic system, in *Lymphangiology*, Földi, M. and Casley-Smith, J. R., Eds., Schattauer, Stuttgart, 1983, 509–518.

35. **McMaster, P. D.,** Lymphatic participation in cutaneous phenomena, *Harvey Lect.*, 37, 227–268, 1942.

36. **McMaster, P. D.,** Conditions in skin influencing interstitial fluid movement, lymph formation and lymph flow, *Ann. N.Y. Acad. Sci.*, 46, 743–787, 1946.

37. **Meyer, F. A. and Silberberg, A.,** The extravascular space; function of the main structural elements, *Bibl. Anat.*, 15, 213–219, 1977.

38. **Mislin, H.,** The lymphangion, in *Lymphangiology*, Földi, M. and Casley-Smith, J. R., Eds., Schattauer, Stuttgart, 1983, 165–176.

39. **Morgan, R. G., Casley-Smith, J. R., Mason, M. R., and Casley-Smith, J. R.,** Complex physical therapy of the lymphoedematous arm, *J. Hand Surg. — British*, 4, 437–492, 1992.

40. **Piller, N. B., Morgan, R. G., and Casley-Smith, J. R.,** Double-blind cross-over trial of O-(β-hydroxy-ethyl)-rutosides (benzo-pyrones) in the treatment of lymphoedema of the arms and legs, *Br. J. Plastic Surg.*, 41, 20–27, 1988.

41. **Renkin, E. M.,** Lymph as a measure of the composition of interstitial fluid, in *Pulmonary Edema*, Fishmann, H. and Renkin, E. M., Eds., Am. Physiol. Soc., 145–159, 1979.

42. **Taylor, A. E.,** Capillary fluid filtration. Starling forces and lymph flow, *Circ. Res.*, 49, 557–575, 1981.

43. **Taylor, A. E.,** The lymphatic edema safety factor: The role of edema dependent lymphatic factors (EDLF), *Lymphology*, 23, 111–123, 1990.

44. **Taylor, A. E., Gibson, W. H., Granger, H. J., and Guyton, A. C.,** The interaction between intracapillary and tissue forces in the overall regulatioin of interstitial fluid volume, *Lymphology*, 6, 192–208, 1973.

45. **Wiederhielm, C. A., Fox, J. R., and Lee, D. R.,** Ground substance mucopolysaccharides and plasma proteins, their role in capillary water balance, *Am. J. Physiol.*, 230, 1121–1125, 1976.

46. **Willoughby, D. A. and Di Rosa, M.,** A unifying concept for inflammation, in *Immunopathology in Inflammation*, Excerpta Med. Int. Cong. Series No. 229, 28–38, 1970.

47. **Yoffey, J. M. and Courtice, F. C.,** *Lymphatics, Lymph and the Lymphomyeloid Complex*, Academic Press, New York, 1970.

Chapter 32

Isolated, Perfused Microvessels

Michael J. Davis, Lih Kuo, William M. Chilian, and Judy M. Muller

CONTENTS

I. INTRODUCTION

Within each organ, the primary site of flow control resides in the vascular segment between arterioles and venules 100 μm in diameter, i.e., microvessels. As discussed in other chapters of this book, this segment of the circulation can usually be made accessible for *in vivo* microscopic studies. However, such studies are inherently limited by the fact that physiologic and pharmacologic stimuli such as pressure, flow, pO_2, agonist concentration, etc. cannot be systematically or independently controlled. For this reason, it is often advantageous to conduct experiments on isolated microvessels that have been dissected free of parenchymal tissue, cannulated, and perfused *in vitro*. In recent years, such studies have provided a wealth of information regarding the unique physiological and pharmacological characteristics of microvessels, confirming and extending early observations that significant regional heterogeneity exists along the vascular tree.[25,46,79]

The methods for study of isolated arterioles were originally described by Duling, Gore et al.[16] in 1981. Detailed descriptions of the dissection and cannulation techniques can be found in their paper and in a subsequent book chapter.[17] The primary purpose of the present chapter is to discuss the types of experiments best suited for isolated microvessel studies and to compare the various procedures and recent modifications of the original techniques.

II. EXPERIMENTS SUITED FOR ISOLATED, PERFUSED MICROVESSELS

For purposes of this chapter, isolated microvessel experiments have been grouped into the following categories: studies of pressure-induced responses; studies of flow-induced responses; bioassay experiments; pharmacology of microvessels; and electrophysiology of microvessels.

A. STUDIES OF PRESSURE-INDUCED RESPONSES

Baez's *in vivo* studies of arterioles in the rat mesoappendix[1] and Johnson's *in vivo* experiments on arterioles in the cat mesentery[41] provided some of the first direct microscopic evidence that the myogenic response existed in the microcirculation. In the 1970s, various tricks were devised[4,13,42] in order to deliver a pure pressure stimulus to microvessels *in vivo*, i.e., to eliminate the confounding influences of flow and metabolites during studies of the myogenic response. These techniques were only partially successful because secondary flow and pressure changes almost inevitably occurred, and because the contributions of local neural reflexes[34] and propagated responses[64] could seldom be excluded. Furthermore, arteriolar pressure measurements were not made in most *in vivo* myogenic studies (see Reference 10 for review), making it difficult to quantitatively compare arteriolar myogenic responses between and within tissues.

Myogenic responses of feed arteries and conduit arteries have long been observed *in vitro* using standard techniques to mount vessels on relatively large glass pipettes or polyethylene tubing.[29,60,68] However, arteries of this size are at best able to maintain a steady-state diameter constant over a limited pressure range. The first studies in which isolated microvessels were shown to demonstrate myogenic responses were published by Jackson and Duling[40] and by Davis and Sikes.[15] Using the techniques described below (Section IV), small (20–30 µm) cheek pouch arterioles were shown to be capable of constricting to nearly 50% of their passive diameter in response to luminal pressure increases; these responses occurred in the absence of flow or extrinsic neural influences.[15] Subsequent myogenic studies using isolated microvessels have tested the rate sensitivity of pressure-induced responses,[15] the role of an intact endothelium,[48] and the existence of longitudinal gradients in myogenic responsiveness.[10]

B. STUDIES OF FLOW-INDUCED RESPONSES

Endothelium-dependent, flow-induced dilation is a common observation in both isolated and *in situ* conduit artery preparations.[61,63] Evidence that it also occurs in the microcirculation was demonstrated by Smiesko et al.[67] and by Koller and Kaley[43] using *in vivo* microscopy. However, in those experiments, it was difficult to establish that the dilation was elicited purely by a change in intraluminal flow.

The first reports of flow-induced responses in isolated microvessels were made by Kuo et al.[51] and by Garcia-Roldan and Bevan.[21] Kuo et al.[51] devised a system to independently control pressure and flow in isolated pig coronary arterioles (64 µm passive i.d.). These arterioles developed 25 to 30% spontaneous tone at a physiologic pressure and dilated in a graded manner to progressive increases in luminal flow. The highest flow rates produced a 20 to 25% dilation, in contrast to 5 to 10% dilations previously shown in larger vessels that had been constricted with agonists.[63] Responsiveness of isolated coronary arterioles to flow was completely abolished by endothelial denudation, while myogenic responses in the same vessels were unaffected. In subsequent studies, Kuo et al.[49] demonstrated that flow-induced dilation in their preparation was mediated by endothelial production of nitric oxide (or a related compound), and that a dynamic interaction with myogenic responses could occur. In isolated, perfused rat cremaster arterioles, Koller et al.[45] recently performed similar experiments while changing perfusate viscosity and concluded that the arteriolar dilation to flow might be a mechanism designed to regulate wall shear stress. The response of rat cremaster arterioles to flow was endothelium dependent, but was mediated in part by nitric oxide and in part by a prostaglandin.

Bevan and colleagues[3,21,22] have demonstrated in several small artery preparations (mostly from rabbit) that dilation *or* constriction can occur in response to flow, depending on the state of initial vascular tone. The constriction appears to be endothelium-independent, while the dilation has both endothelium dependent and independent components.[22] A few of these observations have been made in microvessels,[21] but most have been made in small arteries[3,22] and are reminiscent of similar endothelium-independent constrictions to flow observed in larger vessels.[36,65] The variability in results from different tissues and vessel sizes points to the need for additional studies of flow-induced responses of microvessels under carefully controlled conditions.

C. BIOASSAY EXPERIMENTS

Protocols using two isolated, perfused microvessels connected in series by a short glass pipette (50×1000 μm) have been used to test the release and transferable nature of endothelial-derived products from microvessels. The experimental designs are similar to those used in studies of large vessels *in vitro*.[31,62]

Kuo et al.[49] showed that, when a denuded coronary arteriole (80 μm i.d.) was perfused downstream from a second arteriole with intact endothelium, both arterioles dilated in a graded manner to increasing flow. However, perfusion at the same flow rates in the opposite direction resulted in dilation only of the arteriole with intact endothelium. This was taken as evidence that a transferable, endothelium-derived dilator was released in response to flow. This experiment also suggested that the contribution of (possible) hyperpolarizing signals conducted from arteriolar endothelium to smooth muscle was negligible in that preparation. The reasoning for this was as follows: if flow-induced dilation of the intact arteriole were due in part to action of an endothelium-derived relaxing factor and in part to a conducted hyperpolarization from the endothelium, then removal of the endothelium should have attenuated the magnitude of the flow-induced response; however, the dilation of the downstream, denuded arteriole in those experiments was nearly identical in magnitude to that of the arteriole with intact endothelium.

Davis[9] used a similar experimental configuration to study the release of an as-yet-unidentified factor from isolated cutaneous venules, a factor that inhibits spontaneous vasomotion. Falcone and Meininger (personal communication) recently studied pairs of isolated rat cremaster arterioles and venules perfused in series to determine the action of arteriolar endothelium-derived products on venules.

It should be mentioned in this context that use of isolated microvessels in bioassay experiments greatly increases the technical difficulties associated with successful cannulation. In addition, the technique as applied to microvessels is inherently less flexible than that used for larger vessels; for example, it would be very difficult to estimate the half-life of transferable factors from microvessels because the length of the interconnecting pipette cannot be easily adjusted as it can in experiments with larger vessels.[62]

D. MICROVESSEL PHARMACOLOGY

This is perhaps the most common use of the isolated microvessel technique. Elegant experiments have been conducted by a number of groups to quantitate dose-response relationships of microvessels to pharmacologic agonists. Many of these experiments have been performed on vessels that would otherwise be inaccessible to study with *in vivo* techniques. For example, Dacey and colleagues[7,8,71] have published a series of studies on isolated cerebral arterioles (<20 μm i.d.) in which pH, pO_2, pressure, and other physiological parameters were carefully controlled while agonist responses were measured. Likewise, Edwards[18] and Ito et al.[39] have studied agonist sensitivity of isolated renal afferent and efferent arterioles (<15 μm i.d.).

Isolated microvessel experiments are particularly well suited to pharmacological studies for a number of reasons. First, agonist responses are relatively robust and often preserved even when spontaneous tone, myogenic responses, and flow-induced responses are compromised (see Section VI). Second, agonists can be applied abluminally or intraluminally, e.g., to test for endothelial permeability barriers.[54] Third, agonist responses can be quantitated without secondary changes in pressure and/or flow. Such changes could potentially enhance or mask agonist responses under *in vivo* conditions. For example, it is well known that the initial wall stress of an arteriole can profoundly determine reactivity to an agonist.[25] If an agonist is applied topically to a large area of an *in vivo* microvascular preparation, biphasic responses of small arterioles might be observed that are not directly caused by the agonist but as a result of secondary changes in arteriolar pressure (and consequently wall stress). Similar secondary effects could potentially occur as a result of shear stress changes if the microvessel being studied is sensitive to that stimulus.

E. MICROVASCULAR MECHANICS

Studies of classical muscle mechanics in small blood vessels have been primarily conducted using the myograph system devised by Mulvany and Halpern.[28] This system employs fine tungsten wires (d ≈ 35 μm) that are inserted into the lumen of a vessel and connected to a microforce transducer. Mechanical studies are then performed under isometric or isotonic conditions with the vessel pulled into an elliptical cross-sectional geometry. Due to the size of the wires, this method is limited to vessels approximately 90 μm i.d. or greater. The vascular segments are not perfused and are generally too large or too traumatized to develop spontaneous tone. This is the state-of-the-art technique for studying small artery mechanics, but it has not yet been scaled down for use with microvessels.

Very few mechanical studies of microvessels have been performed *in vitro*. Notable exceptions are studies from Duling's laboratory and from Gore's laboratory. Greensmith and Duling[26] quantitated the phenomenon of intimal buckling that occurs when isolated hamster cheek pouch arterioles undergo progressive constriction. Sleek and Duling[66] measured the myofilament realignment that occurred in the medial layer under the same conditions. In those two studies, agonists were used to constrict the arterioles by a predetermined amount. Jackson and Duling[40] quantitated myogenic responsiveness of 70 μm cheek pouch arterioles at different levels of agonist-induced tone. Davis and Gore[14] determined the maximal active length-tension relationship of consecutive branching orders of cheek pouch arterioles by activating them with norepinephrine and KCl. More recently, Davis has performed isotonic[12] and isobaric[78] quick-release experiments on isolated cheek pouch arterioles to measure maximal velocity of shortening of arteriolar smooth muscle. The latter experiments require a somewhat elaborate set-up that is described in Section IV of this chapter.

F. ELECTROPHYSIOLOGY

The isolated microvessel preparation is a potentially powerful tool that could be used in conjunction with electrophysiological techniques. Unfortunately, this combination of techniques has not been well exploited.

To probe the electrical basis of the myogenic response, Harder and colleagues[29,30] made extensive measurements of smooth muscle membrane potential with intracellular microelectrodes in arteries and small arteries as a function of luminal pressure. Their consistent finding was that a progressive increase in pressure over the myogenic range of a vessel was associated with progressive depolarization. Due to movement artifacts associated with each pressure step, it was virtually impossible to maintain acceptable membrane potential recordings while pressure was changing. It is likely that such movement artifacts will be an even greater problem when this technique is applied to microvessels.

Hirst and Neild[35] developed an isolated guinea pig submucosal arteriole preparation to measure electrical coupling between arteriolar smooth muscle cells. The preparation has been used extensively by Neild and Suprenant[58] to study neuromuscular transmission in submucosal arterioles (30–60 μm o.d.) and to identify neurotransmitters and cotransmitters in that preparation. Although this preparation is quite elegant, the arterioles are neither cannulated nor pressurized, and it remains to be determined the extent to which the experimental findings would be altered at physiological pressures.

III. EQUIPMENT AND PROCEDURES

A general diagram of the system we use for isolated microvessel experiments is shown in Figure 1. The discussion that follows will focus on aspects of the equipment and procedures not previously discussed in other reviews.

A. SOLUTIONS

We typically study isolated microvessels in a physiological salt solution buffered with MOPS (morpholinopropanesulfonic acid), although other buffer systems have been and could be used.[10,36] A detailed description of the MOPS solution is given by Duling et al.[16] We always use highly purified or double-distilled water to prepare all solutions. Small amounts of EGTA are important, probably to chelate residual heavy metal ions that may be present (E. VanBavel, personal communication).

The bath solutions for dissection and cannulation contain 0.5 to 1.0 g% albumin, as albumin appears to exert a protective effect while the vessel is being manipulated. The dissection solution must be precooled to 4°C, so its pH is appropriately adjusted to be 7.4 when it reaches that temperature. Albumin is added to all intraluminal solutions to maintain endothelial cell integrity.[36] The type of albumin used is critical. Some investigators[14,16] use Sigma Fraction V albumin that has been extensively dialyzed and lyophilized prior to use; for convenience, we now use a purified version obtained commercially (US Biochemicals #10856). Unpurified albumin may contain high levels of free fatty acids that can vasoconstrict[56,73] or vasodilate[2] microvessels and possibly interfere with physiological responses. We find no effect of the albumin listed above on basal tone when it is added to the 37°C bath solution surrounding pig coronary arterioles.

B. DISSECTION TECHNIQUES

For excellent and thorough discussions of dissection techniques and microsurgical instrument preparation, the reader is referred to previous works.[16,17] We currently use curved Moria forceps (Fine Science Tools, cat. #11399-87) for dissection, 5/45 Dumont forceps

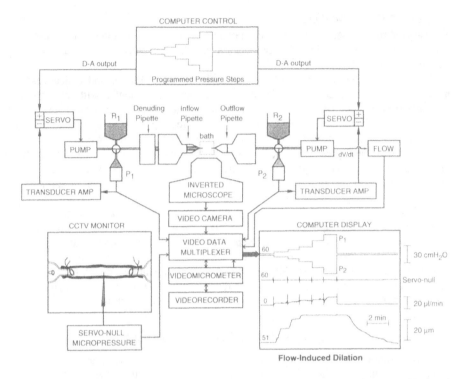

Figure 1 Diagram of system used to study pressure- and flow-induced responses of isolated microvessels. The system uses videomicroscopy to measure vessel inner diameter. Detail in lower left corner shows schematic of cannulating pipettes, denuding pipette (partially withdrawn from cannulating pipette tip), and servo-nulling pipette. Pressures in the two cannulating pipettes can be controlled from moveable reservoirs (R1, R2) or via pumps that are under computer control. When the system operates in pressure-control mode, two servo-control amplifiers are used to maintain constant pressure in the pumps. In perfusion experiments (sample traces shown at lower right), flow rate is controlled by changing pressure (P1, P2) simultaneously in equal and opposite directions. Flow is proportional to the output of a differentiator that measures the rate of pump displacement. All analog signals are fed through a video data multiplexer into a computer interface (not shown). Computer programs to drive experimental protocols are written in LabView 2 and run on a Macintosh Quadra computer.

(cat. #11251-35) for cannulation, and Moria iridectomy scissors (FST cat. #15396-00) for fine cutting. The scissors can typically be used with very little additional sharpening, thus avoiding the complicated procedure described by Duling et al.[16] for preparation of this instrument. We use three different sets of scissors and forceps for gross dissection, fine dissection, and extra-fine dissection, respectively, with the most delicate and finely sharpened tools being reserved only for the final dissection step. As stated by Duling and Rivers,[17] a high-quality dissection scope (e.g., Zeiss or Wild, preferably with Greenough optics for better stereo vision) equipped with a foot-focusing attachment (Unislide, #VB4015P40J) is essential for preparing vessels under ≈80 μm i.d.

C. PIPETTE SYSTEMS AND CANNULATION METHODS

Since this topic was last reviewed,[17] two cannulation systems have come into widespread use. The original system described by Duling et al.[16] was adapted from the concentric, V-track pipette device developed by Burg and Orloff for perfusion of renal tubules.[5] This will be referred to as the Burg system (see Figure 2A). With the other technique, to which

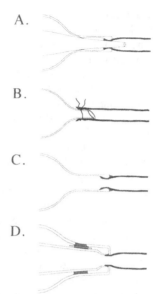

Figure 2 Diagram illustrating different cannulation methods used for microvessels. Panel A: Burg method, using concentric holding and cannulating pipettes. Panel B: Halpern method, using ophthalmic suture. Panel C: Fibrin glue method used for small arteries (vertical hatching indicates glue). Panel D: Vacuum method used for small arteries (vertical hatching indicates where epoxy is placed to center the pipettes). Small tube in between inner and outer pipettes allows vacuum to be applied to tip of outer pipette and hold the vessel end in place.

we refer as the Halpern method, each vessel end is sutured to a single cannulating pipette; that method is based on Osol and Halpern's technique for studying small arteries[60] and was adapted for microvessels by Kuo et al.[50]

Pipettes for cannulating microvessels are fashioned from thin glass tubing on a microforge. We prefer thin-walled Drummond N-51A glass (0.0775-in. o.d., 0.0705-in. i.d.). This glass can be rapidly tapered and broken back to minimize tip resistance, which is important for perfusion experiments. Standard micropipette pullers alone do not provide sufficient control of pipette tip shape to be adequate for most isolated microvessel studies. For detailed procedures for fashioning Burg-type pipettes, the reader is again referred to the chapter by Duling and Rivers.[17] It should be noted that the shape of the cannulating pipettes described in that chapter are slightly different (i.e., tapered) from those in the original description given by Duling et al.[16] We presume (based on our own experience[14]) that better seals at the vessel-pipette interface are obtained with tapered cannulation pipettes.

For the Halpern method (Figure 2B), the shape of the cannulating pipette is generally similar to the holding pipette described for the Burg system by Duling and Rivers.[17] Our final step after manufacture is to break the tip back at a slight angle using forceps and to heat-polish it so that its outer diameter is approximately 50 to 75% of the passive inner diameter of the vessel to be cannulated. The pipette is then bent to an angle of 30 to 45° (using the microforge) near the base of its final taper so that it can be positioned parallel to the bottom of the cannulation chamber. This greatly facilitates manual cannulation and visibility of the microvessel.

The original Halpern apparatus for pressurizing small arteries was designed with a pinch-clamp to hold the vessel at one end, while the other end was tied to a cannulating pipette that was fixed to a micrometer assembly for adjustment of vessel length.[27] A later version of that system allowed the vessel to be cannulated at both ends.[72] The original design would most likely be awkward for use with microvessels. The pipette holders cannot be easily removed for cleaning (see Section VI), and the vessel cannot be positioned near the chamber bottom for use with the high-quality microscope objectives that are required for visualizing small arterioles.

We have modified a Burg V-track system (IVM Instruments, San Antonio, TX; Jim White Instruments, Bradbury Park, MD) for use with the Halpern cannulation technique.

The pipette holders are virtually identical to the standard Burg holders (the two middle holders). The vessel is cannulated just above the bottom surface of the chamber with a single pipette and ligated using 12-O (15 μm) suture (ASSI, #7V43 12/O N-NS). It is then lowered so that it just barely clears the glass surface, allowing oil-immersion objectives to be used on an inverted microscope. A smaller-diameter rear pipette that moves concentrically on the V-track can optionally be used to mechanically denude the microvessel endothelium (see Kuo et al.[48]) after measurements on the intact vessel have been made. The two V-track pipette systems are mounted on manipulators (Narishige, #MN-1) and attached to a baseplate onto which the vessel chamber is mounted. The baseplate is critical for our procedure because the vessel is cannulated under a dissecting microscope and then the entire assembly (vessel, pipettes, chamber, manipulators, and baseplate) is transferred to the stage of the inverted microscope. Additional manipulators (e.g., for servo-null measurements or side-branch experiments) can be easily added to the baseplate after the vessel is mounted onto the inverted microscope.

We use several special pipettes and pipette-making techniques for our experiments. The denuding pipette is made from Drummond R-6 glass (0.047-in. o.d., 0.040-in. i.d.). It has an unpolished, flared tip and a very long and thin flexible shaft (≈1 cm) to allow it to pass around the 30 to 45° bend near the tip of the cannulating pipette. The outer tip diameter is adjusted to be just slightly smaller than the inner tip diameter of the cannulating pipette. Additional information regarding the mechanical denuding procedure is given in Kuo et al.[48] For experiments in which microvessels will be perfused at different flow rates with minimal intraluminal pressure change (see Section IV), the hydraulic resistances of the two cannulating pipettes must be balanced. We assume, for pipettes of similar geometry, that electrical resistance is a good indicator of hydraulic resistance. We make 8 to 10 cannulating pipettes at a time and measure the electrical resistance of each using a bridge circuit (Leader Electronics, #LCR #740). The pipettes are grouped into pairs with similar resistances and the pipette in each pair with the lower resistance is subjected to additional heat-polishing under the microforge until the two resistances are very closely matched. The pipettes are then siliconized by connecting them to a vacuum and by dipping the tips in 7% dimethyl dichlorosilane dissolved in spectroanalyzed chloroform, then in spectroanalyzed acetone.

The rate-limiting step in successfully preparing an isolated microvessel for study will nearly always be at the dissection or the cannulation step. With the Burg method, the major limiting factor is the quality of the dissection, the cleanliness of the vessel ends, or the extent of crimping of the ends; these factors are determined primarily by the skill of the dissector and by the quality of the microsurgical instruments. Vessels down to 15 μm (maximal passive i.d.) can be studied with this method, although physiological responses may be somewhat diminished as compared to the side-branch method (see below and Reference 10). With the Halpern method, the limiting factor will most likely be the cannulating skill and patience of the investigator. We routinely cannulate and perfuse 40 to 50 μm (maximal passive i.d.) arterioles using this method, with up to a 90% success rate (depending on the skill of the dissector). It could probably work down to ≈30 μm vessels with a lower success rate.

A modification we have made for myogenic studies on smaller vessels using the Halpern method is called the side-branch configuration.[15] A parent vessel with a smaller side-branch is dissected, but only the parent vessel is cannulated. The side-branch is positioned parallel to the chamber bottom and ligated with 12-O suture. After the chamber is mounted onto the inverted microscope and the parent vessel is pressurized, a third manipulator is attached to the baseplate. A holding pipette (made from R-6 glass) is positioned so that its tip rests near the side-branch just distal to the tie. Strong suction from a 50-ml syringe is then applied to this holding pipette to draw up the end of the side-branch (distal to the ligature). The length of the parent vessel is adjusted to remove any slack, followed by adjustment of the third holding pipette to remove slack from the side-branch. This method allows pressure-induced responses of very small arterioles (<15 μm i.d.) to be studied, while only requiring that the larger parent vessels be cannulated. It greatly reduces the amount of surgical trauma that would occur if the side-branch were directly cannulated. To prevent myogenic responses of the parent vessel from influencing the response of the side-branch vessel, the parent vessel is intentionally overstretched (longitudinally) before connecting the holding pipette to the side-branch. This method can also be used in conjunction with the Burg cannulation technique.[14] It is useful for mechanical and pharmacological studies, but not for studies in which the side-branch vessel must be perfused.

For perfusion experiments, additional tests can be performed after cannulation to ensure that balanced sets of perfusion pipettes perform as expected. After the vessel is set up, but before it has developed spontaneous tone, the pressure at each end can be changed in equal and opposite directions, starting from the same initial pressure (see Figure 1). The vessel will respond passively to pressure at this time and diameter will change accordingly if a significant change in pressure at the vessel midpoint occurs (this test can also be performed at the end of the experiment with the vessel in calcium-free solution and nitroprusside present to abolish tone). When the vessel has spontaneous tone, the pipette resistance balance can be checked by noting the vascular response to a flow step in one direction and then to an identical step in the opposite direction (see Figure 3). We find that a dilation to flow in one direction, followed by a constriction to the same flow rate in the opposite direction, is usually associated with an imbalance in the two pipette resistances. Of course, the best check is to directly measure pressure at the vessel midpoint during a flow step using a servo-null pipette. We don't use this procedure routinely, but we performed several tests with it when we set up our original experiments[51] and we still use it occasionally when we test a new protocol. Servo-null measurements are notoriously difficult to make *in vivo*, but are quite simple to make with isolated vessels because relatively large-tip (2 to 3 μm) servo-nulling pipettes can be used and because the vessel wall is usually clearly defined, making it simple to puncture with a sharp tip. Increasing the pressures simultaneously at both vessel ends aids in confirmation that the tip is in the lumen and free of obstructions. We use a third micromanipulator for servo-null measurements, which is mounted to the same baseplate as the manipulators for the cannulating pipettes. This manipulator has a hydraulic control for the fine movements that are required. As shown in Figure 1 (lower right), midpoint pressure is virtually constant as the pressures on the two ends of the matched cannulating pipettes are simultaneously altered in equal and opposite directions.

It should be mentioned that at least two other cannulation techniques have been developed for use with small arteries (Figure 2C and D). These methods were specifically designed to perfuse vessels at high (near-physiological) flow rates by minimizing pipette resistance. Sipkema and colleagues[37] use fibrin glue to secure vessels (d = 300 mm) to the inside edge of a relatively large pipette (pipette i.d. ≈ vessel maximal passive o.d.). During the cannulation procedure, an inner, concentric pipette is advanced into the vessel lumen (similar to the Burg method) to hold the vessel end loosely in place against the outer pipette while the glue is applied. Some glue then creeps up into and around the tip of the outer pipette. After the glue bonds, the inner pipette is withdrawn, allowing the vessel to be perfused via the outer pipette that has a relatively low access resistance (see Figure 2C). A somewhat similar method was devised by VanBavel et al.[75] and by Giezeman,[23] in which the end of a small artery (D = 100–300 mm) is pinched longitudinally between inner and outer pipette tips and held in place using a strong (>200 mmHg) vacuum applied to the space between the two concentric pipettes (see Figure 2D). Both of these methods

A.

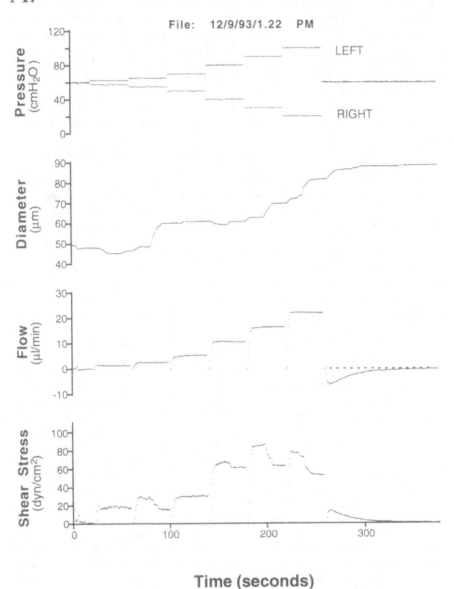

Time (seconds)

Figure 3 Examples of flow-induced responses of a first-order arteriole isolated from hamster cheek pouch. In panel A, the pressure on the left side of the system is raised in steps, while pressure on the right side is simultaneously lowered (flow from left to right). The arteriole constricts slightly at low flow rates, then dilates at high flow rates. To verify that the diameter changes are caused by flow rather than by pressure, the identical sequence of pressure steps is repeated but with flow in the opposite direction. Nearly identical diameter changes are observed (although in both cases, the vessel does not recover within 2 min after flow ceases). This confirms that pipette resistances are balanced. Flow was measured as described in the text, and the overshoots observed after pressures are equalized are artifacts of the differentiator (dotted lines indicate true zero flow). Shear stress was calculated on-line, based on vessel diameter, flow rate, and fluid viscosity (see Reference 59 for equation).

B.

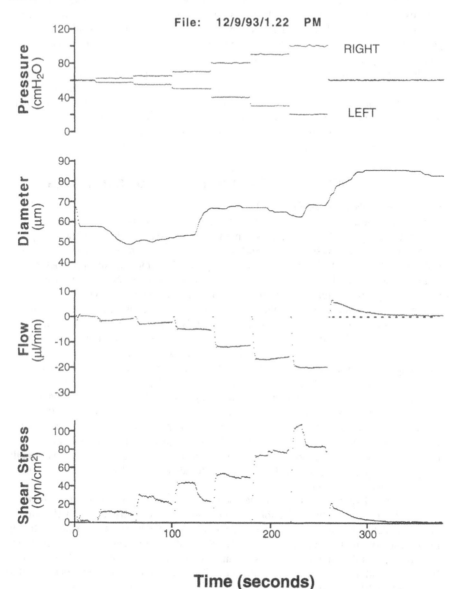

Figure 3 *Continued.*

allow vessels to be perfused via relatively large pipettes so that higher and possibly more physiological flow rates can be achieved. However, it remains to be seen if these methods can be scaled down to work successfully with microvessels.

D. CHAMBERS AND MICROSCOPES

Chamber design is not critical for most applications. We use a lucite chamber similar to that described by Duling et al.,[16] with a 50-µm thick glass coverslip glued into the bottom with silicone compound (Dow Corning, RTV #734). This thickness is critical for calcium imaging experiments in which UV transmissive, oil-immersion objectives with low working distances are used (e.g., Nikon 40× CF-fluor, Zeiss 40× axiostigmat); even with this coverslip, we are barely able to focus on the upper surface of a 120-µm arteriole touching the chamber bottom. The chamber that we use for *in vitro* studies is water-jacketed and, when necessary, it is covered with Saran Wrap during an experiment to minimize evaporation and/or control bath pO_2.

The type of microscope used for isolated microvessel experiments is not critical, but a high-quality, fixed-stage inverted scope is recommended (Leitz, Nikon, Olympus, Zeiss). This allows a wider variety of objectives to be used and eliminates the problem of moisture from the 37°C bath solution condensing on objectives, a problem that will occur on upright microscopes (this can still happen to short-working-distance condensers on an inverted microscope).

IV. EXPERIMENTAL MEASUREMENTS AND TECHNIQUES

A. DIMENSION MEASUREMENTS

Dimensional measurements in isolated microvessel experiments have been discussed by Duling and Rivers.[17] We will address some issues not raised in their review.

In our experience, vessels under ≈60 µm require manual tracking methods, such as with a Colorado Video 321 videomicrometer, to accurately measure inner diameter. This results from the fact that it is difficult to sufficiently clear connective tissue from small vessels to permit internal diameter tracking by automated devices. We use a videomicrometer in conjunction with standard videomicroscopic techniques. Computer and microscope-based image enhancement methods can be useful for visualizing very small arterioles and for measuring wall thickness. We have used differential interference contrast (DIC) microscopy in conjunction with a Zeiss 63× (1.25 n.a.) strain-free oil-immersion objective, but this technique only works well on vessels <30 µm i.d. and requires a nonstandard condenser system. For the condenser, we adapted a Zeiss 55× (0.8 n.a.) UO water-immersion objective by installing a variable aperture in its back focal plane. The sharp taper of that objective allows it to be positioned just above the upper surface of the cannulated microvessel. The technique has proved useful for continuous quantitation of wall buckling in small arterioles, where measurements of both intimal and medial layers are required. Strange and Spring[70] used similar DIC techniques to optically section through isolated, perfused renal tubules to determine cell volume changes under various osmotic conditions.

For vessels larger than 100 µm, it may be feasible to track inner and/or outer diameter using video methods. This is possible when the vessel wall is sufficiently thick to allow more complete removal of connective tissue. For example, we were able to automatically track vasomotion in isolated bat wing venules (i.d. = 100 µm) with the technique developed by Neild[57] and which is now commercially available (Diamtrak©, Montech Pty. Ltd., Australia). For a discussion of other automated techniques, the reader is referred to Intaglietta and Hammersen,[38] to Halpern et al.,[27] and to a recent paper by Magers and Faber.[53] However, our attempts to adapt commercially available tracking methods to isolated microvessels have been unsuccessful. With small vessels, automated diameter tracking devices lock onto connective tissue elements that inevitably remain attached after dissection, or else they switch unpredictably between tracking inner and outer diameter as the microvessel constricts. It is possible to remove more of the connective tissue surrounding small vessels and obtain an improved image and improved tracking, but vessel viability is usually sacrificed in the process.

VanBavel et al.[74] describes an interesting method to automatically monitor vessel diameter. Under epi-illumination, the vessel is slowly perfused with FITC-labeled albu-min, and the fluorescence signal coming from the whole vessel at relatively low magnification is then measured continuously using a photomultiplier tube. If the vessel remains in focus (which is not usually a problem at low magnification), the photomultiplier output is proportional to the cross-sectional area (CSA) of the vessel lumen and can be converted to diameter after a calibration procedure is performed at the end of each experiment. The relationship between CSA and diameter is valid over a limited range of diameters and is adequate for use with small arteries. The technique may not be as accurate for microvessels that can close completely under a variety of experimental conditions.[10,40] Also, long-term FITC fluorescence emission may impair normal arteriolar responsiveness.[44]

B. PRESSURE CONTROL

Several methods are available for controlling pressure in isolated microvessel experiments.

The simplest method of pressure control is to cannulate one end of the microvessel, flush out any remaining blood elements, secure the other end with suture, and connect the cannulating pipette to a vertically adjustable reservoir. We prefer to cannulate both vessel ends and connect them to separate reservoirs because a greater number of protocols and checks can subsequently be performed. For example, leaks in the system can be checked by pressurizing the vessel from one pipette and measuring pressure through the other pipette using a pressure transducer.

Duling et al.[16] used a three-way valve to connect both a reservoir and a micrometer syringe to the cannulating pipette because the syringe allowed very rapid changes in pressure to be applied. VanBavel[74] used compressed air and a pressure regulator to provide the pressure head for a saline reservoir. Both of these methods work well.

We have recently developed a computer-controlled system to manipulate pressure at both ends of an isolated microvessel (see Figure 1, top). The pipette ends are pressurized from reservoirs during the set-up and equilibration period, and then connected to hydraulic pumps (Ling Dynamic Systems, #V203) identical to those used in servo-null micropressure systems. The pumps are driven by servo-control amplifiers, with power amplifiers in each output stage. The input for each servo-amplifier is set by a computer, while the feedback signal comes from the output of a pressure transducer amplifier that monitors pressure applied by the pump. We initially tested the frequency response of this system using a servo-nulling pipette inserted into a small side-branch arteriole.[15] With 30-µm or greater diameter cannulating pipettes, the frequency response was flat nearly to 30 Hz and therefore capable of delivering periodic waveforms or rapid pressure steps to the microvessel. Since the servo-controller can be driven by the computer, an infinite and complex variety of pressure step sequences can be applied. This system has been successfully used to perform a number of different protocols on arterioles.[11,12,15]

C. PERFUSION EXPERIMENTS

Several methods are also available to perfuse isolated microvessels for the study of flow-induced responses.

The system described by Kuo et al.[51] was designed to set up and maintain a constant-pressure differential across the vessel. This system has both advantages and disadvantages. A primary advantage is that no large pressure transients occur at the level of the microvessel when flow is initiated. If pressure transients were to occur, then myogenic responses could potentially interfere with or mask flow-induced responses. Kuo's system also allows different combinations of flow and pressure steps to be applied, and this feature has been used recently to determine the interaction between flow-induced and pressure-induced responses of arterioles.[49] A disadvantage of the system used by Kuo et al.[51] is that it is difficult to determine the flow rates that correspond to a given series of pressure gradients. Kuo et al.[51] calibrated their system using a separate series of experiments in which red blood cells were perfused through passive vessels in order to measure flow velocity at the same series of pressure gradients used in their previous experiments. That calibration method was cumbersome because it required an additional set of experiments using the same-size vessel and same set of pipettes. The computer-controlled modification of Kuo's system described above gets around this problem by continuously monitoring the rate at which one of the hydraulic pumps is displaced during a perfusion experiment; pump displacement rate is converted to flow rate after a simple one-time calibration procedure using calibrated microliter tubes. This allows continual flow measurements to be made during subsequent experiments (see Figure 3).

A fundamental disadvantage with the constant-pressure-differential technique is that, as significant changes in microvessel diameter occur in response to flow, the overall resistance of the system changes, and thus flow rate changes. For example, if a vessel dilates in response to flow and vessel resistance comprises the major fraction of the total system resistance, total resistance will fall significantly while the pressure gradient remains constant; this will produce a secondary increase in flow rate. We don't usually find this effect to be significant (see Figure 3), however, probably because we use the Halpern cannulation technique in which the pipette resistances comprise the major fraction of total system resistance. The effect could be greater in systems where pipette resistances are relatively small.[37,75]

A second type of perfusion set-up would be one in which flow rate is maintained constant by varying the pressure gradient. A system that could potentially be used for this type of experiment is commercially available (Living Systems, Burlington, VT, #PS-200). It was designed for use with small arteries and uses a syringe pump to pressurize the artery. A pressure transducer is interposed between the pump and the vessel end, and a servo-control amplifier receives a feedback signal from the transducer and uses it to adjust the flow rate in the syringe. As described here, the system operates in constant-pressure mode, but it can be switched to operate in constant flow-mode. The system can be configured with one pump and an outflow reservoir, or with two pumps in a push-pull arrangement. Koller et al.[45] have used the former configuration to study flow-induced responses in rat gracilis and cremaster arterioles. Bevan and colleagues[21] have used the latter configuration extensively to study responses of rabbit small arteries. A potential advantage of the syringe-based system is that constant flow rates can be maintained, although it is not clear if studies published to date have actually performed constant-flow experiments. A disadvantage of the push-pull configuration is that pressure transients can potentially occur at the level of the vessel if inflow and outflow resistances are not balanced or if the pumps are not driven precisely in phase. In small arteries, this may not be as much of a problem because a pressure gradient (at the front of the syringe pumps) of 5 to 10 mmHg is sufficient to generate flow rates that produce a vascular response.[21] In microvessels, however, one would be advised to initially monitor pressure at the vessel midpoint using a servo-nulling system (at least in preliminary experiments) to ensure that large pressure transients do not occur.

D. FLUORESCENCE IMAGING EXPERIMENTS

A few laboratories have recently begun using isolated microvessel systems to quantitate changes in Fura-2 fluorescence (and other ion-sensitive dyes) in microvascular endothelium or smooth muscle. Video imaging systems are generally needed for these types of experiments because microvessels contain more than one cell type (i.e., fluorescence signals from endothelium and smooth muscle may interfere with one another) and because slight movement artifacts can potentially cause problems. In addition, in most experiments of this nature, one would want to continuously monitor vessel diameter using a video system.

Some examples of microvessel imaging experiments are studies by Falcone et al.[19] of flow-induced changes in endothelial cell calcium and diameter in rat cremaster arterioles, and studies by Meininger et al.[55] of pressure-induced changes in arteriolar diameter and smooth muscle calcium. Curry's laboratory[33] has a particularly elaborate set-up in which photometry and fluorescence imaging measurements can be made on the same vessel. They perfuse mesenteric capillaries and venules *in situ*, but their techniques are quite similar in many respects to those used in isolated microvessel experiments *in vitro*. Yuan et al.[77] have applied some of the same methods to isolated coronary venules.

One particular problem to be aware of in quantitative fluorescence experiments concerns the requirement for selective loading of either the endothelial or smooth muscle layer with fluorescent dyes. If smooth muscle calcium is to be measured in relatively large vessels (> 80 μm), the entire wall (including the intima) can be loaded using Fura-2 AM via the bath because contamination of smooth muscle fluorescence signals by endothelial cell fluorescence will probably be negligible. However, if one desires to measure only endothelial cell calcium changes, then it is necessary to selectively load the endothelial layer, probably by applying Fura-2 from the luminal side. Falcone et al.[19] devised a procedure to do this and details can be found in their paper.

V. CONSIDERATION OF TISSUES AND SPECIES

A. VESSEL SIZE, LENGTH, AND BRANCHING PATTERN

Isolated microvessels from a variety of tissues have now been successfully studied. Examples include arterioles from cheek pouch,[40] testis,[16] skeletal muscle,[19] heart,[49] brain,[7] mesentery,[69] and kidney,[18] venules from skin,[9] heart,[47] and lymphatics from mesentery.[78]

The majority of isolated microvessel studies are conducted on vessels taken from thin tissues or from those tissues from which microvessels can be easily dissected. This is one reason for the extensive number of studies that have been performed using hamster cheek pouch vessels. Another example of this would be the small penetrating cerebral arterioles studied by Dacey and Duling,[7] which can rather easily be extracted from the surface of the cortex with minimal trauma. We[50] devised a method to facilitate dissection of arterioles embedded deep in tissues such as the heart. Our original plan to study subendocardial arterioles was hampered by the lack of contrast between the arterioles and the surrounding subendocardial parenchymal tissue, so we formulated an ink-gelatin mixture that was liquid at room temperature and could be easily perfused into the coronary arterial system of a warm heart and would solidify when the heart was cooled to 4°C for dissection (see Reference 50 for details). This greatly enhanced the contrast between the vessel and the parenchymal tissue, and facilitated identification of small side branches. The method has also been used to dissect and isolate coronary venules.[77]

Another factor that limits a successful microvessel experiment is the length of the unbranched vessel segment available for study. For cannulations using the Burg procedure, the rule of thumb used by Duling and Rivers[17] was that segment lengths should be 8 to 10 times the vessel diameter, because a length equivalent to 2 to 3 diameters will be traumatized at each vessel end during cannulation. In many tissues, an unbranched segment of this length may be difficult to locate and this is especially true of arterioles <60 μm i.d. In the hamster cheek pouch, many such segments can be located, while in the pig heart one may need to search for an hour or more to find an unbranched segment of adequate length. On the other hand, if it is feasible to tie off side-branches, a longer segment with one or even two branches can be used. This will most likely increase the probability of obtaining a viable vessel, because in our experience, side branches as small as 10 μm i.d. can be carefully ligated (i.e., without applying torque to the parent vessel) without compromising the reactivity of the parent vessel even near the branch site.

B. ANIMAL SPECIES

Isolated microvessels have been obtained from many animal species including rat, hamster, bat, pig, rabbit, dog, and man. In most cases, it is probably desirable or even imperative to use the same species from which *in vivo* data have been previously obtained. As a rule, we suggest that microvessels be obtained from fresh tissue rather than from slaughterhouse tissues. If this requirement cannot be met, then every effort should be made to immediately cool the slaughterhouse tissue samples to 4°C and perform the dissections as quickly as possible at that temperature.

Occasionally, the specific protocol or vessel type may determine what species is used. For example, we examined the subendocardial circulation of several species before concluding that the pig might be the best source for subendocardial arterioles. Edwards[18] made extensive use of rabbits to study afferent and efferent arterioles because dissection of connective tissue from around those arterioles was apparently easier in the rabbit than in the rat (the species most often used for renal micropuncture); it should be noted, though, that Ito et al.[39] have recently adapted the method for rat vessels.

VI. CRITERIA FOR ASSESSING MICROVESSEL VIABILITY

It is essential that each laboratory establish a set of criteria with which to assess the viability of their isolated microvessel preparations. The criteria will vary with the type and size of the vessel used and possibly with the type of experimental protocol to be performed. If possible, a good starting point is to use the same criteria that have been adopted in the literature for *in vivo* microcirculatory studies on that vessel type. For example, hamster cheek pouch vessels studied *in vivo* typically develop 30 to 40% spontaneous tone, show two different patterns of vasomotion, exhibit myogenic responses, and respond to changes in bath pO_2. With the possible exception of the latter response, all of these phenomena are observed in a high-quality isolated cheek pouch arteriole preparation.[10]

In the absence of previous *in vivo* data, criteria for viability can be determined based on the hierarchy of responses used by other laboratories studying isolated microvessels. We find that myogenic and flow-induced responses are usually the most fragile, followed by development of normal, spontaneous vasomotion, then spontaneous tone, and finally pharmacologic reactivity. For example, it is quite common to set up an isolated arteriole that does not show myogenic responses but that develops spontaneous tone and responds to norepinephrine. On the other hand, a vessel that shows good myogenic responses will almost certainly respond to KCl and phenylephrine. Within the category of pharmacologic reactivity, we find that the response to KCl is typically lost before the response to α-agonists (provided that α-adrenoreceptors are present), and we have yet to see an isolated microvessel that does not respond to endothelin. It is uncertain where oxygen sensitivity fits into this hierarchy because we only occasionally observe oxygen responses in isolated cheek pouch arterioles that are reactive in all other respects; in contrast, Fredericks and Lombard[20] typically observe oxygen responses in small arteries that show only weak myogenic responses.

It is not clear to what extent, if any, normal pharmacologic responses are altered in vessels that have lost myogenic or flow-induced responses; that is, is quite possible that valuable pharmacologic information can be obtained from isolated microvessels that have lost physiologic responses. For example, renal afferent arterioles possess robust myogenic responses *in vivo*,[6,24] yet most isolated afferent arterioles show little or no myogenic responsiveness[18,76] even though they respond well to agonists. The same is true of myogenic responses in isolated cerebral arterioles[7] as compared to *in vivo* cerebral arterioles.[32]

Several factors may interfere with the normal reactivity of isolated microvessels. Excessive pulling or stretching during dissection or cannulation will usually cause irreparable damage to an arteriole. Likewise, the slightest nick by scissors or forceps in the outer wall during dissection will produce damage. Excessive bleeding or clotting of the vessel ends during dissection also seems to reduce reactivity. In general, the shorter the time spent dissecting and cannulating an arteriole, the higher the chances of obtaining a viable vessel.

Whenever gelatin solutions are used to facilitate vessel identification, vessel reactivity must be checked. For example, we tested for alterations in both myogenic and endothelium-dependent responses after we perfused the pig coronary system with ink-gelatin.[49] Any glues or adhesives that are used during cannulation[37] or in the chamber must be tested. We have removed all metal pieces (even stainless steel ones) from pipette holders, chambers, pumps, or perfusion lines, as these can become corroded and possibly leak metal ions.[52] For this reason, we do not use needle hubs in our system, but rather pieces of flanged PE-190 tubing to connect the pipette holders to stopcocks and PE-90 tubing to interconnect PE-190 tubing.

We find that many small but important details are overlooked by those who are new to isolated microvessel techniques. For example, three-way valves must be opened to atmosphere before connecting or disconnecting tubes coming from cannulation pipettes. Microvessels do not tolerate even transient exposure to air when transferring them from dissection to cannulation chambers, and they are quite susceptible to osmotic changes in the bath solution due to evaporation. We also find that some microvessels (e.g., cheek pouch arterioles) do not tolerate rapid increases in temperature; our standard procedure for these vessels is to raise bath temperature from 22 to 37°C over the course of an hour at the beginning of an experiment.

Microvessels often fail to develop spontaneous tone because small leaks in the system have not been detected and the vessels are being chronically dilated by flow. These leaks can occur not only from untied side-branches, but also from loose connections to valves and pipette holders. If this problem is suspected, we suggest connecting the pipette system using plugged (heat-polished) pipettes, pressurizing the entire system, then systematically closing off parts of the system while monitoring pressure with a transducer. We find that pressure transducers often have small leaks and may require rigorous tightening or even custom gaskets to prevent leaks. Whenever possible, we use Hamilton 3-way valves rather than disposable stopcocks.

Finally, the importance of a thorough, daily cleaning of the entire pipette, perfusion, and chamber system cannot be overemphasized. We completely disassemble our pipette holders after each experiment, wash each piece with distilled water, followed by 10% Contrad (soap) in distilled water, a 33% ETOH/H_2O rinse, and a distilled water rinse, after which each piece is blown dry with compressed air or nitrogen. The same procedure is followed daily for the vessel chamber. The dissection chamber is also cleaned daily, rinsed with distilled water, and finally with 100% ETOH and allowed to air dry. The reservoirs, pumps, and all tubing and valves are flushed daily with several rinses of near-boiling distilled water. Transducers are flushed or cleaned daily. We typically re-use cannulation pipettes for several experiments, but these are also cleaned daily by applying a vacuum to the back end and dipping the tip first in distilled water, then in spectroanalyzed acetone, then allowing them a few minutes to air-dry with continued suction. If they are used for more than 1 week, they are re-siliconized. If any debris builds up on the tip, it is soaked for 1 to 2 h in 2 N HCl solution, followed by the normal cleaning procedure.

If we experience problems on several consecutive days with vessels that fail to develop spontaneous tone or lose responsiveness to pressure and flow, the whole perfusion system is usually broken down and cleaned, all the PE tubing is replaced, and a new layer of Sylgard is poured into the dissection chamber. If bicarbonate solutions have been used, it is necessary to periodically clean many of the system components with dilute HCl followed by extensive distilled water rinses.

VII. PRACTICAL ISSUES TO CONSIDER

A. COST

The cost of a basic system similar to ours is estimated to be just over $55,000 at current prices (apart from the expense of a chart recorder or data-acquisition system). An approximate breakdown of costs would be: inverted scope, $25,000; manipulators, $2000; V-track system, $2500; pipette holders, $2000; surgical instruments, $500; suture, $250; microforge, $5000; videomicrometer, $2000; video camera, $1000; videomonitor, $500; dissection chamber, $500; dissection scope, $5000; fiber-optic light source, $1000; cooled circulator, $2000; bath circulator, $1000; VCR, $500. Machining costs would probably come to an additional $4000 for a baseplate, manipulator attachments, etc. Our system is only practical if one has access to a complete machine shop because several custom pieces and adapters need to be constructed. As an alternative, many components for a complete Halpern-style system are commercially available from Living Systems (Burlington, VT).

B. PERSONNEL

A visit to a laboratory experienced in the above techniques is imperative if one intends to set up an isolated microvessel laboratory. A primary reason for this is that the actual procedures for dissection and cannulation must be learned first-hand since many of the procedural steps cannot be adequately described. Another reason is that there are a large number of subtle details that are inevitably overlooked in a review of this nature. Ideally, one should arrange to spend 2 to 3 weeks in a laboratory during which time an experienced dissector and cannulator would be available to devote several days to pilot experiments on the particular vessel type and size to be studied (a visit for less than 1 week is probably not sufficient). We recommend that the principal investigator master the isolated microvessel technique before introducing it to others in his/her laboratory. This helps to ensure that quality control standards start high and remain high.

ACKNOWLEDGMENTS

We are grateful to Judy Davidson for editing and proofreading the manuscript. We also acknowledge the contributions of Dr. A. Goodman, who designed and constructed many of the electronic components used in our perfusion system, including the videomicrometer, the analog data multiplexer, servo-control amplifiers, power amplifiers, and the computer interface.

REFERENCES

1. **Baez, S.,** Bayliss response in the microcirculation, *FASEB J.,* 27, 1410–1415, 1968.
2. **Bassett, J. E. and Dacey, R. G., Jr.,** Dilation of intracerebral arterioles *in vitro* by fatty acid contamination in bovine serum albumin, *Microvasc. Res.,* 34, 256–259, 1987.
3. **Bevan, J. A. and Joyce, E. H.,** Comparable sensitivity of flow contraction and relaxation to Na reduction may reflect flow-sensor characteristics, *Am. J. Physiol.,* 263(Heart Circ. Physiol. 32), H182–H187, 1992.
4. **Bouskela, E. and Wiederhielm, C. A.,** Microvascular myogenic reaction in the wing of the intact unanesthetized bat, *Am. J. Physiol.,* 237(Heart Circ. Physiol. 6), H59–H65, 1979.
5. **Burg, M. B. and Orloff, J.,** Control of fluid absorption in the renal proximal tubule, *J. Clin. Invest.,* 47, 2016–2024, 1968.
6. **Carmines, P. K., Inscho, E. W., and Gensure, R. C.,** Arterial pressure effects on preglomerular microvasculature of juxtamedullary nephrons, *Am. J. Physiol.,* 258(Renal. Fluid. Electrolyte. Physiol. 27), F94–F102, 1990.

7. **Dacey, R. G., Jr. and Duling, B. R.,** A study of rat intracerebral arterioles: methods, morphology and reactivity, *Am. J. Physiol.*, 243(Heart Circ. Physiol. 12), H598–H606, 1982.

8. **Dacey, R. G., Jr. and Duling, B. R.,** Effect of norepinephrine on penetrating arterioles of rat cerebral cortex, *Am. J. Physiol.*, 246(Heart Circ. Physiol. 15), H380–H385, 1984.

9. **Davis, M. J.,** Spontaneous contractions of isolated bat wing venules are inhibited by lumenal flow, *FASEB J.*, 6, A2072, 1992 (Abstr.).

10. **Davis, M. J.,** Myogenic response gradient in an arteriolar network, *Am. J. Physiol.*, 264(Heart Circ. Physiol. 33), H2168–H2179, 1993.

11. **Davis, M. J. and Davidson, J.,** Responses of hamster cheek pouch arterioles to pulsatile pressure *in vitro*, *FASEB J.*, 7, A8827, 1993 (Abstr.).

12. **Davis, M. J. and Davidson, J.,** Unloaded shortening velocity of vascular smooth muscle in myogenically active arterioles, *FASEB J.*, 7, A757, 1993 (Abstr.).

13. **Davis, M. J., Gilmore, J. P., and Joyner, W. L.,** Responses of pulmonary allograft and cheek pouch arterioles in the hamster to alterations in extravascular pressure in different oxygen environments, *Circ. Res.*, 49, 133–140, 1981.

14. **Davis, M. J. and Gore, R. W.,** Length-tension relationship of maximally activated arterioles, *Phys. Med. Biol.*, 33, 350, 1988.

15. **Davis, M. J. and Sikes, P. J.,** Myogenic response of isolated arterioles: Test for a rate-sensitive mechanism, *Am. J. Physiol.*, 259(Heart Circ. Physiol. 28), H1890–H1900, 1990.

16. **Duling, B. R., Gore, R. W., Dacey, R. G., Jr., and Damon, D. N.,** Methods for isolation, cannulation, and *in vitro* study of single microvessels, *Am. J. Physiol.*, 241(Heart Circ. Physiol. 10), H108–H116, 1981.

17. **Duling, B. R. and Rivers, R. J.,** Isolation, cannulation, and perfusion of microvessels, in *Microcirculatory Technology*, Baker, C. H. and Nastuk, W. L., Eds., Academic Press, New York, 1986, 265–280.

18. **Edwards, R. M.,** Segmental effects of norepinephrine and angiotensin II on isolated renal microvessels, *Am. J. Physiol.*, 244(Renal Fluid Elec.Physiol. 13), F526–F534, 1983.

19. **Falcone, J. C., Kuo, L., and Meininger, G. A.,** Endothelial cell calcium increases during flow-induced dilation in isolated arterioles, *Am. J. Physiol.*, 264(Heart Circ. Physiol. 33), H653–H659, 1993.

20. **Fredricks, K. T. and Lombard, J. H.,** Mechanisms mediating the inhibition of resting tone and contractile responses by reduced PO_2 in skeletal muscle and cerebral resistance arteries, *FASEB J.*, 6(4), A971, 1992 (Abstr.).

21. **Garcia-Roldan, J. L. and Bevan, J. A.,** Flow-induced constriction and dilation of cerebral resistance arteries, *Circ. Res.*, 66, 1445–1448, 1990.

22. **Gaw, A. J. and Bevan, J. A.,** Flow-induced relaxation of the rabbit middle cerebral artery is composed of both endothelium-dependent and -independent components, *Stroke*, 24, 105–109, 1993.

23. **Giezeman, M. J. M. M.,** *Static and Dynamic Pressure-Volume Relations of Isolated Blood Vessels*, (thesis), University of Amsterdam, The Netherlands, 1992, 1–125.

24. **Gilmore, J. P., Cornish, K. G., Rogers, S. D., and Joyner, W. L.,** Direct evidence for myogenic autoregulation of the renal microcirculation in the hamster, *Circ. Res.*, 47, 226–230, 1980.

25. **Gore, R. W.,** Wall stress: A determinant of regional differences in response of frog microvessels to norepinephrine, *Am. J. Physiol.*, 222, 82–91, 1972.

26. **Greensmith, J. E. and Duling, B. R.,** Morphology of the constricted arteriolar wall: Physiological implications, *Am. J. Physiol.*, 247(Heart Circ. Physiol. 16), H687–H698, 1984.

27. **Halpern, W., Mongeon, S. A., and Root, D. T.,** Stress, tension, and myogenic aspects of small isolated extraperenchymal rat arteries, in *Smooth Muscle Contraction*, Stephens, N. L., Ed., Marcel Decker, New York, 1984, 427–456.

28. **Halpern, W., Mulvany, M. J., and Warshaw, D. M.,** Mechanical properties of smooth muscle cells in the walls of arterial resistance vessels, *J. Physiol.*, 275, 85–101, 1978.

29. **Harder, D. R.,** Pressure-induced myogenic activation of cat cerebral arteries is dependent on intact endothelium, *Circ. Res.*, 60, 102–107, 1987.

30. **Harder, D. R., Gilbert, R., and Lombard, J. H.,** Vascular muscle cell depolarization and activation in renal arteries on elevation of transmural pressure, *Am. J. Physiol.*, 253(Renal Fluid Elec. Physiol. 22), F778–F781, 1987.

454

31. **Harder, D. R., Sanchez-Ferrer, C., Kauser, K., Stekiel, W. J., and Rubanyi, G. M.,** Pressure releases a transferable endothelial contractile factor in cat cerebral arteries, *Circ. Res.*, 65, 193–198, 1989.

32. **Harper, S. L., Bohlen, H. G., and Rubin, M. J.,** Arterial and microvascular contributions to cerebral cortical autoregulation in rats, *Am. J. Physiol.*, 246(Heart Circ. Physiol. 15), H17–H24, 1984.

33. **He, P., Pagakis, S. N., and Curry, F. E.,** Measurement of cytoplasmic calcium in single microvessels with increased permeability, *Am. J. Physiol.*, 258(Heart Circ. Physiol. 27), H1366–H1374, 1990.

34. **Henriksen, O.,** Local nervous mechanism in regulation of blood flow in human subcutaneous tissue, *Acta Physiol. Scand.*, 97, 385–391, 1976.

35. **Hirst, G. D. S. and Neild, T. O.,** An analysis of excitatory junctional potentials recorded from arterioles, *J. Physiol.*, 280, 87–104, 1978.

36. **Hoogerwerf, N.,** *Responses of Peripheral Arteries to Physical Stimuli and the Role of the Endothelium: Studies on Isolated Rabbit Arteries,* thesis, University of Amsterdam, The Netherlands, 1993, 7–125.

37. **Hoogerwerf, N., Van der Linden, P. J. W., Westerhof, N., and Sipkema, P.,** A new mounting technique for perfusion of isolated small arteries: The effects of flow and oxygen on diameter, *Microvasc. Res.*, 44, 49–60, 1992.

38. **Intaglietta, M. and Hammersen, F.,** Measurement of diameter in microvascular studies, in *Microcirculatory Technology,* Baker, C. H. and Nastuk, W. L., Eds., Academic Press, New York, 1986, 137–148.

39. **Ito, S., Arima, S., Ren, Y. L., Juncos, L. A., and Carretero, O. A.,** Endothelium-derived relaxing factor/nitric oxide modulates angiotensin II action in the isolated microperfused rabbit afferent but not efferent arteriole, *J. Clin. Invest.*, 91, 2012–2019, 1993.

40. **Jackson, P. A. and Duling, B. R.,** Myogenic response and wall mechanics of arterioles, *Am. J. Physiol.*, 257(Heart Circ. Physiol. 26), H1147–H1155, 1989.

41. **Johnson, P. C.,** Autoregulatory responses of cat mesenteric arterioles measured *in vivo*, *Circ. Res.*, 22, 199–212, 1968.

42. **Johnson, P. C. and Intaglietta, M.,** Contributions of pressure and flow sensitivity to autoregulation in mesenteric arterioles, *Am. J. Physiol.*, 231, 1686–1698, 1976.

43. **Koller, A. and Kaley, G.,** Endothelium regulates skeletal muscle microcirculation by a blood flow velocity-sensing mechanism, *Am. J. Physiol.*, 258(Heart Circ. Physiol. 27), H916–H920, 1990.

44. **Koller, A., Messina, E. J., Wolin, M. S., and Kaley, G.,** Effects of endothelial impairment on arteriolar dilator responses *in vivo*, *Am. J. Physiol.*, 257(Heart Circ. Physiol. 26), H1485–H1489, 1989.

45. **Koller, A., Sun, D., and Kaley, G. K. W.,** Role of shear stress and endothelial prostaglandins in flow- and viscosity-induced dilation of arterioles *in vitro*, *Circ. Res.*, 72, 1276–1284, 1993.

46. **Krauss, S. L., Dodge, J. T., and Bevan, J. A.,** Magnitude of beta-adrenoceptor-mediated responses of dog epicardial coronary arteries: Inverse relation to diameter, *Am. J. Physiol.*, 263(Heart Circ. Physiol. 32), H1422–H1429, 1992.

47. **Kuo, L., Arko, F., Chilian, W. M., and Davis, M. J.,** Coronary venular responses to flow and pressure, *Circ. Res.*, 72, 607–615, 1993.

48. **Kuo, L., Chilian, W. M., and Davis, M. J.,** Coronary arteriolar myogenic response is independent of endothelium, *Circ. Res.*, 66, 860–866, 1990.

49. **Kuo, L., Chilian, W. M., and Davis, M. J.,** Interaction of pressure- and flow-induced responses in porcine coronary resistance vessels, *Am. J. Physiol.*, 261(Heart Circ. Physiol. 30), H1706–H1715, 1991.

50. **Kuo, L., Davis, M. J., and Chilian, W. M.,** Myogenic activity in isolated subepicardial and subendocardial coronary arterioles, *Am. J. Physiol.*, 255(Heart Circ. Physiol. 24), H1558–H1562, 1988.

51. **Kuo, L., Davis, M. J., and Chilian, W. M.,** Endothelium-dependent, flow-induced dilation of isolated coronary arterioles, *Am. J. Physiol.*, 259(Heart Circ. Physiol. 28), H1063–H1070, 1990.

52. **Lew, M. J., Delashaw, J. B., Segal, S. S., and Duling, B. R.,** Salt solutions elute vasoactive concentrations of heavy metals from hypodermic needles, *Fed. Proc.*, 46(4), 1532, 1987 (Abstr.).

53. **Magers, S. and Faber, J. E.,** Real-time measurement of microvascular dimensions using digital cross-correlation image processing, *J. Vasc. Res.*, 29, 241–247, 1992.

455

54. **Matsuki, T., Hynes, M. R., and Duling, B. R.,** Comparison of conduit vessel and resistance vessel reactivity: Influence of intimal permeability, *Am. J. Physiol.*, 264(Heart Circ. Physiol. 33), H1251–H1258, 1993.
55. **Meininger, G. A., Zawieja, D. C., Falcone, J. C., Hill, M. A., and Davey, J. P.,** Calcium measurement in isolated arterioles during myogenic and agonist stimulation, *Am. J. Physiol.*, 261(Heart Circ. Physiol. 30), H950–H959, 1991.
56. **Muller, J. M., Laughlin, M. H., and Myers, P. R.,** Vasoactivity of isolated coronary arterial microvessels: Influence of albumin, *Microvasc. Res.*, 46, 107–115, 1993.
57. **Neild, T. O.,** Measurement of arteriole diameter changes by analysis of television images, *Blood Vessels*, 26, 48–52, 1989.
58. **Neild, T. O., Shen, K. Z., and Surprenant, A.,** Vasodilatation of arterioles by acetylcholine released from single neurones in the guinea-pig submucosal plexus, *J. Physiol.*, 420, 247–265, 1990.
59. **Olesen, S. P., Clapham, D. E., and Davies, P. F.,** Haemodynamic shear stress activates a K⁺ current in vascular endothelial cells, *Nature*, 331, 168–170, 1988.
60. **Osol, G. and Halpern, W.,** Myogenic properties of cerebral blood vessels from normotensive and hypertensive rats, *Am. J. Physiol.*, 249(Heart Circ. Physiol. 18), H914–H921, 1985.
61. **Pohl, U., Holtz, J., Busse, R., and Bassenge, E.,** Crucial role of endothelium in the vasodilator response to increased flow *in vivo*, *Hypertension*, 8, 37–44, 1986.
62. **Rubanyi, G. M., Lorenz, R. R., and Vanhoutte, P. M.,** Bioassay of endothelium-derived relaxing factor(s): Inactivation by catecholamines, *Am. J. Physiol.*, 249(Heart Circ. Physiol. 18), H95–H101, 1985.
63. **Rubanyi, G. M., Romero, J. C., and Vanhoutte, P. M.,** Flow-induced release of endothelium-derived relaxing factor, *Am. J. Physiol.*, 250(Heart Circ. Physiol. 19), H1145–H1149, 1986.
64. **Segal, S. S. and Duling, B. R.,** Propagation of vasodilation in resistance vessels of the hamster: Development and review of a working hypothesis, *Circ. Res.*, 61, II-20–II-25, 1987.
65. **Shimoda, L., Norins, N., and Madden, J. A.,** A reliable system to electronically adjust pressure and flow independently in an isolated blood vessel, *FASEB J.*, 6(5), A1843, 1992 (Abstr.).
66. **Sleek, G. E. and Duling, B. R.,** Coordination of mural elements and myofilaments during arteriolar constriction, *Circ. Res.*, 59, 620–627, 1986.
67. **Smiesko, V., Lang, D. J., and Johnson, P. C.,** Dilator response of rat mesenteric arcading arterioles to increased blood flow velocity, *Am. J. Physiol.*, 257(Heart Circ. Physiol. 26), H1958–H1965, 1989.
68. **Speden, R. N.,** The use of excised, pressurized blood vessels to study the physiology of vascular smooth muscle, *Experientia*, 41, 1026–1028, 1985.
69. **Stekiel, W. J., Contney, S. J., and Lombard, J. H.,** Small vessel membrane potential, sympathetic input, and electrogenic pump rate in SHR, *Am. J. Physiol.*, 250(Cell Physiol. 19), C547–C556, 1986.
70. **Strange, K. and Spring, K. R.,** Methods for imaging renal tubule cells, *Kidney Int.*, 30, 192–200, 1986.
71. **Takayasu, M. and Dacey, R. G., Jr.,** Spontaneous tone of cerebral parenchymal arterioles: A role in cerebral hyperemic phenomena, *J. Neurosurg.*, 71, 711–717, 1989.
72. **Tesfamariam, B., Halpern, W., and Osol, G.,** Effects of perfusion and endothelium on the reactivity of isolated resistance arteries, *Blood Vessels*, 22, 301–305, 1985.
73. **Van Beek, J. H. G. M., Bouma, P., and Westerhof, N.,** Coronary resistance increase by nondefatted albumin in saline-perfused rabbit hearts, *Am. J. Physiol.*, 259(Heart Circ. Physiol. 28), H1606–H1608, 1990.
74. **VanBavel, E., Giezeman, M. J. M. M., Mooij, T., and Spaan, J. A. E.,** Influence of pressure alterations on tone and vasomotion of isolated mesenteric small arteries of the rat, *J. Physiol.*, 436, 371–383, 1991.
75. **VanBavel, E., Mooij, R., Giezeman, M. J. M. M., and Spaan, J. A. E.,** Cannulation and continuous cross-sectional area measurement of small blood vessels, *J. Pharmacol. Methods*, 24, 219–227, 1990.
76. **Yuan, B. H., Robinette, J. B., and Conger, J. D.,** Effect of angiotensin II and norepinephrine on isolated rat afferent and efferent arterioles, *Am. J. Physiol.*, 258(Renal Fluid Elec.Physiol. 27), F741–F750, 1990.

77. **Yuan, Y., Chilian, W. M., Granger, H. J., and Zawieja, D. C.,** Permeability to albumin in isolated coronary venules, *Am. J. Physiol. Heart Circ. Physiol.,* 265(Heart Circ. Physiol. 34), H543–H552, 1993.

78. **Zawieja, D. C., Davis, M. J., and Granger, H. J.,** Effects of transmural distension on the contractile activity of isolated rat mesenteric collecting lymphatics, *Physiologist,* 32, 1577–1570, 1989.

79. **Zweifach, B. W. and Metz, D. B.,** Regional differences in response of terminal vascular bed to vasoactive agents, *Am. J. Physiol.,* 182, 155–165, 1955.

Chapter 33

Microvascular Architecture and Networks

Peter Gaehtgens

CONTENTS

I. INTRODUCTION: WHY NETWORKS?

In the recent literature, it is increasingly recognized that many features of microvascular physiology cannot be accounted for on the basis of the simplified architectural models that have previously been used to describe the vascular pattern of the terminal circulation. Furthermore, observations of the response, to various stimuli, of total blood flow or substrate exchange between blood and tissue seen in whole-organ studies cannot often be extrapolated to the capillary level.[3,12] For instance, the magnitude and time course of muscle blood flow upon exercise is not precisely reflected by the changes of blood flow seen in individual capillaries.[14]

There is, furthermore, a second category of observations that require an explanation incorporating vascular architecture and functional behavior of complex vascular units rather than single-vessel elements. A number of observations, particularly under pathophysiological conditions, suggest, on the whole-organ level, a substantial discrepancy between changes of blood flow and changes of tissue metabolism. In order to reconcile such observations with the fundamental concepts of cardiovascular physiology, the possibility has been suggested that microvascular blood flow may be, under specific circumstances, redistributed within a given vascular architecture, and redistribution effects may be associated with variation of overall substrate (e.g., oxygen) extraction in the face of constant perfusion rates.[2,11] In other words, a given microvascular system may show, even with the same overall perfusion, quantitatively different exchange characteristics. Under such circumstances, the existence of a "shunt" circulation is often invoked; and it is now recognized that this must be interpreted in a functional rather than morphological sense.

Such observations have led to the concept that specific functions of the microcirculation may not be reflected, under all possible circumstances, by the specific behavior of identifiable single-vessel elements, but may result from the "concerted action" of entire microvascular units or networks. The overall behavior of such networks is thus not determined by the simple arithmetic sum of the individual constituting microvessel segments, but also by the way these are interconnected and the mode by which local responses are integrated within such systems.

0-8493-4870-6/95/$0.00+$.50

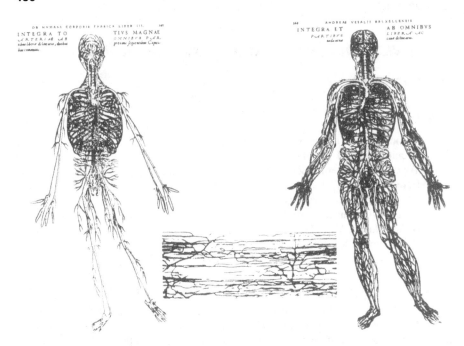

Figure 1 Schematic representation of the arterial (left) and venous (right) "macro"-vessels and the typical "micro"-vessel arrangement in skeletal muscle (middle). While the large conduit vessels are genetically determined, the microvessel pattern is not, and varies between tissues in a characteristic fashion.

The term "microvascular networks" therefore describes the morphological and topological basis of recognizable physiological functions or pathophysiological deviations thereof. In this sense, it is applicable to all terminal vascular systems independent of their specific architecture. By introducing the term, it is recognized that specific functions of the microcirculation are not necessarily supported exclusively by specific and anatomically identified structures. Therefore, morphological properties of single vascular segments, as well as their architectural arrangement and topology, and the integration of individual response characteristics determine the behavior of the network as a unit.

Different tissues can be identified not only by their specific parenchymal characteristics, but also by the typical architecture of the supplying microvascular systems. This is not only true for the system of true capillaries, but applies to all microvessel segments located within the parenchyma. While the design of the extraparenchymal conduit "macro"-vessels appears to be controlled by a genetically fixed program, the architectural arrangement of the terminal "micro"vascular bed depends on control mechanisms exerted by the surrounding tissues and adapted to local and potentially specific needs (Figure 1).

In the present context, a more detailed analysis of microvascular architecture is of interest only insofar as network hemodynamics and thus the hydrodynamic conditions under which blood flows through the terminal vessels are affected. The simplest architectural model of the microcirculation is that of a symmetric branching system consisting of not only equivalent, but identical parallel pathways between feeding artery and draining vein. This model is frequently used in textbook descriptions of the circulation in which total vascular resistance, mean capillary blood flow velocities, or total capillary surface areas available for exchange are estimated. It is also the model classically used by Adolf Fick (1888)[7] to estimate the distribution of pressure in the circulation (Figure 2).

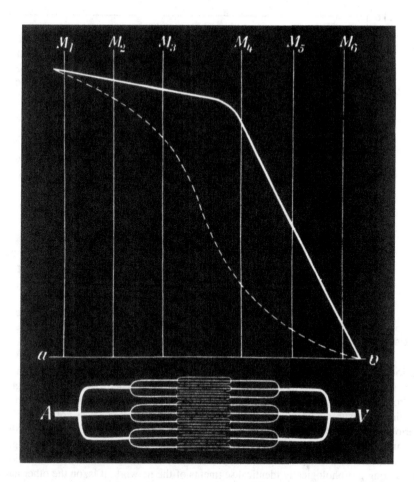

Figure 2 Symmetric network schema of the vascular system used by Fick[7] for calculation of pressure decay along the vessel tree. While obviously not realistic in an anatomical sense, such models are frequently used for an estimation of hemodynamic features of the circulation.

While useful for an overall approach, this model is in fact obviously erroneous. This is not only clear from a direct inspection of the vascular arrangement in the many tissues, but also from the measurement of hydrodynamic parameters at the level of the true capillaries: there, a significantly wider distribution of capillary pressures has been found by direct measurement than is assumed in Fick's estimation.[23] This is also the result of model calculations based on morphological analysis of complete mesenteric networks (Figure 3). Such results indicate that pressure differences are significantly greater between neighboring capillaries than between the arterial and venous end of a single capillary vessel. This suggests that the equilibrium of fluid exchange, if at all present, is provided between neighboring vessels rather than through a filtration/reabsorption balance along a single microvascular pathway. Although similar data are not available for many different tissues, the existing ones clearly show pronounced heterogeneity at the capillary level.

The same finding also shows that the pressure decay occurring between inflow artery and the capillaries supplied is quite different along individual arterio-venous pathways, demonstrating that pathway conductance is far from uniformly distributed. This does not invalidate the generally accepted concept that pressure drop is greatest in the precapillary

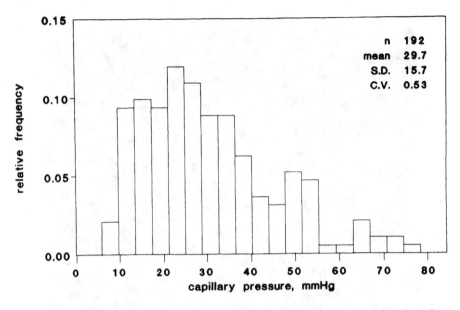

Figure 3 Frequency distribution of capillary pressure as obtained from calculations based on the morphology of a complete mesenteric vessel network. The wide distribution of pressures reflects the wide dispersion of conductances along single arterio-venous pathways.

arterioles, but it goes to show that the specific anatomic arrangement, as well as differences in vascular tone between "parallel" precapillary resistance vessels, play a significant role for the behavior of the complex network. It is therefore not so very surprising that direct measurements of microvascular tone within a limited "class" of precapillary arterioles (with a rather narrow distribution of resting diameters) in skeletal muscle show substantial differences in vascular smooth muscle tone (Figure 4). While it is of great interest, on one hand, to identify the reasons for such wide distributions of the functional state among morphologically identical segments of the network, it is, on the other hand, obviously very important to understand the mechanisms whereby single-vessel responses are integrated within the network to yield the overall system response.

II. ARCHITECTURE AND TOPOLOGY

In principle, microvascular networks may be divided into an arterial and venous subnetwork, using the "true" capillaries as the dividing line. The architecture of the two subnetworks and, in addition, the connection between them may be separately evaluated. While this approach may appear straightforward, it requires, in practice, additional definitions of the "true capillary", since in many beds, such as in the mesentery, several vessel segments (between bifurcations) along a single arteriovenous pathway show practically identical morphology. Therefore, additional features such as the flow at vascular branch points (diverging or converging) can be used and, in the topological sense, the distinction between arterial and venous subnetworks is then made according to the flow distribution rather than vessel morphology.[15]

For the purpose of the present description, the following more specific features of microvascular architecture are of particular relevance:

1. The classical structure of microvascular subsystems is that of a bifurcating tree that in the simplest case, is symmetrical ("strictly symmetric branching"), but in most real networks shows some degree of nonsymmetry (Figure 5). The functional consequences

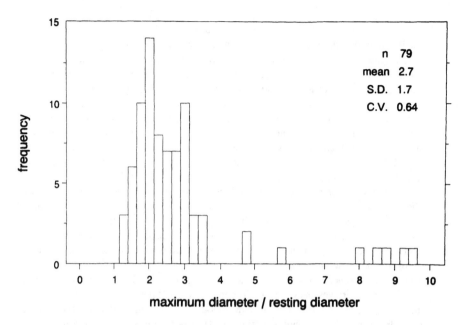

Figure 4 Frequency histogram of vascular tone in arterioles of the resting spinotrapezius muscle of the rat. Tone is expressed here as the ratio of maximal vessel diameter (after maximal dilation with papaverine) and resting diameter.

of these differences with respect to the nonuniformity of network hemodynamics are immediately obvious: in the extreme case of the "ladder"-type arrangement ("strictly asymmetric branching"), the most terminal capillaries are far from being parallel and thus will show a most pronounced heterogeneity in terms of, e.g., intravascular and

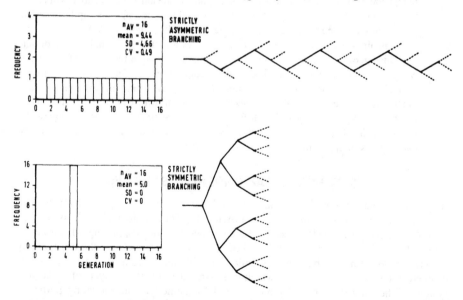

Figure 5 Schematic representation of two extreme types of an arteriolar vessel tree feeding a number of capillaries (dashed lines). Capillary pressure distribution would be rather uniform in the symmetric pattern (bottom), but extremely nonuniform in the asymmetric case (top).

driving pressure, hematocrit, or, if unidirectional oxygen exchange is assumed along the length of the pathways, oxygen tension or saturation. Thus, even tree-like topological structures can exhibit substantial heterogeneity, unless specific adjustments of single-segment conductivity are provided. The latter may then, however, be subject to different control mechanisms, and the overall performance of such systems may, as a consequence, be highly variable.

2. The existence, at various levels of the vascular tree, of vessel segments that represent connecting links, or anastomoses, between parallel vascular pathways. Arteriolar-arteriolar connections are present in many tissues and constitute the basis of the so-called "meshes" ("modules," "arcading," or "arcuate" vessel systems) found in the coronary microcirculation, skeletal muscle, skin, intestinal wall, and mesentery.[1,8,22] The functions of arterio-arterial connections are not very well understood. Obviously, they may serve to equalize pressure at a given level of the tree, thus providing a more uniform input pressure for the more distal vessel trees supplying the capillaries.[16] The pressure drop across such connecting arteriolar anastomoses may be rather small such that even minor readjustments of the resistance distribution may lead to flow reversal or oscillatory flow directions.

3. Even in the absence of the typical arcading arrangement, the branching pattern of pre- and post-capillary vessels varies in different tissues, and the alternative arterio-venous pathways that may be taken by, e.g., a red blood cell transiting a microvascular network may therefore exhibit a wide variation of pathway length and a variable number of branch points. As a result, vessel segments with similar morphological or geometrical characteristics (e.g., diameter) are not necessarily parallel elements in the context of the entire network. This is one of the reasons why the sum of volume flow rates in individual sections of the microcirculation, e.g., "all arterioles with diameters between 15 and 20 μm" or "all A3-vessels," is not necessarily the same, although mass balance is of course preserved. Therefore, it may be useful to define so-called "complete flow cross-sections," i.e., the sum of all vessel elements of a tree that carry the total flow.

4. Independent of the specific structure of the arteriolar and venular subnetworks, the connection of the feeding and draining microvessel trees through the capillary system proper may be quite variable. This is quite frequently demonstrated by systems that show a pair-like arrangement of feeding arterioles and draining venules, and, despite this close geographical association, only a limited overlap in the group of capillaries connected to these two vessels. The mode of connection can, for instance, be directly appreciated from fluorescence angiograms of the human retina, in which the passage of the injected dye through a feeding sector artery is followed by dye appearance in two neighboring veins, but at rather different appearance times. In most microvascular networks, the blood fed into the capillary system by one arteriole is drained by at least two venules of approximately similar dimensions.

III. TOPOLOGICAL ORDERING SCHEMES

As a result of the existence of such architectural features, the topological characteristics of microvascular networks may differ substantially. The topological analysis of such networks can be performed by using different ordering schemes, among which the so-called Horton-Strahler scheme[6,13,18,21] and the generation scheme[15] are the most widely used (Figure 6). While both schemes permit a quantifiable assessment of the architecture of interest, the generation scheme, which was introduced for the analysis of the airway system of the lung,[20] is generally more useful for hemodynamic modeling purposes. However, it cannot without additional modifications be applied to systems exhibiting arterio-arterial connections (arcade systems), and substantial limitations also result from the presence of a rete mirabile.

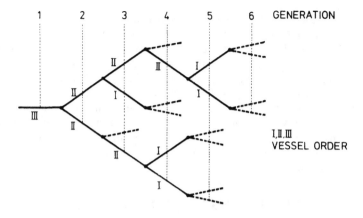

Figure 6 Schematic representation of two ordering nomenclatures to be used for a topological analysis of arteriolar or venular trees: the Horton-Strahler scheme (roman numbers) and the generation scheme (arabic numbers).

IV. HETEROGENEITY OF MICROVASCULAR NETWORKS

As a result of architectural and topological features, a substantial heterogeneity can be found in most microvascular beds. In principle, this is meant to say that most of the hemodynamic, rheological, and functional parameters that can be measured in a terminal vascular bed show a variability which by far exceeds that resulting from measurement errors. Experimental data from most tissues exhibit coefficients of variation that range up to 60 to 80%.[4,10] Typical examples were already given in Figures 3 and 4, but better known and functionally more relevant are the histograms of pO_2 that are also used for the analysis of tissue supply conditions in clinical applications. The dispersion of tissue pO_2 that is seen in such recordings is, however, not only due to intrinsic morphological and supply heterogeneity of the microcirculation, but also to the conditions of measurement (e.g., variation of the position of the measuring electrode relative to the microvessels, etc.). It is, on the basis of such measurements, in general also very difficult to differentiate between morphological and functional causes of heterogeneity, unless variation of the experimental conditions can be achieved that is the case in the experiment but not always in the clinical patient.

An additional source of heterogeneity is due to the temporal variation of microcirculatory perfusion that results from both systemic influences, mediated through the autonomic nervous system and local vasomotion within the arteriolar tree. While single-vessel rhythmicity that results from the action of localized pacemaker cells is to some degree synchronized between connected vessel segments by signal conduction, nonsynchronous rhythmicity may be observed between neighboring regions within one tissue. Therefore, the fluctuations that can even be seen in overall measurements of blood flow (such as during laser Doppler measurements from the skin) represent the net result of the underlying local oscillations that under different circumstances may show enhancement or attenuation resulting from varying synchronization. Nonsynchronous fluctuations of flow between microvessels of a given network will, of course, lead to temporal heterogeneity that may be superimposed onto the spatial heterogeneity resulting from vascular architecture and/or vascular tone.

Of particular clinical interest is the occurrence of enhanced heterogeneity in microcirculatory systems that are under normal conditions well adapted to the specific needs of the tissue. This means that the metabolic state of the tissue may not be adequately assessed by the analysis of, e.g., the outflowing venous blood that represents a mixture of outflows from tissue regions which may be very heterogeneously supplied. As a result, a relatively high mixed venous oxygen saturation can be found despite severe local tissue hypoxia.[2,11] The mechanisms underlying such enhanced heterogeneities, which have for instance been seen in peripheral arterial disease, in various forms of shock (e.g., hypovolemic or septic) or during disseminated intravascular coagulation, are presently not very well understood. Aside from failure of the normal control mechanisms adapting local supply to local demand, microembolization of single arterio-venous pathways by platelet aggregates or poorly deformable leukocytes have been discussed to play a major role. As a consequence, the state of a tissue cannot be assessed by the measurement of a specific parameter in any one tissue location, but only by an estimate of parameter dispersion within the tissue.

V. INTEGRATING CONTROL MECHANISMS

In view of the anatomical and topological characteristics of microvascular networks, it is almost surprising that, normally, tissue supply is remarkably well adapted to metabolic demand. According to the classical theory, this is due to the local control of vascular smooth muscle tone by mediator/metabolites released according to metabolic activity from the tissue cells. While this concept is still generally acceptable, it needs to be modified and complicated in view of the many observations demonstrating mechanisms that appear to act independently of local metabolic activity. Among these, endothelium-dependent, myogenic, and neurogenic mechanisms are particularly prominent. In addition, metabolic signals from the surrounding tissue will only be able to reach the intraparenchymal blood vessels, and even maximal dilatation of these vessels would not be sufficient to generate the maximal flow rates observed. It is therefore evident that:

- Mechanisms must be present whose integrating action leads to a coordinated response of complex microvascular units or networks.
- Mechanisms of communication along the vascular tree are required to allow for a response also of those upstream vessels that cannot be reached by intraparenchymal signals.

A. FLOW-DEPENDENT VASODILATION

Dilation of small precapillary arterioles due to exposure to a local metabolic signal causes an increase of local conductance. The resulting increase of flow rate will lead to an increased wall shear stress in the upstream arterioles. This mechanical signal is recognized by the endothelium and leads to the release of mediators (EDRF, prostanoids), causing dilatation. This sequence of events thus generates an ascending vasodilation that allows upstream (and extraparenchymal) vessels to participate in the response. Obviously, the response is terminated as soon as the primary metabolic signal is turned off.

B. CONDUCTED VASCULAR RESPONSES

Local stimulation of small arterioles has been shown to result in dilator or constrictor responses that spread significantly beyond the primary site of stimulation.[17] This appears to be the result of direct conduction of an electrotonic signal along the vascular walls, from endothelial to smooth muscle cells,[5] and may involve a vessel length of several millimeters. Since the conduction also overcomes branching points, an extended microvascular tree may participate in a response to a stimulus that was primarily restricted to a very confined site. There is evidence that this type of reaction can also be evoked from the true capillaries and lead to diameter adjustments in all of the arterioles feeding the capillary system.[9]

C. INTEGRATED RESPONSES DUE TO SPECIFIC VESSEL ARRANGEMENT

In many tissues, feeding arterioles and draining venules are typically found in a paired fashion. The immediate vicinity between these vessels allows diffusible signals to reach the feeding arteriole of a network from which it is removed via the draining vein.[19] As a result of this kind of architecturally determined communication, vascular responses may be spreading into network compartments that have not been primarily exposed to the vasoactive principles generating the original response.

Obviously, every control mechanism that leads to an adjustment of smooth muscle tone in response to a change of the mechanical state of the vessel (e.g., by alteration of the distending force or the surface shear stress) will automatically act as an integrating mechanism. For example, a change of vascular diameter in any constituent vessel segment within a network will cause a redistribution of pressure and flow which, in turn, will elicit a readjustment of conductance in all other vessels of the network. Besides the above-described flow-dependent mechanism, myogenic adjustment of smooth muscle tone will be relevant here. Therefore, it is evident that the presence of such integrating mechanisms, under normal conditions, supports the coordination of vascular responses throughout a given microvascular network — even beyond the limits of the microcirculation. It is therefore quite conceivable that disturbances of any of these mechanisms, under conditions of pathology, will attenuate or even eliminate the appropriate reaction that is required to meet the metabolic demand of the tissue. The existence of overperfusion and underperfusion in closely neighboring tissue areas under such conditions, and the resulting enhancement of supply heterogeneity is thus a typical pathophysiological phenomenon.

REFERENCES

1. **Baez, S.,** Skeletal muscle and gastrointestinal microvascular morphology, in *Microcirculation,* Vol. 1, Kaley, G. and Altura, B. M., Eds., University Park Press, Baltimore, 1977, 69–74.
2. **Benner, K. U., Gaehtgens, P., and Schickendantz, S.,** Hemodynamic and functional consequences of intravascular platelet aggregation in skeletal muscle, *Microvasc. Res.,* 9, 310–316, 1976.
3. **Chien, S.,** Symposium on the correlation of microcirculation and macrocirculation, *Int. J. Microcirc. Clin. Exp.,* 1, 347–425, 1982.
4. **Damon, D. H. and Duling, B. R.,** Evidence that capillary perfusion heterogeneity is not controlled in striated muscle, *Am. J. Physiol.,* 249, H386–H392, 1985.
5. **Davis, P. F.,** Current concepts of vascular endothelial and smooth muscle cell communication, *Surv. Synth. Pathol. Res.,* 4, 357–373, 1985.
6. **Fenton, B. R. and Zweifach, B. W.,** Microcirculatory model relating geometrical variation to changes in pressure and flow rate, *A Biomed. Eng.,* 9, 303–321, 1981.
7. **Fick, A.,** Über den Druck in den Blutkapillaren, *Pflügers Arch. ges Physiol.,* 42, 482–488, 1888.
8. **Frasher, W. G. and Wayland, H.,** A repeating modular organization of the microcirculation of cat mesentery, *Microvasc. Res.,* 4, 62–76, 1972.
9. **Gaehtgens, P., Tigno, X. T., Thies, K., and Ley, K.,** Is there a retrograde control of arteriolar tone originating from capillaries?, in *Funktionsanalyse Biologischer Systeme,* Vol. 19, Grote, J. and Witzleb, E., Eds., Fischer, Stuttgart, 1989, 87–95.
10. **Gaehtgens, P.,** Why networks?, *Int. J. Microcirc. Clin. Exp.,* 11, 123–132, 1992.
11. **Gaehtgens, P., Benner, K. U., and Schickendantz, S.,** Nutritive and non-nutritive blood flow in canine skeletal muscle after partial microembolization, *Pflügers Arch. ges Physiol.,* 361, 183–189, 1976.
12. **Honig, C. R. and Gayeski, T. E. J.,** Correlation of O_2-transport on the macro and micro scale, *Int. J. Microcirc. Clin. Exp.,* 1, 367–381, 1982.
13. **Horton, R. E.,** Erosional development of streams and their drainage basins: Hydrophysical approach to quantitative morphology, *Geol. Soc, Am. Bull.,* 56, 275–370, 1945.
14. **Hudlicka, O., Zweifach, B. W., and Tyler, K. R.,** Capillary recruitment and flow velocity in skeletal muscle after contraction, *Microvasc. Res.,* 23, 201–213, 1982.

15. **Ley, K., Pries, A. R., and Gaehtgens, P.,** Topological structure of rat mesenteric microvessel networks, *Microvasc. Res.,* 32, 315–332, 1986.
16. **Mayrovitz, H. N.,** Hemodynamic significance of microvascular arteriolar anastomosing, in *Microvascular Networks,* Popel, A. S. and Johnson, P. C., Eds., Karger, Basel, 1986, 197–209.
17. **Segal, S. S. and Duling, B. R.,** Flow control among microvessels coordinated by intercellular conduction, *Science,* 234, 868–870, 1986.
18. **Strahler, A. N.,** Hypsometric (area-altitude) analysis of erosional topography, *Geol. Soc. Am. Bull.,* 63, 1117–1142, 1952.
19. **Tigno, X. T., Ley, K., Pries, A. R., and Gaehtgens, P.,** Venulo-arteriolar communication and propagated response: A possible mechanism for local control of blood flow, *Pflügers Arch. ges Physiol.,* 414, 450–456, 1989.
20. **Weibel, E. R.,** *Morphometry of the Human Lung,* Springer, Berlin, 1963.
21. **Wiedeman, M. P.,** Blood flow through terminal arterial vessels after denervation of the bat wing, *Circ. Res.,* 22, 83–89, 1968.
22. **Zweifach, B. W.,** *Functional Behaviour of the Microcirculation,* Charles C. Thomas, Springfield, IL, 1961.
23. **Zweifach, B. W.,** Quantitative studies of microcirculatory structure and function. I. Analysis of pressure distribution in the terminal vascular bed in cat mesentery, *Circ. Res.,* 34, 843–857, 1974.

Chapter 34

Vascular Smooth Muscle Cells

Lars M. Rasmussen, Jens L. Andresen, and Thomas Ledet

CONTENTS

I. INTRODUCTION

Arterial smooth muscle cells are responsible for maintaining both arterial tension by contraction-relaxation and blood-vessel integrity by proliferation, migration, and synthesis of extracellular matrix. In a normal blood vessel, smooth muscle cells respond by contraction or relaxation to blood pressure-regulating factors derived from the blood or produced locally in overlaying endothelial cells, thereby determining the tone of the vessel.[79] Vascular smooth muscle cells do, however, play other roles than merely being responder cells determining vascular tone; proliferative, migrative and synthetic properties of these cells are key functions during the development of blood vessels and in the maintenance of normal vessel integrity, but also in many pathological situations. Thus, accumulation of vascular smooth muscle cells and their matrix is one hallmark of fibrous atherosclerotic plaques[99] and restenotic lesions after arterial injury.[30,84,118] In addition, hypertension is associated with structural alterations in the wall of small arteries.[9,41] In diabetic angiopathy, vascular smooth muscle cells in both small and large vessels seem to be involved, since altered biochemical composition and structural properties of the extracellular matrix has been reported.[61,94,95]

Since smooth muscle cells are key players in the pathogenesis of these common and severe arterial diseases, it is not surprising that large amounts of information about arterial smooth muscle cells are available. Recent reviews cover some areas in comprehensive ways,[13,48,104,105,114] whereas in the present chapter we will give a short overview and some contemporary details about important aspects of the physiology and pathophysiology of the vascular smooth muscle cell.

II. ASPECTS ON DIFFERENTIATION AND PHENOTYPIC DIVERSITIES

Although the classical smooth muscle cell is defined as one cell type, the microscopic appearance are very diverse, depending on the temporal and spatial position of the cells. Vascular cells in the fetal arteries, in the atherosclerotic plaques, and in the tunica media of normal arteries share common feature, as they express the cytoskeletal protein α-smooth muscle cell actin. Nevertheless, they have different ultrastructure, and phenotypic properties, such as different expression of certain cytokine receptors, contractile proteins, and extracellular matrix components.[104,105,114] The cells in fetal arteries and cells in atherosclerotic plaques have a fibroblast-like appearance often referred to as the synthetic

0-8493-4870-6/95/$0.00+$.50

phenotype, whereas the phenotype of cells from normal tunica media is often called contractile.[13,114] Recently, Simons et al. were able to show that the rate of restenosis after atherectomy was strongly related to the phenotypic state of the smooth muscle cells in the removed atherosclerotic tissue. *In situ* hybridization for non-muscle myosin was used as a differentiation marker to determine the phenotype of the cells in this study.[109] The phenotypic state of the cells may therefore determine if the smooth muscle cells have the potential to start formation of intimal lesions and fibrous plaques. Consequently, it may be important to understand the regulatory mechanisms determining the phenotypic properties of vascular smooth muscle cells. One way of gaining insight into the regulation of the vascular smooth muscle cell phenotypes comes from studies of developing fetal arteries. Vascular smooth muscle cells derived from embryonic or newborn rats grown *in vitro* have an epitheloid appearance and are capable of proliferation without the presence of serum, probably because of high autocrine production of platelet-derived growth factor (PDGF) and the presence of PDGF-receptors on these cells when compared to cells from adult animals.[105,107] Interestingly, these capacities of fetal cells resemble the functions of cells harvested from balloon-injured rat carotid arteries, indicating that those from developing arteries share important growth features with cells from injured arteries.[117] In an attempt to find genes expressed in smooth muscle cells derived from newborn rats, thereby characterizing the "synthetic" smooth muscle cell phenotype common for newborn and injured cells, Giachelli et al.[31] have cloned genes by differential screening of a rat cDNA library derived from newborn rat aortas. This technique allows cloning of genes predominantly expressed in one cell population and not in another. With this methodology, they found the bone-related protein osteopontin to be expressed mainly in the fetal cells[31] and reported later that also PDGF-B, tenascin, and alpha(1)-I collagen genes are found with increased expression in the cells from newborn rats.[106]

Another approach to study the regulation of phenotypic properties of smooth muscle cells is by using freshly harvested smooth muscle cells from normal rat arteries. These cells go through an adaptation to *in vitro* conditions where the cells change from a highly differentiated contractile phenotype to a more fibroblast-like synthetic phenotype.[13,114] This phenomenon has been used as a model to study the shift in phenotype, which by these authors is believed to occur in a similar fashion also *in vivo* in situations when cells are recruited to participate in different pathological processes. Several characteristics of phenotypic modulation have been described using this model, and some insights into mechanisms that regulate this process have been obtained. It seems that extracellular matrix components interfere with the phenotypic shift since cells grown on the basement membrane component laminin do not go through the phenotypic shift, but stay in the highly differentiated form.[42]

Although information about the characteristics of different vascular smooth muscle phenotypes have been gained using these techniques, almost nothing is known about the regulation of the differentiation processes. A major breakthrough in the understanding of skeletal muscle cell development could, however, be extrapolated to the regulation mechanisms of smooth muscle cell differentiation. The differentiation of skeletal muscle cells has been shown to be driven by the expression of members of a large family of basic helix-loop-helix transcription factors, now designated as the MyoD family.[22,113] When expressed in mesenchymal cells, these proteins will bind to promotor regions in skeletal muscle cell specific genes, turning the transcription on, thereby making the cells into a skeletal muscle. Recently, sequence analysis of the smooth muscle cell specific gene, α-smooth muscle cell actin, revealed that the promotor of this gene contains a consensus region for the binding of proteins of the basic helix-loop-helix family, the so called "E-box".[86] Moreover, gel-shift analyses with smooth muscle cell nuclear extracts have indicated that proteins binding to this area are present in vascular smooth muscle cells. Transfection experiments have indicated that vascular smooth muscle cells contain endogenous, still unknown genes of this family that could be of importance in the differentiation of smooth muscle cells.[86,116]

III. REGULATION OF PROLIFERATION

Smooth muscle proliferation is a key event in disease such as atherosclerosis,[98] hypertension,[18,64,103] and restenosis after both angioplasty or bypass grafting.[14,19,37,39,63,76,84,112,121] A wealth of information has therefore accumulated concerning the regulation of smooth muscle proliferation and emphasis in this area has been on the effects of peptide growth factors on cultured smooth muscle cells. In recent years, however, focus has shifted to include the regulation of cell division by vasoreactive factors, intracellular signal transduction mechanisms, and the design of specific inhibitors of vascular smooth muscle cell division.

Among peptide factors known to stimulate proliferation of vascular smooth muscle cells *in vitro*, are platelet-derived growth factor (PDGF),[3,47,49,83,89,97,100] insulin-like growth factor I, (IGF-I),[3,10,24,87,88] growth hormone,[59] and fibroblast growth factors (FGFs).[34,35,119] Several of these factors have also been shown, *in vivo*, to be involved in the proliferative events leading to formation of intimal lesions after experimentally induced injuries. In the arterial balloon injury model in rats, medial smooth muscle cell proliferation and migration is induced by stripping off the endothelium and injuring the underlying smooth muscle cells. In this model, the proliferation of the medial smooth muscle cells was reduced by infusion of antibodies to basic FGF.[65] In contrast, antibodies to PDGF inhibited the migratory response, but failed to lower proliferation significantly.[28]

Other substances, primarily known for functions not related to cell proliferation, like the thrombogenic enzyme thrombin[4,36,53,77] and the vasoconstrictor angiotensin II,[69] are now also known to stimulate smooth muscle cell proliferation *in vitro*. Moreover, it has been shown that the increment of PDGF mRNA expression in arterial smooth muscle cells after balloon catheter denudation can be interrupted by reduction of the proteolytic activity of circulating thrombin.[85] Furthermore, infusion of inhibitors of the angiotensin-converting enzyme (ACE) into experimental animals reduces migration and proliferation of the smooth muscle cells at the site of injury.[90,91] It is of interest that PDGF and FGF seem to be potent vasoconstrictors.[6] Since angiotensin II, PDGF, and FGF have a parallel signal transducing pathway with intracellular activation of proteinkinase C and release of Ca^{2+},[7,32,33,38,54] it is possible that the effect is more dependent upon the phenotypic "settings" of the SMCs than the precise nature of the active factor.

For some time, heparin has been known to inhibit smooth muscle cell proliferation both *in vitro* and *in vivo* in animals with experimentally induced arterial injuries.[5,16,27,46,67] Recently, the nitric oxide (NO) generating vasodilators[29,55] and atrial natriuretic peptide (ANP)[1,12] have also been shown to possess inhibitory effects on smooth muscle cells at least *in vitro*. Interestingly, both the receptors for NO and ANP have guanylate cyclase activity, and it is therefore likely that an increase in the level of cGMP in smooth muscle cells decreases proliferation.

Many of the various substances mentioned are believed to be synthesized and secreted locally by the smooth muscle cells or by the endothelial cells, and may exert their effects via an autocrine/paracrine mechanism. *In situ* hybridization experiments have revealed that IGF-I, PDGF, FGF, and TGF-β mRNA are expressed in normal rat aortas[101] and in increased amounts in injured arteries.[72,73] Moreover, the smooth muscle cells are able to synthesize both PDGF,[71,107,108,117] IGF-I,[23,89] and FGFs[35,119] *in vitro*. Apart from injury, hemodynamic conditions can change the expression of growth factors in the vascular smooth muscle cells. Occlusion of the right femoral artery in adult rats resulted in a strongly increased IGF-I immunoreactivity in the tunica media of the contralateral, left femoral artery, probably due to the increased vascular load.[40] In another series of experiments, the

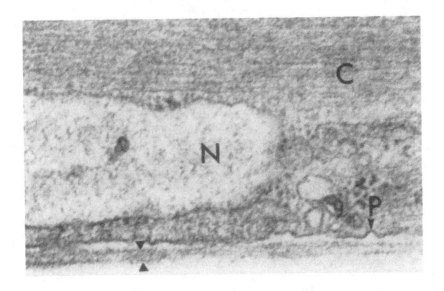

Figure 1 Electron micrograph of arterial smooth muscle cells. Arrows indicate the basement membrane surrounding each individual cell; (N) nucleus, (C) cytoplasma, and (P) plasma membrane.

level of TGF-β mRNA was increased up to 300% in aortas from hypertensive rats as compared with normotensive rats.[101]

The pathophysiological importance of vascular smooth muscle cell proliferation in several arterial diseases, combined with the increasing knowledge about mechanisms behind vascular cell proliferation, has led to several attempts to make drugs designed to inhibit smooth muscle cell proliferation. Fusion of recombinant growth factors with toxins is one approach where delivery of cytotoxins to specific cell surface receptors, abundantly expressed on the surface of proliferating smooth muscle cells, is a way of overcoming the problem with normal tissue being otherwise affected. It was possible to decrease neointimal proliferation[15,57,66] after linking bFGF to saporin, a ribosome inactivator, and subsequently administering this complex to rats after balloon catheter denudation. Also, antisense nucleotide technology has been successfully used in growth inhibitory substances. By using antisense oligonucleotides to target specific genes associated with smooth muscle division, such as proliferating cell nuclear antigen c-myb and c-myc, it has been possible to inhibit growth *in vitro*.[8,111] Recently, this technique was also used *in vivo* by Simons et al.,[110] who used oligonucleotides targeting c-myb, a protooncogene expressed in proliferating smooth muscle cells.[11] The oligonucleotide was solubilized in a pluronic solution that instantly gelled on contact with tissues at 39°C. After the induction of vascular injury, intimal lesions were almost nonexistent in the treated animals.

IV. INTERACTIONS WITH THE EXTRACELLULAR MATRIX

To understand vessel wall behavior under normal and pathological conditions, it is necessary to know the regulation and composition of the extracellular matrix produced by smooth muscle cells. The presence of a remarkable thick basement membrane is a unique feature of the smooth muscle cell (Figure 1). This structure has recently been isolated and shown to contain classical markers such as laminin, type IV collagen, fibronectin, chondroitin sulfate, and heparan sulfate proteoglycan.[43-45] It was shown that the synthesis of basement membrane from rabbit aortic smooth muscle cell cultures is regulated by factors in serum from patients with diabetes mellitus and growth hormone.[60,93] The function of the basement membrane around the smooth muscle cell is unknown. However, the presence of very charged molecules, such as chondroitin sulfate and heparan sulfate, is compatible with the concept of a basement membrane with a very important regulatory function of the flow of molecules to the smooth muscle cells. It is of interest that under certain pathological conditions, the amount of type IV collagen, a basement membrane marker, is increased, which is shown in a study of aorta from persons with diabetes mellitus, whereas type V collagen was unchanged.[95]

A large proportion of the vessel wall is occupied by the various types of collagens — in particular, type I and type III. On rabbit aortic smooth muscle cell cultures, it has been shown that the production of type I collagen and fibronectin is increased after addition of human growth hormone, whereas insulin led to reduced amounts of the two matrix components.[62] Tissue culture studies have shown that the production of type III collagen is reduced in the presence of extracellular matrix and the analysis indicated that basic fibroblast growth factor is at least partly responsible for the effect of the matrix.[74] However, slot-blot mRNA analysis demonstrated no effect on the synthesis of type I collagen. The extracellular matrix seems to be of importance for the transition of smooth muscle cells from a contractile to a synthetic state. It has been demonstrated on freshly isolated smooth muscle cells that the attachment, spreading, and proliferation is promoted on type I collagen matrix as well as on fibronectin. Moreover, the type I collagen was as efficient as fibronectin in promoting the transition of the cells into the synthetic phenotype without the presence of mitogens. It is remarkable that the synthetic peptide GRGDSP (Gly-Arg-Gly-Arp-Ser-Pro) and the peptide KDGEA (Lys-Arg-Gly-Glu-Ala) interfered little with the attachment, spreading, and phenotypic modulation of the cells. The peptide KDGEA contains the recognition sequence of the $\alpha2\beta1$ integrin in type I collagen. However, the phenotypic modulation was counteracted by an anti-$\beta1$ integrin antibody, indicating that the type I collagen promotes the phenotypic transition by interacting with a cell surface receptor ($\beta1$ integrin family). Elastin and laminin were shown to suppress the attachment and spreading of the smooth muscle cells and to maintain the cells in the contractile phenotype.[115] The presence of proteoglycans in the extracellular matrix may be of significant importance for the metabolism of the cells due to the very charged glycosaminoglycan chains that can bind a variety of substances. It has been demonstrated that monkey smooth muscle cells produce a large versican-like chondroitin sulfate proteoglycan, which can be regulated by PDGF and TGF-β.[102] The presence of both growth factors leads to an increase in the amount of glycoprotein core as well as an increase in glycosaminoglycan chain length. In a later report from the same group, it was shown that bovine aortic smooth muscle cells synthesized two populations of small chondroitin/dermatan sulfate proteoglycan (biglycan/decorin). It was demonstrated that the bovine smooth muscle cells expressed an mRNA transcript for both biglycan and decorin. Biglycan from the smooth muscle cell seems to be a single proteoglycan species, whereas endothelial cells synthesize two forms with different molecular weights. It is noteworthy that the production of decorin was correlated to the expression of type I collagen, which is known to interact specifically with decorin.[52]

The extracellular matrix seems to be of importance for the migration and adhesion of the smooth muscle cells, both under normal and pathological conditions. In a tissue culture system, it has been demonstrated that smooth muscle cells migrate over surfaces coated with fibronectin, laminin, vitronectin, and type I and IV collagen. However using blocking antibodies specific to different integrin complexes, it was shown that smooth muscle cell adhesion to fibronectin, laminin, and type I and IV collagen was exclusively dependent on the function $\beta1$ integrins, whereas there was no contribution from the $\alpha_v\beta_3$ integrin. Immunofluorescent staining demonstrated that during the early phase of the smooth muscle cell migration, the $\beta1$ integrins organized rapidly into focal plaques that gradually covered the cell's basal surface, whereas the β3 receptor remained concentrated at all times at the cell's margins. The attachment of human vascular smooth muscle cells to both collagen type VI and fibrillin was studied in a tissue culture system. Intact collagen type VI was capable of mediating cell attachment and partial spreading, as well as the triplehelical and noncollagenous domains at reduced levels. Fibronectin was found to be a modulator of the intact collagen type VI mediated attachment.[20] Fibrillin, a 350-kDa extracellular matrix glycoprotein, which recently has been shown to be the mutated gene in Marfan Syndrome,[25,75] was also tested for its ability to mediate cell attachment. Purified fibrillin-containing microfibrils support the vascular smooth muscle cell adhesion, as does both pepsin-resistant and pepsin-sensitive domains of the fibrillin. These analyses indicated that the cell-matrix interaction involves integrin cell surface receptors containing the β1 subunit.[56]

Extracellular matrix accumulation has been investigated on porcine smooth muscle cell cultures after addition of combinations of various mitogenic cytokines. The two matrix components, elastin and collagen type I, were measured. TGF-β1 mediated matrix production was significantly reduced when either basic fibroblast growth factor or TGF-α was added. However, IGF-1 was a weak additive with respect to elastin production. It is noteworthy that the effect on matrix accumulation was not directly related to the proliferative state of the cell.[21]

Recently, it has been demonstrated that freshly harvested smooth muscle cells derived from injured arteries synthesize significantly larger amounts of connective tissue components as compared to cells from normal arteries.[96] This increase could at least partly be ascribed to local production of TGF-β. Moreover, it was shown that the size of the intimal lesion was reduced after application of neutralizing TGF-β antibodies.[120]

The circumstantial evidence obtained in various tissue culture systems with arterial smooth muscle cells is compatible with the concept of an extracellular matrix that is not an inert filling-up substance between the cells, but necessary for the modulation and response of the vessel wall under normal and pathological conditions. The extracellular matrix acts as a storage for hormones, a structure containing sequences for the various integrins, and a regulator of the phenotypic state of smooth muscle cells. All of these are essential for the vessel wall function.

V. INTERACTIONS WITH MACROPHAGES

The arterial wall is normally inhabited by endothelial and smooth muscle cells; however, during the development of atherosclerotic plaques and in arteritis, leukocytes from the bloodstream enter the vascular wall. The close contact with the arterial smooth muscle cells[51] opens the possibility of an interaction with extravasated leukocytes, which may be important in the formation of fibrous atherosclerotic plaques.

A recent study of the cellular components of human aortas from both atherosclerosis-predisposed and -resistant areas indicated that macrophage infiltration is followed by phenotypic alterations in the surrounding smooth muscle cells. This was evidenced by smooth muscle cells that became desmin positive and contained well-developed endoplasmic reticulum.[2] Observations made by Liptay et al. and Jaeger et al., in atherosclerotic pulmonary[68] and renal arteries,[50] confirmed the presence of macrophages in the lesions. The macrophages often were surrounded by vascular smooth muscle cells with high production of extracellular matrix components. These observations were made by in situ hybridization and support the concept that macrophages may interfere with vascular smooth muscle cells. It looks as if macrophages may secrete factors capable of influencing matrix production in vascular smooth muscle cells. It is therefore noteworthy that conditioned medium from cultured macrophages increased the production of a connective tissue component, dermatan sulfate proteoglycan, when tested on cultured vascular smooth muscle cells.[26] Using activity-neutralizing antibodies against several factors, the increased proteoglycan production could at least partly be ascribed to secretion of interleukin-1 by the macrophages. A better understanding of the interaction between the extravasated leukocytes and the smooth muscle cells in the arterial wall may throw light on important mechanisms, which initiates the development of the fibrous plaque.

VI. GENE THERAPY

Vascular smooth muscle cells, as target cells for gene transfer techniques with the aim of applying therapy to both genetic and acquired diseases, is currently under investigation. Lynch et al.[70] investigated the possibility of expressing genes in arterial cells with the intention of substituting genetically defective genes in certain genetic diseases. Most studies in this area have, however, focused on the possibility of expressing proteins capable of influencing local homeostasis in the vascular wall itself. By introduction of an eukaryotic expression vector which encodes PDGF B by direct gene transfer to normal porcine iliofermoral arteries, Nabel et al.[81] were able to show, for the first time, that overproduction of this growth factor in normal arteries stimulates cell proliferation and the formation of intimal lesions *in vivo*. Later, the same group obtained similar results, using local overexpression of bFGF.[82] This powerful technique provides a tool to study *in vivo* and *in situ* the influence of peptide factors in vascular biology. A futuristic application of gene transfer methodology may be in the design of inhibitors of the development of atherosclerotic and restenotic lesions, using gene transfer of vectors, containing genes coding for inhibitors of proliferation or matrix production. These methods are, however, still beset with major technical difficulties; the level of gene transfer efficiency is poor, which restricts the production of active factor. Finally, it is difficult to administer the plasmids to the cells, without producing cell injury.[17,58,70,78,80,81]

Although still encumbered with technical difficulties, transfer of genes into vascular cells may provide us with greater knowledge of vascular biology and may provide a tool for treatment of arterial diseases.

REFERENCES

1. **Abell, T. J., Richards, A. M., Ikram, H., Espiner, E. A., and Yandle, T.,** Atrial natriuretic factor inhibits proliferation of vascular smooth muscle cells stimulated by platelet derived growth factor, *Biochem. Biophys. Res. Commun.*, 160, 1392–1396, 1989.
2. **Babaev, V. R., Bobryshev, Y. V., Sukhova, G. K., and Kasantseva, I. A.,** Monocyte/macrophage accumulation and smooth muscle cell phenotypes in early atherosclerotic lesions of human aorta, *Atherosclerosis*, 100, 237–248, 1993.
3. **Banskota, N. K., Taub, R., Zellner, K., and King, G. L.,** Insulin, insulin-like growth factor I and platelet-derived growth factor interact additively in the induction of the protoncogene c-myc and cellular proliferation in cultured bovine smooth muscle cells, *Mol. Endocrin.*, 3, 1183–1190, 1989.
4. **Bar-Shavit, R., Benezra, M., Eldor, A., Hy-Am, E., Fenton, J. W., II, Wilner, G. D., and Vlodavsky, I.,** Thrombin immobilized to extracellular matrix is a potent mitogen for vascular smooth muscle cells: Nonenzymatic mode of action, *Cell Regul.*, 1, 453–463, 1990.
5. **Benitz, W. E., Lessler, D. S., Coulson, J. D., and Bernfield, M.,** Heparin inhibits proliferation of fetal vascular smooth muscle cells in the absence of platelet derived growth factor, *J. Cell. Physiol.*, 127, 1–7, 1986.
6. **Berk, B. C., Alexander, R. W., Brock, T. A., Gimbrone, M. A., and Webb, C. R.,** Vasoconstriction: A new activity for platelet derived growth factor, *Science*, 232, 87–90, 1986.
7. **Berridge, M., Heslop, J. P., Irvine, R. F., and Brown, K. D.,** Inositol triphosphate formation and calcium mobilization in Swiss 3T3 cells in response to platelet-derived growth factor, *Biochem. J.*, 222, 195–201, 1984.

8. **Biro, S., Fu, Y., Yu, Z., and Epstein, S.,** Inhibitory effects of antisense oligodeoxynucleotides targeting c-myc mRNA on smooth muscle cell proliferation and migration, *Proc. Natl. Acad. Sci. U.S.A.*, 90, 654–658, 1993.

9. **Bondjers, G., Glukhova, M., Hansson, G. K., Postnov, Y. V., Reidy, M. A., and Schwartz, S. M.,** Hypertension and atherosclerosis. Cause and effect, or two effects with one unknown cause?, *Circulation*, 84, V-2–16, 1991.

10. **Bornfeldt, K. E., Gidlöf, R. A., Wasteson, A., Lake, M., Skottner, A., and Arnqvist, H. J.,** Binding and biological effects of insulin, insulin analogues and insulin-like growth factors in rat aortic smooth muscle cells. Comparison of maximal, growth promoting activities, *Diabetologia*, 34, 307–313, 1991.

11. **Brown, K. E., Kindy, M. S., and Sonnenshein, G. E.,** Expression of the c-myb protooncogene in bovine vascular smooth muscle cells, *J. Biol. Chem.*, 267, 4625–4630, 1992.

12. **Cahill, P. A. and Hassid, A.,** Differential antimitogenic effectiveness of atrial natriuretic peptides in primary versus subcultured rat aortic smooth muscle cells: Relationship to expression of ANF-C receptors, *J. Cell. Physiol.*, 154, 28–38, 1993.

13. **Campbell, G. R., Campbell, J. H., Manderson, J. A., Horrigan, S., and Rennick, R. E.,** Arterial smooth muscle. A multifunctional mesenchymal cell, *Arch. Pathol. Lab. Med.*, 112, 977–986, 1988.

14. **Casscells, W.,** Migration of smooth muscle and endothelial cells. Critical events in restenosis, *Circulation*, 86, 723–729, 1992.

15. **Casscells, W., Lappi, D. A., Olwin, B. B., Wai, C., Siegman, M., Speir, E. H., Sasse, J., and Baird, A.,** Elimination of smooth muscle cells in experimental restenosis: Targeting of fibroblast growth factor receptors, *Proc. Natl. Acad. Sci. U.S.A.*, 89, 7159–7163, 1992.

16. **Castellot, J. J., Jr., Wright, T. C., and Karnovsky, M. J.,** Regulation of vascular smooth muscle cell growth by heparin and heparan sulfates, *Semin. Thromb. Hemost.*, 12, 489–503, 1987.

17. **Chapman, G. D., Lim, C. S., Gammon, R. S., Culp, S. C., Desper, J. S., Baumann, R. P., Swain, J. L., and Stack, R. S.,** Gene transfer into coronary arteries of intact animals with a percutaneous ballon catheter, *Circ. Res.*, 71, 27–33, 1992.

18. **Chobanian, A. V.,** The influence of hypertension and other hemodynamic factors in atherogenesis, *Prog. Cardiovasc. Dis.*, 26, 177–196, 1983.

19. **Clagett, G. P.,** Intimal hyperplasia and restenosis after carotid endarterectomy, *J. Vasc. Surg.*, 10, 577–579, 1989.

20. **Clyman et al.,** Beta 1 and beta 3 integrins have different roles in the adhesion and migration of vascular smooth muscle cells on extracellular matrix, *Exp. Cell Res.*, 200, 272–284, 1992.

21. **Davidson, J. M., Zoia, O., and Liu, Ji-Min,** Modulation of transforming growth factor-beta 1 stimulated elastin and collagen production and proliferation in porcine vascular smooth muscle cells and skin fibroblasts by basic fibroblast growth factor, transforming growth factor-α, and insulin-like growth factor-I, *J. Cell. Phys.*, 155, 149–156, 1993.

22. **Davis, R. L., Weintraub, H., and Lassar, A. B.,** Expression of a single transfected cDNA converts fibroblasts to myoblasts, *Cell*, 51, 987–1000, 1987.

23. **Delafontaine, P., Lou, H., and Alexander, R. W.,** Regulation of insulin-like growth factor I messenger RNA levels in vascular smooth muscle cells, *Hypertension*, 18, 742–747, 1991.

24. **Dempsey, E. C., Stenmark, K. R., McMurtry, I. F., O'Brien, R. F., Voelkel, N. F., and Badesch, D. B.,** Insulin-like growth factor I and protein kinase C activation stimulate pulmonary artery smooth muscle cell proliferation through separate but synergistic pathways, *J. Cell. Physiol.*, 144, 159–165, 1990.

25. **Dietz, H. C., Cutting, G. R., Pyeritz, R. E., Maslen, C. L., Sakai, L. Y., Corson, C. M., Puffenberger, E. G., Hannosh, A., Nanthakumar, E. J., and Cukristin, S. M.,** Marfan syndrome cuased by recurrent *de novo* missense mutation in the fibrillin gene, *Nature*, 352, 337–339, 1991.

26. **Edwards, I. J., Wagner, W. D., and Owens, R. T.,** Macrophage secretory products selectively stimulate dermatan sufate proteoglycan production in cultured arterial smooth muscle cells, *Am. J. Pathol.*, 136, 609–621, 1990.

27. **Fager, G., Hansson, G. K., Ottosson, P., Dahllöf, B., and Bondjers, G.,** Human arterial smooth muscle cells in culture. Effects of platelet-derived growth factor and heparin on growth *in vitro*, *Exp. Cell. Res.*, 176, 319–335, 1988.

28. **Ferns, G. A. A., Raines, E. W., Sprugel, K. H., Motani, A. S., Reidy, M. A., and Ross, R.,** Inhibition of neointimal smooth muscle accumulation after angioplasty by an antibody to PDGF, *Science*, 253, 1129–1132, 1991.

29. **Garg, U. C. and Hassid, A.,** Nitric oxide-generating vasodilators and 8-bromo-cyclic guanosine monophosphate inhibit mitogenesis and proliferation of cultured rat vascular smooth muscle cells, *J. Clin. Invest.*, 83, 1774–1777, 1989.

30. **Garratt, K. N., Edwards, W. D., Kaufmann, U. P., Vlietstra, R. E., and Holmes, D. R.,** Differential histopathology of primary atherosclerotic and restenotic lesions in coronary arteries and saphenous vein bypass grafts: Analysis of tissue obtained from 73 patients by directional atherectomy, *J. Am. Coll. Cardiol.*, 17, 442–448, 1990.

31. **Giachelli, C., Bae, N., Lombardi, D., Majesky, M., and Schwartz, S. M.,** Molecular cloning and characterization of 2B7, a rat mRNA which distinguishes smooth muscle cell phenotypes *in vitro* and is identical to osteopontin, *Biochem. Biophys. Res. Commun.*, 177, 867–873, 1991.

32. **Gospodariwicz, D., Neufeld, G., and Schweigerer, L.,** Fibroblast growth factor, *Mol. Cell Endocrin.*, 46, 187–206, 1986.

33. **Gospodarowicz, D., Neufeld, G., and Schweigerer, L.,** Molecular and biological characterization of fibroblast growth factor, an angiogeneic factor which also controls the proliferation and differentiation of mesoderm and neuroectoderm derived cells, *Cell. Differ.*, 19, 1–17, 1986.

34. **Gospodarowicz, D.,** Isolation and characterization of acidic and basic fibroblast growth factor, in *Methods in Enzymology. Peptide Growth Factors*, Vol. 147B, Academic Press, Orlando, FL, 1987, 106–117.

35. **Gospodarowicz, D., Ferrara, N., Haaparanta, T., and Neufeld, G.,** Basic fibroblast growth factor: Expression in cultured bovine vascular smooth muscle cells, *Eur. J. Cell Biol.*, 46, 144–151, 1988.

36. **Graham, D. J. and Alexander, J. J.,** The effects of thrombin on bovine aortic endothelial and smooth muscle cells, *J. Vasc. Surg.*, 11, 307–313, 1990.

37. **Gravanfis, M. B. and Roubin, G. S.,** Histopathological phenomena at the site of percutaneous transluminal coronary angioplasty: The Problem of restenosis, *Hum. Pathol.*, 20, 477–485, 1989.

38. **Haebnicht, A. J. R., Glomset, J. A., King, W. C., Nist, C., Mitchell, C. D., and Ross, R.,** Early changes in phosphatidylinositol and arachidonic acid metabolism in quiescent swiss 3T3 cells stimulated to divide by platelet-derived growth factor, *J. Biol. Chem.*, 256, 12329–12335, 1981.

39. **Hanke, H., Strohschneider, T., Oberhoff, M., Betz, E., and Karsch, R.,** Time course of smooth muscle cell proliferation in the intima and media of arteries following experimental angioplasty, *Circ. Res.*, 67, 651–659, 1990.

40. **Hansson, H. A., Jennische, E., and Skottner, A.,** IGF-I expression in blood vessel varies with vascular load, *Acta Physiol. Scand.*, 129, 165–169, 1987.

41. **Heagerty, A. M., Aalkjaer, C., Bund, S. J., Korsgaard, N., and Mulvany, M. J.,** Small artery structure in hypertension. Dual processes of remodeling and growth, *Hypertension*, 21, 391–397, 1993.

42. **Hedin, U., Bottger, B. A., Forsberg, E., Johansson, S., and Thyberg, J.,** Diverse effects of fibronectin and laminin on phenotypic properties of cultured arterial smooth muscle cells, *J. Cell Biol.*, 107, 307–319, 1988.

43. **Heickendorff, L. and Ledet, T.,** Arterial basement-membrane-like material isolated and characterized from rabbit aortic myomecial cells in culture, *Biochem. J.*, 211, 397–404, 1983.

44. **Heickendorff, L. and Ledet, T.,** The carbohydrate components of arterial basement-membrane-like material. Studies on rabbit aortic myomedial cells in culture, *Biochem. J.*, 211, 735–741, 1983.

45. **Heickendorff, L. and Ledet, T.,** Glycosaminoglycans of arteial basement membrane-like material from cultured rabbit aortic myomedial cells, *Biochim. et Biophys. Acta*, 798, 276–282, 1984.

46. **Hoover, R. L., Rosenberg, R., Haering, W., and Karnovsky, M. J.,** Inhibition of rat arterial smooth muscle cell proliferation by heparin, *Circ. Res.*, 47, 578–583, 1980.

47. **Hwang, D. L., Latus, L. J., and Lev-Ran, A.,** Effects of platelet-contained growth factors (PDGF, EGF, IGF-I and TGF-β) on DNA synthesis in porcine aortic smooth muscle cells in culture, *Exp. Cell Res.*, 200, 358–360, 1992.

48. **Hüttner, I., Kocher, O., and Gabbiana, G.,** Endothelial and smooth muscle cells, in *Diseases of the Arterial Wall*, Camilleri, J. P., Berry, C. L., Fiessinger, J. N., and Bariety, J., Eds., Springer Verlag, London, 1989, 3–41.

49. **Inui, H., Kondo, T., and Inagami, T.,** Platelet-derived growth factor AA homodimer stimulates protein synthesis rather than DNA synthesis in vascular smooth muscle cells from spontaneously hypertensive rats but not from normotensive rats, *Biochem. Biophys. Res. Commun.*, 188, 524–530, 1992.

50. **Jaeger, E., Rust, S., Roessner, A., Kleinhans, G., Buchholz, B., Althaus, M., Rauterberg, J., and Gerlach, U.,** Joint occurrence of collagen mRNA containing cells and macrophages in human atherosclerotic vessels, *Atherosclerosis*, 31, 55–68, 1991.

51. **Jonasson, L., Holm, J., Skalli, O., Bondjers, G., and Hansson, G. K.,** Regional accumulations of T cells, macrophages, and smooth muscle cells in the human atherosclerotic plaque, *Arteriosclerosis*, 6, 131–138, 1986.

52. **Järveläinen, H. T., Kinsella, M. G., Wight, T. N., and Sandel, L. J.,** Differential expression of small chondroitin/dermatan sulfate proteoglycans, PG-I/biglycan and PG-II/decorin, by vascular smooth muscle and endothelial cells in culture, *J. Biol. Chem.*, 266, 27274–2281, 1991.

53. **Kanthou, C., Parry, G., Wijelath, E., Kakkar, V. V., and Demoliou-Mason, C.,** Thrombin-induced proliferation expression of platelet-derived growth factor-A chain gene in human vascular smooth muscle cells, *FEBS Lett.*, 314, 143–148, 1992.

54. **Kariya, K., Kawahara, Y., Tsuda, T., Fukuzaki, H., and Takai, Y.,** Possible involvement of protein kinase C in platelet-derived growth factor stimulated DNA synthesis in vascular smooth muscle cells, *Atherosclerosis*, 63, 251–255, 1987.

55. **Kariya, K., Kawahara, Y., Araki, S., Fukuzaki, H., and Takai, Y.,** Antiproliferative action of cyclic GMP-elevating vasodilators in cultured rabbit aortic smooth muscle cells, *Atherosclerosis*, 80, 143–147, 1989.

56. **Kielty, C. M., Whittaker, S. P., Grant, M. E., and Shuttleworth, C. A.,** Attachment of human vascular smooth muscle cells to intact microgibrillar assemblies of collagen VI and fibrillin, *J. Cell Sci.*, 103, 445–451, 1992.

57. **Lappi, D. A., Martineau, D., and Baird, A.,** Biological and chemical characterization of basic FGF-saporin mitotoxin, *Biochem. Biophys. Res. Commun.*, 160, 917–923, 1989.

58. **Leclerc, G., Gal, D., Takeshita, S., Nikol, S., Weir, L., and Isner, J. M.,** Percutaneous arterial gene transfer in a rabbit model. Efficiency in normal and balloon-dilated atherosclerotic arteries, *J. Clin. Invest.*, 90, 936–944, 1992.

59. **Ledet, T.,** Growth hormone stimulating the growth of arterial medial cells *in vitro*, *Diabetes*, 25, 1011–1017, 1976.

60. **Ledet, T. and Heickendorff, L.,** Growth hormone effect on accumulation of arterial basement membrane-like material studied on rabbit aortic myomedial cell cultures, *Diabetologia*, 28, 922–927, 1985.

61. **Ledet, T., Heickendorff, L., and Rasmussen, L. M.,** Cellular mechanisms of diabetic large vessel disease, in *The International Textbook of Diabetes Mellitus*, Alberti, K. G. M. M., DeFronzo, R. A., Keen, H., and Zimmet, P., Eds., 1992.

62. **Ledet, T. and Vuust, J.,** Arterial procollagen type I, and type III, and fibronectin: effects of diabetic serum, glucose, insulin, ketone, and growth hormone studied on rabbit aortic myomedial cell cultures, *Diabetes*, 29, 964–970, 1980.

63. **Libby, P., Schwartz, D., Brogi, E., Tanaka, H., and Clinton, S. K.,** A cascade model for restenosis. A special case of atherosclerosis progression, *Circulation*, 86(Suppl. III), III-47–III-52, 1992.

64. **Lichtenstein, A. H., Brecher, P., and Chobanian, A. V.,** Effects of deoxycorticosterone-salt hypertension on cell ploidy in the rat aorta, *Hypertension*, 8(Suppl. II), II-50–II-54, 1986.

65. **Lindner, V. and Reidy, M. A.,** Proliferation of smooth muscle cells after vascular injury is inhibited by an antibody against basic fibroblast growth factor, *Proc. Natl. Acad. Sci. U.S.A.*, 88, 3739–3743, 1991.

66. **Lindner, V., Lappi, D. A., Baird, A., Majack, R. A., and Reidy, M. A.,** Role of basic fibroblast growth factor in vascular lesion formation, *Circ. Res.*, 68, 106–113, 1991.

67. **Lindner, V., Olson, N. E., Clowes, A. W., and Reidy, M. A.,** Inhibition of smooth muscle cell proliferation in injured rat arteries, *J. Clin. Invest.*, 90, 2044–2049, 1992.

68. **Liptay, M. J., Parks, W. C., Mecham, R. P., Roby, J., Kaiser, L. R., Cooper, J. D., and Botney, M. D.,** Neointimal macrophages colocalize with extracellular matrix gene expression in human atherosclerotic pulmonary arteries, *J. Clin. Invest.*, 91, 588–594, 1993.

69. **Lyall, F., Morton, J. J., Lever, A. F., and Cragoe, E. J.,** Angiotensin II activates Na^+-H^+ exchange and stimulates growth in cultured vascular smooth muscle cells, *J. Hypertens.*, 6(Suppl. 4), S438–S441, 1988.

70. **Lynch, C. M., Clowes, M. M., Osborne, W. R. A., Clowes, A. W., and Miller, D.,** Long-term expression of human adenosine deaminase in vascular smooth muscle cells of rats: A model for gene therapy, *PNAS*, 89, 1138–1142, 1992.

71. **Majesky, M. W., Benditt, E. P., and Schwartz, S. M.,** Expression and developmental control of platelet-derived growth factor A-chain and B-chain/Sis genes in rat aortic smooth muscle cells, *Proc. Natl. Acad. Sci. U.S.A.*, 85, 1524–1528, 1988.

72. **Majesky, M. W., Reidy, M. A., Bowen-Pope, D. F., Hart, C. E., Wilcox, J. N., and Schwartz, S. M.,** PDGF ligand and receptor gene expression during repair of arterial injury, *J. Cell Biol.*, 111, 2149–2158, 1990.

73. **Majesky, M. W., Lindner, D. R., Twardzik, D. R., Schwartz, S. M., and Reidy, M. A.,** Production of transforming growth factor-β1 during repair of arterial injury, *J. Clin. Invest.*, 88, 904–910, 1991.

74. **Majors, A. and Ehrhart, L. A.,** Basic fibroblast growth factor in the extracellular matrix suppresses collagen synthesis and Type III procollagen mRNA levels in arterial smooth muscle cell cultures, *Artheroscler. Thromb.*, 13, 680–686, 1991.

75. **Maslen, C. L., Corson, G. M., Maddox, B. K., Glanville, R. W., and Sakai, L. Y.,** Partial sequence of a candidate gene for the Marfan syndrome, *Nature*, 352, 334–337, 1991.

76. **McBride, W., Lange, R. A., and Hillis, L. D.,** Restenosis after successful coronary angioplasty, *N. Engl. J. Med.*, 318, 1734–1737, 1988.

77. **McNamara, C. A., Sarembock, I. J., Gimple, L. W., Fenton, J. W., II, Coughlin, S. R., and Owens, G. K.,** Thrombin stimulates proliferation of cultured rat aortic smooth muscle cells by a proteolytically activated receptor, *J. Clin. Invest.*, 91, 94–98, 1993.

78. **Miller, A. D., Clowes, M. M., Osborne, W. R. A., Clowes, A. W., and Miller, A. D.,** Long-term expression of human adenosine deaminase in vascular smooth muscle cells of rats: A model for gene therapy, *PNAS*, 89, 1138–1142, 1992.

79. **Mulvany, M. J. and Alkjaer, C.,** Structure and function of small arteries, *Physiol. Rev.*, 70, 921–961, 1990.

80. **Nabel, E. G., Plautz, G., and Nabel, G. J.,** Transduction of a foreign histocompatibility gene into the arterial wall induces vasculitis, *PNAS*, 89, 5157–5161, 1992.

81. **Nabel, E. G., Yang, Z., Liptay, S., San, H., Gordon, D., Haudenschild, C. C., and Nabel, G. J.,** Recombinant platelet-derived growth factor B gene expression in porcine arteries induces intimal hyperplasia *in vivo*, *J. Clin. Invest.*, 91, 1822–1829, 1993.

82. **Nabel, E. G., Yang, Z., Plautz, G., Forough, R., Zhan, X., Haudenschild, C. C., Macaig, T., and Nabel, G. J.,** Recombinant fibroblast growth factor-1 promotes intimal hyperplasia and angiogenesis in arteries *in vivo*, *Nature*, 362, 844–846, 1993.

83. **Nemeck, G. M., Coughlin, S. R., Handley, D. A., and Moskowitz, M. A.,** Stimulation of aortic smooth muscle cell mitogenesis by serotinin, *Proc. Natl. Acad. Sci. U.S.A.*, 83, 674–678, 1986.

84. **Nobuyoshi, M., Kimura, T., Ohishi, H., Horiuchi, H., Nosaka, H., Hamasaki, N., Yokoi, H., and Kim, K.,** Restenosis after percutaneous transluminal coronary angioplasty: Pathologic observations in 20 patients, *J. Am. Coll. Cardiol.*, 17, 433–439, 1991.

85. **Okazaki, H., Majesky, M. W., Harker, L. A., and Schwartz, S. M.,** Regulation of platelet-derived growth factor ligand and receptor gene expression by α-thrombin in vascular smooth muscle cells, *Circ. Res.*, 71, 1285–1293, 1992.

86. **Owens, G. K., Shimizu, R., Thompson, M., McNamara, C., and Blank, R. S.,** Transcriptional regulation of the smooth muscle alpha actin promotor: Evidence for involvement of helix-loop-helix factors, *J. Cell. Biochem.*, 16A, p.5, A 011, 1992.

87. **Pfeifle, B., Ditshuneit, H. H., and Ditshuneit, H.,** Binding and biological actions of insulin-lik growth factors on huma arterial smooth muscle cells, *Horm. Metabol. Res.*, 14, 409–414, 1982.

88. **Pfeifle, B., Boeder, H., and Ditshuneit, H.,** Interaction of receptors for insulin-like growth factor I, platelet-derived growth factor, and fibroblast growth factor in rat aortic cells, *Endocrinology*, 120, 2251–2258, 1987.

89. **Pfeifle, B., Hamann, H., Fussganger, H., and Ditshuneit, H.,** Insulin as a growth regulator of arterial smooth muscle cells: Effect of insulin on IGF-I, *Diabet. Metab.*, 13, 326–330, 1987.

90. **Powell, J. S., Clozel, J., Müller, R. K. M., Kuhn, H., Hefti, F., Hosang, M., and Baumgartner, H. R.,** Inhibitors of angiotensin-converting enzyme prevent myointimal proliferation after vascular injury, *Science*, 245, 186–188, 1989.

91. **Prescott, M. F., Webb, R. L., and Reidy, M. A.,** Angiotensin-converting enzyme inhibitor versus angiotensin II, AT_1 receptor antagonist, *Am. J. Pathol.*, 139, 1291–1296, 1991.

92. **Rasmussen, H. and Barret, P.,** Calcium messenger systems: An integrated view, *Physiol. Rev.*, 63, 938–984, 1984.

93. **Rasmussen, L. M. and Ledet, T.,** Diabetic serum enhances synthesis of basement membrane-like material in cultures of rabbit smooth muscle cells, *APMIS*, 96, 77–83, 1988.

94. **Rasmussen, L. M. and Heickendorff, L.,** Accumulation of fibronectin in aortae from diabetic patients. A quatitative immunohistochemical and biochemical study, *Lab. Invest.*, 61, 440–446, 1989.

95. **Rasmussen, L. M. and Ledet, T.,** Collagen alterations in diabetic aortas. Changes in basement membrane collagen content and in the total collagen susceptibility to cyanogen bromide solubilization, *Diabetologia*, 36, 445–453, 1993.

96. **Rasmussen, L. M., Wolf, Y., and Ruoslahti, E.,** Vascular smooth muscle cells derived from balloon injured rat aortas display a matrix producing phenotype, associated with enhanced TGF-β activity, submitted.

97. **Ross, R., Glomset, J. A., Kariya, B., and Harker, L.,** A platelet dependent serum factor that stimulates the proliferation of arterial smooth muscle cells, *Proc. Natl. Acad. Sci. U.S.A.*, 71, 1207–1210, 1974.

98. **Ross, R.,** The pathogenesis of atherosclerosis — an update, *N. Engl. J. Med.*, 314, 488–502, 1986.

99. **Ross, R.,** The pathogenesis of atherosclerosis: A perspective for the 1990s, *Nature*, 362, 801–809, 1993.

100. **Rutherford, R. B. and Ross, R.,** Platelet factors stimulates fibroblasts and smooth muscle cells quiescent in plasma serum to proliferate, *J. Cell. Biol.*, 69, 196–203, 1976.

101. **Sarzani, R., Brecher, P., and Chobanian, A. V.,** Growth factor expression in aorta of normotensive and hypertensive rats, *J. Clin. Invest.*, 83, 1404–1408, 1989.

102. **Schönherr, E., Järveläinen, H. T., Sandel, L. J., and Wight, T. N.,** Effects of platelet-derived growth factor and transforming growth factor-β1 on the synthesis of a large versican-like chondroitin sulfate proteoglycan by arterial smooth muscle cells, *J. Biol. Chem.*, 266, 17640–17647, 1991.

103. **Schwartz, S. M., Campbell, G. R., and Campbell, J. H.,** Developmentally regulated production of platelet-derived growth factor-like molecules, *Circ. Res.*, 58, 427–444, 1986.

104. **Schwartz, S. M., Heimark, R. L., and Majesky, M. W.,** Developmental mechanisms underlying pathology of arteries, *Physiol. Rev.*, 70, 1177–1209, 1990.

105. **Schwartz, S. M., Foy, L., Bowen-Pope, D. F., and Ross, R.,** Derivation and properties of platelet-derived growth factor-independent rat smooth muscle cells, *Am. J. Pathol.*, 136, 1417–1428, 1990.

106. **Schwartz, S. M. and Giachelli, C. M.,** Smooth muscle diversity, *VIIth Int. Symp. of the Biology of Vascular Cells*, San Diego, 1992, 2.

107. **Seifert, R. A., Schwartz, S. M., and Bowen-Pope, D. F.,** Developmentally regulated production of platelet-derived growth factor-like molecules, *Nature*, 311, 669–671, 1984.

108. **Sejersen, T., Betsholtz, C., Sjölund, M., Heldin, C. H., Westermark, B., and Thyberg, J.,** Rat skeletal myoblasts and arterial smooth muscle cells express the gene for the A chain but not the gene for the B chain (c-sis) of platelet-derived growth factor (PDGF) and produce a PDGF-like protein, *Proc. Natl. Acad. Sci. U.S.A.*, 83, 6844–6848, 1986.

109. **Simons, M. Leclerc, G., Safian, R. D., Isner, J. M., Weir, L., and Baim, D. S.,** Relation between activated smooth-muscle cells in coronary-artery lesions and restenosis after atherectomy, *N. Engl. J. Med.*, 328, 608–613, 1993.

110. **Simons, M., Edelman, E. R., DeKeyser, J., Langer, R., and Rosenberg, R. D.,** Antisense c-myb oligonucleotides inhibit intimal arterial smooth muscle cell accumulation *in vivo, Nature*, 359, 67–70, 1992.

111. **Speir, E. and Epstein, S. E.,** Inhibition of smooth muscle cells proliferation by an antisense oligodeoxynucleotide targetting the messenger RNA encoding proliferating cell nuclear antigen, *Circulation*, 86, 538–547, 1992.

112. **Steele, P. M., Chesebro, J. H., Stanson, A. W., Holmes, D. R., Dewanjee, M. K., Badimon, L., and Fuster, V.,** Balloon angioplasty. Natural history of the pathophysiological response to injury in a pig model, *Circ. Res.*, 57, 105–112, 1985.

113. **Tapscott, S. J. and Weintraub, H.,** MyoD and the regulation of myogenesis by helix-loop-helix proteins, *J. Clin. Invest.*, 87, 1133–1138, 1991.

114. **Thyberg, J., Hedin, U., Sjoelund, M., Palmberg, L., and Bottger, B. A.,** Regulation of differentiated properties and proliferation of arterial smooth muscle cells, *Arteriosclerosis*, 10, 966–990, 1990.

115. **Yamamoto, M., Yamamoto, K., and Noumura, T.,** Type I collagen promotes modulation of cultured rabbit arterial smooth muscle cells from a contractile to a synthetic phenotype, *Exp. Cell Res.*, 204, 121–129, 1993.

116. **VanNeck, J. W., Medina, J. J., Onnekink, C., Van der Vent, P. F., Bloemers, H. P., and Schwartz, S. M.,** Basic fibroblast growth factor has a differential effect on MyoD conversion of cultured aortic smooth muscle cells from newborn and adult rats, *Am. J. Pathol.*, 143, 269–282, 1993.

117. **Walker, L. N., Bowen-Pope, D. F., Ross, R., and Reidy, M. A.,** Production of platelet-derived growth factor-like molecules by cultured arterial smooth muscle cells accompanies proliferation after arterial injury, *PNAS*, 83, 7311–7315, 1986.

118. **Waller, B. F., Pinkerton, C. A., Orr, C. M., Slack, J. D., VanTassel, J. W., and Peters, T.,** Marphological observations late after clinically successful coronary balloon angioplasty, *Circulation*, 83(Suppl. I), I28–41, 1991.

119. **Winkles, J. A., Friesel, R., Burgess, W. H., Howk, R., Mehlman, T., Weinstein, R., and Maciag, T.,** Human vascular smooth muscle cells both express and respond to heparin-binding growth factor I (endothelial cell growth factor), *Proc. Natl. Acad. Sci. U.S.A.*, 84, 7124–7128, 1987.

120. **Wolf, Y. G., Rasmussen, L. M., and Ruoslahti, E.,** Antibodies against transforming growth factor-β1 suppress intimal hyperplasia in a rat model, *J. Clin. Invest.*, 93, 1172–1178, 1994.

121. **Zierler, R. E., Bandyk, D. F., Thiele, B. L., and Strandness, D. E.,** Carotid artery stenosis following endarterectomy, *Arch. Surg.*, 117, 1408–1415, 1982.

INDEX